Every Decker book is accompanied by a CD-ROM.

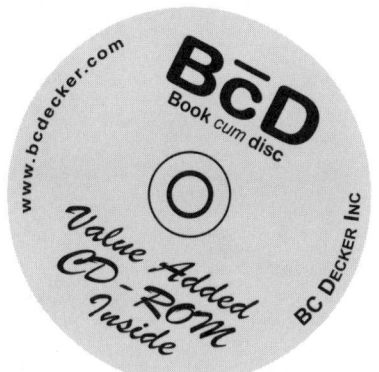

BC Decker Inc is committed to providing high-quality electronic publications that complement traditional information and learning methods.

Tinnitus: Theory and Management is accompanied by a dual-platform CD-ROM, which features the complete text and full-color illustrations. The fully searchable PDF files facilitate the exploration of need-to-know information. The disc is also ideal for printing pertinent information necessary for patient education.

The book and disc are sold only as a package; neither are available independently, and no prices are available for the items individually. We trust you will find the book/CD package invaluable and invite your comments and suggestions.

Access information. Acquire knowledge. Please visit www.bcdecker.com for a complete list of titles in your discipline. Our innovative approach to meeting the informational needs of healthcare professionals ensures that Decker products belong in your library and on your computer.

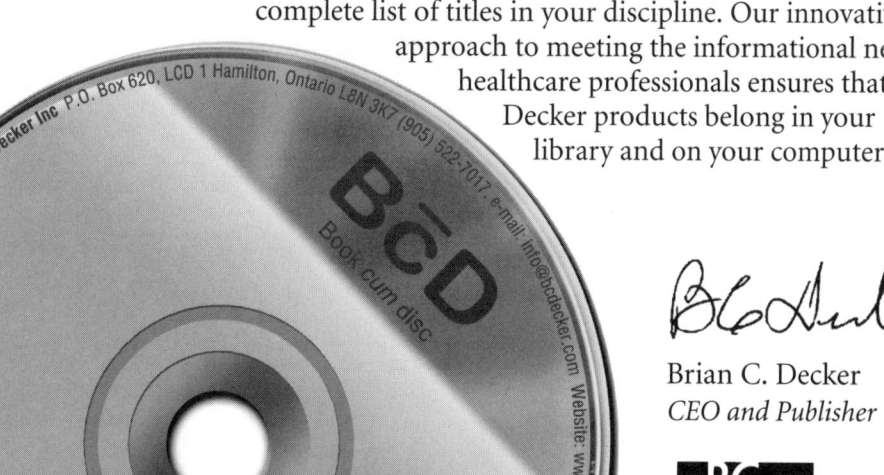

Brian C. Decker
CEO and Publisher

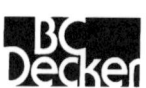

Tinnitus:
Theory and Management

Tinnitus: Theory and Management

James B. Snow Jr, MD
Former Director
National Institute on Deafness and
Other Communication Disorders
National Institutes of Health
Bethesda, Maryland
Professor Emeritus
University of Pennsylvania
Philadelphia, Pennsylvania

2004
BC Decker Inc
Hamilton • London

BC Decker Inc
P.O. Box 620, L.C.D. 1
Hamilton, Ontario L8N 3K7[Decker Logo]
Tel: 905-522-7017; 800-568-7281
Fax: 905-522-7839; 888-311-4987
E-mail: info@bcdecker.com
www.bcdecker.com

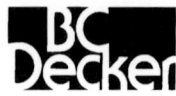

© 2004 BC Decker Inc

All rights reserved. No part of this publication may be reproduced, stored in a retrieval system, or transmitted, in any form or by any means, electronic, mechanical, photocopying, recording, or otherwise, without prior written permission from the publisher.

04 05 06 07/ WPC /9 8 7 6 5 4 3 2 1

ISBN 1-55009-243-X
Printed in the United States of America

SALES AND DISTRIBUTION

United States
BC Decker Inc
P.O. Box 785
Lewiston, NY 14092-0785
Tel: 905-522-7017; 800-568-7281
Fax: 905-522-7839; 888-311-4987
E-mail: info@bcdecker.com
www.bcdecker.com

Canada
BC Decker Inc
20 Hughson Street South
P.O. Box 620, LCD 1
Hamilton, Ontario L8N 3K7
Tel: 905-522-7017; 800-568-7281
Fax: 905-522-7839; 888-311-4987
E-mail: info@bcdecker.com
www.bcdecker.com

Foreign Rights
John Scott & Company
International Publishers' Agency
P.O. Box 878
Kimberton, PA 19442
Tel: 610-827-1640
Fax: 610-827-1671
E-mail: jsco@voicenet.com

Japan
Igaku-Shoin Ltd.
Foreign Publications Department
3-24-17 Hongo
Bunkyo-ku, Tokyo, Japan 113-8719
Tel: 3 3817 5680
Fax: 3 3815 6776
E-mail: fd@igaku-shoin.co.jp

UK, Europe, Scandinavia, Middle East
Elsevier Science
Customer Service Department
Foots Cray High Street
Sidcup, Kent
DA14 5HP, UK
Tel: 44 (0) 208 308 5760
Fax: 44 (0) 181 308 5702
E-mail: cservice@harcourt.com

Singapore, Malaysia,Thailand, Philippines, Indonesia, Vietnam, Pacific Rim, Korea
Elsevier Science Asia
583 Orchard Road
#09/01, Forum
Singapore 238884
Tel: 65-737-3593
Fax: 65-753-2145

Australia, New Zealand
Elsevier Science Australia
Customer Service Department
STM Division
Locked Bag 16
St. Peters, New South Wales, 2044
Australia
Tel: 61 02 9517-8999
Fax: 61 02 9517-2249
E-mail: stmp@harcourt.com.au
www.harcourt.com.au

Mexico and Central America
ETM SA de CV
Calle de Tula 59
Colonia Condesa
06140 Mexico DF, Mexico
Tel: 52-5-5553-6657
Fax: 52-5-5211-8468
E-mail: editoresdetextosmex@
 prodigy.net.mx

Argentina
CLM (Cuspide Libros Medicos)
Av. Córdoba 2067 - (1120)
Buenos Aires, Argentina
Tel: (5411) 4961-0042/(5411) 4964-0848
Fax: (5411) 4963-7988
E-mail: clm@cuspide.com

Brazil
Tecmedd
Av. Maurílio Biagi, 2850
City Ribeirão Preto – SP – CEP:
 14021-000
Tel: 0800 992236
Fax: (16) 3993-9000
E-mail: tecmedd@tecmedd.com.br

Notice: The authors and publisher have made every effort to ensure that the patient care recommended herein, including choice of drugs and drug dosages, is in accord with the accepted standard and practice at the time of publication. However, since research and regulation constantly change clinical standards, the reader is urged to check the product information sheet included in the package of each drug, which includes recommended doses, warnings, and contraindications. This is particularly important with new or infrequently used drugs. Any treatment regimen, particularly one involving medication, involves inherent risk that must be weighed on a case-by-case basis against the benefits anticipated. The reader is cautioned that the purpose of this book is to inform and enlighten; the information contained herein is not intended as, and should not be employed as, a substitute for individual diagnosis and treatment.

This book is dedicated to Robert Warne Wilson, patron of the arts and biomedical science, whose generous support over the last decade has contributed to unprecedented progress in tinnitus research.

Contents

Preface — xi
Contributors — xiii

INTRODUCTION

1. Overview: Suffering from Tinnitus — 1
   Robert A. Dobie, MD

2. Decreased Sound Tolerance — 8
   Pawel J. Jastreboff, PhD, ScD, and Margaret M. Jastreboff, PhD

3. Epidemiology of Tinnitus — 16
   Howard J. Hoffman, MA, and George W. Reed, PhD

Editorial Commentary — 42
   James B. Snow Jr, MD

THEORETICAL BASES

4. Molecular Biology of Hearing and Tinnitus — 43
   Allen F. Ryan, PhD, and Lina M. Mullen, PhD

5. Peripheral Processes Involved in Tinnitus — 52
   Alfred L. Nuttall, PhD, Mary B. Meikle, PhD, and Dennis R. Trune, PhD, MBA

6. Otoacoustic Emissions and Tinnitus — 69
   Brenda L. Lonsbury-Martin, PhD, and Glen K. Martin, PhD

Editorial Commentary — 79
   James B. Snow Jr, MD

7. Animal Models of Tinnitus — 80
   David B. Moody, PhD

8. The Neurophysiological Model of Tinnitus — 96
   Pawel J. Jastreboff, PhD, ScD

Editorial Commentary — 107
   James B. Snow Jr, MD

9. Somatic Tinnitus   108
   Robert A. Levine, MD

10. Sensory Nuclei in Tinnitus   125
    Susan E. Shore, PhD

Editorial Commentary   140
   James B. Snow Jr, MD

11. Neural Correlates of Tinnitus   141
    James A. Kaltenbach, PhD, Jinsheng Zhang, PhD, and Mark A. Zacharek, MD

12. The Limbic System and Tinnitus   162
    Anthony T. Cacace, PhD

13. The Auditory Cortex and Tinnitus   171
    Jos J. Eggermont, PhD

14. Cortical Plasticity and Tinnitus   189
    Christoph E. Schreiner, PhD, MD, and Steven W. Cheung, MD

Editorial Commentary   203
   James B. Snow Jr, MD

MANAGEMENT

Evaluation of the Patient with Tinnitus

15. Otologic Evaluation   205
    P. Ashley Wackym, MD, and David R. Friedland, MD, PhD

16. Audiologic Assessment   220
    James A. Henry, PhD

17. Tinnitus Questionnaires   237
    Craig W. Newman, PhD, and Sharon A. Sandridge, PhD

18. Imaging Tinnitus   255
    Alan H. Lockwood, MD, Robert F. Burkard, PhD, and Richard J. Salvi, PhD

Editorial Commentary   265
   James B. Snow Jr, MD

Treatment of the Patient with Tinnitus

19. Clinical Trials and Drug Therapy for Tinnitus — 266
Robert A. Dobie, MD

20. Antidepressant Therapy for Tinnitus — 278
Shannon K. Robinson, MD, Erik S. Viirre, MD, PhD, and Murray B. Stein, MD

Editorial Commentary — 294
James B. Snow Jr, MD

21. Tinnitus Retraining Therapy — 295
Pawel J. Jastreboff, PhD, ScD, and Margaret M. Jastreboff, PhD

22. Role of Hearing Aids in Management of Tinnitus — 310
Jacqueline B. Sheldrake, RHAD, BSHAA, and Margaret M. Jastreboff, PhD

23. Psychological Treatments for Tinnitus — 314
Richard S. Tyler, PhD, William Noble, PhD, John P. Preece, PhD,
Camille C. Dunn, PhD, Shelley A. Witt, MA

Editorial Commentary — 324
James B. Snow Jr, MD

24. Electrical Suppression of Tinnitus — 326
Jay T. Rubinstein, MD, PhD, and Richard S. Tyler, PhD

Editorial Commentary — 336
James B. Snow Jr, MD

25. Veterans and Tinnitus — 337
James A. Henry, PhD, Martin A. Schechter, PhD, Raymond T. Regelein,
and Kyle C. Dennis, PhD

Editorial Commentary — 356
James B. Snow Jr, MD

Index — 357

Preface

Great progress has been made in the last decade in research on tinnitus and the development of theoretic concepts regarding the initiation, generation, and perpetuation of the percept of tinnitus. Tinnitus is a symptom that is associated with virtually all diseases and disorders affecting the auditory system and can arise from a lesion in any part of the auditory system. Interestingly, tinnitus can also arise in the absence of other apparent abnormalities of the auditory system. Many of the causes of tinnitus are well known, such as intense sound and ototoxic drugs, but the mechanisms and sites of its production are less certain. This book is designed to present a comprehensive view of the current state of the art of basic and clinical tinnitus research. The authors of each chapter were chosen on the basis of their personal contributions to the knowledge underlying the subject matter of the chapter and their recognition as intellectual leaders in that aspect of research. The aim has been to review the literature critically and present the subject in a scientifically rigorous manner based on the experience of the authors.

Three chapters introduce the reader to the clinical aspects of tinnitus, the closely related subject of decreased sound tolerance, and the epidemiology of tinnitus. The current theoretic basis of tinnitus is presented in 11 chapters that address discoveries and concepts from the inner ear to the auditory cortex and the limbic and autonomic nervous systems and encompass somatosensory modulation, analogy to phantom limb pain, neural plasticity, and much more. The evaluation of the patient with tinnitus is presented in four chapters covering otologic and audiologic considerations, accession to and outcome measures of clinical trials, and brain imaging. The final seven chapters address treatment options for patients with tinnitus, including drug trials and therapy, antidepressant therapy, tinnitus retraining therapy, the role of hearing aids, psychological methods of therapy, electrical suppression of tinnitus, and the management of tinnitus in the American veteran population.

After groups of chapters, I have made comments that I hope will help the reader understand the significance and interrelationship of the information in the various chapters. The authors of the chapters and I hope that readers will find this book interesting, enjoyable, and stimulating.

James B. Snow Jr, MD
September 1, 2004

Contributors

Robert F. Burkard, PhD
Department of Otolaryngology
University at Buffalo
Buffalo, New York

Anthony T. Cacace, PhD
Department of Neurology
The Neurosciences Institute and the Advanced
  Imaging Research Center
Albany Medical College
Albany, New York

Steven W. Cheung, MD
Department of Otolaryngology–Head and Neck
  Surgery
University of California–San Franciso
San Francisco, California

Kyle C. Dennis, PhD
Audiology and Speech Pathology Service
Veterans Affairs Central Office
Washington, District of Columbia

Robert A. Dobie, MD
Department of Otolaryngology
University of California–Davis
Sacramento, California

Camille C. Dunn, PhD
Department of Otolaryngology–Head and Neck
  Surgery
University of Iowa Hospitals and Clinics
Iowa City, Iowa

Jos J. Eggermont, PhD
Departments of Physiology and Biophysics and
  Psychology
University of Calgary
Calgary, Alberta, Canada

David R. Friedland, MD, PhD
Department of Otolaryngology and
  Communication Sciences
Medical College of Wisconsin
Milwaukee, Wisconsin

James A. Henry, PhD
Department of Otolaryngology–Head and Neck
  Surgery
Oregon Health and Science University
Portland, Oregon

Howard J. Hoffman, MA
Division of Scientific Programs
National Institute on Deafness and Other
  Communication Disorders (NIDCD), National
  Institutes of Health (NIH)
Bethesda, Maryland

Margaret M. Jastreboff, PhD
Department of Otolaryngology
Emory University
Atlanta, Georgia

Pawel J. Jastreboff, PhD, ScD
Department of Otolaryngology
Emory University
Atlanta, Georgia

James A. Kaltenbach, PhD
Department of Otolaryngology
Wayne State University
Detroit, Michigan

Robert A. Levine, MD
Department of Neurology
Harvard Medical School
Boston, Massachusetts

Brenda L. Lonsbury-Martin, PhD
Department of Otolaryngology
University of Colorado Health Sciences Center
Denver, Colorado

Alan H. Lockwood, MD
Department of Neurology and Nuclear Medicine
University at Buffalo
Buffalo, New York

Glen K. Martin, PhD
Department of Otolaryngology
University of Colorado Health Sciences Center
Denver, Colorado

Mary B. Meikle, PhD
Department of Otolaryngology–Head and Neck Surgery
Oregon Health and Science University
Portland, Oregon

David B. Moody, PhD
Departments of Otolaryngology and Psychology
University of Michigan
Ann Arbor, Michigan

Lina M. Mullen, PhD
Departments of Surgery and Otolaryngology
University of California–San Diego
La Jolla, California

Craig W. Newman, PhD
Head and Neck Institute
Cleveland Clinic Foundation
Cleveland, Ohio

William Noble, PhD
Department of Psychology
University of New England
Armidale, New South Wales, Australia

Alfred L. Nuttall, PhD
Department of Otolaryngology–Head and Neck Surgery
Oregon Health and Science University
Portland, Oregon

John P. Preece, PhD
Department of Communicative Disorders
University of Rhode Island
Providence, Rhode Island

George W. Reed, PhD
Department of Medicine
University of Massachusetts School of Medicine
Worcester, Massachusetts

Raymond T. Regelein
Veterans Affairs Regional Office
Portland, Oregon

Shannon K. Robinson, MD
Department of Psychiatry
University of California–San Diego
San Diego, California

Jay T. Rubinstein, MD, PhD
Department of Otolaryngology and Biomedical Engineering
University of Iowa
Iowa City, Iowa

Allen F. Ryan, PhD
Department of Surgery
University of California–San Diego
La Jolla, California

Richard J. Salvi, PhD
Department of Communicative Disorders and Sciences
University at Buffalo
Buffalo, New York

Sharon A. Sandridge, PhD
Head and Neck Institute
Cleveland Clinic Foundation
Cleveland, Ohio

Martin A. Schechter, PhD
Audiology and Speech Pathology Service
Veterans Affairs Medical Center
Portland, Oregon

Christoph E. Schreiner, PhD, MD
Department of Otolaryngology
University of California–San Francisco
San Francisco, California

Jacqueline B. Sheldrake, RHAD, BSHAA
The Tinnitus and Hyperascusis Centre
London, United Kingdom

Susan E. Shore, PhD
Department of Otolaryngology
University of Michigan
Ann Arbor, Michigan

Murray B. Stein, MD
Department of Psychiatry
University of California–San Diego
La Jolla, California

Dennis R. Trune, PhD, MBA
Department of Otolaryngology–Head and Neck Surgery
Oregon Health and Science University
Portland, Oregon

Richard S. Tyler, PhD
Department of Otolaryngology
University of Iowa
Iowa City, Iowa

Erik S. Viirre, MD, PhD
Department of Surgery
University of California–San Diego
San Diego, California

P. Ashley Wackym, MD
Department of Otolaryngology and Communication Sciences
Medical College of Wisconsin
Milwaukee, Wisconsin

Shelley A. Witt, MA
Department of Otolaryngology–Head and Neck Surgery
University of Iowa
Iowa City, Iowa

Mark A. Zacharek, MD
Department of Otolaryngology
Wayne State University
Detroit, Michigan

Jinsheng Zhang, PhD
Department of Otolaryngology
Wayne State University
Detroit, Michigan

CHAPTER 1

Overview: Suffering from Tinnitus

Robert A. Dobie, MD

Tinnitus is a sensation—specifically, a sound—that sometimes causes suffering. In this chapter, tinnitus is defined, along with its causes and associations; the sounds that patients with tinnitus hear (sensation) are discussed, and the ways in which tinnitus sometimes affects people (suffering) are described. Finally, the natural history of tinnitus, a subject about which very little is known, is discussed briefly.

WHAT IS TINNITUS?

McFadden defined tinnitus as a conscious experience of sound that originates in the head of its owner, in other words, without an external acoustic source.[1] Most audiologists and otolaryngologists would accept this definition but would then divide it into two categories: objective and subjective tinnitus. Objective tinnitus is produced by an internal acoustic source activating the cochlea (and then the auditory pathways of the brain) by air and/or bone conduction. Objective tinnitus (by definition) can be heard by another person. For example, a vascular tumor of the middle ear may produce a pulsatile or rushing sound, synchronous with the heartbeat, which is audible to the patient and to a physician who places one end of a stethoscope tube in the ear of the patient and the other in his or her own ear. Subjective tinnitus, on the other hand, can be heard only by the patient and is usually considered to have no acoustic source and thus no associated movements of the cochlear fluids or partitions.

One problem with this common usage is that some internal acoustic sources may produce sounds that are not audible to anyone except the patient. One could finesse this issue by redefining objective tinnitus to include sounds that potentially would be audible to another person, perhaps with amplification or with a middle ear microphone (many clinicians use the term in this way). A better approach, one followed in this chapter, may be to use the term *somatosound*, meaning "body sound," for all sounds with internal acoustic sources, whether or not they are audible to outsiders, and to reserve the term *tinnitus* for a sensation of sound in the absence of any acoustic source (in other words, *tinnitus* is used where many others would use *subjective tinnitus*).

WHAT CAUSES TINNITUS?

Brief spontaneous tinnitus, lasting seconds to minutes, is a nearly universal sensation. Temporary tinnitus, lasting minutes to hours, occurs routinely after noise exposures that are sufficiently intense and/or prolonged to cause temporary injury to the ear (eg, a firecracker explosion near the ear or attending a rock concert). Our concern, however, is with chronic tinnitus that is present frequently or continuously. As is discussed in Chapter 3, "Epidemiology of Tinnitus," chronic tinnitus is quite common; it occurs in men and women, in the young and old, and in people from all walks of life. Although it is more common in men, the elderly, blue-collar workers, and people with certain common health problems (arthritis, hypertension, varicose veins, and arteriosclerosis),[2] all of these associations are probably explained by one simple correlation: the worse one's hearing is, the more likely one is to have tinnitus (Figure 1-1).[3] It does not seem to matter very much whether the hearing problem is in the middle ear (conductive hearing loss) or in the inner ear (sensorineural hearing loss) or which otologic disorder has caused the hearing loss.

In the United States, as in other developed nations, most hearing loss develops gradually during middle or old age, without any identifiable cause or association other than advancing years. Age-related hearing loss,

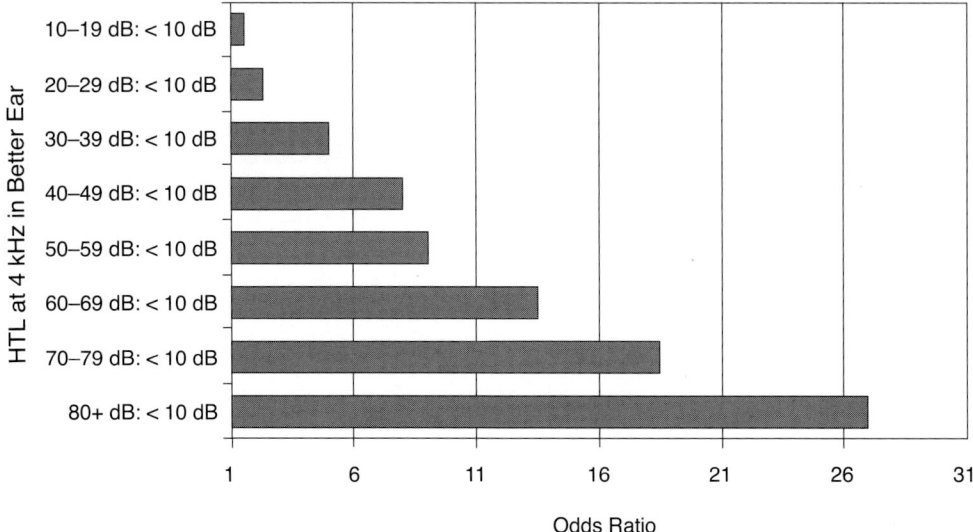

FIGURE 1-1. Bar graph showing how the odds of having tinnitus increase as hearing threshold level (HTL) at 4 kHz increases in the United Kingdom National Study of Hearing. Because the prevalence of tinnitus in people with 4 kHz thresholds less than 10 dB (the reference group) was about 1%, the odds ratios in this case are very close to the actual prevalence rates in percent. Reproduced with permission from Coles R.[3]

often called presbycusis, occurs whether or not people have had significant noise exposure, ear infections, or any other specific ear disease. It continues to progress throughout the life span and is usually more severe in men than in women of the same age. Thus, the prevalence of tinnitus may be expected to be higher in men and to increase with increasing age, and that is indeed what is uniformly found in epidemiologic surveys.

These same surveys generally show that the next most important risk factor for hearing loss and tinnitus, after age and gender, is excessive noise exposure. Noise-induced hearing loss is a dose-related phenomenon: although there is considerable variability in susceptibility across individuals, it is generally true that the louder the noise and the longer the exposure, the more hearing loss can be expected. People who have regular and prolonged noise exposure, usually at work, begin to be at risk of developing permanent hearing loss and tinnitus at levels of about 85 dBA (85 dB on the A scale); at this level of noise, most people would notice the need to speak very loudly or even to shout to converse at arm's length. Outside the workplace, the most important source of harmful noise exposure is recreational shooting. Any noise exposure that causes temporary tinnitus or muffled hearing can, if repeated regularly, cause permanent hearing loss and tinnitus. The US Occupational Safety and Health Administration regulates noise exposure for most US workers and requires annual audiometry, worker education, and use of hearing protection devices.

Many ear disorders other than noise-induced and age-related hearing loss cause hearing loss and tinnitus. For example, sensorineural hearing loss can be caused by infections, genetic mutations, some drugs used to fight infection and cancer, and head injuries. Conductive hearing loss is often caused by chronic ear infections or otosclerosis, a hereditary middle ear disease.

A few people who deny any hearing loss, including some who have completely normal hearing by ordinary clinical audiometry, complain of tinnitus. Although many clinicians postulate that such patients have subtle inner ear damage, I am unaware of any evidence that their ears are any different from those of healthy young adults who do not notice tinnitus. Perhaps some people are just unusually aware of and attentive to low-level sounds that are actually there for the listening in many, if not most, normal adult ears. Fowler introduced the concept of "subaudible" tinnitus; this apparent oxymoron refers to tinnitus that is not heard until one listens for it.[4] Heller and Bergman found that 94% of their normal-hearing adult subjects, all of whom initially denied tinnitus, reported sounds (usually buzzing, ringing, or humming) when placed in a soundproof booth and asked to listen for them.[5] Levine and colleagues reported a lower rate of tinnitus (35%) induced by simply placing normal subjects in an audiometric booth, but a similar proportion (37%) reported previously unnoticed tinnitus that was apparent only on contracting neck or jaw muscles (see Chapter 9, "Somatic Tinnitus").[6] Only 28% did not notice tinnitus in the booth. Of course, all of these subjects were adults, and even the youngest adults hear less well than children at frequencies beyond those conventionally used in audiometry (above 8 kHz).

Thus, it may be true that almost all tinnitus (excluding "somatosounds" or "objective tinnitus") is associated with some degree of hearing loss. But if, as one is tempted to conclude, "hearing loss causes tinnitus," how does it do so, and why does not everyone with hearing loss notice tinnitus? These questions of mechanism and pathophysiology are discussed in Chapters 4 through 14.

WHAT DOES TINNITUS SOUND LIKE?

Patients who complain of tinnitus usually describe their sounds as similar to those reported by normal subjects placed in a soundproof booth: most use words such as ringing, buzzing, humming, and whistling; some mention hissing, crickets, roaring, falling water, and a variety of other descriptions.[5] Just as the prevalence of tinnitus is related to the presence and severity of hearing loss rather than to particular otologic disorders, the quality of tinnitus is generally unrelated to specific diagnosis and is thus of little diagnostic use. One exception is the tinnitus of Meniere's disease, which is usually described as low pitched or roaring. In classic cases of Meniere's disease, this correlates with low-frequency hearing loss, but in early cases, when the audiogram may be normal between vertigo spells, a history of roaring tinnitus may be a clue to diagnosis. Of course, patients who describe pulsatile sounds, particularly if synchronous with the heartbeat, should be suspected of having somatosounds caused by vascular lesions in or near the ear.

Patients can be asked to compare their tinnitus sounds with tones and noises produced by audiometric equipment. This process is called matching (see Chapter 16, "Audiologic Assessment"). Most report that their tinnitus pitch is closest to tones or noises with central frequencies above 3 kHz.[7] Pitch judgments are rather variable on retesting, and octave errors are frequent.[1] Nevertheless, match frequency correlates, in general, with hearing loss severity and configuration (Figure 1-2).[3,8] When a tone or noise of about the right pitch is varied in intensity until it is just as loud as the patient's tinnitus, the matching intensity is usually found to be less than 10 dB above the patient's threshold at that frequency.[7]

Tinnitus is often maskable, that is, it can be rendered inaudible in the presence of external sounds, and this phenomenon has been exploited therapeutically; wearable masking devices were first widely available in the 1980s but seem less popular in recent years. Tinnitus masking is different in many respects from masking of external sounds. In some cases, a noise that initially totally masked the tinnitus may need to be gradually increased in intensity to prevent the tinnitus from becoming audible. In other cases, tinnitus may remain inaudible for a period of time after the masking noise has been turned off (this is called residual inhibition). Perhaps most strikingly, unilateral tinnitus may be masked by noises presented to the opposite ear, even at levels that are much too low to cross over and stimulate the cochlea of the "affected" ear. None of these phenomena have been

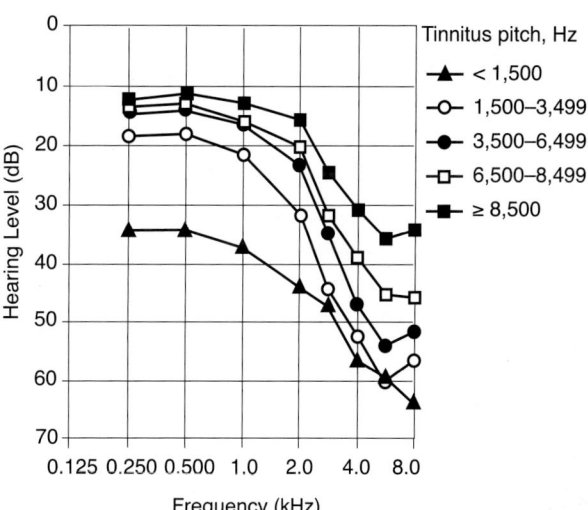

FIGURE 1-2. Patients with low-pitched tinnitus (< 1,500 Hz) tend to have much more severe hearing losses, especially in the low frequencies, than do patients with higher-pitched tinnitus. Mean right ear thresholds are shown for each tinnitus pitch group. Reproduced with permission from Henry JA et al.[8]

shown to have any diagnostic significance, although the proponents of masking therapy sometimes rely on them to guide their prescriptions and to predict treatment outcome.

Patients may describe tinnitus as heard in either ear, in both ears, or simply in the head. Left ear tinnitus is slightly more common than right ear tinnitus. Although serious otologic disorders such as acoustic tumors are usually associated with unilateral tinnitus, the prevalence of unilateral tinnitus in the general population is so high that the converse is certainly not true (most cases of unilateral tinnitus are not associated with life-threatening otologic disease).

HOW DOES TINNITUS AFFECT PEOPLE?

Fortunately, most people with chronic tinnitus are not too bothered by it. Many people never seek medical attention for their tinnitus, and many who see a physician want only to know that their tinnitus is not a harbinger of serious disease or impending deafness; such patients can almost always be reassured after appropriate diagnostic evaluation (see Chapter 16, "Audiologic Assessment"). Parenthetically, this evaluation and reassurance should never be cursory or dismissive; Stouffer and Tyler found that even after otologic evaluation, most patients were still concerned that their tinnitus was "a symptom of a much worse disease" or that they "might go deaf because of [their] tinnitus."[9]

On the other hand, many patients (tinnitus "sufferers") are very much bothered by their tinnitus. They may say that it is annoying, intrusive, upsetting, and distracting and even that it prevents them from carrying out certain activities in their daily lives (in other words, that it causes disability or handicap). The distinction between the sound of tinnitus (sensation) and the impact that tinnitus may have on a person (suffering) is important because they are essentially independent phenomena.

Although tinnitus sufferers often describe their tinnitus as very loud, their matching levels are not significantly different from those measured for patients with nonbothersome tinnitus, that is, they are usually less than 10 dB sensation level. In fact, it is impossible to predict from tinnitus sensation—its loudness, pitch, and quality—whether a person will be a tinnitus sufferer or will be someone who, like most people with tinnitus, forgets about it most of the time and denies any effect on mood or activities. In this respect, reaction to tinnitus is somewhat like reaction to unwanted external noise. Even very soft sounds—a dripping faucet, for example—can be very annoying, not because of the sound itself (the sensation) but rather for cognitive and psychological reasons ("The landlord won't return my calls requesting repair," "The plumber is going to charge too much," or "It just won't stop") that lead to suffering.

Tyler and Baker asked 97 tinnitus sufferers (members of a tinnitus self-help group) to list the difficulties that they had as a result of their tinnitus.[10] They received 72 responses, and most listed 4 or more problems. The most frequently reported problems were as follows:

1. Getting to sleep (57% of respondents)
2. Persistence of tinnitus (49%)
3. Understanding speech (38%)
4. Despair, frustration, or depression (36%)
5. Annoyance, irritation, or inability to relax (35%)
6. Poor concentration or confusion (33%)

Most other descriptive studies of tinnitus suffering have come to similar conclusions (reviewed by Stouffer and Tyler[9]): self-reported tinnitus problems tend to cluster into the categories of sleep (1, above), hearing (3), emotion (4 and 5), and concentration (6).

The persistence of tinnitus (2) seems to be a special case. Many patients state that their tinnitus is not particularly unpleasant except for the fact that, like a dripping faucet, it will not go away. Indeed, when my patients who have had tinnitus for years are asked if they would be satisfied with a treatment that would be guaranteed to make the tinnitus go away 6 months later, most admit that this would be entirely satisfactory. Tinnitus, unlike pain (but perhaps like paresthesia), is not inherently very unpleasant; it causes suffering in large part because of the meanings that people attach to it, for example, "It is a sign of serious disease," "I am going to go deaf," "It will get worse," or "I cannot control it" (Glass and Singer found that "loss of control" was an important factor in determining whether an external noise was perceived to be aversive[11]). These concerns can make it difficult for some people to ignore their tinnitus (ie, it becomes intrusive), leading to the typical problems with sleep, concentration, and emotion.

The hearing difficulties that tinnitus sufferers report are considered by most experts to be attributable to their hearing loss rather than to the tinnitus per se. Stouffer and Tyler state that "it seems likely that patients confuse the effects of tinnitus on speech understanding with the effects of hearing loss on speech understanding."[9] Bosman points out that most tinnitus matches to frequencies well above those most important for speech understanding[12]; thus, even if the tinnitus interfered with hearing external sounds in that spectral region, it would be difficult to explain tinnitus-related speech understanding problems based on conventional notions of speech acoustics. If there were any such direct effects of tinnitus on audibility, they should be reflected in the audiogram, and one would expect some patients to demonstrate improved audiograms on days when their tinnitus is absent or reduced; this appears not to have been reported. On the other hand, one report by Newman and colleagues suggests that tinnitus patients do worse on difficult speech tests than do patients with similar audiograms but no tinnitus.[13] Perhaps this is due to distraction and irritability making it difficult to concentrate, as suggested by Tyler and Baker.[10]

Many tinnitus sufferers, and some people who have no tinnitus, complain of difficulty tolerating external sounds of even moderate intensity (see Chapter 2, "Decreased Sound Tolerance").

Why do some people with tinnitus become tinnitus sufferers, whereas most do not? We have seen that the nature of the tinnitus sensation (loudness, pitch, quality) does not predict suffering, nor does the severity of hearing loss or its etiology (one possible exception: patients with Meniere's disease report more distress than other patients).[9] Retrospective studies suggest that psychological factors present before the onset of tinnitus may be very important. Many, if not most, patients with really bothersome tinnitus are found to have a major depressive disorder,[14] and about half of depressed tinnitus patients reported that they had had episodes of depression before they ever noticed tinnitus.[15] It seems likely that people who have had prior problems with depression,[16] and possibly with anxiety disorders,[17] are more likely to become tinnitus sufferers than are people who have not had such problems (see Chapter 23, "Psychological Methods of Therapy for Tinnitus").

Of course, people with tinnitus cannot simply be divided into two groups: those who suffer and those who do not. I find it useful to think of a pyramid with multiple levels: the base of the pyramid is formed by the people who are not concerned about their tinnitus, the next level includes people who just want to be checked to be sure that they do not have serious ear or brain disease, and the higher levels are composed of the people with progressively more severe problems with tinnitus in their daily lives. The highest levels include a very small number of people with very severe problems.

Some people with tinnitus commit suicide, but it is difficult to conclude that tinnitus "causes" suicide. Lewis and colleagues studied 6 of their own patients and reviewed the 22 other cases that they found in the literature.[18] Most were male, elderly, socially isolated, and depressed—classic warning signs for suicide with or without tinnitus. Any clinician seeing tinnitus patients should be aware of these associations and should promptly treat or refer patients who are clinically depressed (see Chapter 20, "Antidepressant Therapy for Tinnitus").

WHAT IS THE NATURAL HISTORY?

Patients frequently ask their physicians whether their tinnitus will get better, get worse, or stay the same. Unfortunately, there has been far too little good research to guide the answers. Retrospective clinic-based studies asking tinnitus patients how their tinnitus has changed over time tend to suggest that more patients get worse than get better[19] but are flawed by selection bias (patients whose tinnitus has improved spontaneously are much less likely to seek care and will not be counted). Population-based retrospective studies could provide useful information, but none of these studies appears to have inquired about changes over time (see Chapter 3, "Epidemiology of Tinnitus").

Two prospective clinical studies suggest that more patients get better than get worse,[20,21] but these studies have their own pitfalls. First, all patients had received at least brief counseling, and many had been more extensively treated, so these changes over time cannot be considered to be truly "natural history." Second, just as with retrospective clinical studies, selection bias is a problem: if some patients have spontaneous fluctuations of severity and if patients are more likely to seek care when they are more symptomatic, apparent spontaneous improvement after the first visit will be overrepresented (and spontaneous exacerbation underrepresented) in the data. Students of statistics will recognize this as the problem of regression to the mean.

One population-based longitudinal study of 153 elderly Swedes who had been followed from age 70 to age 79 found, as expected, that the prevalence of continuous or occasional tinnitus increased from age 70 (31%) to age 79 (44%).[22] Interestingly, 11 of 15 patients who had reported continuous tinnitus at age 70 reported only occasional tinnitus or no tinnitus by age 79, suggesting that some elderly patients experience spontaneous remissions or improvements. Unfortunately, this study did not attempt to measure tinnitus severity, so it is of little help in counseling patients who are really bothered by their tinnitus.

Even more striking is the lack of data pertaining to prognostic factors. We simply do not know how to predict which patients are likely to do well and which patients will do poorly without treatment. One could guess that factors such as age, gender, educational level, initial severity, and duration might predict outcome, but that would be conjecture.

Lacking better research data on natural history, most clinicians will fall back on clinical lore and their own clinical experience. Vernon recommends that tinnitus that is present for 2 years or more be considered permanent.[23] My own experience suggests that after 1 year, major spontaneous changes are infrequent, but that, over time, people are more likely to get better (suffer less), even without any treatment other than brief counseling, than to get worse.

IMPLICATIONS FOR TREATMENT

Sensation and suffering are different attributes of tinnitus, and most treatments aim to attack one or the other. Obviously, the ideal treatment would eliminate tinnitus altogether, that is, the sensation would be gone. Even if that did not make the patient an altogether happy person, there would no longer be any suffering that could be blamed on tinnitus, and the therapist could claim success. Unfortunately, no treatment has been shown to achieve that goal frequently or even more often than placebo treatment.

Changing the tinnitus sensation, for example, by making it less loud, might seem a worthy goal, but as we have seen, even very soft tinnitus can be associated with severe suffering. If the tinnitus is less loud, but the patient still cannot sleep, work, or play, has anything really been accomplished? Masking devices and hearing aids (see Chapter 22, "Role of Hearing Aids in Management for Tinnitus") are treatments aimed at the tinnitus sensation (making the tinnitus less audible, at least during the time in which the device is worn). In my opinion, the success or failure of such treatments should be measured in terms of the reduction in suffering, not the change in sensation.

Conversely, some treatments aim squarely at tinnitus suffering and make no attempt to change the tinnitus sensation. If they succeed in this goal, allowing the tinnitus sufferer to join the multitude of people who have tinnitus but do not care, why should we care whether the sensation—loudness, pitch, and quality—has changed?

This does not necessarily mean that treatments aimed at tinnitus suffering are better than those aimed at tinnitus sensation. It does mean that unless tinnitus sensation can be completely eliminated—an elusive goal—the outcomes of treatment should be measured in terms of reduction of suffering. Here we have a problem: there is so far no consensus among clinicians or clinical scientists on the best ways to measure tinnitus suffering (see Chapter 17, "Tinnitus Questionnaires"). This makes it more difficult to assess and compare the various treatments that have been tried.

Our lack of knowledge about the natural history of tinnitus sensation and suffering means that we can never rely on uncontrolled observations of treatment effects. There is really no substitute at this time for randomized clinical trials. Our lack of understanding of prognostic factors means that we will not be able to strengthen these trials by stratification (ensuring that patients with good or bad prognoses are equally represented in the different treatment groups). These issues are discussed in Chapter 19, "Clinical Trials and Drug Therapy for Tinnitus."

SUMMARY

Salient conclusions are as follows:
1. Tinnitus sensation and tinnitus suffering are different and largely independent phenomena.
2. Most tinnitus is associated with hearing loss (usually age related or noise induced in the United States).
3. The sounds described by tinnitus sufferers do not differ from those described by people who are not bothered by their tinnitus.
4. Tinnitus sufferers are often found to have current major depressive disorder.
5. Tinnitus sufferers frequently describe difficulties with sleep, concentration, and emotion; they also complain of hearing difficulties, which are, in most cases, attributable to their coexisting hearing loss.
6. Our lack of understanding of the natural history of tinnitus makes randomized clinical trials essential to prove the value of treatments for tinnitus.

REFERENCES

1. McFadden D. Tinnitus: facts, theories, and treatments. Washington (DC): National Academy Press; 1982.
2. Brown SC. Older Americans and tinnitus: a demographic study and chartbook. GRI monograph series a, number 2. Washington (DC): Gallaudet University; 1990.
3. Coles R. Medicolegal issues. In: Tyler RS, editor. Tinnitus handbook. San Diego (CA): Singular Publishing; 2000. p. 399–417.
4. Fowler EP Jr. Nonvibratory tinnitus, factor underlying subaudible and audible tinnitus. Arch Otolaryngol 1948;47:29.
5. Heller MF, Bergman M. Tinnitus aurium in normally hearing persons. Ann Otol Rhinol Laryngol 1953;62:73–93.
6. Levine RA, Abel M, Cheng H. Somatic tinnitus in nonclinical subjects and the profoundly deaf. In: Patuzzi R, editor. Proceedings of the Seventh International Tinnitus Seminar. Perth (Australia): University of Western Australia; 2002. p. 99–102.
7. Reed GF. An audiometric study of two hundred cases of subjective tinnitus. Arch Otolaryngol 1960;71:94–104.
8. Henry JA, Meikle M, Gilbert A. Audiometric correlates of tinnitus pitch. In: Hazell J, editor. Proceedings of the Sixth International Tinnitus Seminar. London: The Tinnitus and Hyperacusis Centre; 1999. p. 51–7.
9. Stouffer JL, Tyler RS. Characterization of tinnitus by tinnitus patients. J Speech Hear Disord 1990;55:439–53.
10. Tyler RS, Baker LJ. Difficulties experienced by tinnitus sufferers. J Speech Hear Disord 1983;48:150–4.
11. Glass DC, Singer JE. Behavioral after-effects of unpredictable and uncontrollable aversive events. Am Sci 1972;60:457–65.
12. Bosman AJ. Tinnitus assessment and its relation to rehabilitation. In: Patuzzi R, editor. Proceedings of the Seventh International Tinnitus Seminar. Perth (Australia): University of Western Australia; 2002. p. 143–6.
13. Newman CW, Wharton JA, Shivapuja BG, Jacobson GP. Relationships among psychoacoustic judgments, speech understanding ability, and self-perceived handicap in tinnitus subjects. Audiology 1994;33:47–60.
14. Sullivan MD, Katon WJ, Dobie RA, et al. Disabling tinnitus: association with affective disorder. Gen Hosp Psychiatry 1988;10:285–91.
15. Dobie RA, Katon WJ, Sullivan MD, Sakai CS. Tinnitus, depression, and aging. In: Goldstein JC, Kashima HK, Kooperman CF, editors. Geriatric otolaryngology. Toronto: BC Decker Inc; 1989. p. 45–8.
16. Zoger S, Svedlund J, Holgers KM. Is there a relationship between depressive disorder and the severity of tinnitus? In: Patuzzi R, editor. Proceedings of the Seventh International Tinnitus Seminar. Perth (Australia): University of Western Australia; 2002. p. 229–30.
17. Zoger S, Svedlund J, Holgers KM. Psychiatric profile of tinnitus patients with high risk of severe and chronic tinnitus. In: Patuzzi R, editor. Proceedings of the Seventh International Tinnitus Seminar. Perth (Australia): University of Western Australia; 2002. p. 306–7.
18. Lewis JE, Stephens SD, McKenna L. Tinnitus and suicide. Clin Otolaryngol 1994;19:50–4.
19. Stouffer JL, Tyler RS, Kileny PR, Dalzell LE. Tinnitus as a function of duration and etiology: counseling implications. Am J Otol 1991;12:188–94.
20. Holgers KM, Erlandsson SI, Barrenas ML. Predictive factors for the severity of tinnitus. Audiology 2000;39:284–91.
21. Andersson G, Vretblad P, Larsen HC, Lyttkens L. Longitudinal follow-up of tinnitus complaints. Arch Otolaryngol 2001;127:175–9.
22. Rubinstein B, Osterberg T, Rosenhall U. Longitudinal fluctuations in tinnitus as reported by an elderly population. J Audiol Med 1992;1:149–55.
23. Vernon JA. Is the claimed tinnitus real and is the claimed cause correct? In: Reich GE, Vernon JA, editors. Proceedings of the Fifth International Tinnitus Seminar. Portland (OR): American Tinnitus Association; 1996. p. 395–6.

CHAPTER 2

Decreased Sound Tolerance

Pawel J. Jastreboff, PhD, ScD, Margaret M. Jastreboff, PhD

Decreased sound tolerance is a recognized medical affliction, but it is rarely seriously addressed as a problem. Its negative impact on the patient's life is not appreciated and is frequently ignored. For years, the most common approach to decreased sound tolerance was the use of ear protection and avoidance of loud or specific, intrusive sounds. This approach, which was intuitively implemented and overused by patients, contributed to worsening of the problem instead of the expected relief. Many patients affected by tinnitus also complain of decreased sound tolerance, and often decreased sound tolerance is the more disturbing of the two symptoms. Fortunately, with growing interest in tinnitus, decreased sound tolerance is attracting more attention, and some advances have been made in understanding this problem.

DEFINITIONS

For years, two terms, *hyperacusis* and *phonophobia*, have been used in the literature to describe abnormal sensitivity or reactions to sound. They were not carefully defined and are frequently used interchangeably, resulting in unnecessary confusion. There is no generally accepted definition for decreased sound tolerance, although a variety of terms have been proposed, with hyperacusis used most frequently. Some descriptions of hyperacusis included oversensitive hearing, hearing with unusually low thresholds, exceptionally acute sense of hearing, abnormal acuteness of hearing owing to increased irritability of the sensorineural mechanisms, or collapse of loudness tolerance.[1-3] Descriptions of phonophobia include an overwhelming fear of sound or aversive reactions to sounds. According to *Stedman's Concise Medical Dictionary*,[2] hyperacusis is defined as "abnormal acuteness of hearing due to increased irritability of the sensory neural mechanism. SYN auditory hyperesthesia," and hyperesthesia is defined as "abnormal acuteness of sensitivity to touch, pain, or other sensory stimuli."[2] According to the *American Heritage Dictionary*, hyperesthesia is defined as "an abnormal or pathological increase in sensitivity to sensory stimuli, as of the skin to touch or the ear to sound."[4] It has been recognized that decreased sound tolerance might reflect physical discomfort or be related to fear of sound.[5] It is common for individuals with hearing impairment and individuals with normal hearing to experience decreased sound tolerance, contradicting statements that hyperacusis and phonophobia are related to exceptionally sensitive hearing abilities.

Several clinical observations lead to the conclusion that decreased sound tolerance and its severity are complex issues that involve more than the auditory system. Considering principles of auditory neuroscience, it can be concluded that the limbic and autonomic nervous systems are equally important as the peripheral and central parts of the auditory system in the phenomena related to decreased sound tolerance. Therefore, it is proposed that the definition of hyperacusis be an abnormally high level of sound-induced neuronal activity occurring within the auditory pathways owing to an abnormal amplification of sound-evoked neural signals. Hyperacusis manifests at the behavioral level as an experience of physical discomfort resulting from an exposure to moderate, or even weak, sound that would not evoke a similar reaction in the average person.[6,7] The discomfort strictly depends on the physical characteristics of a sound (its spectrum and intensity). The limbic and autonomic nervous systems are activated only secondarily owing to the abnormal activity within the auditory pathways. The functional connections with the auditory system are not changed (Figure 2-1).

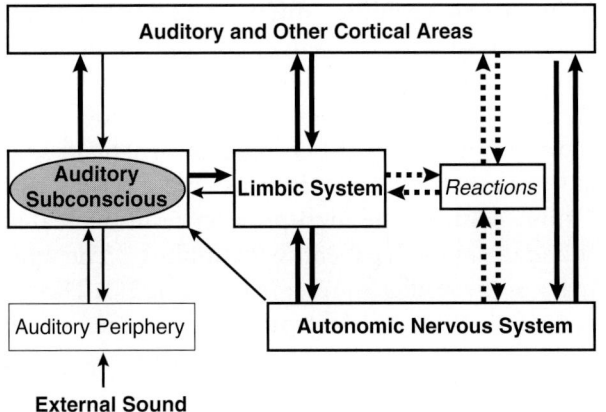

FIGURE 2-1. Neural systems and mechanisms involved in hyperacusis. Gray oval indicates the primary brain area responsible for hyperacusis. The thickness of arrows and boxes indicates the strength of activation. Dashed arrows indicate the interactions between various systems in the nervous system and reactions.

Most individuals who are diagnosed with hyperacusis, as well as some individuals without hyperacusis, express a negative attitude toward sound. Frequently, they avoid sound in general or specific sounds; others have fearful reactions or choose a particular sound environment. In the past, all of these behaviors were labeled as phobic, and patients were considered phonophobic. Treatments commonly implemented for phobias were rarely helpful in patients considered phonophobic; in addition, many of them strongly objected to the concept that they were afraid of sound(s). Frequently, very specific sounds or situations associated with sound were reported as causing discomfort or annoyance, leading to their strong dislike, hate, and, consequently, avoidance of sound.

Because of these observations, a new term, misophonia, was proposed from the Greek: *miso*, meaning hate or strong dislike.[6,7] This term describes an overall negative attitude to sound, including fear of sound (phonophobia). Misophonia reflects an abnormally strong reaction of the limbic and autonomic nervous systems to sound without abnormally high activation of the auditory system (Figure 2-2). Whereas in the case of hyperacusis, the strength of the reaction depends on the physical characteristics of a sound; in misophonia, this link is not direct, and the strength of reaction depends on the patient's previous experience with a given sound (or type of sound), the context in which the sound is presented, and the patient's psychological profile. Either a traumatic experience or repetitive negative association can enhance misophonia and result in a lifelong aversion.

There is no relationship between hyperacusis and/or misophonia with the threshold of hearing. Both problems can be present in individuals with normal hearing or with hearing loss. Hyperacusis and misophonia can also coexist with recruitment, a cochlear phenomenon associated with hearing loss and referring to an unusually rapid growth of loudness as the intensity of a tone is increased.[8] There is no functional link between hyperacusis and recruitment.

Although there are individuals with only hyperacusis or misophonia, in clinical practice, decreased sound tolerance is most frequently a combination of these problems.

METHODS OF EVALUATION

Although there is no consensus regarding a protocol for the evaluation of decreased sound tolerance, there is general agreement that a careful history and pure-tone loudness discomfort levels (LDLs) provide a reasonable estimation of the problem. Variations in the protocol for evaluation of LDLs are based on the types of sounds used, for example, continuous or pulsed, pure-tone, or narrowband noise.[9–11] Auditory brainstem responses have also been proposed for the estimation of LDLs.[12] Our preference is for a modification of a commonly used procedure[13] to minimize the ef-

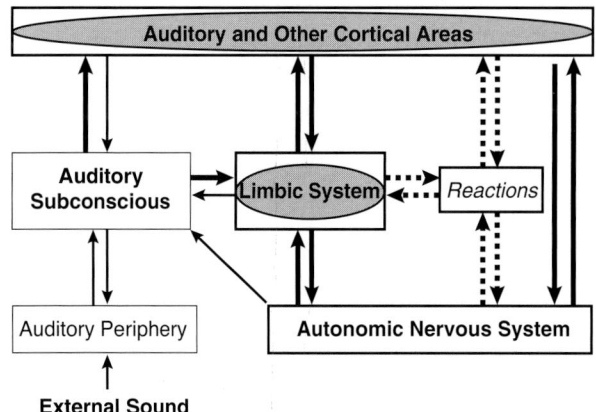

FIGURE 2-2. Neural systems and mechanisms involved in misophonia. *Gray ovals* indicate the primary brain areas responsible for misphonia. *Dashed arrows* indicate interactions between various systems in the nervous system and reactions.

fects of the misophonic component and, therefore, test predominantly the extent of the hyperacusis. During testing, patients have control over the maximal sound intensity to which they will be exposed and can stop the evaluation at any time.[14] As patients become familiar with the procedure, the anxiety and concerns that they may have had about the estimation of the LDLs decrease. Each patient receives a specific set of instructions regarding the test procedure. The measurements of LDLs are performed twice using short pure tones, with the initial intensity below the threshold of hearing and increased in 5 dB (or typically 1 dB) increments. It is common for patients with misophonia to have the first set of measurements be 10 to 15 dB lower than the second set. This protocol does not ensure complete elimination of the misophonic component; it does decrease the misophonic impact on final estimation of the LDLs. As a result, the measurements are more stable, that is, there is high test–retest repeatability.

A detailed interview is needed to determine the relative contribution of hyperacusis and misophonia to the overall problem of decreased sound tolerance. Reported normative data are not uniform, and there is substantial individual variability even while using one method of measuring LDLs[15] when proper control for misophonia is not carried out. It is advisable to consider the possible presence of hyperacusis when average LDL values are lower than 90 to 100 dB HL. Several studies indicate that normal LDLs are in the range of 90 to 110 dB SPL, with varied results related to the specific method used for testing, for example, stimuli of pure tones, warble tone, noise and presentation via free field, insert earphones, and headphones.[9,13–15] The results tend to cluster within 95 to 110 dB SPL for frequencies from 500 to 8,000 Hz, which correspond to approximately 90 to 100 dB HL.[13,14,16]

Although average values of LDLs provide some guidelines for diagnosis, patients' complaints do not simplistically correlate with the values of LDLs. Some patients with normal LDLs exhibit strong reactions to everyday sounds that are accepted by others in their surroundings. Other patients with LDLs in the range of 90 dB HL do not report any noticeable impact of these sounds on their life. Another group may have LDLs in the range of 20 to 40 dB HL, and even though they report problems of decreased sound tolerance, they are, nevertheless, able to tolerate some louder sounds than indicated by their LDLs, for example, the normal level of speech.

Many patients exhibit a different level of tolerance to various sounds, which does not correspond to the physical characterization of these sounds, that is, their spectrum and overall intensity. The most recent results from a group of 149 consecutive patients seen at Emory University Tinnitus and Hyperacusis Center confirm the high prevalence of decreased sound tolerance in patients with tinnitus.[17] The summary of the results is presented in Table 2-1. The average of LDLs for patients reporting problems with sound tolerance was 81.7 dB HL, whereas for all other patients, it was 102.0 dB HL.

Patients with significant hyperacusis typically develop misophonia as well. Because LDLs represent an estimation of the sum of hyperacusis and misophonia, as expected, the average LDLs for patients with hyperacusis, some of whom had misophonia as well, were the lowest in our patient population.[17] Note that LDL values tend to be around 80 dB HL for patients exhibiting some problems with decreased sound tolerance, suggesting 80 to 85 dB HL as the indicator for the need for sound tolerance treatment.

PREVALENCE AND EPIDEMIOLOGY

The prevalence of decreased sound tolerance in the general population is not well documented. The only study on randomly selected subjects, by Fabijanska and

TABLE 2-1. Decreased Sound Tolerance and Loudness Discomfort Level in a Population of 149 Consecutive Patients

Diagnosis	Percentage of Population	LDL (dB HL)
DST (with or without tinnitus)	66.4	82.2
DST (no tinnitus)	2.7	85.0
Misophonia (with or without hyperacusis)	57.0	81.9
Misophonia (no hyperacusis)	28.9	92.8
Hyperacusis (with or without misophonia)	32.9	73.5
Hearing loss and hyperacusis	17.4	75.6

DST = decreased sound tolerance; LDL = loudness discomfort level.
All subgroups, except second, represent data from patients with or without tinnitus.[17]

colleagues, showed that 15.3% of 10,349 questioned individuals reported decreased sound tolerance.[18] These results were based exclusively on questionnaires, and the severity of the problem and the need for intervention were not studied. Decreased sound tolerance affects people of all ages, including children.[19–22]

On the basis of the neurophysiological model of tinnitus[23] (see Chapter 8, "The Neurophysiological Model of Tinnitus"), it was reasonable to expect a high prevalence of hyperacusis in a population of patients with tinnitus. Consequently, from 1990, estimation of the LDLs was included in the audiologic assessment of all patients during the initial and follow-up visits to the tinnitus centers at the University of Maryland and Emory University. From the beginning, it became clear that about 40% of patients experience decreased sound tolerance.[24] Approximately 30% of them required specific treatment for hyperacusis.[6,14,25] This observation has been confirmed by other centers.[18,26–31]

At present, there appears to be a consensus that decreased sound tolerance affects a substantial proportion of tinnitus patients. This is in contrast to some reports in the literature stating that only 0.3% of patients with tinnitus have symptoms of hyperacusis.[3] The results presented in Table 2-1 indicate that 66.4% of patients with tinnitus exhibited some degree of decreased sound tolerance, with 32.9% requiring specific treatment for hyperacusis. Therefore, assuming that approximately 30% of patients with tinnitus require treatment for hyperacusis, considering that 86% of hyperacusis patients reported tinnitus,[32] and accepting that approximately 4% of the general population have clinically significant tinnitus, it is possible to extrapolate using Bayesian probability theory ($0.3 \times 4\% = 1.2\%$, $100\% - 86\% = 14\%$, $1.2\% \times 0.14 = 0.168\%$, and $1.2\% + 0.168\% = 1.4\%$) that significant hyperacusis probably exists in at least 1.4% of the general population, and decreased sound tolerance affects a proportion twice as large. This assessment might be very conservative if the findings of Fabijanska and colleagues[18] are confirmed.

Finally, because increased gain within the auditory pathways will enhance an already existing low level of tinnitus-related neuronal activity and consequently may cause it to cross the threshold of detection, individuals with hyperacusis may have a tendency to develop tinnitus. On the other hand, decreasing this gain should reduce the tinnitus signal. For some patients, tinnitus and hyperacusis may be considered the double manifestation of the same internal phenomenon. Therefore, it was postulated that, in some cases, hyperacusis might be a pretinnitus state.[23]

There is a rather common opinion that hyperacusis occurs only or predominantly in individuals with normal hearing. Contrary to this belief, our results show that 52.9% of patients requiring treatment for hyperacusis have a hearing loss.[17]

In 91 patients with hearing loss, 62.6% reported decreased sound tolerance, 57.0% were diagnosed with misophonia, and 29.7% were diagnosed with hyperacusis.[17] Of those with hearing loss, 72.5% had high-frequency hearing loss, 5.5% conductive hearing loss, and 22.0% other types of hearing loss.

ETIOLOGY AND POSSIBLE MECHANISMS

In the majority of patients with hyperacusis, the cause is unknown. Hyperacusis has been linked to sound exposure, particularly impulse noise, head injury, stress, and medications.[6,29,33,34] A specific study of 187 patients aimed at predisposing and triggering factors for decreased sound tolerance revealed that the most common factors were recent onset of tinnitus, followed by stress, acute sound exposure, chronic sound exposure, and long-term dislike of sound.[35] Notably, 69% of the patients were linked to nonauditory triggers.

Hyperacusis and misophonia can appear in individuals with normal hearing or various types of hearing loss. These phenomena are not related to recruitment, which results from the elevated threshold of hearing and is governed by purely peripheral mechanisms caused by a loss of outer hair cells (OHCs) in the cochlea. On the other hand, the mechanisms of hyperacusis can be not only peripheral but also central or mixed. Misophonia always involves only central mechanisms.

At the peripheral level, it is possible to speculate that the abnormal enhancement of the vibratory signals within the cochlea by the OHCs might result in overstimulation of inner hair cells (IHCs) and, subsequently, in hyperacusis.[23] Indeed, in some cases, it is possible to observe high amplitude of distortion-product otoacoustic emissions reflecting a high level of OHC activity and responses evoked by low-level primaries.[36] An abnormally steep growth function has been reported as well.[37] Other possible peripheral mechanisms of hyperacusis might involve dysfunction of the mechanisms controlling the decrease of the amplification produced by OHCs when the sound level increases or abnormally high amplification provided by OHCs. Indeed, in some patients, there is an indication of inappropriate function of the OHC system, as evaluated by distortion-product otoacoustic emissions. The involvement of the efferent medial olivocochlear bundle has been proposed,[38] but the results are not conclusive.[39] The finding that reduced LDLs are not associated with the threshold of the stapedial reflex[28,29] suggests that the IHC system is not involved.

Central mechanisms of hyperacusis might involve the increase of the sensitivity of neurons in the central auditory pathways (dorsal cochlear nuclei, inferior colliculi) after decreased auditory input.[40–44] Research in animals has shown that damage to the cochlea or decrease of the auditory input results in a decrease in the threshold of response in a substantial proportion of neurons in the ventral cochlear nucleus and inferior colliculus.[45] Studies with evoked potentials demonstrate the abnormal increase in the gain in the auditory pathways after such manipulations.[46] Some medical conditions can be linked to the central processing of signals and modification of the level of neuromodulators, for example, in depression, as factors inducing or enhancing hyperacusis. Moreover, serotonin has been implicated in hyperacusis,[47] and a case report indicated that selective serotonin reuptake inhibitors might be helpful in the treatment of hyperacusis.[48]

The postulate of autonomic gain control can explain why hyperacusis sometimes emerges after removal of bilateral cerumen or stapedectomy. Both procedures result in a rapid increase in input to the auditory system, which was compensating for the previous lower level of sound reaching the cochlea by overamplification. The presence of asymmetric hyperacusis[14] suggests peripheral mechanisms because central mechanisms would more likely act similarly on both sides.

Mechanisms of misophonia could involve enhancement of the functional links between the auditory and limbic systems at the cognitive and subconscious levels.[23] Alternatively, a high level of tonic activation of the limbic and autonomic nervous systems may result in strong behavioral reactions to moderate sounds.[49,50] As mentioned above, most frequently, significantly decreased sound tolerance results from a combination of both hyperacusis and misophonia.

HYPERACUSIS AND MISOPHONIA AS A PROBLEM

Decreased sound tolerance can strongly affect patients' lives, and it can be an even more debilitating problem than tinnitus. Whereas tinnitus may affect sleep, attention, quiet recreational activities, work, family interaction, and life enjoyment and make social contact less rewarding, hyperacusis can completely stop individuals from exposure to even a slightly louder environment. Therefore, it prevents them from working, interacting socially, attending concerts or sports events, driving a car, etc. Sometimes high-pitched or children's voices are mentioned as particularly unpleasant. Sounds from moving china and from using vacuum cleaners, hair dryers, and lawn mowers, as well as many other everyday events, can be very intrusive. In extreme cases, patients do not leave their homes, and the issues of sound preoccupy their lives and the lives of their families. Misophonia can have very similar effects, and because misophonia is inevitable in all cases with significant hyperacusis, it further enhances the effects of hyperacusis and increases the focus on avoidance of any sound. It is a natural tendency to plug the ears to exclude unpleasant sounds, which unfortunately makes decreased sound tolerance worse, frequently inducing anxiety, obsessive tendencies, and depression. Therefore, application of hearing conservation measures is detrimental.

DECREASED SOUND TOLERANCE AS A SYMPTOM OF MEDICAL CONDITIONS

Hyperacusis has been linked to a number of medical conditions, including tinnitus, Bell's palsy, Lyme disease, Williams syndrome, Ramsay Hunt syndrome, stapedectomy, perilymphatic fistula, head injury, migraine, depression, withdrawal from benzodiazepines, cerebrospinal fluid hypertension, and Addison's disease.[14,19,20,48,51–61] Interestingly, 95% of children with Williams syndrome have hyperacusis,[61] suggesting a genetic basis for hyperacusis.

TREATMENT FOR DECREASED SOUND TOLERANCE

Treatment for hyperacusis goes in two contrary directions. First, the most common approach is to advise patients to avoid sound and use ear protection. This is based on reasoning that because patients have become sensitive to sound, this may indicate that they are more susceptible to sound exposure and, consequently, need extra protection. Patients easily embrace this philosophy and start to protect their ears, even to the extent of using earplugs in quiet environments. Unfortunately, this approach actually makes the auditory system even more sensitive and further exacerbates hyperacusis.

The second approach involves the desensitization of patients by exposure to a variety of sounds. The desensitization approach has been promoted for some time with a variety of protocols and types of sounds used, such as the recommendation of using sound with certain frequencies removed, short exposures to moderately loud sound, or prolonged exposures to low-level sounds.[3,25,29,62,63] The introduction of the neurophysiological model of tinnitus and tinnitus retraining therapy (TRT) offered a new approach to hyperacusis (see Chapter 21, "Tinnitus Retraining Therapy"). A significant improvement in hyperacusis patients with TRT has already been reported.[14,30,31,35,64–66] The misophonic component cannot be eliminated by desensitization, and a different approach is implemented in TRT.[17] Although TRT offers only relief of, not a cure for, tinnitus, it can, in some patients, totally eliminate hyperacusis and misophonia, thus providing a cure for these conditions.[67,68] Additionally, because tinnitus and hyperacusis are two manifestations of the same internal mechanisms of increased gain within the auditory pathways in some patients, the improvement in hyperacusis results in improvement in tinnitus as well. Moreover, the elimination of hyperacusis decreases general anxiety and stress, which, in combination with proper counseling, greatly facilitates tinnitus habituation.

REFERENCES

1. Dorland's illustrated medical dictionary. 26th ed. Philadelphia: WB Saunders; 1974.
2. Stedman's concise medical dictionary. 26th ed. Baltimore: Williams & Wilkins; 1997.
3. Vernon J, Press L. Treatment for hyperacusis. In: Vernon JA, editor. Tinnitus treatment and relief. Boston: Allyn and Bacon; 1998. p. 223–7.
4. The American heritage dictionary. 3rd ed. Boston: SoftKey International; 1994.
5. Jastreboff PJ, Gray WC, Mattox DE. Tinnitus and hyperacusis. In: Cummings CW, Fredrickson JM, Harker LA, et al, editors. Otolaryngology head and neck surgery. St. Louis: Mosby; 1998. p. 3198–222.
6. Jastreboff PJ, Jastreboff MM. Tinnitus and hyperacusis. In: Snow JB, Ballenger JJ, editors. Ballenger's otorhinolaryngology head and neck surgery. Hamilton (ON): BC Decker; 2003. p. 456–75.
7. Jastreboff MM, Jastreboff PJ. Hyperacusis. Audiology On-line June 2001. Available at: http://www.audiologyonline.com (accessed April 20, 2004).
8. Moore BCJ. An introduction to the psychology of hearing. 3rd ed. San Diego (CA): Academic Press; 1995.
9. Cox RM, Alexander GC, Taylor IM, Gray GA. The contour test of loudness perception. Ear Hear 1997;18:388–400.
10. Ricketts TA, Bentler RA. The effect of test signal type and bandwidth on the categorical scaling of loudness. J Acoust Soc Am 1996;99:2281–7.
11. Hawkins DB, Walden BE, Montgomery A, Prosek RA. Description and validation of an LDL procedure designed to select SSPL90. Ear Hear 1987;8:162–9.
12. Thornton ARD, Farrell G, McSporran EL. Clinical methods for the objective estimation of loudness discomfort level (LDL) using auditory brainstem responses in patients. Scand Audiol 1989;18:225–30.
13. Hood JD, Poole JP. Tolerable limit to loudness: its clinical and physiological significance. J Acoust Soc Am 1966;40:47–53.
14. Jastreboff PJ, Jastreboff MM, Sheldrake JB. Audiometrical characterization of hyperacusis patients before and during TRT. In: Hazell J, editor. Proceedings of the Sixth International Tinnitus Seminar. London: Tinnitus and Hyperacusis Centre; 1999. p. 495–8.
15. Byrne D, Dirks D. Effects of acclimatization and deprivation on non-speech auditory abilities. Ear Hear 1996;17(3 Suppl):29S–37S.
16. Stephens SD, Anderson C. Experimental studies on the uncomfortable loudness level. J Speech Hear Res 1971;14:262–70.
17. Jastreboff MM, Jastreboff PJ. Decreased sound tolerance and tinnitus retraining therapy (TRT). Aust N Z J Audiol 2002;21:74–81.
18. Fabijanska A, Rogowski M, Bartnik G, Skarzynski H. Epidemiology of tinnitus and hyperacusis in Poland. In: Hazell J, editor. Proceedings of the Sixth International Tinnitus Seminar. London: Tinnitus and Hyperacusis Centre; 1999. p. 569–71.
19. Oen JM, Begeer JH, Staal-Schreinemachers A, Tijmstra T. Hyperacusis in children with spina bifida; a pilot-study. Eur J Pediatr Surg 1997;7 Suppl 1:46.
20. Klein AJ, Armstrong BL, Greer MK, Brown FR. Hyperacusis and otitis media in individuals with

Williams syndrome. J Speech Hear Disord 1990; 55:339–44.
21. Jastreboff MM, Jastreboff PJ. Tinnitus retraining therapy in treating tinnitus and hyperacusis in children [abstract 966]. In: Santi PA, editor. Abstracts of the Twenty-Fifth Annual Midwinter Research Meeting of the Association for Research in Otolaryngology. Mt. Royal (NJ): Association for Research in Otolaryngology; 2002. p. 254.
22. Jastreboff MM, Jastreboff PJ. Hyperacusis in children. Audiology On-line. November 2001. Available at: http://www.audiologyonline.com/askexpert (accessed April 20, 2004).
23. Jastreboff PJ. Phantom auditory perception (tinnitus): mechanisms of generation and perception. Neurosci Res 1990;8:221–54.
24. Jastreboff PJ, Gold SL, Gray WC. Neurophysiological approach to tinnitus and hyperacusis patients [abstract]. In: Abstracts of the Seventeenth Annual Midwinter Research Meeting of the Association for Research in Otolaryngology. Des Moines (IA): Association for Research in Otolaryngology; 1994. p. 9.
25. Jastreboff PJ, Jastreboff MM. Tinnitus retraining therapy (TRT) as a method for treatment of tinnitus and hyperacusis patients. J Am Acad Audiol 2000;11:156–61.
26. Lux-Wellenhof G. Treatment history of incoming patients to the Tinnitus & Hyperacusis Centre in Frankfurt/Main. In: Hazell J, editor. Proceedings of the Sixth International Tinnitus Seminar. London: Tinnitus and Hyperacusis Centre; 1999. p. 502–6.
27. Pilgramm M, Rychlick R, Lebisch H, et al. Tinnitus in the Federal Republic of Germany: a representative epidemiological study. In: Hazell J, editor. Proceedings of the Sixth International Tinnitus Seminar. London: Tinnitus and Hyperacusis Centre; 1999. p. 64–7.
28. Coles RRA, Sood SK. Hyperacusis and phonophobia in tinnitus patients. Br J Audiol 1988;22:228.
29. Hazell JWP, Sheldrake JB. Hyperacusis and tinnitus. In: Aran J-M, Dauman R, editors. Tinnitus 91. Proceedings of the Fourth International Tinnitus Seminar. Amsterdam: Kugler Publications; 1992. p. 245–8.
30. Gold SL, Frederick EA, Formby C. Shifts in dynamic range for hyperacusis patients receiving tinnitus retraining therapy (TRT). In: Hazell J, editor. Proceedings of the Sixth International Tinnitus Seminar. London: Tinnitus and Hyperacusis Centre; 1999. p. 297–301.
31. Gold SL, Formby C, Frederick EA, Suter C. Shifts in loudness discomfort level in tinnitus patients with and without hyperacusis. In: Patuzzi R, editor. Proceedings of the Seventh International Tinnitus Seminar. Perth (Australia): The University of Western Australia; 2002. p. 170–2.
32. Anari M, Axelsson A, Elies W, Magnusson L. Hypersensitivity to sound—questionnaire data, audiometry and classification. Scand Audiol 1999;28:219–30.
33. Jastreboff PJ, Jastreboff MM. Tinnitus retraining therapy for patients with tinnitus and decreased sound tolerance. Otolaryngol Clin North Am 2003;36:321–36.
34. Reich GE, Griest SE. A survey of hyperacusis patients. In: Aran J-M, Dauman R, editors. Tinnitus 91. Proceedings of the Fourth International Tinnitus Seminar. Amsterdam: Kugler Publications; 1992. p. 249–53.
35. Hazell JWP, Sheldrake JB, Graham RL. Decreased sound tolerance: predisposing/triggering factors and treatment outcome following tinnitus retraining therapy (TRT). In: Patuzzi R, editor. Proceedings of the Seventh International Tinnitus Seminar. Perth (Australia): The University of Western Australia; 2002. p. 255–61.
36. Jastreboff PJ, Mattox DE. Treatment of hyperacusis by aspirin [abstract]. In: Popelka GR, editor. Abstracts of the Twenty-First Annual Midwinter Research Meeting of the Association for Research in Otolaryngology. Mt. Royal (NJ): Association for Research in Otolaryngology; 1998. p. 52.
37. Hesse G, Masri S, Nelting M, Brehmer D. Hypermotility of outer hair cells: DPOAE findings with hyperacusis patients. In: Hazell J, editor. Proceedings of the Sixth International Tinnitus Seminar. London: Tinnitus and Hyperacusis Centre; 1999. p. 342–4.
38. Collet L, Veuillet E, Bene J, Morgon A. Effects of contralateral white noise on click-evoked emissions in normal and sensorineural ears: towards an explanation of the medial olivocochlear system. Audiology 1992;31:1–7.
39. Khalfa S, Veuillet E, Grima F, et al. Hyperacusis assessment: relationship with tinnitus. In: Hazell J, editor. Proceedings of the Sixth International Tinnitus Seminar. London: Tinnitus and Hyperacusis Centre; 1999. p. 128–32.
40. Salvi RJ, Wang J, Powers N. Rapid functional reorganization in the inferior colliculus and cochlear nucleus after acute cochlear damage. In: Salvi RJ, Henderson D, Fiorino F, Colletti V, editors. Auditory system plasticity and regeneration. New York: Thieme Medical Publishers; 1996. p. 275–96.
41. Gerken GM, Simhadri-Sumithra R, Bhat KHV. Increase in central auditory responsiveness during continuous

tone stimulation or following hearing loss. In: Salvi RJ, Henderson D, Hamernik RP, Colletti V, editors. Basic and applied aspects of noise-induced hearing loss. New York: Plenum Publishing Corporation; 1986. p. 195–211.
42. Gerken GM, Saunders SS, Paul RE. Hypersensitivity to electrical stimulation of auditory nuclei follows hearing loss in cats. Hear Res 1984;13:249–59.
43. Sasaki CT, Kauer JS, Babitz L. Differential [^{14}C]2-deoxyglucose uptake after deafferentation of the mammalian auditory pathway—a model for examining tinnitus. Brain Res 1980;194:511–6.
44. Gerken GM. Central denervation hypersensitivity in the auditory system of the cat. J Acoust Soc Am 1979;66:721–7.
45. Boettcher FA, Salvi RJ. Functional changes in the ventral cochlear nucleus following acute acoustic overstimulation. J Acoust Soc Am 1993;94:2123–34.
46. Gerken GM. Alteration of central auditory processing of brief stimuli: a review and a neural model. J Acoust Soc Am 1993;93:2038–49.
47. Marriage J, Barnes NM. Is central hyperacusis a symptom of 5-hydroxytryptamine (5-HT) dysfunction? J Laryngol Otol 1995;109:915–21.
48. Gopal KV, Daly DM, Daniloff RG, Pennartz L. Effects of selective serotonin reuptake inhibitors on auditory processing: case study. J Am Acad Audiol 2000;11:454–63.
49. Jastreboff PJ. The neurophysiological model of tinnitus and hyperacusis. In: Hazell J, editor. Proceedings of the Sixth International Tinnitus Seminar. London: Tinnitus and Hyperacusis Centre; 1999. p. 32–8.
50. Jastreboff PJ. Optimal sound use in TRT—theory and practice. In: Hazell J, editor. Proceedings of the Sixth International Tinnitus Seminar. London: Tinnitus and Hyperacusis Centre; 1999. p. 491–4.
51. Adour KK, Wingerd J. Idiopathic facial paralysis (Bell's palsy): factors affecting severity and outcome in 446 patients. Neurology 1974;24:1112–6.
52. Fallon BA, Nields JA, Burrascano JJ, et al. The neuropsychiatric manifestation of Lyme borreliosis. Psychiatr Q 1992;63:95–117.
53. Nields JA, Fallon BA, Jastreboff PJ. Carbamazepine in the treatment of Lyme disease-induced hyperacusis. J Neuropsychiatry Clin Neurosci 1999;11:97–9.
54. Wayman DM, Pham HN, Byl FM, Adour KK. Audiological manifestations of Ramsay Hunt syndrome. J Laryngol Otol 1990;104:104–8.
55. McCandless GA, Goering DM. Changes in loudness after stapedectomy. Arch Otolaryngol 1974;100:344–50.
56. Fukaya T, Nomura Y. Audiological aspects of idiopathic perilymphatic fistula. Acta Otolaryngol Suppl (Stockh) 1988;456:68–73.
57. Waddell PA, Gronwall DMA. Sensitivity to light and sound following minor head injury. Acta Neurol Scand 1984;69:270–6.
58. Vingen JV, Pareja JA, Storen O, et al. Phonophobia in migraine. Cephalalgia 1998;18:243–9.
59. Lader M. Anxiolytic drugs: dependence, addiction and abuse. Eur Neuropsychopharmacol 1994;4:85–91.
60. Henkin RI, Daly RL. Auditory detection and perception in normal man and in patients with adrenal cortical insufficiency: effect of adrenal cortical steroids. J Clin Invest 1968;47:1269–80.
61. Nigam A, Samuel PR. Hyperacusis and Williams syndrome. J Laryngol Otol 1994;108:494–6.
62. Valente M, Goebel J, Duddy D, et al. Evaluation and treatment of severe hyperacusis. J Am Acad Audiol 2000;11:295–9.
63. Vernon JA. Pathophysiology of tinnitus: a special case—hyperacusis and a proposed treatment. Am J Otol 1987;8:201–2.
64. Wolk C, Seefeld B. The efects of managing hyperacusis with maskers (noise generators). In: Hazell J, editor. Proceedings of the Sixth International Tinnitus Seminar. London: Tinnitus and Hyperacusis Centre; 1999. p. 512–4.
65. McKinney CJ, Hazell JWP, Graham RL. Changes in loudness discomfort level and sensitivity to environmental sound with habituation based therapy. In: Hazell J, editor. Proceedings of the Sixth International Tinnitus Seminar. London: Tinnitus and Hyperacusis Centre; 1999. p. 499–501.
66. Bartnik G, Fabijanska A, Rogowski M. Our experience in treatment of patients with tinnitus and/or hyperacusis using the habituation method. In: Hazell J, editor. Proceedings of the Sixth International Tinnitus Seminar. London: Tinnitus and Hyperacusis Centre; 1999. p. 415–7.
67. Jastreboff PJ. Categories of the patients and the treatment outcome. In: Hazell J, editor. Proceedings of the Sixth International Tinnitus Seminar. London: Tinnitus and Hyperacusis Centre; 1999. p. 394–8.
68. Jastreboff PJ, Jastreboff MM. Tinnitus retraining therapy. In: Baguley D, editor. Perspectives in tinnitus management. New York: Thieme Medical Publishers; 2001. p. 51–63.

CHAPTER 3

Epidemiology of Tinnitus

Howard J. Hoffman, MA, George W. Reed, PhD

In this chapter, we review recent epidemiologic studies of risk factors for tinnitus, the perception of ringing, buzzing, or other noise in the ears or head without an external source of sound. We supplement the available epidemiologic literature with new analyses based on two large, nationally representative health interview surveys from the United States and a recent health examination survey conducted in one county (Nord Trøndelag) in central Norway.

For those who are not well acquainted with the field of epidemiologic research, it is natural to wonder what is epidemiology? In an early treatment of the scope, principles, and methods of epidemiology in 1927, Frost stated that epidemiology is

> essentially a collective science, and its progress is largely dependent upon that which has been made in other fields ... Epidemiology must also draw upon statistical method and theory, because even the simplest of quantitative descriptions must be stated statistically... Usage has extended the meaning of epidemiology beyond its original limits, to denote not merely the doctrine of epidemics but a science of broader scope in relation to the mass-phenomena of diseases in their usual or endemic as well as their epidemic occurrences.[1]

The etymology of the word epidemiology is instructive: *epi* means either on or about, *demos* is the people or population, and *logy* means "the study of." Hence, in broad terms, epidemiology can be defined "as the study of the distribution of a disease or a physiological condition in human populations and of factors that influence this distribution."[2] Another definition of epidemiology is "the study of the distribution and determinants of health-related events in specified populations and the application of this study to control health problems."[3] This rewording of the definition clarifies the purpose of epidemiologic research, which is to provide knowledge to improve health and prevent disease.

A further distinction, reflecting historical developments, divides the subject into "descriptive" and "analytic" epidemiology. Szklo and Nieto refer to descriptive epidemiology as the examination of available data to investigate how rates (usually concerning mortality) vary according to demographic variables (eg, those available in censuses). When the rates are not uniform according to person, time, and place, the epidemiologist seeks to identify high-risk groups for prevention purposes and to generate hypotheses about causal factors.[4] These authors define analytic epidemiology as the assessment of hypotheses of association between suspected risk factor exposures and health outcomes. The techniques for assessment of associations in analytic epidemiology can be applied equally to (1) experimental studies using populations or groups of individuals as units in clinical trials and (2) observational studies that use individuals as the unit for analysis in (prospective) cohort, case-control, or cross-sectional study designs.[4] In this chapter, our focus is primarily on the use of analytic epidemiologic techniques for observational studies of potential risk factors for tinnitus.

METHODS AND SOURCES OF DATA

In addition to citing data from published studies on the epidemiology of tinnitus, we analyzed available public use data sets from the National Health Interview Survey (NHIS). This survey has been conducted by the National Center for Health Statistics on a continuing basis since 1957 and is designed to assess the health status of the civilian, noninstitutionalized population of the United States. Participants are selected randomly through a complex multistage probability sampling design and are interviewed in their own homes.[5] The US Bureau of the Census employs and trains the interviewers who conduct the field work for the NHIS. Response rates have routinely been between 94 and 98% each year.[6] To ensure that estimates are representative of the population by sex, race or ethnicity, and residence, weights are provided as part of the public use data set. All statistical estimates are subject to concerns about bias and variability. Weights are used in the analysis to reduce bias from the particular sample of respondents who participated in the survey. Weights, together with additional information about the primary sampling units (cities, counties, etc) in the sampling design, are also used to provide appropriate estimates of variability, which are crucial for statistical significance testing and derivation of confidence intervals (CIs).

In 1990–1991, the NHIS conducted the third periodic supplement on hearing ability in the United States. Previous survey supplements on hearing were conducted in 1971 and 1977. The interviewed sample for 1990–1991 consisted of 93,237 randomly selected households (239,663 persons); the noninterview rate for households was 4.4%, of which 2.7% were refusals, and the remainder were due primarily to failure to locate the residents at home.[7] For this chapter, we analyzed data from the 1990 Hearing Supplement to the NHIS, sponsored by the National Institute on Deafness and Other Communication Disorders (NIDCD), National Institutes of Health. The tinnitus questions were replaced with questions on the cause of hearing loss in the 1991 Hearing Supplement. When possible, all adults in the household participated in the interview; however, proxy responses were accepted for family members who were not at home during the interview. In addition, proxy responses were required for all children and family members who were physically or mentally incapable of responding to questions. In reviewing estimates of tinnitus prevalence with and without proxy respondents, we found significantly lower prevalence when proxy responses were used. Therefore, we chose to use only self-reported information and exclude proxy responses. This decision results in a loss of information on 31.7% ($n = 27,364$) of the subjects, excluded because of proxy or unknown respondent source, but we are ensured of more uniform quality of ascertainment.

We also analyzed another large US survey, the 1994–1995 Disability Supplement to the NHIS, for information about tinnitus. Although not one of the four federal offices that initially planned this survey, NIDCD joined the research consortium and was invited to suggest questions relating to the prevalence of sensory impairment. Because of overlapping interests in disability issues among the sponsoring offices, a decision was made to merge the interests into one survey to be carried out over 2 years.[8] The data we analyzed for this chapter are based on one question about chronic tinnitus ("ringing, roaring, or buzzing in the ears or head now that has lasted for at least 3 months"). Three months is the NHIS-specified time period for a "chronic" condition. This question was part of the Disability Supplement Phase I screening questionnaire conducted concurrently with the NHIS core questionnaire in 1994 and 1995. The core questionnaire contains sociodemographic information and questions on chronic health conditions and use of health services. The Disability Supplement contained sections on (a) sensory, communication, and mobility problems; (b) medical conditions such as cerebral palsy and autism; (c) ability to perform activities of daily living (eg, bathing or showering, dressing, eating without help) and instrumental activities (eg, preparing meals, shopping, managing money); (d) functional limitations (eg, unable to lift 10 pounds or walk a quarter of a mile): (e) mental health; (f) services and benefits received; (g) special health needs of children; and (h) early child development. In 1994, 45,705 households (116,179 persons) participated in the NHIS core questionnaire, for a 94.1% response rate.[9] In 1995, changes were made in the NHIS survey design, including oversampling of Hispanic persons for the first time; interviews were conducted in 39,239 households (102,467 persons), for a 93.8% response rate.[10] The combined 1994–1995 Disability Supplement Phase I data set contains information on 197,558 persons (including 57,553 children), or 90.4% of the persons represented in the NHIS core survey for the 2 years. We excluded children and adults less than 20 years old and proxy respondents to the 1994–1995 NHIS core questionnaire, which left a total of 99,435 subjects for analysis. A longitudinal follow-up study was conducted after 1 year (Disability Supplement Phase II) for a subset of the 1994–1995 NHIS sample that included persons with disabilities identified in the Phase I screening questionnaire. Phase II did not address tinnitus and was not analyzed for this report.

The third data set we analyzed is the Nord Trøndelag Hearing Loss Study, an ancillary component of the Nord Trøndelag Health Survey (in Norwegian: Helseundersøkelsen I Nord Trøndelag [HUNT]). HUNT was conducted for the first time in 1984–1986 as a general health screening study for the population of Nord Trøndelag county, was repeated in 1995–1997, and is planned to be repeated every 10 years in the future. The Nord Trøndelag Hearing Loss Study was conducted in 1996–1998 and enrolled 51,975 adults aged 20 to 101 years (mean age 50.2 years; SD 17.0). Valid audiometric and questionnaire data were obtained for 62% of the eligible population.[11] Participation was slightly less than 50% for the youngest subjects (less than 35 years old), many of whom were not then living in the county, although it was their permanent residence. For subjects 50 to 80 years old, the participation rate varied from 75 to 87%. Some of the results from this study, including a detailed description of the audiometric procedures, have been published.[11]

STATISTICAL ANALYSIS

Statistical significance has been determined using chi-square statistics for categorical data. Differences in means for continuous data were evaluated with Student's *t*-test. For more detailed analyses, we used the odds ratio (OR) to provide an estimate of relative risk. The OR was introduced originally by Cornfield, who showed that, under suitable conditions, it can be used in retrospective studies to provide an estimate of relative risk.[12] The uses of ORs have mushroomed since Cornfield's original article, to the point that it is now the standard measure for estimation in epidemiologic studies, whether for simple univariate comparisons of one exposure variable and one response variable or for more general multivariable logistic regression models.[13] In this chapter, we also use generalized estimating equations to perform logistic regression analysis involving correlated observations, that is, for the sibling cohorts in the familial analyses of the Nord Trøndelag data.[14]

We used *Stata* programs to perform analyses of the sibling data and the *SAS* package of computer programs for most of the other analyses.[15,16] *SUDAAN* was used to obtain corrected estimates of variability based on the complex sampling designs of the two US NHIS surveys.[17]

CLASSIFICATION OF TINNITUS

One of the first nationally representative studies including questions on tinnitus was the 1960–1962 National Health Examination Survey (NHES), which examined 6,672 adults, 18 to 79 years old, who were selected in a probability sample from the civilian, noninstitutionalized population of the United States. After the 1960s, the scope of the recurrent NHES was enlarged to include dietary and nutritional information, and the survey was renamed the National Health and Nutrition Examination Survey (NHANES). These are multipurpose surveys that include a household questionnaire and a general health examination conducted in mobile examination units or trailers. These surveys always have included audiometric testing for at least a portion of the subjects involved. For the 1960–1962 NHES, air-conduction, pure-tone audiometric thresholds were obtained at 0.5, 1, 2, 3, 4, and 6 kHz in each ear. Leske published results from this survey showing that 32% of the subjects had experienced ringing (tinnitus) in their ears or had been bothered by other funny noises at some time over the past few years.[18] However, only 5.6% of subjects considered their tinnitus severe. Furthermore, mild tinnitus did not increase markedly with age, whereas the prevalence of severe tinnitus increased from 3.0% in subjects 18 to 24 years to 11.5% in subjects 65 to 74 years old. Leske also demonstrated a close connection between hearing impairment, whether from subjective report or measured threshold levels, and severe tinnitus.[18] The prevalence of mild tinnitus did not vary much by hearing level (poor, fair, or good hearing).

One implication for epidemiologic research from this early study is that tinnitus questions must be worded carefully and, ideally, should ascertain severity. There are a number of ways to accomplish these goals; our review of the literature suggests that most epidemiologic studies of tinnitus have used different phrasing of questions but were designed to distinguish mild, occasional ringing in the ears from troubling, longer-lasting tinnitus.

There are few additional reports using health examination data and audiometric thresholds from NHANES. Cooper reported results from NHANES I, 1971–1975, showing a slightly greater prevalence for black versus white race,[19] and some data from NHANES were summarized in a survey of sociodemographic variables and tinnitus.[20] The primary reason for the lack of more studies is that hearing (audiometric) testing on a general sample of adults in the United States was not repeated after 1975 until recently. The current NHANES 1999–2004 is testing hearing in adults 20 to 69 years of age and is also asking about tinnitus, but data collection is ongoing, and complete study results of audiometric data are not yet available.

A summary of several studies focusing on tinnitus severity was published by Holgers and colleagues.[21] The authors included information on reliability, correlation to audiometric thresholds, psychological factors (eg, depression), and general health status from several instruments. The focus was to determine characteristics distinguishing tinnitus that interferes with working capacity from less severe forms.

A more formal approach to the rating of tinnitus severity has been proposed recently by McCombe and colleagues.[22] These authors distinguish grade I (slight) tinnitus, which is not "troubling," from grade II (mild) and grade III (moderate) tinnitus, which may or may not interfere with sleep but is unlikely to interfere with working capacity. The authors suggest that the majority of people suffering from tinnitus should fall into these two intermediate categories. Grade IV (severe) tinnitus is described as almost always heard by the subject and rarely, if ever, masked. It leads to disturbed sleep patterns and can interfere with the ability to carry out usual daily activities. Worst of all, grade V (catastrophic) tinnitus is so severe that there are usually associated psychological problems.[22] This classification should be valuable for planning future studies to elicit better information about the subjective complaint of tinnitus.

DEFINITE AND POSSIBLE RISK FACTORS

In Table 3-1, we list several risk factors for tinnitus previously identified in the biomedical literature. These include age,[23] a number of drugs or medications,[24] and otologic diseases such as otosclerosis,[25] otitis media,[26,27] presbycusis,[27,28] sudden deafness,[29] Meniere's disease,[30,31] and vestibular schwannoma (acoustic neuroma).[32,33] Tinnitus has also been associated with hypo- and hyperthyroidism[34,35] and cardiovascular[36] and cerebrovascular disease.[37,38] Explanation of how these conditions may result in tinnitus is beyond the scope of this chapter. Except for age and presbycusis, these conditions probably account for a relatively small proportion of subjects reporting tinnitus.

Instead of focusing on underlying disease or conditions associated with tinnitus, we are concerned with the strength of association between tinnitus and a number of risk factors commonly ascertained in population-based studies, including age, sex, race or ethnicity, socioeconomic measures, and many others.

Two environmental factors that have been extensively studied in relation to the risk of tinnitus are exposure to loud noise (impulsive or continuous) and head or neck trauma and injuries.[28,39,40]

Table 3-1 lists a number of possible risk factors in addition to those considered definite or well established, including possible associations between tinnitus and lifestyle or behavioral factors such as cigarette smoking and alcohol consumption. General health status, as reported by the subject, is a simple summary measure included in nearly all large health interview or examination surveys. This subjective assessment of health status can be considered a generalized risk factor or, in other contexts, a codependent outcome measure.

TABLE 3-1. Factors Associated with Tinnitus

Definite Risk Factors

Age

Cardiovascular and cerebrovascular disease

Drugs or medications
    Salicylate analgesics, nonsteroidal anti-inflammatory drugs, antibiotics, cardiac medications, "loop" diuretics, chemotherapeutic agents

Ear infections/inflammation

Head or neck trauma and injury

Hyper- and hypothyroidism

Loud noise exposure

Meniere's disease

Otosclerosis

Presbycusis

Sudden deafness

Vestibular schwannoma (acoustic neuroma)

Possible Risk Factors

Alcohol

Anxiety

Depression

Familial inheritance

Geographic region

Health status—fair or poor

Heavy weight or high body mass index

Limited education

Low height

Low socioeconomic status

Low weight or low body mass index

Rural residence

Smoking (cigarettes)

Self-report of hearing loss is another subjective measure that may be even more intimately related to tinnitus. Socioeconomic disadvantage, as manifested by limited education, low income, and occupation or employment subject to increased noise exposure, may also play an important role in increasing the risk of tinnitus. In addition, a number of anthropometric measures reflecting long-term nutritional status may be associated with tinnitus, for example, low height and/or low weight or low body mass (ponderal) index. Alternatively, a high body mass index (BMI) tending toward obesity may be a risk factor. Increased risk for tinnitus may be found in certain geographic regions, reflecting different cultural and environmental influences. Living in a rural setting may implicate both occupational (eg, farming) and leisure-time (eg, shooting or hunting) pursuits as predisposing risk factors for tinnitus. One potentially large and relatively unexplored association is whether familial (genetic inheritance or shared environmental exposure) factors are associated with increased risk of tinnitus. Finally, what is the relationship between anxiety and depression and the risk of tinnitus; are these mental conditions predisposing risk factors or codependent outcome measures?

INCIDENCE OF TINNITUS

Few studies have examined tinnitus incidence, that is, the number of new cases of tinnitus occurring in a specified time interval (typically 1 year). A notable exception is the Beaver Dam, Wisconsin Hearing Loss Study, which calculated tinnitus incidence by comparing each subject's report of tinnitus in the baseline study and then again at the 5-year follow-up interview and examination. After excluding subjects with tinnitus at baseline, subjects who reported tinnitus (defined as moderate or severe and/or causing trouble sleeping) in the 5-year follow-up study represented new, "incident" cases of tinnitus.[36] The incidence of tinnitus in subjects who were 48 to 92 years old at baseline over the 5-year interval until follow-up examination was 5.7%, which corresponds roughly to 1.14% per year.

A few studies have attempted to address this question with a retrospective study design. One example is the interview study conducted in 1998–1999 in Germany by Pilgramm and colleagues, who reported that the yearly incidence of new, chronic tinnitus for subjects 10 years and older was 0.33%.[41] The 1990 US NHIS Hearing Supplement provides another example because participants were asked how old they were when they first began suffering from tinnitus. From these reports, we can estimate the incidence of bothersome tinnitus in the United States for persons of different ages and varying time intervals. In young adults less than 30 years of age with tinnitus, 53% reported an onset in the last 5 years. Multiplying this percentage by the number of young adults reporting bothersome tinnitus, we can crudely estimate the 5-year incidence to be 2.6%. Similar calculations for persons aged 30 to 49 years led to a slightly greater incidence of 2.9% in this age range. However, the incidence nearly doubles at older ages: 4.3% for persons aged 50 to 69 years and 5.1% for persons 70 or more years of age. The latter two estimates are close to the 5.7% incidence over 5 years shown in the more carefully designed prospective study in Beaver Dam, WI.

PREVALENCE WITH AGE

Tinnitus prevalence is a measure of how many people in a defined population have tinnitus at any given time or over an interval of time. It includes tinnitus of relatively recent onset (eg, in the last 6 months) and tinnitus that has been present for 5, 10, 20, or more years. The United Kingdom National Study of Hearing investigated different definitions of tinnitus in their pilot phase before deciding to use "prolonged spontaneous" tinnitus, defined as lasting for more than 5 minutes and occurring not only after loud sounds.[42] In contrast, Axelsson and Ringdahl defined tinnitus as an "ear noise that occurs often or always and sounds like a peep, chirping, roaring, wind blowing in the trees, etc."[43] Published findings from these two postal surveys on the prevalence of tinnitus are compared in Table 3-2 with newly analyzed results from two large national health interview surveys in the United States and two population-based health examination surveys, one conducted in Beaver Dam, WI, and the other in Nord Trøndelag, Norway. Information was obtained only for adults; children were not questioned about tinnitus in these studies. The results are displayed as age-specific percent prevalence of tinnitus in 10-year age groups with two summary measures, the prevalence for those aged ≥ 50 years and for adults aged ≥ 20 years.

The UK and Gothenburg, Sweden, studies were conducted in the 1980s, and both relied on mailed

TABLE 3-2. Prevalence of Self-Reported Tinnitus in Adults by Decade of Life from Several Population-Based, Epidemiologic Studies

Age, yr	United Kingdom National Study of Hearing* (1980–1986), %	Gothenburg, Sweden† (1989), %	US NHIS Hearing Supplement‡ (1990), %	US NHIS Disability Supplement§ (1994–1995), %	Beaver Dam, WI Hearing Loss Study‖ (1993–1995), %	Nord Trøndelag, Norway Hearing Loss Study# (1996–1998), %
20–29	5.7	7.5	5.1	1.4	—	9.8
30–39	7.4	5.8	6.0	2.0	—	9.6
40–49	9.9	8.9	7.2	3.7	—	11.8
50–59	12.5	18.6	10.1	5.7	7.3	16.9
60–69	16.3	20.3	13.0	7.9	10.1	20.2
70–79	14.4	21.3	12.6	9.4	8.7	24.0
≥ 80	13.6	—	14.1	8.3	5.5	22.9
Age ≥ 50	14.2	20.1	12.1	7.6	8.2	20.1
Total adult	10.2	14.2	8.4	4.4	—	15.1
No. in study	34,050	2,556	59,343	99,435	3,737	47,410

*Postal questionnaire in Cardiff, Glasgow, Nottingham, and Southampton; age groups were 17–30, 31–40, 41–50, and so on. Tinnitus was defined as "prolonged spontaneous tinnitus" that lasts for more than 5 minutes and occurs not only after loud sounds.[44]
†Mailed questionnaire with blinded response (no follow-up of nonresponders). Tinnitus was defined as an ear noise that occurs often or always and sounds like a peep, chirping, roaring, wind blowing in the trees, etc.[43]
‡The United States National Health Interview Survey (US NHIS) is a household survey with personal interviews of noninstitutionalized civilians from randomly chosen areas constituting a nationally representative sample. Tinnitus was defined as having been bothered by ringing in the ears or other funny noises in the head in the past 12 months.[7]
§The 1994–1995 US NHIS Disability Supplement, Phase I, was an impairment and disability screening questionnaire.[9,10] Chronic tinnitus was defined in the interview as "now having a ringing, roaring or buzzing in the ears that has lasted for at least three months."
‖Personal interviews in the study clinic prior to conduct of the hearing examination. Significant tinnitus was defined as "buzzing, ringing, or noise in the ears in the past year of at least moderate severity and/or tinnitus that caused difficulty in falling asleep."[36]
#Self-administered questionnaires filled out in study clinics prior to the hearing examination.[11] Tinnitus was defined as "bothered by ringing in the ears."

questionnaires.[43,44] As mentioned, the definition of tinnitus was different in the two studies, which, unfortunately, seems to be the rule in epidemiologic investigations, and methods of follow-up for nonresponders also differed. Despite differences in definition and follow-up, the age trends reported in the prevalence of tinnitus were similar, although it was slightly higher in Sweden (14.2%) than in the United Kingdom (10.2%).

The two US national health interview surveys conducted in 1990 and 1994–1995 were household surveys conducted as face-to-face interviews in the subject's home. The question asked in the 1990 survey was "At any time over the past 12 months, have you ever noticed ringing in the ears, or have you been bothered by other funny noises in your ears or head."[7] If the subject answered "yes," follow-up questions inquired (a) whether the ringing or funny noises occurred all the time, every few days, or less often and (b) whether the person was bothered quite a bit, just a little, or not at all by the ringing or funny noises. For the purposes of the present analysis, tinnitus is defined as "yes" to the first question and "yes" to being bothered. In the 1994–1995 survey, the tinnitus question asked was "Do you now have ringing, roaring, or buzzing in the ears that has lasted for at least 3 months?" The age trends for prevalence of tinnitus are similar for the 1990 US survey and the UK and Swedish surveys. The 1994–1995 US survey prevalence for chronic tinnitus is considerably lower than in the 1990 US survey, in which a more inclusive question about bothersome tinnitus occurring over the past 12 months was asked.

The last two columns of Table 3-2 are derived from two hearing examination studies, one in Beaver Dam, WI, and the other in Nord Trøndelag, Norway.[11,36] The Beaver Dam study recruited only subjects above the age of 48 for the hearing examination, whereas the Norwegian study included all adults age 20 years or more. In the Beaver Dam study, a more restrictive definition of tinnitus was used: "a buzzing, ringing, or noise in the ears in the past year of at least moderate severity and/or tinnitus that caused difficulty falling asleep."[36] The Norwegian study included four questions on tinnitus, but in this comparison, we defined tinnitus by a "yes" response to the general question, "Are you bothered by ringing in your ears?" The age trends in Norway are nearly the same as that reported for Sweden, with an overall adult prevalence of tinnitus of 15.1% in Nord Trøndelag compared with 14.2% in Gothenburg. The age trend in Beaver Dam is similar to the other studies because the prevalence increases up to age 60 to 69, remains high between 70 and 79 years, and then declines for the oldest age group ≥ 80 years. Yet the more restrictive definition of tinnitus in the Beaver Dam study resulted in a lower estimated prevalence among subjects ≥ 50 years of age, 8.2%, which is similar to the prevalence of 7.6% found for chronic tinnitus in the 1994–1995 US NHIS Disability Supplement.

RISK FACTORS OR ASSOCIATED CHARACTERISTICS

Although several risk factors for tinnitus are well accepted by researchers in the field, others have been examined in only a few studies, sometimes with conflicting results. In Table 3-3, we show the frequencies of 37 selected characteristics, available from the two US surveys and the Norwegian study, to examine whether these factors are increased or decreased for subjects with tinnitus. To the extent possible, we listed the characteristics included in all three studies. However, we also exploited the opportunity to examine characteristics available from one of these three studies that were not available in the other two. For example, several questions about impairments in other senses (vision, balance, olfaction, and taste) were asked in the 1994–1995 US Disability Survey that were not asked in the other two studies. Also, the Norwegian study included several questions potentially related to hearing loss, such as frequent exposure to impulse noise and hospitalization for head

TABLE 3-3. Percentage of Adult Subjects with Selected Characteristics and Statistical Significance, p Value*, of Differences by Report of Tinnitus

	US NHIS Hearing Supplement (1990)			US NHIS Disability Supplement (1994–1995)			Nord Trøndelag, Norway Hearing Loss Study (1996–1998)		
	Bothersome Tinnitus			Chronic Tinnitus			Bothersome Tinnitus		
Characteristics	No	Yes	p value	No	Yes	p value	No	Yes	p value
No. of respondents	50,310	7,267		95,003	4,432		40,164	7,153	
Mean age, yr	45.8	53.4	<.0001	44.9	57.5	<.0001	48.5	55.0	<.0001
Male sex	38.0	41.0	<.0001	47.5	53.1	<.0001	46.3	54.4	<.0001
Hispanic	8.2	5.6	<.0001	9.3	6.5	<.0001			
Black, non-Hispanic	13.3	11.8	.0001	11.1	7.0	<.0001			
White, non-Hispanic	75.6	80.6	<.0001	75.1	83.4	<.0001			
Education, < 12 yr (not high school graduate)	22.0	31.9	<.0001	18.2	28.7	<.0001	68.3	77.6	<.0001
Income, < $20,000 annually	34.7	49.4	<.0001	26.4	41.0	<.0001	56.1	64.7	<.0001
US Northeast	21.6	15.3	<.0001	20.8	16.4	.0105			
US Midwest	24.9	26.5	.0036	24.4	24.6	NS			
US South	32.5	35.6	.0084	34.0	34.8	NS			
US West	21.0	22.5	.0494	20.9	24.2	.0009			

(Table continues on next page)

TABLE 3-3. Continued

Characteristics	US NHIS Hearing Supplement (1990) Bothersome Tinnitus			US NHIS Disability Supplement (1994–1995) Chronic Tinnitus			Nord Trøndelag, Norway Hearing Loss Study (1996–1998) Bothersome Tinnitus		
	No	Yes	p value	No	Yes	p value	No	Yes	p value
Occupational noise exposure				40.1	46.0	< .0001	39.4	50.9	< .0001
Military service veteran	14.0	20.7	< .0001	14.9	28.9	< .0001			
Health status, "fair" or "poor"	12.0	29.4	< .0001	12.1	35.6	< .0001	17.5	29.6	< .0001
Low height[†]	8.1	8.5	NS	8.3	8.3	NS	8.9	13.4	< .0001
Low weight[‡]	11.3	10.6	NS	9.7	9.0	NS	9.5	11.0	< .0001
Low body mass index, < 21.0	18.3	15.9	.0001	15.1	10.9	< .0001	8.5	7.1	.0003
High body mass index, > 32.0	7.9	11.5	< .0001	10.5	14.6	< .0001	7.3	8.2	.0179
Serious difficulty seeing (vision)				3.0	12.0	< .0001			
Hearing loss, moderate or worse	7.8	42.2	< .0001	4.1	31.7	< .0001	4.7	18.2	< .0001
Uses hearing aid				1.9	11.9	< .0001	3.1	11.9	< .0001
Dizziness, chronic (3+ mo)				2.1	19.5	< .0001			
Imbalance, chronic (3+ mo)				9.0	33.4	< .0001			
Olfactory (smell) impairment (3+ mo)				1.3	6.9	< .0001			
Gustatory (taste) impairment (3+ mo)				0.5	4.3	< .0001			
Activities of daily living,[§] unable to do one or more				2.6	10.2	< .0001			
Functional limitations,[‖] one or more				12.5	43.2	< .0001			
Frequently depressed or anxious				5.3	21.5	< .0001			
Daily cigarette smoker, ≥ 15 yr							12.1	16.9	< .0001
Alcohol, 15+ drinks last 2 wk							3.2	3.3	NS
Frequently exposed to impulse noise							7.6	16.4	< .0001
Ever played in a band							19.2	15.7	< .0001
Frequent exposure to loud music							26.6	20.5	< .0001
Ever hospitalized for head injury							5.8	9.5	< .0001
Recurrent ear infections (especially childhood)							19.6	28.2	< .0001
Familial hearing loss (sibling or child)							10.9	19.0	< .0001
Hearing examination by doctor, last 5 yr							34.0	49.5	< .0001

NS = not significant.
*p value is the level of statistical significance based on the chi-square probability distribution for categorical data and Student's t probability distribution for mean differences.
[†]Low height was defined as less than 66 inches for US males and less than 61 inches for US females; low height for Norwegians was less than 169 cm for males and less than 156 cm for females. These cut points correspond approximately to 10th percentiles for the respective sex and nationality group.
[‡]Low weight was defined as less than 145 pounds for US males and less than 115 pounds for US females; low weight for Norwegians was less than 69 kg for males and less than 56.5 kg for females. These cut points correspond approximately to 10th percentiles for the respective sex and nationality group.
[§]The activities of daily living include a list of six activities that, owing to impairment or health problems, results in the need for help from another person with these personal care needs: bathing, eating, dressing, getting up or out of bed or chairs, using the toilet, and getting around inside the home.
[‖]Functional limitation refers to difficulties with any of the following: lifting 10 pounds (eg, a full bag of groceries), walking up 10 steps without resting, walking a quarter of a mile (about three city blocks), standing for about 20 minutes, bending down from a standing position to pick up an object from the floor (eg, a shoe), reaching up over the head or reaching out as if to shake someone's hand, using fingers to grasp or handle something such as picking up a glass from a table or holding a pen or pencil.

injury, that are not typically included on general purpose health surveys. Many of these additional variables are of interest either as possible risk factors for tinnitus or as codependent outcome measures.

Reviewing the data in Table 3-3, we observe that most of the characteristics have significantly different frequencies, depending on whether the subjects have tinnitus. The more salient of these factors, found in all three of the studies, are mean age (6 to 12 years greater for the tinnitus group), male sex, less than a high school education, lower income, occupational noise exposure, general health status reported as "fair" or "poor," higher BMI, and reported hearing loss of a moderate or higher degree. Many of these characteristics have been reported in earlier studies.[20,43–46] The excess of males with tinnitus has not been consistently reported. Most epidemiologic studies have found either similar prevalence for males and females[20,41,46–48] or slightly increased rates for females.[43,45] Nondahl and colleagues reported a slightly higher prevalence of tinnitus in men in their cohort of older subjects, but, after adjusting for other explanatory factors in a multivariate logistic model, women had a significantly increased OR of 1.38 (95% CI 1.06–1.80).[36] This result implies that at least one of the other factors in the multivariate model (eg, hearing loss, cardiovascular disease, or a history of head injury) was more closely associated with men because there was no significantly greater risk for women in the univariate comparison.

In the Norwegian study, we also examined whether daily cigarette smoking or frequent use of alcohol is associated with tinnitus. There was a statistically significant association between tinnitus and long-term daily cigarette smoking but no apparent association with the consumption of alcohol. Some noise exposure variables in the Norwegian study, namely, "ever played in a band" and "frequent exposure to loud music," showed significant associations but in a manner opposite to expectation, that is, increased frequencies among subjects without tinnitus. This effect is probably due to the fact that mostly younger (< 35 years of age) subjects reported having played in a band or frequent exposure to loud music and that the percentages shown in this table are not age adjusted. Recurrent ear infections, mostly from childhood, were also associated with tinnitus. In addition, familial hearing loss in a sibling or child was associated with tinnitus.

TRENDS IN TINNITUS PREVALENCE BY AGE AND SEX

Table 3-4 shows tinnitus prevalence for different levels of potential risk factors across four age groups, separately for males and females, using the 1990 Hearing Supplement data. Subsequent to completing univariate analyses (seeking statistical associations for each factor separately, as in Table 3-3), it is common practice in epidemiologic studies to examine cross-classifications of key variables (bivariate tables). Because 1990 was also a census year in the United States, we included population estimates for each age and sex combination in the first row of Table 3-4. Using the prevalence figures in the second row and multiplying by the population count in the first row for each age and sex category produces an estimate of nearly 15 million adults with bothersome tinnitus in the United States in 1990. The number of adults with bothersome tinnitus has probably increased somewhat since 1990 owing to increases in mean age and population growth over the past decade. Ries reported an estimate of 18.5 million persons 3 years of age and older in the civilian, noninstitutionalized US population reporting ringing in the ears over the previous 12 months.[7] Our estimate is different because we analyzed only adults who self-reported bothersome tinnitus (proxy responses provided by spouses or parents for their children were excluded).

Of the 15 million adults with bothersome tinnitus, about one-quarter (27%) were seniors 65 or more years of age. However, more than two-fifths (41%) were under 45 years of age. More young adults than seniors are affected by tinnitus despite the twofold increase in prevalence for seniors. This age pattern distribution distinguishes tinnitus from hearing impairment per se. In Figure 3-1, the age-specific prevalence of tinnitus and two categories of reported hearing impairment ("any trouble hearing" and "a lot of trouble hearing in one or both ears") are displayed. The patterns for the hearing impairment follow a typical exponential-like trajectory with age, as do measures of hearing impairment based on pure-tone thresholds.[49–51] In contrast, tinnitus prevalence plateaus between 65 and 74 years of age and then gradually declines.

Sex- and age-specific trends in tinnitus prevalence are shown in Figure 3-2, based on the 1994–1995 Disability Survey to the US NHIS. As mentioned previously, tinnitus was defined for this

TABLE 3-4. Percent Prevalence* of Bothersome Tinnitus, Stratified by Age and Sex, and Percentage of Each Characteristic in the Adult Population, Based on the 1990 Hearing Supplement to the National Health Interview Survey

	Population n (%)	18–24 yr		25–44 yr		45–64 yr		65+ yr	
		Male	Female	Male	Female	Male	Female	Male	Female
1990 US adult population (number in thousands)	181,447	12,242	12,781	39,298	40,760	22,324	24,261	12,414	17,367
Prevalence, %		4.3	5.2	5.8	6.2	10.6	9.5	12.3	13.9
Race/ethnicity									
Hispanic	(8.1)	3.2	4.4	3.6	6.3	7.8	8.9	12.4	11.9
Black, non-Hispanic	(10.7)	1.5	3.2	4.5	6.7	8.4	11.9	14.5	15.6
White, non-Hispanic	(78.2)	5.2	5.7	6.4	6.3	11.2	9.3	12.2	13.9
Other, non-Hispanic	(3.0)	1.5	5.1	4.0	3.7	6.2	8.3	8.6	8.3
Sociodemographic variables									
Education (completed)									
< 12 yr	(22.5)	3.9	8.1	5.9	8.6	14.1	14.2	13.8	17.0
12 years (high school graduate)	(37.6)	3.9	4.0	6.3	6.1	9.3	8.9	12.2	12.7
> 12 yr	(39.9)	4.8	5.1	5.5	5.8	9.5	7.0	10.6	10.2
Household income (annual)									
< $10,000	(12.3)	6.2	6.2	12.5	11.5	22.7	22.6	17.0	18.6
$10,000–19,999	(18.1)	4.6	6.9	8.3	7.8	15.6	12.9	15.4	15.9
$20,000–34,999	(21.5)	3.5	3.8	5.5	6.3	11.6	8.0	10.1	11.9
$35,000+	(32.0)	3.9	3.6	4.8	4.9	7.7	6.3	10.1	8.9
Unknown	(16.1)	1.5	4.2	3.4	4.7	7.7	8.0	9.2	11.1
Metropolitan statistical area (MSA)									
Central city	(32.3)	3.8	4.9	5.3	6.7	9.8	8.7	11.2	12.9
Not central city	(45.9)	3.3	5.1	5.4	5.8	10.0	9.0	11.0	13.0
Non-MSA	(21.8)	6.8	5.9	7.8	6.6	12.9	11.6	15.8	16.6
Health and hearing status variables									
General health status									
Excellent	(32.8)	3.5	2.6	3.4	3.2	5.9	4.0	6.6	6.3
Very good	(28.7)	4.3	5.3	6.2	5.3	8.8	6.6	9.6	10.7
Good	(24.9)	6.3	7.2	8.1	8.9	9.3	9.2	11.6	13.1
Fair	(9.5)	4.1	9.6	13.1	15.2	18.9	20.2	18.3	20.4
Poor	(3.8)	10.7	30.3	20.8	30.4	28.8	30.0	22.2	27.3
Hearing trouble (self-report)									
None	(85.9)	3.1	3.9	3.8	4.8	5.4	6.7	5.8	8.8
Yes	(11.2)	35.9	41.8	30.4	40.2	32.5	35.5	22.9	29.0
Unknown	(2.9)	6.6	8.2	8.6	11.0	19.8	19.4	21.6	17.1
Gallaudet Hearing Scale									
No problem hearing	(88.5)	3.1	3.9	3.8	4.8	5.4	6.7	5.8	8.8
Understands whispers	(2.6)	38.9	18.8	21.8	35.6	29.9	29.8	16.5	21.7
Cannot hear whispering	(5.3)	29.2	47.0	35.2	40.4	29.7	34.2	21.9	28.9
Cannot hear normal voice	(2.8)	54.1	73.3	35.3	54.8	39.4	47.2	26.7	33.6
Cannot hear shouting	(0.7)	—	—	37.2	45.3	42.6	32.2	26.4	30.1

*Estimates of prevalence are based on self-report of tinnitus only (not spousal report or other respondent) and are weighted to represent the US civilian, noninstitutionalized adult population.

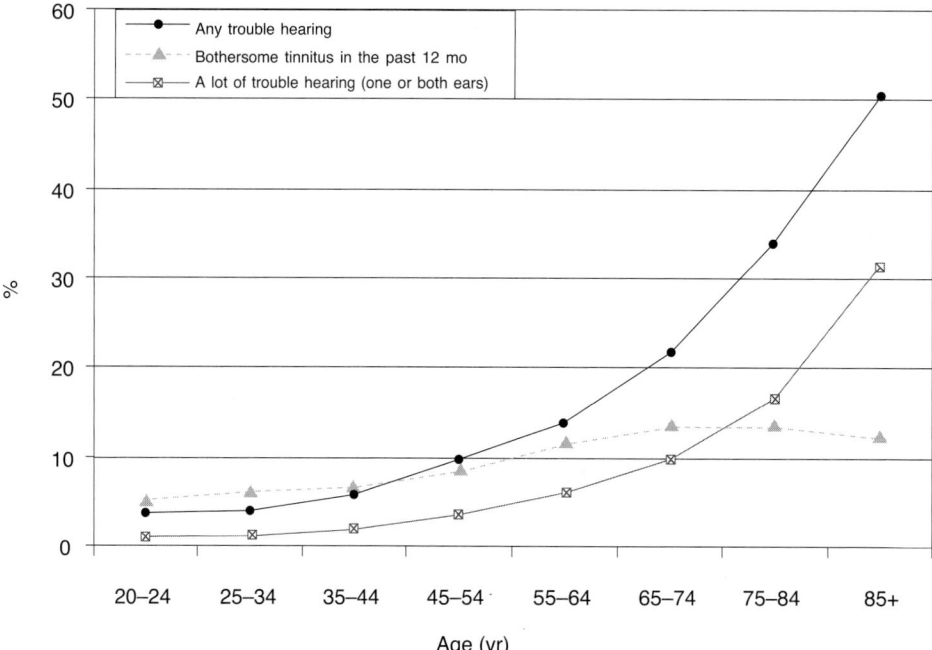

FIGURE 3-1. Prevalence (%) of self-reported hearing loss ("a lot of trouble hearing" or "any trouble hearing") and bothersome tinnitus by age, based on the 1990 US National Health Interview Survey Hearing Supplement.

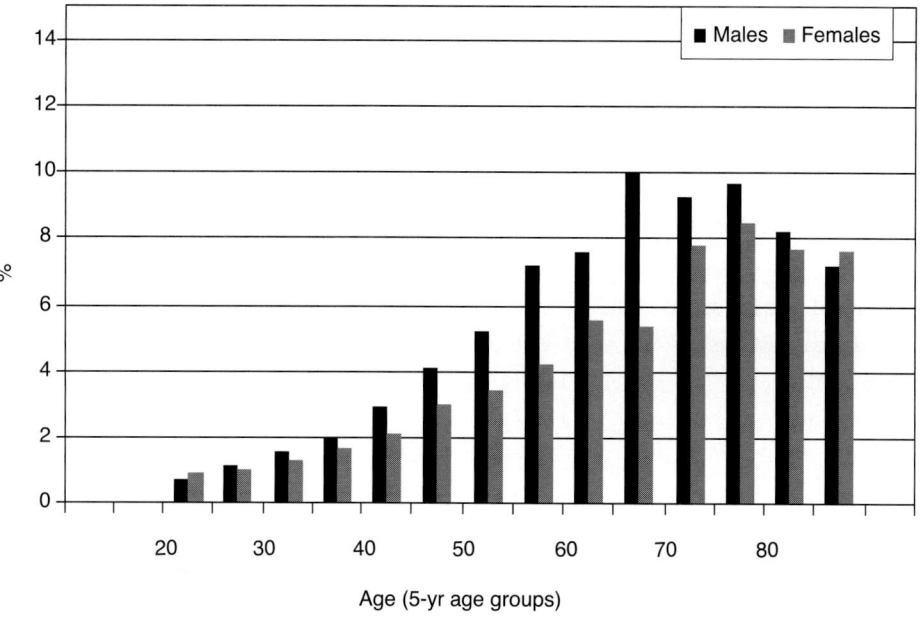

FIGURE 3-2. Age- and sex-specific prevalence (%) of chronic tinnitus (ringing, roaring, or buzzing in the ears or head now that has lasted for at least 3 months) based on the 1994–1995 US National Health Interview Survey Disability Supplement.

survey as a chronic condition (tinnitus that has lasted for at least 3 months). The overall age trends for males and females are similar to those shown in Figure 3-1. Beginning about age 30, however, males have a steeper rise, and the prevalence remains higher for males until age 85. The difference between the age trends for males and females is statistically significant ($p < .0001$). This difference is attributable to the clear separation in prevalence from age 40 to 79 and to the number of respondents in the survey (almost 100,000). What might account for the different prevalences for males and females? One obvious suggestion, based on the ages involved, is that men were much more likely to have been exposed to high levels of environmental noise, whether through work and occupational environment or leisure-time activities. Strong associations between occupational noise exposure and tinnitus have been well documented.[52–57]

There are also consistent age-specific trends in tinnitus prevalence across differing levels of education and in annual household income, shown in Table 3-4. Higher educational and income levels are associated with lower prevalence of bothersome tinnitus within each of the four age categories. Overall, the prevalence of bothersome tinnitus increases 178% as age increases; in the youngest age group (combining sexes), the prevalence is 4.8%, whereas for the oldest, it is 13.3%. The relative increase in tinnitus prevalence across levels of education (< 12 versus > 12 years) or income (< $10,000 versus $35,000+) is significant for each age category but somewhat larger for older persons, 65 or more years of age. The effect of sex is much weaker and less consistent in these data from the 1990 US NHIS Hearing Supplement. There is a lower prevalence of bothersome tinnitus in persons of urban residence who live in metropolitan statistical areas (MSAs), as defined by the US Census Bureau, compared with persons living in the non-MSA of the United States. The relative increase in prevalence for non-MSA, compared with MSA, is greatest for younger adults. For example, non-MSA adults 18 to 24 years old have about a 50% higher prevalence of tinnitus, whereas non-MSA adults 65 or more years old have a 33% higher prevalence, respectively, for the same-age adults in an MSA (central city and not central city combined).

Much larger differences in the prevalence of bothersome tinnitus are shown in Table 3-4 for variables relating to the general health of respondents and, particularly, to their reported hearing loss. Approximately 3.1% of young adults with excellent health report bothersome tinnitus, whereas senior adults, also of excellent health, have a prevalence of about 6.4%. However, if health status is reported as "poor," then 25.9% and 25.3% of young adults and seniors, respectively, have bothersome tinnitus. Young adults who report having trouble hearing have an even higher prevalence of bothersome tinnitus, 39.2% (sexes combined), whereas seniors who report trouble hearing have a lower prevalence (26.1%) of bothersome tinnitus.

The 1990 US NHIS Hearing Supplement included a self-rating scale, the Gallaudet Hearing Scale, to assess the degree of hearing impairment because pure-tone hearing threshold testing could not be included in this household survey. Age- and sex-specific prevalences of bothersome tinnitus are shown in Table 3-4 for varying levels of hearing impairment according to the Gallaudet scale. The results confirm a strong association between the prevalence of bothersome tinnitus and the level of hearing impairment. For example, tinnitus prevalence across all categories was about 26% for adults with mild hearing loss ("usually hears and understands whispering from across a quiet room without seeing the speaker's face") and approximately 35% for adults with moderate to severe hearing loss ("cannot hear or understand what a person says without seeing his face if that person is talking in a normal voice from across a quiet room") and then falls off slightly to about 31% for adults with still greater hearing loss ("cannot hear or understand shouting across a quiet room").

ODDS RATIOS FOR RISK OF TINNITUS

To study tinnitus risk associations in more detail, we used logistic regression analysis to estimate ORs with 95% CIs (Table 3-5). ORs are calculated with respect to a "reference" (or baseline) category for each potential risk factor; for example, for sex, female is the reference category. The OR for males, with respect to females, is 1.49 for chronic tinnitus, based on the US NHIS Disability Supplement data, and 1.39 for bothersome tinnitus, based on the Nord Trøndelag, Norway Hearing Loss Study. Both ORs are highly statistically significant; the 95% CIs exclude 1.00 and are relatively narrow, ranging between 1.32 and 1.60. Hence, in these studies, males are nearly 50% more likely to have reported chronic tinnitus or bothersome tinnitus. Because all ORs in this table are adjusted for age and sex, these are age-adjusted ORs for male sex.

The ORs for age for the US and Norwegian studies in Table 3-5 demonstrate a much greater effect of age in the US study. This is largely a result of the differing definitions of tinnitus used in the two studies. Chronic tinnitus in the US study has a lower prevalence overall compared with bothersome tinnitus in the Norwegian study, and this difference is particularly marked for the reference group chosen for age, adults 20 to 24 years old. Although the ORs for the various age groups shown are very different between the two studies, the pattern is similar. ORs for age in both studies increase monotonically until maxima are

TABLE 3-5. Tinnitus Risk (Odds Ratios Adjusted for Age and Sex and 95% Confidence Intervals) by Selected Characteristics in the US National Health Interview Survey Disability Supplement and Nord Trøndelag, Norway Hearing Study

	US NHIS Disability Supplement (1994–1995)			Nord Trøndelag, Norway Hearing Study (1996–1998)		
	Respondents, %	OR*	95% CI	Respondents, %	OR†	95% CI
No. in study	99,435			47,410		
Age, yr						
20–24	8.3	1.00	—	6.1	1.00	—
25–34	21.7	1.24	0.99–1.55	15.7	1.05	0.91–1.22
35–44	22.0	2.12	1.67–2.68	19.6	1.09	0.95–1.26
45–54	16.1	3.62	2.92–4.50	21.2	1.68	1.46–1.93
55–64	11.8	5.75	4.61–7.16	14.4	2.22	1.93–2.55
65–74	11.7	7.25	5.83–9.00	13.9	2.71	2.36–3.12
75–84	6.8	7.82	6.23–9.82	7.8	3.22	2.78–3.72
≥ 85	1.7	6.94	5.27–9.14	1.2	2.72	2.16–3.44
Sex						
Male	41.1	1.49	1.39–1.60	47.5	1.39	1.32–1.46
Female	58.9	1.00	—	52.3	1.00	—
Race/ethnicity						
Hispanic	8.9	0.89	0.78–1.02			
Black, non-Hispanic	11.0	0.73	0.64–0.82			
White, non-Hispanic	76.0	1.00	—			
Other, non-Hispanic	4.2	0.86	0.71–1.04			
Education, yr						
≤ 8 (grade school)	8.8	1.64	1.43–1.87	35.0	1.19	1.09–1.29
9–11 (some high school)	10.8	1.49	1.32–1.68	34.6	1.02	0.93–1.12
12 (high school graduate)	36.0	1.35	1.23–1.49	9.6	1.03	0.91–1.16
13–15 (some college)	22.3	1.30	1.15–1.47	12.7	0.89	0.79–0.99
≥ 16 (college graduate/plus)	22.0	1.00	—	8.0	1.00	—
Annual income						
$0–9,999	10.8	2.46	2.16–2.80	22.7	0.95	0.87–1.04
$10,000–19,999	17.2	1.74	1.55–1.96	25.9	1.22	1.12–1.33
$20,000–34,999	22.4	1.55	1.33–1.70	25.6	1.12	1.03–1.22
$35,000–49,999	15.2	1.20	1.06–1.37	8.0	1.15	1.03–1.29
$50,000+	20.4	1.00	—	3.2	1.00	—
Region of the country, US						
Northeast	20.6	1.00	—			
Midwest	24.6	1.29	1.08–1.55			
South	33.9	1.35	1.13–1.62			
West	20.9	1.58	1.31–1.91			
Occupation						
Professional	9.8	1.00	—			
Managerial or administrative	8.6	0.82	0.68–0.99			
Technical or sales	18.7	0.83	0.70–0.98			
Transportation	4.1	1.02	0.84–1.23			
Service (plus police and firefighters)	8.7	1.11	0.92–1.33			
Farming, forestry, fishing	1.5	1.13	0.82–1.56			
Skilled or unskilled workers	9.2	1.18	1.00–1.39			

(Table continues on next page)

TABLE 3-5. Continued

	US NHIS Disability Supplement (1994–1995)			Nord Trøndelag, Norway Hearing Study (1996–1998)		
	Respondents, %	OR*	95% CI	Respondents, %	OR†	95% CI
Military service veteran						
No	85.1	1.00	—			
Yes	14.9	1.34	1.19–1.42			
Health status						
Excellent	30.4	0.52	0.47–0.58			
Very good	29.3	0.73	0.67–0.80	12.7	0.67	0.62–0.74
Good	26.0	1.00	—	45.5	1.00	—
Fair	10.1	1.78	1.61–1.97	13.5	1.53	1.43–1.64
Poor	4.2	2.89	2.58–3.23	0.7	1.89	1.48–2.41
Body mass index (weight in kg/height in m^2)						
≤ 22.0 (thin)	22.6	0.96	0.86–1.07	15.6	1.03	0.94–1.12
> 22.0 and ≤ 24.5	23.2	1.00	—	21.7	1.00	—
> 24.5 and ≤ 27.0	20.1	1.00	0.90–1.11	23.3	1.03	0.95–1.11
> 27.0 and ≤ 30.0	17.1	1.15	1.04–1.29	24.0	1.11	1.03–1.20
> 30.0 (obese)	17.0	1.46	1.32–1.62	15.4	1.12	1.03–1.22
Smoking cigarettes						
Never smoked daily				43.1	1.00	—
Smoked daily: < 5 yr				3.3	1.20	1.03–1.41
Smoked daily: 5–14 yr				12.6	1.25	1.15–1.36
Smoked daily: ≥ 15 yr				33.7	1.26	1.19–1.34
Alcohol						
No drinks last 2 wk				36.7	1.00	—
< 5 drinks last 2 wk				36.6	0.87	0.82–0.93
5–14 drinks last 2 wk				23.5	0.90	0.84–0.97
≥ 15 drinks last 2 wk				3.2	0.96	0.82–1.13
Hearing loss, self-reported						
None or no trouble hearing	94.5	1.00	—	85.4	1.00	—
A little or slight hearing loss				7.9	2.74	2.53–2.97
A lot (cannot hear normal conversation)	5.3	7.14	6.46–7.88	4.2	3.69	3.34–4.08
Severe (cannot hear loud noises)	0.2	6.88	4.63–10.2	2.5	5.49	4.85–6.20

*Odds ratio for chronic tinnitus.
†Odds ratio for bothersome tinnitus.

achieved for adults 75 to 84 years, followed by a slight decline for adults 85+ years old.

Age- and sex-adjusted race and ethnicity ORs are also shown for the United States in Table 3-5. As seen previously in Table 3-3, non-Hispanic whites are more likely to report chronic tinnitus; the other race and ethnic groups all have reduced ORs (ranging from 0.73 to 0.89) compared with the reference group, non-Hispanic whites. However, only the difference for non-Hispanic blacks achieves statistical significance, that is, the 95% CI excludes (is less than) 1.00. Despite this finding based on a sample of nearly 100,000 respondents, race and ethnicity in the United States do not appear to be strongly related to the risk of tinnitus.[19,20]

The risk of tinnitus by differing levels of education and income, adjusting for age and sex, is also shown in Table 3-5. The reference category for each is the highest level, namely, 16+ years of education and $50,000+ annual income. In the United States, there is a clear gradient of increasing ORs for lower levels of education and lower levels of income. Nearly every estimate is statistically significantly different from not only the reference group but also from adjacent levels of income (or education). No such consistent results are evident in the Norwegian study, although for education, the highest and only statistically significant OR is for the lowest level (grade school or less). Several caveats should be mentioned; for example, the educational system in Norway does not conform precisely to the US categories listed. Also, the income levels reported for Nord Trøndelag are even more disparate from the US measure; they refer only to that portion of income used to calculate pensions. Nevertheless, the implication is that education and income are not as closely related to tinnitus risk in Norway.

We also examined region in the United States—Northeast, Midwest, South, and West—for differences in tinnitus, adjusting for age and sex (see Table 3-5). The ORs show that relative to the reference region, the Northeast, the other three all have significantly increased ORs. The largest OR is for the West region, which, in turn, is significantly increased over the other three regions. Why there should be more than 50% greater odds of chronic tinnitus in the West compared with the Northeast is unknown. It may relate to increased noise exposure due to certain recreational activities (hunting and shooting may be more common) or to unidentified lifestyle or occupational differences.

Risk for chronic tinnitus according to different occupational groups in the United States is shown in Table 3-5. The reference occupational group, "professionals," heads the category. Two occupational groups, managerial or administrative (OR 0.82; CI 0.68–0.99) and technical or sales (OR 0.83, CI 0.70–0.98), have a reduced risk of chronic tinnitus after adjusting for age and sex. Most of the other occupational groups have practically the same risk as the professional group, with ORs that are just above 1.00 and CIs overlapping 1.00. The exception occurs for skilled or unskilled workers who have an OR of 1.18 (CI 1.00–1.39) that is statistically significant. In a separate comparison in Table 3-5, prior military service or veteran's status is associated with a significantly greater risk of chronic tinnitus (OR 1.34; CI 1.19–1.42).

General health status, as reported by subjects in both the US and Norwegian studies, has a strong, consistent relationship to tinnitus. There is a gradient such that excellent or very good health has a reduced risk of tinnitus compared with the reference category (good health), whereas fair or poor health is associated with significantly increased ORs. Subjects reporting poor health had nearly a threefold risk of chronic tinnitus in the United States (OR 2.89; CI 2.58–3.23) and about a twofold risk of bothersome tinnitus in Norway (OR 1.89; CI 1.48–2.41).

The pattern of tinnitus risk in the United States and Nord Trøndelag is similar as a function of BMI, or Quetelet's ponderal index.[58] Within each study sample, body mass index (weight in kilograms divided by the square of height in meters) was classified into five ascending groups, with 15 to 24% of subjects in each category. Rather than use exact quintiles varying by sex and country, we chose the following fixed categories: ≤ 22.0, > 22.0 to ≤ 24.5, > 24.5 to ≤ 27.0, > 27.0 to ≤ 30.0, and > 30.0. Subjects in the first BMI group are lean or thin, whereas those in the highest group are fat or obese.[58,59] The second BMI group (> 22.0 to ≤ 24.5) was chosen as the reference category. In the US and Norwegian studies, significantly increased ORs were found for the two highest BMI groups. The highest BMI group in the US study had an OR for chronic tinnitus of 1.46 (CI 1.32–1.62), whereas in the Norwegian study, the highest BMI group for bothersome tinnitus had an OR of 1.12 (CI 1.03–1.22).

Only in the Norwegian study did we have information available to examine whether daily cigarette smoking and frequent alcohol use are associated with bothersome tinnitus. There was a significantly increased OR for daily smoking of cigarettes; for example, the OR was 1.26 (CI 1.19–1.34) for daily smoking of cigarettes for 15 or more years. With age and sex adjustment, the ORs were of similar magnitude for daily smoking of shorter time intervals (< 15 years) as well. There was no increase in OR, however, for more frequent drinking in the past 2 weeks. Instead, moderate drinking of less than or equal to one drink a day was associated with a 10 to 15% reduction in the risk of tinnitus.

Finally, we compared the risk of tinnitus with the report of hearing trouble in the US and Norwegian studies. In the Norwegian study, there was a steadily increasing risk of tinnitus associated with increasing hearing impairment, culminating in an OR of 5.49 (95% CI 4.85–6.20) for subjects with severe hearing loss. The pattern for chronic tinnitus was similar for the United States, with an OR of 7.14 (95% CI 6.46–7.88) for subjects who could not hear or understand normal conversation from across a quiet room if not looking at the speaker.

MULTIVARIATE LOGISTIC MODELS FOR CHRONIC TINNITUS IN THE UNITED STATES

After examining associations for different levels within risk variables separately, it is natural to inquire whether adjusting for more factors than just age and sex would eliminate some of the associations found in Table 3-5. We report these multivariate analyses for the 1994–1995 US NHIS Disability Supplement data in Table 3-6.

Two multivariate models are shown alongside each other. Model I excludes variables that might be considered codependent outcome variables for chronic tinnitus, namely general health status and reported hearing loss. To simplify the table, not all variables were included in the analysis; however, the ORs shown in Table 3-6 can be compared with the corresponding age- and sex-adjusted ORs in Table 3-5. By comparing ORs for model I of Table 3-6 with those in Table 3-5, we find that the association with education is the most affected. Although all of the levels of education remain significantly increased compared with the reference category of ≥ 16 years (college graduate or more education), there is no longer a marked gradient. In contrast, the gradient of increasing ORs with decreasing annual income is still present in model I, as it was in the age- and sex-adjusted analysis in Table 3-5. All of the other variables—age, sex, region, and military service veteran—either remained unchanged or were somewhat attenuated in the model I multivariate logistic model; however, the interpretation of effects or associations with these factors remains unchanged.

The expanded multivariate logistic analysis, labeled model II in Table 3-6, includes general health status and reported hearing loss among the variables used to adjust all of the rest simultaneously. If we consider both of these variables as possible predictive risk factors, then most of the ORs shown in the age- and sex-adjusted univariate analyses of Table 3-5 are considerably reduced in Table 3-6. The significant ORs for differing levels of education have all been eliminated, except for the lowest category (≤ 8 years), which now has lower risk. In comparison with the model I multivariately adjusted OR, the excess risk for males has been reduced by half (OR 1.17; CI 1.07–1.28). The highest ORs for specific age groups also are reduced by about half; for example, for subjects 75 to 84 years old, the OR decreased from 7.35 to 3.60. Level of annual income does remain important, and the gradient effect is still present, but the ORs are reduced considerably. Region of the country is one of the few variables not much changed in the model II multivariate logistic regression analysis. This suggests that whatever accounts for regional differences is not associated with the other variables included in this model. Military service veterans have a slightly reduced OR of 1.29 (CI 1.17–1.43), but this factor also is not much affected by the other variables in the multivariate model.

MULTIVARIATE LOGISTIC MODELS FOR BOTHERSOME TINNITUS IN NORD TRØNDELAG

In Table 3-7, we show multivariate models using the Nord Trøndelag data, which included several factors, such as occupational noise exposure, report of hospitalization for head injury, and lifestyle factors (eg, daily cigarette smoking) that were not available in either US study. Because the Norwegian study measured hearing thresholds in each ear, we replaced the subjective report of hearing trouble with an objective measure of hearing impairment. The multivariate analysis is performed separately for each sex. We thought that this approach was necessary because some of the factors examined—loud noise exposure at work, more frequent exposure to impulse noise, and hospitalization for head injuries—were much more common for males. We were interested in learning whether these factors are associated with tinnitus in women and in men. The findings confirm that these factors operate at about the same level of risk for both men and women, despite being less frequent exposures for women. Also, daily cigarette smoking represents about a 20% significantly greater risk of tinnitus for both men and women.

The effect of age is much reduced in this multivariate analysis. There is still a significantly greater risk of tinnitus for men aged 45 to 54 years (OR 1.30; 95% CI 1.06–1.60). However, for men aged 75 to 84 years (OR 0.71; 95% CI 0.55–0.92) and 85+ years (OR 0.54; 95% CI 0.35–0.83), there is a significantly reduced risk of tinnitus. Another way to describe this effect is to say that aging (> 75 years) in men is "protective" against tinnitus, a term that can be applied whenever the OR is significantly less than 1.0. The greater risk of tinnitus for men around the age of 50

TABLE 3-6. Risk of Chronic Tinnitus Estimated by Multivariately Adjusted Odds Ratios and 95% Confidence Intervals for Two Logistic Regression Models ("Excluding" versus "Including" Health Status and Reported Hearing Loss) in the US National Health Interview Survey Disability Supplement, 1994–95

	Multivariate Model I (excludes health status and reported hearing loss)		Multivariate Model II (includes health status and reported hearing loss)	
	OR	95% CI	OR	95% CI
Age, yr				
20–24	1.00	—	1.00	—
25–34	1.41	1.12–1.77	1.23	0.98–1.55
35–44	2.55	2.01–3.24	1.93	1.52–2.44
45–54	4.30	3.45–5.37	2.85	2.29–3.56
55–64	6.17	4.92–7.72	3.77	3.01–4.72
65–74	6.99	5.59–8.74	4.08	3.25–5.12
75–84	7.35	5.81–9.29	3.60	2.82–4.61
≥ 85	6.51	4.93–8.60	2.43	1.81–3.28
Sex				
Male	1.33	1.22–1.46	1.17	1.07–1.28
Female	1.00	—	1.00	—
Education, yr				
≤ 8 (grade school)	1.30	1.13–1.49	0.85	0.74–0.98
9–11 (some high school)	1.22	1.08–1.38	0.89	0.78–1.02
12 (high school graduate)	1.19	1.08–1.31	1.02	0.92–1.12
13–15 (some college)	1.16	1.04–1.31	1.05	0.93–1.18
≥ 16 (college graduate/plus)	1.00	—	1.00	—
Annual income				
$0–9,999	2.30	2.01–2.63	1.56	1.36–1.78
$10,000–19,999	1.63	1.45–1.84	1.22	1.08–1.39
$20,000–34,999	1.42	1.26–1.60	1.20	1.06–1.36
$35,000–49,999	1.16	1.02–1.32	1.05	0.92–1.20
$50,000+	1.00	—	1.00	—
Region of the country, US				
Northeast	1.00	—	1.00	—
Midwest	1.26	1.07–1.49	1.20	1.03–1.39
South	1.28	1.08–1.51	1.16	1.00–1.35
West	1.58	1.33–1.87	1.48	1.26–1.72
Military service veteran				
No	1.00	—	1.00	—
Yes	1.41	1.28–1.56	1.29	1.17–1.43
Health status				
Excellent			0.58	0.52–0.65
Very good			0.79	0.72–0.87
Good			1.00	—
Fair			1.63	1.46–1.80
Poor			2.36	2.10–2.65
Hearing loss, self-reported				
None or slight trouble hearing			1.00	—
A lot (cannot hear normal conversation)			5.92	5.37–6.53
Serious (cannot hear loud noises)			6.08	4.04–9.15

TABLE 3-7. Risk of Bothersome Tinnitus Estimated by Multivariately Adjusted Odds Ratios and 95% Confidence Intervals for Males and Females Separately in the Nord Trøndelag, Norway Hearing Loss Study, 1996–1998

	Males (n = 22,467)			Females (n = 24,850)		
	%	Adjusted OR	95% CI	%	Adjusted OR	95% CI
Age, yr						
20–24	5.6	1.00	—	6.6	1.00	—
25–34	15.7	0.82	0.66–1.02	15.8	1.02	0.82–1.26
35–44	19.5	0.95	0.77–1.17	19.7	0.95	0.77–1.18
45–54	21.8	1.30	1.06–1.60	20.7	1.13	0.92–1.39
55–64	14.8	1.15	0.92–1.43	14.0	1.17	0.94–1.46
65–74	14.4	0.91	0.72–1.15	13.5	0.98	0.78–1.23
75–84	7.1	0.71	0.55–0.92	8.4	0.96	0.75–1.23
85+	1.1	0.54	0.35–0.83	1.4	0.75	0.53–1.07
Loud noise exposure at work						
No, never	36.6	1.00	—	79.4	1.00	—
< 5 h/wk	21.9	1.05	0.94–1.18	10.1	1.06	0.92–1.23
5–15 h/wk	16.5	1.37	1.22–1.54	5.0	1.71	1.45–2.03
> 15 h/wk	25.0	1.70	1.53–1.87	5.6	1.59	1.36–1.86
Impulse noise, frequent exposure						
No	71.9	1.00	—	96.1	1.00	—
Yes	15.9	1.78	1.61–1.96	1.1	1.73	1.25–2.40
Maybe	12.2	1.44	1.28–1.61	2.8	1.16	0.91–1.46
Hearing loss, $PTA_{0.5,1,2,4}$ worse ear						
≤ 25 dB	69.6	1.00	—	78.6	1.00	—
> 25 dB and ≤ 40 dB	17.2	2.84	2.55–3.16	12.7	2.78	2.45–3.15
> 40 dB	13.1	4.18	3.66–4.77	8.8	5.40	4.67–6.24
Ever hospitalized for head injury						
No	90.6	1.00	—	95.0	1.00	—
Yes	8.4	1.43	1.26–1.62	4.4	1.50	1.26–1.79
Maybe	1.0	1.42	1.01–1.99	0.6	1.27	0.78–2.10
Health status						
Very good	18.3	0.78	0.68–0.88	16.9	0.65	0.56–0.76
Good	63.6	1.00	—	62.3	1.00	—
Fair or "not so good"	17.0	1.28	1.14–1.43	20.1	1.58	1.42–1.77
Poor	1.1	1.50	1.04–2.16	0.8	1.64	1.04–2.57
Smoked cigarettes daily						
No, never	40.8	1.00	—	51.8	1.00	—
Yes, for 0 to < 5 yr	3.4	1.26	1.00–1.58	3.7	1.22	0.96–1.55
Yes, for ≥ 5 and < 15 yr	13.3	1.22	1.07–1.38	13.9	1.31	1.15–1.50
Yes, for ≥ 15 yr	42.5	1.19	1.09–1.30	30.6	1.21	1.09–1.33

PTA = pure-tone average.

may be attributable to noise exposure that is not entirely "explained" by the noise exposure variables included in the multivariate model. Also, a large amount of the overall reduction in ORs for age groups is likely due to the improved measure of hearing loss included in the model (namely, pure-tone average

[PTA] of 0.5, 1, 2, and 4 kHz, worse ear). Why there should be a reduced risk of tinnitus, or protective effect, in men aged ≥ 75 years when all of the other variables are included in the multivariate model is not clear. A decline in tinnitus prevalence in the oldest subjects has been found in many other epidemiologic studies.[36,44] For women, none of the ORs by age group are significant, although the pattern is similar to that discussed for men.

INFLUENCE OF FAMILIAL AND OTHER SELECTED RISK FACTORS ON TINNITUS

To our knowledge, almost nothing is known about familial (either genetic or shared environment) risk of tinnitus. Some recent studies, however, have begun to demonstrate familial effects on adult age-related hearing loss (presbycusis).[60–62] In addition, recent studies using animal models (inbred strains of mice) have shown genetic influences on individual susceptibility to noise, as well as correlation to age-related hearing loss in the same animal models.[63,64] Petersen and colleagues were able to show a statistically significant heritability ($h^2 = 0.39$) for tinnitus in a sample of 544 monozygotic and same-sex dizygotic elderly (≥ 70 years old) female twins who participated in the fourth wave of the Longitudinal Study of Aging Danish Twins.[65] However, no significant heritability for tinnitus could be shown for the sample of 412 monozygotic and same-sex dizygotic elderly (≥ 70 years old) male twins in this Danish cohort; instead, among the males, long-term exposure to occupational noise was the main risk factor for their tinnitus.[65]

One of the principal goals of the Nord Trøndelag, Norway Hearing Loss Study was to investigate familial effects on hearing loss. A unique personal number system exists in Norway that makes the usually difficult task of linking close family members in cohort studies much easier. Based on this linkage, we have explored whether male (or female) siblings of tinnitus sufferers have an increased risk of bothersome tinnitus after adjusting for several other well-known risk factors. In these comparisons, we analyzed only the 3,936 males with at least one male sibling and the 3,442 females with at least one female sibling (Table 3-8).

Two models, one univariate and the other multivariate (adjusting for all of the other variables listed in the table), are shown separately for males and females. Because the cohorts with siblings were younger on average (mean age was 38 years for females and 40 years for males) compared with the total sample (mean age was 50 years), we collapsed the oldest age groups into ≥ 65 years. For subjects ≥ 45 years old, there is a greater risk of tinnitus in the univariate models for each sex, but after adjusting for all of the variables in the multivariate model, age is a nonsignificant factor for tinnitus. The only exception is for men ≥ 65 years in the multivariate model, in which the OR for age was significantly reduced. Having ever worked in a noisy environment for 5 or more hours per week is significantly associated with bothersome tinnitus for males and females in univariate and multivariate models. Similarly, frequent exposure to impulse noise (eg, explosions, shooting) was significantly associated with tinnitus across all models. Having been hospitalized for a head injury was significant for males in the univariate analysis but not otherwise. Likewise, daily cigarette smoking for 15 or more years was significant for males in the univariate analysis but not otherwise.

Two of the strongest risk factors from the US studies, general health status and hearing loss, are also the strongest risk factors for these sibling cohorts. Fair or poor health status is associated with greater risk of bothersome tinnitus for males and females in both univariate and multivariate analyses. As in Table 3-7, rather than use reported hearing trouble here, we chose to substitute the degree of hearing impairment in the worse ear based on the air-conduction PTA of thresholds at 0.5, 1, 2, and 4 kHz. This has the advantage of replacing a "report" measure by a more reliable, objective measure. Compared with subjects with normal hearing ($PTA_{0.5,1,2,4} \leq 25$ dB), those with mild hearing loss ($PTA_{0.5,1,2,4} > 25$ dB and ≤ 40 dB) have a high risk of bothersome tinnitus, the multivariately adjusted OR is 4.04 (95% CI 3.00–5.43) for males and 3.64 (95% CI 2.28–5.81) for females. The association between bothersome tinnitus and moderate or worse hearing loss ($PTA_{0.5,1,2,4} > 40$ dB) is even stronger.

Although these results are informative, the critical comparison for the question of familial association of tinnitus is the variable "male (or female) sibling with tinnitus." In the two univariate comparisons, the ORs for bothersome tinnitus are increased about twofold for both male siblings (OR 2.22; 95% CI 1.81–2.72) and female siblings (OR 1.81; 95% CI 1.35–2.44). Even after including all of the other potent variables in the multivariable model, the familial

TABLE 3-8. Tinnitus Risk Estimated by Univariate, Unadjusted, and Multivariately Adjusted Odds Ratios and 95% Confidence Intervals in Logistic Regression Models for Two Subgroups, Males with at least One Male Sibling and Females with at least One Female Sibling, in the Nord Trøndelag, Norway Hearing Loss Study, 1996–1998

	Males (n = 3,936)					Females (n = 3,442)				
		Univariate Model		Multivariate Model			Univariate Model		Multivariate Model	
	%	Unadjusted OR	95% CI	Adjusted OR	95% CI	%	Unadjusted OR	95% CI	Adjusted OR	95% CI
Age, yr										
20–24	6.9	1.00	—	1.00	—	9.4	1.00	—	1.00	—
25–34	26.3	0.94	0.60–1.48	0.81	0.53–1.23	33.6	1.18	0.74–1.89	0.98	0.62–1.56
35–44	35.2	1.01	0.65–1.57	0.71	0.47–1.09	36.6	0.91	0.56–1.46	0.68	0.42–1.10
45–54	21.9	1.45	0.92–2.28	0.77	0.49–1.19	13.8	1.75	1.05–2.93	1.04	0.61–1.75
55–64	6.4	2.12	1.24–3.63	0.60	0.34–1.05	4.5	1.35	0.67–2.72	0.73	0.35–1.52
≥ 65	3.2	2.97	1.59–5.56	0.45	0.23–0.89	2.2	2.85	1.29–6.31	0.57	0.25–1.30
Loud noise exposure at work										
No, never	29.9	1.00	—	1.00	—	75.2	1.00	—	1.00	—
< 5 h/wk	27.8	1.15	0.86–1.54	1.02	0.77–1.36	12.5	1.02	0.69–1.50	1.03	0.71–1.51
5–15 h/wk	17.9	1.74	1.28–2.37	1.31	0.97–1.77	5.7	2.90	1.88–4.47	2.72	1.80–4.12
> 15 h/wk	24.4	2.82	2.14–3.72	1.78	1.36–2.33	6.6	2.37	1.56–3.62	1.95	1.30–2.91
Impulse noise, frequent exposure										
No	69.5	1.00	—	1.00	—	95.5	1.00	—	1.00	—
Yes	15.2	2.93	2.26–3.76	2.08	1.63–2.63	1.4	4.22	1.86–9.58	3.64	1.67–7.94
Maybe	14.3	2.03	1.54–2.68	1.51	1.51–1.97	3.1	1.78	0.96–3.29	1.15	0.62–2.13
Sibling with tinnitus										
No	82.9	1.00	—	1.00	—	88.7	1.00	—	1.00	—
Yes, male sibling	17.1	2.22	1.81–2.72	1.86	1.48–2.33					
Yes, female sibling						11.3	1.81	1.35–2.44	1.75	1.27–2.42
Hearing loss, PTA$_{0.5,1,2,4}$ worse ear										
≤ 25 dB	87.4	1.00	—	1.00	—	94.2	1.00	—	1.00	—
> 25 dB and ≤ 40 dB	8.9	5.09	3.81–6.81	4.04	3.00–5.43	3.7	4.72	2.92–7.63	3.64	2.28–5.81
> 40 dB	3.7	7.46	4.92–11.3	5.60	3.64–8.62	2.2	10.6	5.88–19.1	9.26	5.31–16.2
Ever hospitalized for head injury										
No	91.5	1.00	—	1.00	—	95.8	1.00	—	1.00	—
Yes	8.5	1.44	1.03–2.00	1.19	0.86–1.63	4.2	1.29	0.74–2.25	1.09	0.63–1.91

(Table continues on next page)

TABLE 3-8. Continued

		Males (n = 3,936)					Females (n = 3,442)			
		Univariate Model		Multivariate Model			Univariate Model		Multivariate Model	
	%	Unadjusted OR	95% CI	Adjusted OR	95% CI	%	Unadjusted OR	95% CI	Adjusted OR	95% CI
Health status										
Very good	21.7	0.64	0.49–0.85	0.78	0.59–1.02	23.9	0.45	0.31–0.64	0.51	0.35–0.74
Good	62.8	1.00	—	1.00	—	59.2	1.00	—	1.00	—
Fair or "not so good"	14.5	1.96	1.50–2.57	1.37	1.06–1.78	16.3	2.03	1.55–2.65	1.90	1.43–2.54
Poor	1.0	6.66	3.14–14.1	4.68	2.32–9.45	0.7	5.24	2.13–12.9	4.06	1.59–10.4
Smoked cigarettes daily										
No, never	50.5	1.00	—	1.00	—	50.4	1.00	—	1.00	—
Yes, for < 15 years	19.9	1.25	0.96–1.64	1.19	0.92–1.54	22.5	1.25	0.92–1.69	1.26	0.93–1.70
Yes, for ≥ 15 years	29.6	1.60	1.27–2.00	1.17	0.92–1.48	27.1	1.29	0.98–1.72	1.15	0.85–1.56

PTA = pure-tone average.

factor remains at nearly the same level, about an 80% increased risk of bothersome tinnitus; the multivariately adjusted OR for male siblings is 1.86 (95% CI 1.48–2.33) and for female siblings is 1.75 (95% CI 1.27–2.42). These analyses suggest that there are important familial associations in tinnitus risk that cannot be attributed to measured hearing loss, noise exposure, or general health status, all of which were included in the multivariate model. Still unmeasured shared environmental factors could be responsible, but genetic factors also deserve consideration as a possible explanation for these findings.

AGE VERSUS HEARING LOSS AS RISK OF TINNITUS

Some earlier epidemiologic studies, notably the study by Chung and colleagues on a large sample of 33,168 noise-exposed workers in British Columbia, Canada, suggested that once there is proper accounting for hearing loss, age is no longer a risk factor for tinnitus.[48] Because we also had available a very large sample of measured hearing levels in the Nord Trøndelag study,[11,51] we revisited this issue. Figure 3-3 is similar to the figure Chung and colleagues used to demonstrate their conclusion that only degree of hearing loss is truly related to tinnitus, not age. This figure displays the prevalence (%) of tinnitus versus hearing loss (PTA of 0.5, 1, 2, and 4 kHz, worse ear) in 5 dB steps. Each age category is a separate curve in the figure. The curves are smoothed by third-degree polynomial (cubic) fits to the raw percentages. If age added no information beyond hearing loss, then the curves could be superimposed on top of each other, with only sampling variation or measurement error contributing to differences, which was the pattern that Chung and colleagues observed. A different pattern emerges from this Norwegian population of unscreened adults for men and women. As age group (cohort) increases, the relationship between tinnitus prevalence (%) and hearing level is shifted to the right and becomes less steep. Hence, for each age cohort, there is a relationship between tinnitus prevalence and hearing loss, but these relationships change systematically as age increases, that is, older cohorts have lower tinnitus prevalence for any given level of hearing impairment. This pattern may be attributable to an effect of "aging" or, conceivably, to an effect of

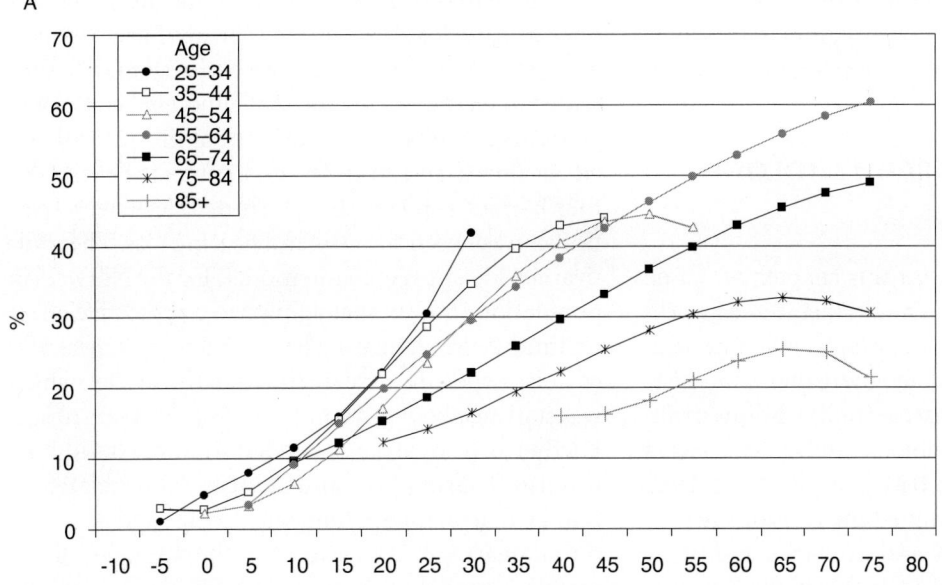
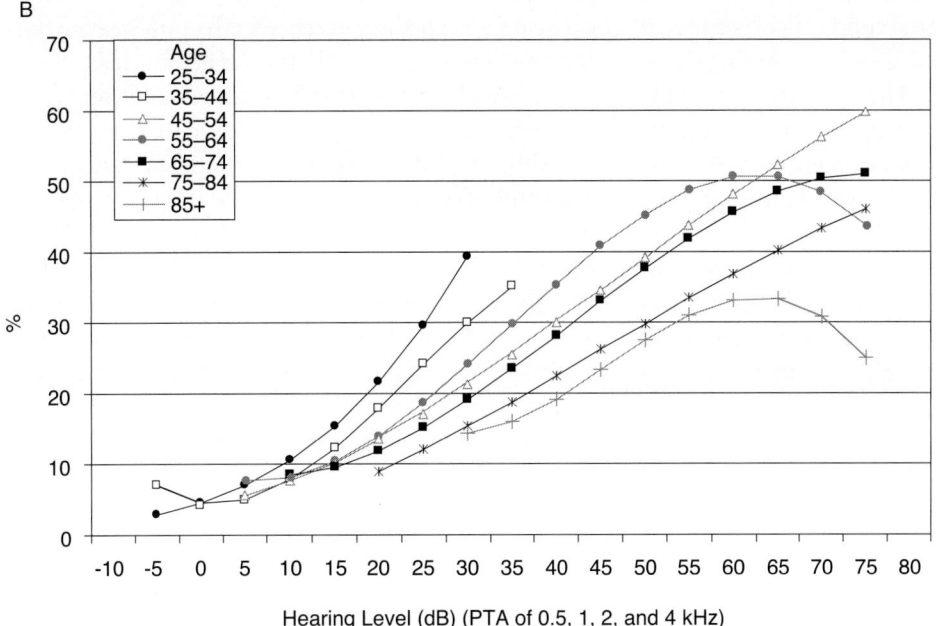

FIGURE 3-3. Age-specific prevalence (%) of tinnitus by pure-tone average (PTA) hearing level in the worse ear for men (*A*) and women (*B*) in the Nord Trøndelag Hearing Loss Study, 1996–1998. Each curve is a separate age cohort smoothed by a third-degree polynomial (cubic) fit.

"cohort." The only way to disentangle aging from cohort effects is through a longitudinal study, which is not available.

These results leave open the question of how much additional information about tinnitus risk is contributed by age after allowance is made for hearing levels. The difference in results between the two studies may be due to the different populations analyzed; one is a sample of only noise-exposed workers, whereas the other is an unscreened sample. Other distinctions were that the results for noise-exposed workers were shown only for tinnitus reported as occurring in the left ear and for hearing loss measured at 4 kHz in the left ear.

TINNITUS IN CHILDREN

We have not presented any information on tinnitus in children because no source of data was available to us. Some articles address tinnitus in childhood and associated risk factors.[26,27] However, much more epidemiologic research in this area remains to be done.

OTHER FINDINGS IN EPIDEMIOLOGIC STUDIES

In reviewing the literature for this chapter, we came across a few publications with results that seemed worth noting, although they were not easy to integrate with the other material. Rather than ignore them, we mention two that reported negative (null) findings from large, well-executed epidemiologic studies. The first of these is a report by Weiss based on the 1960–1962 NHES data set, which examined the relationship between high blood pressure and headache and other symptoms, including tinnitus.[66] In this study, there was no relationship between tinnitus and either systolic or diastolic blood pressure. The second article is a report on oral contraception and ear disease, including tinnitus, by Vessey and Painter.[67] These authors used data from the Oxford–Family Planning Association contraceptive study on 17,032 married women, 25 to 39 years old at recruitment, from 17 family planning clinics across England and Scotland, who were then followed for periods up to 26 years. There was no association (OR 0.9; 95% CI 0.5–1.7) between ever-use of oral contraceptives and tinnitus. Given the negative results of this study, the question of any female-specific risk factors for tinnitus remains open.

SUMMARY

This chapter presents a review of what is known, to date, about the incidence and prevalence of tinnitus. The risk factors and associated characteristics, whether these are etiologic or correlative, of tinnitus have been catalogued. Factors such as general health status, level of hearing loss, and exposure to loud occupational and recreational sounds are highly correlated with the presence and severity of tinnitus across many studies. Although the results presented on familial risk for tinnitus are quite suggestive of an association, the influence of familial and hereditary factors on tinnitus has not yet been established in the scientific literature. This remains an important research goal because other studies are needed to confirm the findings discussed here.

There is a strong suggestion in the literature that once hearing loss is accounted for, age has no association with tinnitus. In fact, the Norwegian data presented in Figure 3-3 suggest that although hearing loss accounts for most of the variance of tinnitus reported in young and middle-aged subjects (especially men), older subjects show a shifted, less steep relationship between tinnitus and hearing loss. The multivariate logistic regression models for the Norwegian population showed that aging had a protective effect on tinnitus when hearing levels and several measures of noise exposure were included in the model, which was statistically significant for males 75+ years of age. Further investigation is needed to understand how tinnitus, hearing loss, and aging are interrelated. It may be that an interaction between age and noise-induced hearing loss measures in the multivariate regression model is responsible for producing the protective association with aging. This is plausible because noise exposure exerts its effect on hearing loss at a much younger age than does presbycusis.

In conclusion, we express our admiration for the breadth and scope of epidemiologic research on tinnitus that has already been accomplished. Although many questions remain to be addressed, future epidemiologic studies have a solid base on which to build. We look forward to studies that will elucidate the etiology of tinnitus and to population-based studies that will reveal other potentially modifiable risk factors. With advances in current treatment options and further understanding of the risk factors and underlying etiology of tinnitus, there is hope for relief from the burden of tinnitus.

ACKNOWLEDGMENTS

The 1990 US NHIS Hearing Supplement was funded in part by an Intra-Agency Agreement between the National Center for Health Statistics (NCHS), Centers for Disease Control and Prevention, Department of Health and Human Services (DHHS), and NIDCD, National Institutes of Health, DHHS. In addition, NIDCD was one of several sponsoring agencies that collaborated with the NCHS on the 1994–1995 NHIS Disability Supplement; NIDCD staff and consultants proposed questions on sensory impairment, including the chronic tinnitus question.

The HUNT is a collaboration between the HUNT Research Centre, Verdal; the Faculty of Medicine, Norwegian University of Science and Technology (NTNU), Trondheim; the Norwegian Institute of Public Health (NIPH or Folkehelsa), Oslo; and Nord Trøndelag County Council. The Nord Trøndelag Hearing Loss Study, which is a part of HUNT, was funded by NIDCD research contract no. N01-DC-6-2104. The Nord Trøndelag county health officer and the community health officers in Levanger and other municipalities provided organizational and other practical support. We thank the Nord Trøndelag Hearing Loss Study team and, particularly, Kristian Tambs, PhD, NIPH, who directed the study, and Hans M. Borchgrevink, MD, Norwegian Medical Research Council, Oslo, Norway, who developed and monitored the audiometric examination protocol.

In addition, we received valuable technical assistance from Ms. May Chiu, Epidemiology and Biostatistics Program, NIDCD, and statistical programming assistance from Ms. Katalin Losonczy, Allied Technology, Inc., Rockville, MD.

REFERENCES

1. Lilienfeld AM. Epidemiology of infectious and non-infectious disease: some comparisons. The first Wade Hampton Frost Lecture. Am J Epidemiol 1973;97:135–47.
2. Lilienfeld AM. Foundations of epidemiology. New York: Oxford University Press; 1976.
3. Last JM. A dictionary of epidemiology. 3rd ed. New York: Oxford University Press; 1995.
4. Szklo M, Nieto FJ. Epidemiology: beyond the basics. Gaithersburg (MD): Aspen Publishers, Inc.; 2000.
5. Massey JT, Moore TF, Parsons VL, Tadros W. Design and estimation for the National Health Interview Survey, 1985–94. Vital and health statistics. Vol 2(110). Hyattsville (MD): National Center for Health Statistics; 1989.
6. Stein REK, Silver EJ. Comparing different definitions of chronic conditions in a national data set. Ambul Pediatr 2002;2:63–70.
7. Ries PW. Prevalence and characteristics of persons with hearing trouble: United States, 1990–91. Vital and health statistics. Vol 10(188). Hyattsville (MD): National Center for Health Statistics; 1994.
8. Russell JN, Hendershot GE, LeClere F, et al. Trends and differential use of assistive technology devices: United States, 1994. Advance data from vital and health statistics; no. 292. Hyattsville (MD): National Center for Health Statistics; 1997.
9. Adams PF, Marano MA. Current estimates from the National Health Interview Survey, 1994. Vital and health statistics. Vol 10(193). Hyattsville (MD): National Center for Health Statistics; 1995.
10. Benson V, Marano MA. Current estimates from the National Health Interview Survey 1995. Vital and health statistics. Vol 10(199). Hyattsville (MD): National Center for Health Statistics; 1998.
11. Tambs K, Hoffman HJ, Borchgrevink HM, et al. Hearing loss induced by noise, ear infections, and head injuries: results from the Nord-Trøndelag Hearing Loss Study. Int J Audiol 2003;42:89–105.
12. Cornfield J. A method of estimating comparative rates from clinical data. Applications to cancer of the lung, breast and cervix. J Natl Cancer Inst 1951;11:1269–75.
13. Kahn HA, Sempos CT. Statistical methods in epidemiology. New York: Oxford University Press; 1989.
14. Hudson JI, Laird NM, Betensky RA. Multivariate logistic regression for familial aggregation of two disorders. I. Development of models and methods. Am J Epidemiol 2001;153:500–5.
15. StataCorp. Stata statistical software: release 8.0. College Station (TX): Stata Corporation; 1996.
16. SAS Institute Inc. SAS/STAT user's guide, version 8. Cary (NC): SAS Institute Inc.; 1996.
17. Shah BV, Barnwell BG, Bieler GS, et al. SUDAAN technical manual. Statistical methods and algorithms used in SUDAAN. Research Triangle Park (NC): Research Triangle Institute; 1996.
18. Leske MC. Prevalence estimates of communicative disorders in the U.S. Language, hearing and vestibular disorders. ASHA 1981;23:229–37.
19. Cooper JC Jr. Health and Nutrition Examination Survey of 1971–75: Part II. Tinnitus, subjective hearing loss, and well-being. J Am Acad Audiol 1994;5:37–43.
20. Brown SC. Older Americans and tinnitus: a demographic study and chartbook. GRI monograph series A, no. 2. Washington (DC): Gallaudet Research Institute; 1990.
21. Holgers K-M, Erlandsson SI, Barrenäs M-L. Predictive factors for the severity of tinnitus. Audiology 2000;39:284–91.
22. McCombe A, Baguley D, Coles R, et al. Guidelines for the grading of tinnitus severity: the results of a working group commissioned by the British Association of Otolaryngologists, Head and Neck Surgeons, 1999. Clin Otolaryngol 2001;26:388–93.
23. Rosenhall U. The influence of ageing on noise-induced hearing loss. Noise Health 2003;5:47–53.
24. Huang MY, Schacht J. Drug-induced ototoxicity. Pathogenesis and prevention. Med Toxicol Adverse Drug Exp 1989;4:452–67.
25. Gristwood RE, Venables WN. Otosclerosis and chronic tinnitus. Ann Otol Rhinol Laryngol 2003;112:398–403.
26. Martin K, Snashall S. Children presenting with tinnitus: a retrospective study. Br J Audiol 1994;28:111–5.
27. Podoshin L, Ben-David J, Teszler CB. Pediatric and geriatric tinnitus. Int Tinnitus J 1997;3:101–3.

28. Rosenhall U, Karlsson A-K. Tinnitus in old age. Scand Audiol 1991;20:165–71.
29. Chiossoine-Kerdel JA, Baguley DM, Stoddart RL, Moffat DA. An investigation of the audiologic handicap associated with unilateral sudden sensorineural hearing loss. Am J Otol 2000;21:645–51.
30. Havia M, Kentala E, Pyykko I. Hearing loss and tinnitus in Meniere's disease. Auris Nasus Larynx 2002;29:115–9.
31. Soderman AC, Bagger-Sjoback D, Bergenius J, Langius A. Factors influencing quality of life in patients with Ménière's disease, identified by a multidimensional approach. Otol Neurotol 2002;33:941–8.
32. Kentala E. Characteristics of six otologic diseases involving vertigo. Am J Otol 1996;17:883–96.
33. Kentala E, Pyykko I. Clinical picture of vestibular schwannoma. Auris Nasus Larynx 2001;28:15–22.
34. Bhatia PL, Gupta OP, Agrawal MK, Mishr SK. Audiological and vestibular function tests in hypothyroidism. Laryngoscope 1977;87:2082–9.
35. Maguchi S, Fukuda S, Chida E, Terayama Y. Myeloperoxidase-antineutrophil cytoplasmic antibody-associated sensorineural hearing loss. Auris Nasus Larynx 2001;28 Suppl:S103–6.
36. Nondahl DM, Cruickshanks KJ, Wiley TL, et al. Prevalence and 5-year incidence of tinnitus among older adults: the epidemiology of hearing loss study. J Am Acad Audiol 2002;13:323–31.
37. Malm J, Kristensen B, Carlberg B, et al. Clinical features and prognosis in young adults with infratentorial infarcts. Cerebrovasc Dis 1999;9:282–9.
38. Sismanis A. Pulsatile tinnitus. Otolaryngol Clin North Am 2003;36:389–402.
39. McFeely WJ Jr, Bojrab DI, Davis KG, Hegyi DF. Otologic injuries caused by airbag deployment. Otolaryngol Head Neck Surg 1999;121:367–73.
40. Folmer RL, Griest SE. Chronic tinnitus resulting from head or neck injuries. Laryngoscope 2003;113:821–7.
41. Pilgramm M, Rychlick R, Lebisch H, et al. Tinnitus in the Federal Republic of Germany: a representative epidemiological study. In: Hazell J, editor. Proceedings of the Sixth International Tinnitus Seminar. London: The Tinnitus and Hyperacusis Centre; 1999. p. 64–7.
42. Coles RRA, Davis AC, Haggard MP. Medical Research Council's Institute of Hearing Research. Epidemiology of tinnitus. CIBA Found Symp 1981;85:16–34.
43. Axelsson A, Ringdahl A. Tinnitus—a study of its prevalence and characteristics. Br J Audiol 1989;23:53–62.
44. Davis AC. Hearing in adults. The prevalence and distribution of hearing impairment and reported hearing disability in the MRC Institute of Hearing Research's National Study of Hearing. London: Whurr Publishers Ltd; 1995.
45. Davis A, Rafaie EA. Epidemiology of tinnitus. In: Tyler RS, editor. Tinnitus handbook. San Diego (CA): Singular Publishing Group; 2000. p. 1–23.
46. Quaranta A, Assennato G, Sallustio V. Epidemiology of hearing problems among adults in Italy. Scand Audiol Suppl 1996;42:9–13.
47. Sindhusake D, Mitchell P, Newall P, et al. Prevalence and characteristics of tinnitus in older adults: the Blue Mountains Hearing Study. Int J Audiol 2003;42:289–94.
48. Chung DY, Gannon RP, Mason K. Factors affecting the prevalence of tinnitus. Audiology 1984;23:441–52.
49. Hinchcliffe R. The threshold of hearing as a function of age. Acustica 1959;9:303–8.
50. Davis AC. The prevalence of hearing impairment and reported hearing disability among adults in Great Britain. Int J Epidemiol 1989;18:911–7.
51. Borchgrevink HM, Tambs K, Hoffman HJ. The Nord-Trøndelag Norway Audiometric Survey 1996–98: unscreened adult high-frequency thresholds, normative thresholds and noise-related socio-acusis. In: Henderson D, Prasher D, Kopke R, et al, editors. Noise induced hearing loss: basic mechanisms, prevention and control. London: Noise Research Network (nRn) Publications; 2001. p. 377–85.
52. Daniell WE, Fulton-Kehoe D, Smith-Weller T, Franklin GM. Occupational hearing loss in Washington State, 1984–1991: II. Morbidity and associated costs. Am J Indust Med 1998;33:529–36.
53. Kowalska S, Sulkowski W. Tinnitus in noise-induced hearing impairment [in Polish]. Med Pr 2001;52:305–13.
54. Palmer KT, Griffin MJ, Syddall HE, et al. Occupational exposure to noise and the attributable burden of hearing difficulties in Great Britain. Occup Environ Med 2002;59:634–9.
55. Phoon WH, Lee HS, Chia SE. Tinnitus in noise-exposed workers. Occup Med (Lond) 1993;43:35–8.
56. Sulkowski W, Kowalska S, Lipowczan A, Prasher D. Tinnitus and impulse noise-induced hearing loss in drop-forge operators. Int J Occup Med Environ Health 1999;12:177–82.
57. Ylikoski ME, Ylikoski JS. Hearing loss and handicap of professional soldiers exposed to gunfire noise. Scand J Work Environ Health 1994;20:93–100.
58. Lean MEJ, Han TS, Seidell JC. Impairment of health and quality of life using new US federal guidelines

for the identification of obesity. Arch Intern Med 1999;159:837–43.
59. Sturm R. Increases in clinically severe obesity in the United States, 1986–2000. Arch Intern Med 2003; 163:2146–8.
60. Karlsson KK, Harris JR, Svartengren M. Description and primary results from an audiometric study of male twins. Ear Hear 1997;18:114–20.
61. Gates GA, Couropmitree NN, Myers RH. Genetic associations in age-related hearing thresholds. Arch Otolaryngol Head Neck Surg 1999;125:654–9.
62. Christensen K, Frederiksen H, Hoffman HJ. Genetic and environmental influences on self-reported reduced hearing among the old and oldest-old. J Am Geriatr Soc 2001;49:1512–7.
63. Davis RR, Newlander JK, Ling X-B, et al. Genetic basis for susceptibility to noise-induced hearing loss in mice. Hear Res 2001;155:82–90.
64. Davis RR, Kozel P, Erway LC. Genetic influences in individual susceptibility to noise: a review. Noise Health 2003;5:19–28.
65. Petersen HC, Andersen T, Frederiksen H, et al. The heritability of tinnitus—a twin study [abstract]. Arhus (Denmark): Nordic Epidemiology Congress; June 2002.
66. Weiss NS. Relation of high blood pressure to headache, epistaxis, and selected other symptoms. The United States Health Examination Survey of Adults. N Engl J Med 1972;287:631–3.
67. Vessey M, Painter R. Oral contraception and ear disease: findings in a large cohort study. Contraception 2001;63:61–3.

EDITORIAL COMMENTARY

Dobie emphasizes the major role of exposure to intense sound in the causation of tinnitus and calls attention to the importance of small arms fire in recreational activities. He makes the distinction between having tinnitus and suffering from tinnitus. Dobie points out that psychological factors, such as depression and anxiety present before the onset of tinnitus, may be the major determinants of whether tinnitus causes suffering. He opines that whether a therapeutic strategy attempts to reduce tinnitus sensation or reduce tinnitus suffering, the outcome should be measured in terms of reduction of tinnitus suffering. Dobie draws attention to our lack of knowledge of the natural history of and prognostic factors in tinnitus and concludes that clinical trials are essential in the evaluation of therapy for tinnitus.

Jastreboff and Jastreboff define hyperacusis as an abnormally high level of neuronal activity in the auditory pathways owing to abnormal amplification of sound-evoked neural signals and misophonia as an abnormally strong reaction of the limbic and autonomic nervous systems to sound without abnormally high activation of the auditory system. They draw a clear distinction between the two conditions based on whether there is abnormal amplification of soundinduced activity in the auditory system. Usually, the two conditions coexist.

Jastreboff and Jastreboff point out that decreased sound tolerance can be associated with tinnitus, stress, or intense sound exposure in individuals with normal hearing or hearing loss. Hyperacusis and misophonia are not related to recruitment. Whereas hyperacusis may have peripheral or central mechanisms responsible for its development, misophonia always involves central mechanisms.

Jastreboff and Jastreboff advocate tinnitus retraining therapy (TRT) for hyperacusis and misophonia and advise against ear protection from sound. In the individual with tinnitus and decreased sound tolerance, TRT is directed first at hyperacusis. The elimination of hyperacusis facilitates habituation to tinnitus.

Hoffman and Reed provide evidence that tinnitus prevalence increases during young adulthood and middle age, levels off between 65 and 74 years of age, and then gradually declines. Although the overall age trends for men and women are similar, the prevalence in men increases more rapidly with age, probably owing to noise exposure, and remains higher until about 85 years of age.

They demonstrate that lower educational attainment and annual income and poorer health status are associated with a higher prevalence of bothersome tinnitus. Noise exposure and head injury are important risk factors for bothersome tinnitus in both men and women.

Hoffman and Reed emphasize the strong association between the prevalence of bothersome tinnitus and the level of hearing impairment. In addressing the issue of the role of aging once there is proper accounting for hearing loss, Hoffman and Reed find that there is a lower prevalence of tinnitus as age cohort increases for any given level of hearing impairment.

They draw attention to the approximately twofold increase in the odds ratios for bothersome tinnitus for male and female siblings, which suggests a familial association owing to shared environmental factors or a genetic basis.

James B. Snow Jr

CHAPTER 4

Molecular Biology of Hearing and Tinnitus

Allen F. Ryan, PhD, Lina M. Mullen, PhD

Because the underlying mechanisms of tinnitus remain obscure,[1] any discussion of the molecular biology of this condition must be speculative. However, we can reasonably assume that the sensation of tinnitus involves at least some of the same molecular substrates that are involved in normal auditory perception. This could include substrates of homeostasis, mechanoelectrical transduction, afferent neurotransmission, and efferent neural processing in the inner ear and/or central auditory pathway. Of course, tinnitus is a disorder of the auditory system. A substantial proportion of tinnitus appears to reflect plastic change in the auditory system. Thus, in addition to genes involved in normal auditory function, those important to other disorders involving neural plasticity may provide clues as to molecular substrates involved in tinnitus. However, to approach the potential molecular mechanisms of tinnitus, we must first comprehend the molecular biology of audition.

MOLECULAR BIOLOGY OF THE COCHLEA

The various tissues of the body express thousands of different genes, most of which are ubiquitously expressed by many or even all cell types. These genes are involved in the routine maintenance of cell structure and survival and are thus termed "housekeeping" genes. A much smaller subset of genes subserves the specific functions of cells. These genes vary with the characteristics of the cell in question. Thus, a nerve cell can be expected to express a very different set of genes than, say, a cartilage cell. The inner ear contains many different cell types and thus expresses a wide variety of specific structural and functional genes, depending on cochlear cell type. Our understanding of the genes that participate in cochlear function is far from complete. However, in recent years, we have identified many such genes through expression studies or by the effects of natural and induced mutations. The survey presented below is necessarily selective but presents the major categories of genes thought to be involved in cochlear function, with important examples of each. We concentrated on those aspects of function that are potentially related to tinnitus: cochlear potassium gradients, hair cell function, and afferent and efferent auditory neurotransmission.

INNER EAR FLUID HOMEOSTASIS

The function of the inner ear depends on the ionic composition and charge of its fluid compartments. The high potassium and low sodium content of endolymph and the positive resting potential of the scala media, which are generated by the stria vascularis, are required for the transduction of pressure differences into electrical potentials within hair cells. The energy stored in the endolymph also powers the active mechanical amplifier of the outer hair cells (OHCs). The ionic environment of the inner ear is also relevant to tinnitus in other ways. Because elevated extracellular potassium can lead to the discharge of neurons, it has been suggested that some forms of tinnitus may be caused by potassium leakage from endolymph into the extracellular fluid surrounding the afferent dendrites of the auditory nerve. This includes the low-frequency tinnitus characteristic of Meniere's disease, which is associated with an imbalance in endolymph homeostasis.

As noted above, differences in the ionic composition between endolymph and perilymph have been shown to play a critical role in inner ear function. It is, therefore, not surprising that genes encoding a number of ion transport proteins are expressed in the inner ear. Of particular interest are the Na, K–adenosine triphosphatase (ATPase) genes because this enzyme appears to be a critical determinant of the composition of perilymph and endolymph.[2,3] This transport enzyme is composed of an α and a β subunit. There are three α and two β subunit isoforms, each encoded by a separate gene, which can combine to form different isozymes.[4] In the stria vascularis, the $α_1$ and $β_2$ isoforms are the only ones expressed. This subunit combination is not found in isolation in any other tissue in the body. The $β_2$ subunit is known to be associated with transporting sodium against a high electrochemical gradient. Thus, for the stria to transport sodium against the highest gradient in the body into endolymph, this unique composition of the enzyme may be required. Other potassium transporters known to be expressed in the stria and critical for its function include the Na-K-Cl cotransporter[5,6] and H, K-ATPase.[7]

Selective ion channels also participate in inner ear fluid regulation. In particular, the KCNQ1 and Isk potassium channels are expressed in the lateral membrane of the marginal cells and allow potassium to exit these cells into endolymph.[8,9] In the absence of the Isk gene, the scala media collapses, resulting in complete deafness.[8]

During the transduction process, potassium enters hair cells from scala media through the transduction channels, driven by the electrochemical gradient between the endolymph and the hair cell cytoplasm. The potassium ions exit the hair cells into the organ of Corti. In OHCs, this is at least in part through KCNQ4 potassium channels on their lateral membranes. Mutations in the gene encoding this channel lead to OHC death.[10] The potassium that exits hair cells appears to be taken up by the supporting cells of the organ via the K-Cl cotransporter Kcc4[11] and to pass through these cells and into the fibrocytes of the spiral ligament through gap junctions containing connexins 26 and 31.[12] Mutations in genes encoding these gap junction proteins lead to deafness.[13–15]

HAIR CELL TRANSDUCTION

The major function of the sensory epithelium of the cochlea is the transduction of mechanical vibrations of the cochlear partition into neuronal impulses in the auditory nerve. The sensory cells of the cochlea (and the vestibular sensory organs) are mechanoreceptors equipped with geometrically arranged sensory stereociliary bundles on the cell surface. Deflection of the ciliary bundle by mechanical force toward the kinocilium (or basal body in the case of the cochlea) is excitatory and in the opposite direction is inhibitory for neural discharges. Deflection of the stereociliary bundle toward the excitatory direction is now known to open transduction channels located on the upper part of the stereocilia.[16–18] The opening of the transduction channels is believed to be mediated by a filamentous structure connecting the tip of the lower stereocilium to the neighboring taller stereociliary surface and is known as the tip-links.[19,20]

Most of the molecules responsible for the hair cell transduction process have yet to be identified. However, some progress has been made in the transduction channel[21,22] and the adaptation motor in vestibular sensory hairs.[23] The precise location of the transduction channels is not yet established. It is believed to be associated with tip-links because the calcium chelator BAPTA (1,2-bis(o-aminophenoxy)ethane-N,N,N′,N′-tetraacetic acid) eliminates transduction current and tip-links.[19] However, Hackney and colleagues used an antibody to amiloride-sensitive sodium channel to label the side of the stereocilia just below the tip-link attachment site, suggesting a possible alternative location.[21] Identification of the gene or genes that encode the channel remains an important goal in hearing science. Mammalian homologs of the MEC family genes of *Caenorhabditis elegans* have been considered as candidates, in part based on the expression of developmental genes in the mechanically sensitive neurons on this species and mammals.[24,25] A recent advance is the identification of a mechanically sensitive ion channel of the transient receptor potential (TRP) superfamily that is required for mechanotransduction in the bristle organ of *Drosophila*, which may also be evolutionarily related to hair cells.[26] Several TRP-like channels in vertebrates are also candidates for hair cell transduction channel components.[27] It is possible that several molecular components contribute to the channel, as is the case for the MEC channel in *C. elegans* mechanoreceptor neurons, which complicates the search.

To retain sustained sensitivity during transient displacement, the vestibular sensory cell must adapt to sustained stimuli. Adaptation of the vestibular sensory cell is thought to be mediated by a "slipping" of tip-link attachment and by an active "tensioning."[28] Readjusting tension of the tip-link is necessary for the adaptation of the vestibular sensory cells.[23,29] This tensioning is suggested to be mediated by 120 kDa myosin motors, which are presumably located in the insertional plaque and run on the surface of the stereociliary actin filaments as guides.[22,23,29] It is not clear whether a similar process occurs in auditory hair cells.

Other channels are also thought to be present at the tips of the hair cell stereocilia. For example, adenosine triphosphate (ATP)-gated channels have been localized to this area.[30] It has been suggested that these channels may modulate the activity of the transduction channel in response to extracellular ATP in endolymph by shunting current away from the channel. Extracellular ATP could itself be generated in response to stress, such as acoustic trauma.[31]

The discoveries of acoustic emissions[32] and the electromechanical activity of dissociated OHCs of mammals[33,34] provided strong support for the concept of active hearing. According to this concept, auditory sensitivity and sharp tuning of the basilar membrane frequency are the result of an active, electromechanical amplification process in OHCs. This motor activity was thought to be driven by multiple molecular motors that are an integral part of the OHC membrane.[35,36] These molecular motors are activated by changes in transmembrane voltage, produced when potassium enters the cell from endolymph on the opening of the transduction channel. In response to transmembrane voltage changes, the motors change shape, resulting in length and/or stiffness changes in the membrane. This process actively amplifies the vibrations of the basilar membrane, resulting in the 40 to 50 dB of threshold shift that has long been associated with the presence of OHCs.[37]

More recently, strong evidence has been obtained to support this hypothesis and to identify the molecular substrate. The molecule responsible for OHC electromotility was identified by Zheng and colleagues, who used a subtractive polymerase chain reaction technique to identify molecules expressed by outer, but not inner, hair cells.[38] Identified clones were expressed in mammalian cells. One such clone produced membrane responses consistent with electromotility, leading to the identification of a member of an anion transporter family that had lost ion transport function. This molecule was termed *prestin*. Later studies by Oliver and colleagues determined the molecule operates when a Cl^- ion enters a pore in the intracellular side of the transmembrane molecule in response to transmembrane voltage change, resulting in a shape change.[39]

A targeted deletion of the prestin gene in mice was found to result in a 40 to 50 dB loss of auditory sensitivity and no otoacoustic emissions,[40] providing convincing evidence that prestin and OHC electromotility are responsible for active cochlear amplification. Mutation of the prestin gene was also recently found to mediate a form of inherited hearing loss in humans with similar effects on hearing.[41]

INNER EAR NEUROTRANSMITTERS

The afferent and efferent (medial and lateral) systems and the innervation patterns of the auditory organ are relatively well established. Although remarkable progress has been made in recent years, our knowledge concerning the inner ear neurochemistry is yet to be complete. Afferent neurotransmission between the cochlear hair cells and spiral ganglion neurons is mediated by an as yet unidentified neurotransmitter. Based on pharmacologic evidence, the strongest candidate for this transmitter is glutamate or a related amino acid. Recently, the expression of messenger ribonucleic acids (mRNAs) encoding glutamate receptors has been detected in spiral ganglion neurons. These include members of the α-amino-3-hydroxy-5-methyl-4-isoazolepropionate (AMPA), N-methyl-D-aspartate (NMDA), and kainate glutamate receptor families.[42–44] These observations strongly support the hypothesis that an excitatory amino acid such as glutamate is one of the cochlear afferent neurotransmitters. Glutamate released from hair cells is thought to be cleared from the synapse by glutamate transporters.[45]

The primary efferent neurotransmitter between the brainstem and the cochlea is thought to be acetylcholine, with other transmitters, including γ-aminobutyric acid (GABA), opioid and other peptides, and possibly ATP, also being involved. Members of several neuronal receptor gene families have been shown to be expressed in the cochlea. Expression of genes encoding nicotinic,[46] muscarinic,[47] and metabotropic[48] acetylcholine receptors; GABA receptors[49]; and ATP receptors[50] has been documented in the cochlea, whereas preproenkephalin mRNA has been found in cochlear and vestibular efferent cell bodies in the brainstem.[51] In particular, the α9 and α10 members of the nicotinic acetylcholine receptor family have been shown to be strongly expressed in OHCs and to match exactly the pharmacology of the OHC response to this transmitter.[52,53] In general, the diversity of receptor and transmitter expression associated with the efferent system matches the complex pharmacology of the inner ear.

ION CHANNELS IN INNER EAR NEURONS

Neurotransmission depends on the action of many ion channels. Within the spiral ganglion, expression of potassium channel genes varies along the length of the cochlea, with apical neurons expressing a preponderance of Kv4.2 subunits, whereas basal turn neurons express higher levels of Kca, Kv1.1, and Kv3.1 subunits.[54] This difference appears to be related to the physiologic characteristics of the neurons. Apical neurons are characterized by long-latency, slowly adapting responses to depolarizing current injection and normally fire slowly in response to low-frequency acoustic stimulation. Basal neurons show short-latency and rapidly adapting responses consistent with their normally rapid firing to high-frequency acoustic stimulation.

OTHER INNER EAR PROTEINS

Genes important for inner ear function have often been highlighted by mutational analysis. An additional paradigm for identifying functionally important proteins is to look for genes whose pattern of expression is limited to the inner ear and to test if these genes are important for inner ear function, creating animal models with nonfunctional mutant versions of these genes. To date, very few genes showing a pattern of expression limited to the inner ear have been reported. Two organ of Corti–specific proteins, OCP I and OCP II, have been identified[55] and cloned.[56] These proteins are involved in ubiquitination of supporting cell proteins, including connexins.[57] Tectorial membrane proteins (tectorins) with little homology to known proteins have also been cloned,[58] and mutations in these genes can lead to deafness.[59] Similarly, mutations in the gene encoding otoanchorin, an inner ear–specific protein expressed at the interface between sensory epithelia and their overlying acellular gels, result in deafness.[60]

MOLECULAR BIOLOGY OF THE CENTRAL AUDITORY SYSTEM

Unlike the inner ear, the central auditory pathway appears to have few unique genes, the expressions of which are confined to central auditory cells. This presumably reflects the reality that the central auditory pathway does not appear to contain unique cell types but rather consists of the same cell types present in other central nervous system pathways and systems.

This said, progress has been made in identifying genes that are expressed in the cells of the central auditory pathway, and some of these appear to be preferentially expressed in this pathway.

CENTRAL AUDITORY NEUROTRANSMITTERS

Several neurotransmitters employed by central auditory neurons have long been known from pharmacologic experiments. More recently, the genes that encode receptors for the transmitters have been identified. Documentation of the expression of these genes in auditory neurons has confirmed the role of specific transmitters and added detailed information regarding receptor distribution and the properties of cellular responses.

Glutamate is the primary, excitatory, afferent neurotransmitter of auditory neurons. Cytochemical studies have demonstrated that virtually all of the many ionotropic and metabotropic gluamate receptor subunit genes are expressed by central auditory neurons. Because neuronal receptors typically require assembly of a number of subunits to produce a functional receptor, this provides an extraordinary potential for response diversity within the central auditory pathway. This said, the AMPA receptor subunits GluR2 and GluR3 tend to dominate ionotropic receptor expression, whereas the NMDA receptor subunit NR1 often dominates the metabotropic receptors in auditory neurons.[61] Expression of glutamate receptors is far from uniform across cell types, however. In some specific neuronal types, other combinations were dominant.[62]

The most important inhibitory neurotransmitters in the central auditory system appear to be GABA and glycine.[63] Considerable diversity in the expression of GABA receptor subunits has been observed in auditory neurons.[64] In contrast, glycine receptors in the adult central auditory pathway appear to consist primarily of the α_1 subunit. Expression of the α_2 to α_4 subunits may be more important during development.[65] An additional modulatory transmitter in the central auditory pathway is serotonin. Serotonin receptors are widespread in auditory nuclei, as they are in many brain regions.[66]

CENTRAL AUDITORY ION CHANNELS

A wide variety of ion channels are expressed by all neurons, including those of the central auditory pathway. However, the neurons of the auditory pathway preferentially express the two isoforms of the Kv3.1 potassium channel.[67] Expression of this channel is associated with neurons that characteristically fire rapid trains of action potentials,[68] as in the transmission of acoustically derived information. In addition, most auditory neurons also express the KCNQ4 K channel, which is also expressed by OHCs. Few cells outside the auditory system express this channel.[69]

GENES MEDIATING NEURAL PLASTICITY

Tinnitus represents a more or less permanent change in auditory perception. It often appears to arise from a peripheral insult or injury and later develops into a self-sustaining characteristic of the central nervous system. It has been compared with the phenomenon of chronic pain, which also begins with a peripheral stimulus but later is thought to move to the central nervous system. Tinnitus thus appears to represent a form of neural plasticity.

The molecular substrates of tinnitus may thus be similar to other forms of neural plasticity, of which the best studied example is memory. Memory appears to be the results of changes in the morphology and biochemistry of neurons and their synapses that are caused by experience. Studies of gene expression during conditioning have documented the expression of many genes involved in synaptic plasticity, including NMDA and calcium channel genes, as well as protein kinase and transcription factor genes presumably involved in gene expression changes.[70,71] Of these, the calcium response element binding protein (CREB) may be of interest because overexpression of CREB in the basolateral amygdala has been shown to enhance fear conditioning.[71,72] Another gene of interest encodes the 65 kDa isoform of glutamate decarboxylase (GAD65), which is involved in GABA synthesis. Learning-specific reductions in expression of this gene have recently been reported.[73] Because GABA is a major inhibitory transmitter of the central auditory pathway, changes in this gene might be speculated to participate in the neuroplasticity associated with tinnitus.

MOLECULAR MECHANISMS OF TINNITUS

There have been no reports of tinnitus that is inherited without hearing loss. All reports of familial tinnitus appear to also involve inherited hearing loss.[74–76] Thus, it seems highly unlikely that tinnitus can be linked to a single gene. Genetics may yet turn out to be a factor in tinnitus susceptibility. However, if several genes were involved, unraveling this would be a complex task. Far more likely than a genetic cause per se is that changes in the expression of genes participate in the processes that underlie tinnitus.

As mentioned above, because we have yet to identify the underlying mechanisms of tinnitus, we can only speculate on its molecular substrates. Tinnitus is often associated with damage to the cochlea. However, it is not a wholly or even primarily peripheral process. It has been speculated that tinnitus can originate in the periphery and then lead to a central process that is independent of the cochlea. If this model is correct, we should look at both peripheral and central substrates.

In the cochlea, disorders resulting in an increase in potassium concentration within the organ of Corti or even Rosenthal's canal could result in increased spontaneous discharge of auditory neurons and tinnitus. Alternatively, over- or underproduction of endolymph could result in static deformation of the basilar membrane, again producing increased spontaneous rate in auditory neurons. Thus, changes in the expression of genes involved in endolymph production, as well as potassium clearance and recycling, could be involved in tinnitus.

It is also possible that increased expression of neuronal receptors by spiral ganglion neurons could lead to an increase in spontaneous activity in the auditory nerve. Independent of any changes in receptor expression, decreases in glutamate clearance from the hair cell or afferent dendrite synapse could also lead to increased discharge of auditory neurons. Mice with a targeted deletion of a glutamate transporter gene show increased susceptibility to noise damage.[77] Finally, changes in the sensitivity and activity of cochlear efferent neurons or their receptors on hair cells and cochlear afferent neurons could create decreased suppression of hair cell and/or auditory nerve neuron activity. For example, a model of interaction between efferent opioid transmitters and cochlear afferent NMDA receptors was recently proposed by Sahley and Nodar.[78]

If tinnitus that is mediated in the central auditory pathway originates as a cochlear process that then alters the central pathway, we might expect the molecular substrates to be similar to those in other forms of neural plasticity. As mentioned above, the gene encoding CREB has been implicated in long-term changes to central nervous system neurons during memory formation. Interestingly, it has recently been demonstrated that CREB expression is up-regulated in central auditory pathways for many months after noise damage to the cochlea.[79]

Changes in the balance of inhibitory and excitatory neurotransmission could lead to the creation of positive feedback loops in the central auditory pathway.[80] It has been suggested that changes in glycine or GABA inhibition, through loss of specific receptors or owing to increased release or uptake, could contribute to tinnitus.[81] Similarly, altered serotonin neurochemistry has been postulated as contributing to tinnitus.[82]

In addition to the root causes of tinnitus, it is important to consider the role of molecular events in its effects on tinnitus patients. The effects of tinnitus vary widely among individuals who experience this condition. The majority of those who, on being surveyed, report tinnitus do not perceive it as a problem. The remainder of tinnitus sufferers, however, consider their condition to range from moderately negative to intolerable, leading to depression and anxiety. Thus, it can be argued that the psychological response to tinnitus may be more important than the tinnitus itself. Treatment with antidepressants has been shown to be effective in ameliorating the negative consequences of tinnitus, even though it does not change the percept.[83] Many of the medications used to treat depression and anxiety target auditory neuronal receptor systems that may participate in tinnitus, and new targets for such medications include others, such as metabotropic glutamate receptors.[84] Finally, a number of genes have been suggested as contributing to susceptibility to psychological disorders that include depression and anxiety.[85–90] It is possible that such genes may also contribute to susceptibility to the negative psychological consequences of tinnitus.

CONCLUSION

Increased knowledge regarding the molecular substrates of hearing, hearing loss, and neural plasticity may help us understand the underlying processes of tinnitus. Genes involved in these processes will also provide new therapeutic targets and may lead to novel treatments. Similarly, understanding genes that contribute to depression and anxiety may also provide new insights into the medical management of tinnitus, independent of the underlying mechanism that produces the sensation.

REFERENCES

1. Baguley DM. Mechanisms of tinnitus. Br Med Bull 2002;63:195–212.
2. Ryan AF, Watts AG. Expression of genes coding for α and β isoforms of Na/K-ATPase in the cochlea of the rat. Cell Molec Neurosci 1991;2:179–87.
3. Fina M, Ryan AF. Expression of mRNAs encoding subunit isoforms of the Na, K-ATPase in the vestibular labyrinth of the rat. Cell Molec Neurosci 1994;5:604–13.
4. Fambrough DM, Lemas MV, Hamrick M, et al. Analysis of subunit assembly of Na, K-ATPase. Am J Physiol 1994;6:579–89.
5. Delpire E, Lu J, England R, et al. Deafness and imbalance associated with inactivation of the secretory Na-K-2Cl co-transporter. Nat Genet 1999;22:192–5.
6. Wangemann P, Liu J, Marcus DC. Ion transport mechanisms responsible for K^+ secretion and the transepithelial voltage across marginal cells of stria vascularis in vitro. Hear Res 1995;84:19–29.
7. Lecain E, Robert JC, Thomas A, Tran Ba Huy P. Gastric proton pump is expressed in the inner ear and choroid plexus of the rat. Hear Res 2000;149:147–54.
8. Vetter DE, Mann JR, Wangemann P, et al. Inner ear defects induced by null mutation of the isk gene. Neuron 1996;17:1251–64.
9. Neyroud N, Tesson F, Denjoy I, et al. A novel mutation in the potassium channel gene KVLQT1 causes the Jervell and Lange-Nielsen cardioauditory syndrome. Nat Genet 1997;15:186–9.
10. Kubisch C, Schroeder BC, Friedrich T, et al. KCNQ4, a novel potassium channel expressed in sensory outer hair cells, is mutated in dominant deafness. Cell 1999;96:437–46.
11. Boettger T, Hubner CA, Maier H, et al. Deafness and renal tubular acidosis in mice lacking the K-Cl co-transporter Kcc4. Nature 2002;416:874–8.
12. Minowa O, Ikeda K, Sugitani Y, et al. Altered cochlear fibrocytes in a mouse model of DFN3 nonsyndromic deafness. Science 1999;285:1408–11.
13. Carrasquillo MM, Zlotogora J, Barges S, Chakravarti A. Two different connexin 26 mutations in an inbred kindred segregating non-syndromic recessive deafness: implications for genetic studies in isolated populations. Hum Mol Genet 1997;6:2163–72.
14. Kelsell DP, Dunlop J, Stevens HP, et al. Connexin 26 mutations in hereditary non-syndromic sensorineural deafness. Nature 1997;387:80–3.

15. Grifa A, Wagner CA, D'Ambrosio L, et al. Mutations in GJB6 cause nonsyndromic autosomal dominant deafness at DFNA3 locus. Nat Genet 1999;23:16–8.
16. Corey DP, Hudspeth AJ. Ionic basis of the receptor potential in a vertebrate hair cell. Nature 1979;281:675–7.
17. Corey DP, Hudspeth AJ. Kinetics of the receptor current in bullfrog saccular hair cells. J Neurosci 1983;3:962–76.
18. Hudspeth AJ. Extracellular current flow and the site of transduction by vertebrate hair cells. J Neurosci 1982;2:1–10.
19. Pickles JO, Comis SD, Osborne MP. Cross-links between stereocilia in the guinea pig organ of Corti and their possible relation to sensory transduction. Hear Res 1984;15:103–12.
20. Assad JA, Shepherd GM, Corey DP. Tip-link integrity and mechanical transduction in vertebrate hair cells. Neuron 1991;7:985–94.
21. Hackney CM, Furness DN, Benos DJ, et al. Putative immunolocalization of the mechanoelectrical transduction channels in mammalian cochlear hair cells. Proc R Soc Lond B Biol Sci 1992;248:215–21.
22. Hudspeth AJ, Gillespie PC. Pulling springs to tune transduction: adaption by hair cells. Neuron 1994;12:1–9.
23. Gillespie PC, Wagner MC, Hudspeth AJ. Identification of a 120 kD hair-bundle myosin located near stereociliary tips. Neuron 1993;31:581–94.
24. Erkman L, McEvilly RJ, Luo L, et al. Role of transcription factors Brn-3.1 and Brn-3.2 in auditory and visual system development. Nature 1996;381:603–6.
25. Ryan AF. Transcription factors and the control of inner ear development. Semin Cell Dev Biol 1997;8:249–56.
26. Walker RG, Willingham AT, Zuker CS. A Drosophila mechanosensory transduction channel. Science 2000;287:2229–34.
27. Mutai H, Heller S. Vertebrate and invertebrate TRPV-like mechanoreceptors. Cell Calcium 2003;33:471–8.
28. Howard J, Hudspeth AJ. Mechanical reaction of the hair bundle mediated adaptation in mechanoelectrical transduction by the bullfrog's saccular hair. Proc Natl Acad Sci U S A 1987;84:3064–8.
29. Sole CK, Derfler BH, Duyk GM, Corey DP. Molecular cloning of myosins from the bullfrog saccular macula: a candidate for the hair cell adaptation motor. Auditory Neurosci 1994;3:63–5.
30. Housley GD, Greenwood D, Ashmore JF. Localization of cholinergic and purinergic receptors on outer hair cells isolated from the guinea-pig cochlea. Proc R Soc Lond B Biol Sci 1992;249:265–73.
31. Housley GD, Kanjhan R, Raybould NP, et al. Expression of the P2X(2) receptor subunit of the ATP-gated ion channel in the cochlea: implications for sound transduction and auditory neurotransmission. J Neurosci 1999;19:8377–88.
32. Kemp DT. Stimulated acoustic emissions from within the human auditory system. J Acoust Soc Am 1978;64:1386–91.
33. Brownell WE, Bader CR, Bertrand D, de Ribaupierre Y. Evoked mechanical responses of isolated cochlear outer hair cells. Science 1985;227:194–6.
34. Kachar B, Brownell WE, Altschuler R, Fex J. Electrokinetic shape changes of cochlear outer hair cells. Nature 1986;322:365–7.
35. Dallos P, Evans BN, Hallworth R. Nature of the motor element in electrokinetic shape changes of cochlear outer hair cells. Nature 1991;350:155–7.
36. Kalinec F, Holley MC, Iwasa KH, et al. A membrane-based force generation mechanism in auditory sensory cells. Proc Natl Acad Sci U S A 1992;89:8671–5.
37. Ryan AF, Dallos P. Absence of cochlear outer hair cells: effect on behavioural auditory threshold. Nature 1975;253:44–6.
38. Zheng J, Shen W, He DZ, et al. Prestin is the motor protein of cochlear outer hair cells. Nature 2000;405:149–55.
39. Oliver D, He D, Klöcker N, et al. Intracellular anions as the voltage sensor of prestin, the outer hair cell motor protein. Science 2001;292:2340–3.
40. Liberman MC, Gao J, He DZ, et al. Prestin is required for electromotility of the outer hair cell and for the cochlear amplifier. Nature 2002;419:300–4.
41. Liu XZ, Ouyang XM, Xia XJ, et al. Prestin, a cochlear motor protein, is defective in non-syndromic hearing loss. Hum Mol Genet 2003;12:1155–62.
42. Ryan AF, Brumm D, Kraft M. Occurrence and distribution of non-NMDA glutamate receptor mRNAs in the cochlea. Neuroreport 1991;2:643–6.
43. Niedzielski AS, Safieddine S, Wenthold RJ. Molecular analysis of excitatory amino acid receptor expression in the cochlea [published erratum appears in Audiol Neurootol 1997;2:231]. Audiol Neurootol 1997;2:79–91.
44. Niedzielski AS, Wenthold RJ. Expression of AMPA, kainate, and NMDA receptor subunits in cochlear and vestibular ganglia. J Neurosci 1995;5:2338–53.
45. Rebillard G, Ruel J, Nouvian R, et al. Glutamate transporters in the guinea-pig cochlea: partial mRNA sequences, cellular expression and functional implications. Eur J Neurosci 2003;17:83–92.

46. Housley CD, Batcher S, Kraft M, Ryan AF. Nicotinic acetylcholine receptor subunits expressed in rat cochlea detected by polymerase chain reaction. Hear Res 1994;75:47–53.
47. Drescher DG, Upadhyay S, Wilcox E, Fex J. Analysis of muscarinic receptor subtypes in the mouse cochlea by means of the polymerase chain reaction. J Neurochem 1992;59:765–7.
48. Eybalin M, Safieddine S. Neurotransmitters and neuro-modulators in the cochlea. Presented at the Inner Ear Neuropharmacology Symposium; 1994 September 14–15; Montpellier, France.
49. Drescher DG, Green GE, Khan KM, et al. Analysis of GABA-A receptor subunits in the mouse cochlea by means of PCR. J Neurochem 1993;61:1167–70.
50. Housley GD, Luo L, Ryan AF. Localization of mRNA encoding the P2X2 receptor subunit of the adenosine 5′-triphosphate-gated ion channel in the adult and developing rat inner ear by in situ hybridization. J Comp Neurol 1998;393:403–14.
51. Ryan AF, Simmons DM, Watts AG, Swanson LW. Enkephalin mRNA production by cochlear and vestibular efferents in the gerbil brainstem. Exp Brain Res 1991;87:259–67.
52. Elgoyhen A, Johnson D, Boulter J, et al. Alpha 9: acetylcholine receptor with novel pharmacological properties expressed in rat cochlear hair cells. Cell 1994;18:705–15.
53. Elgoyhen AB, Vetter DE, Katz E, et al. Alpha10: a determinant of nicotinic cholinergic receptor function in mammalian vestibular and cochlear mechanosensory hair cells. Proc Natl Acad Sci U S A 2001;98:3501–6.
54. Adamson CL, Reid MA, Mo ZL, et al. Firing features and potassium channel content of murine spiral ganglion neurons vary with cochlear location. J Comp Neurol 2002;447:331–50.
55. Thalmann I, Suzuki H, McCourt DW, et al. Partial amino acid sequences of organ of Corti proteins OCP1 and OCP2: a progress report. Hear Res 1993;64:191–8.
56. Chen H, Thalmann I, Adams JC, et al. cDNA cloning, tissue distribution, and chromosomal localization of Ocp2, a gene encoding a putative transcription-associated factor predominantly expressed in the auditory organs. Genomics 1995;27:389–98.
57. Thalmann R, Henzl MT, Killick R, et al. Toward an understanding of cochlear homeostasis: the impact of location and the role of OCP1 and OCP2. Acta Otolaryngol (Stockh) 2003;123:203–8.
58. Legan PK, Rau A, Keen JN, Richardson GP. The mouse tectorins. Modular matrix proteins of the inner ear homologous to components of the sperm-egg adhesion system. J Biol Chem 1997;272:8791–801.
59. Verhoeven K, Van Laer L, Kirschhofer K, et al. Mutations in the human alpha-tectorin gene cause autosomal dominant non-syndromic hearing impairment [published erratum appears in Nat Genet 1999;21:449]. Nat Genet 1998;19:60–2.
60. Zwaenepoel I, Mustapha M, Leibovici M, et al. Otoancorin, an inner ear protein restricted to the interface between the apical surface of sensory epithelia and their overlying acellular gels, is defective in autosomal recessive deafness DFNB22. Proc Natl Acad Sci U S A 2002;99:6240–5.
61. Petralia RS, Wang YX, Zhao HM, Wenthold RJ. Ionotropic and metabotropic glutamate receptors show unique postsynaptic, presynaptic, and glial localizations in the dorsal cochlear nucleus. J Comp Neurol 1996;372:356–83.
62. Schwartz IR, Keh A, Eager PR. Differential postsynaptic distribution of GluRs 1-4 on cartwheel and octopus cell somata in the gerbil cochlear nucleus. Hear Res 2000;147:70–6.
63. Korada S, Schwartz IR. Development of GABA, glycine, and their receptors in the auditory brainstem of gerbil: a light and electron microscopic study. J Comp Neurol 1999;409:664–81.
64. Shiraishi S, Shiraishi Y, Oliver DL, Altschuler RA. Expression of GABA(A) receptor subunits in the rat central nucleus of the inferior colliculus. Brain Res Mol Brain Res 2001;96:122–32.
65. Piechotta K, Weth F, Harvey RJ, Friauf E. Localization of rat glycine receptor alpha1 and alpha2 subunit transcripts in the developing auditory brainstem. J Comp Neurol 2001;438:336–52.
66. Woods CI, Azeredo WJ. Noradrenergic and serotonergic projections to the superior olive: potential for modulation of olivocochlear neurons. Brain Res 1999;836:9–18.
67. Grigg JJ, Brew HM, Tempel BL. Expression of voltage-gated potassium channel genes in auditory nuclei of the mouse brainstem. Hear Res 2000;140:77–90.
68. Gan L, Kaczmarek LK. When, where, and how much? Expression of the Kv3.1 potassium channel in high-frequency firing neurons. J Neurobiol 1998;37:69–79.
69. Kharkovets T, Hardelin JP, Safieddine S, et al. KCNQ4, a K^+ channel mutated in a form of dominant deafness, is expressed in the inner ear and the central auditory pathway. Proc Natl Acad Sci U S A 2000;97:4333–8.
70. Johnston MV. Brain plasticity in paediatric neurology. Eur J Paediatr Neurol 2003;7:105–13.

71. Schafe GE, Nader K, Blair HT, LeDoux JE. Memory consolidation of pavlovian fear conditioning: a cellular and molecular perspective. Trends Neurosci 2001;24:540–6.
72. Josselyn SA, Shi C, Carlezon WA, et al. Long-term memory is facilitated by cAMP response element-binding protein overexpression in the amygdala. J Neurosci 2001;21:2404–12.
73. Pape HC, Stork O. Genes and mechanisms in the amygdala involved in the formation of fear memory. Ann N Y Acad Sci 2003;985:92–105.
74. Oliveira CA, Bezerra R, Araujo MF. Tinnitus in hereditary Meniere's syndrome. Int Tinnitus J 1998;4:131–3.
75. Verstreken M, Declau F, Schatteman I, et al. Audiometric analysis of a Belgian family linked to the DFNA10 locus. Am J Otol 2000;21:675–81.
76. Verstreken M, Declau F, Wuyts FL, et al. Hereditary otovestibular dysfunction and Meniere's disease in a large Belgian family is caused by a missense mutation in the COCH gene. Otol Neurotol 2001;22:874–81.
77. Hakuba N, Koga K, Gyo K, et al. Exacerbation of noise-induced hearing loss in mice lacking the glutamate transporter GLAST. J Neurosci 2000;20:8750–3.
78. Sahley TL, Nodar RH. A biochemical model of peripheral tinnitus. Hear Res 2001;152:43–54.
79. Michler SA, Illing RB. Molecular plasticity in the rat auditory brainstem: modulation of expression and distribution of phosphoserine, phospho-CREB and TrkB after noise trauma. Audiol Neurootol 2003;8:190–206.
80. Gerken GM. Central tinnitus and lateral inhibition: an auditory brainstem model. Hear Res 1996;97:75–83.
81. Suneja SK, Potashner SJ, Benson CG. Plastic changes in glycine and GABA release and uptake in adult brain stem auditory nuclei after unilateral middle ear ossicle removal and cochlear ablation. Exp Neurol 1998;151:273–88.
82. Simpson JJ, Davies WE. A review of evidence in support of a role for 5-HT in the perception of tinnitus. Hear Res 2000;145:1–7.
83. Dobie RA. A review of randomized clinical trials in tinnitus. Laryngoscope 1999;109:1202–11.
84. Gorman JM. New molecular targets for antianxiety interventions. J Clin Psychiatry 2003;64 Suppl 3:28–35.
85. Exton MS, Artz M, Siffert W, et al. G protein beta3 subunit 825T allele is associated with depression in young, healthy subjects. Neuroreport 2003;14:531–3.
86. Sen S, Nesse RM, Stoltenberg SF, et al. A BDNF coding variant is associated with the NEO personality inventory domain neuroticism, a risk factor for depression. Neuropsychopharmacology 2003;28:397–401.
87. Finn DA, Rutledge-Gorman MT, Crabbe JC. Genetic animal models of anxiety. Neurogenetics 2003;4:109–35.
88. Williams NM, Preece A, Spurlock G, et al. Support for genetic variation in neuregulin 1 and susceptibility to schizophrenia. Mol Psychiatry 2003;8:485–7.
89. Tomita H, Shakkottai VG, Gutman GA, et al. Novel truncated isoform of SK3 potassium channel is a potent dominant-negative regulator of SK currents: implications in schizophrenia. Mol Psychiatry 2003;8:524–35.
90. Toulouse A, Rochefort D, Roussel J, et al. Molecular cloning and characterization of human RAI1, a gene associated with schizophrenia. Genomics 2003;82:162–71.

CHAPTER 5

Peripheral Processes Involved in Tinnitus

Alfred L. Nuttall, PhD, Mary B. Meikle, PhD, Dennis R. Trune, PhD

Until relatively recent times, the cochlea and its output via the auditory nerve were the major contenders considered in theories of tinnitus mechanisms.[1,2] However, a prevailing view now is that the cochlea is only one source of tinnitus, the quality of which is modified and/or sustained by central processes.[3] Either scenario requires an understanding of potential cochlear mechanisms in tinnitus.

"FINAL COMMON PATH"

It is clear from the vast body of knowledge about tinnitus in humans that most tinnitus occurs in response to some form of auditory system pathology, the majority of which is usually peripheral in origin.[4] Regardless of the specific type of cochlear dysfunction associated with an individual's tinnitus, the central nervous system (CNS) learns about the peripheral disorder via neural signals (or their lack) traversing the auditory nerve. The auditory nerve can thus be viewed as a "final common path" over which tinnitus-invoking information is conveyed to the centers of perception. The nature of that information in any given pathologic situation is as yet conjectural, and much work is needed to elucidate the underlying tinnitus mechanisms in such disparate conditions as Meniere's disease, noise trauma, and otitis media.

The principle that tinnitus results from functional alteration of a final common path, represented by the auditory nerve, rests on the concept that tinnitus is usually precipitated by hearing loss. It is relatively rare for individuals with normal hearing to develop chronic, severe tinnitus. Further, tinnitus is a common occurrence in those disorders that reduce stimulation of the auditory pathway. The clearest examples are tinnitus resulting from agents known to cause hair cell loss (eg, noise, presbycusis, and ototoxicity). Tinnitus can also occur where hair cells are normal, but normal acoustic stimulation is prevented by conductive hearing loss. Thus, although there may be only one path to the neural centers where tinnitus perceptions are generated, there is a multitude of ways in which that path can be affected.

DEAFFERENTATION AFFECTS THE FINAL COMMON PATH

The absence of normal afferent activity might be as important as the presence of abnormal activity in triggering tinnitus. For example, the CNS may function as a difference detector, actively comparing the level of activity in the auditory nerve with some expected range of values. In that case, unusual alterations of afferent activity in either direction (whether increases or decreases) could be interpreted by the CNS as indicators of unusual peripheral sensations. This concept might explain why people who have not previously experienced tinnitus often report hearing tinnitus for the first time when in a sound-shielded booth.[5]

In this chapter, we chose to focus on three major lines of inquiry regarding cochlear mechanisms in tinnitus. First, data gained from audiometric examination of patients with clinically significant tinnitus indicate a strong linkage between the nature of tinnitus sensations and the extent of peripheral hearing damage. These observations suggest that there is continuing, dynamic interaction between the cochlea and the brain centers involved in tinnitus. Second, clinical observations of ear diseases and disorders provide insights into potential tinnitus-inducing mechanisms. Third, experimental investigation of physiologic, anatomic, and pharmacologic effects of known tinnitus-inducing agents has suggested many possibilities for underlying mechanisms that could account for clinical and behavioral manifestations of tinnitus. The following sections deal with each of these three lines of evidence.

RELATIONSHIPS BETWEEN AUDIOMETRIC DATA AND THE SPECIFIC NATURE OF TINNITUS SENSATIONS

Although there is a high prevalence of both hearing loss and tinnitus within the US population, there is relatively little epidemiologic information relating the nature of the hearing losses to specific tinnitus characteristics. To address this, a consideration is made of data from more than 1,000 individuals with clinically significant tinnitus seen at the Tinnitus Clinic of the Oregon Health and Science University. These patients were tested to quantify the perceptual aspects of tinnitus, such as its pitch and localization.[6] Audiometric tests confirmed that most patients had sensorineural hearing loss and permitted comparisons between their hearing losses and associated tinnitus.

Tinnitus Pitch

There is a strong association between the pitch of tinnitus and the frequency range of abnormal hearing.[7] Patients with low-pitched tinnitus usually have the greatest amount of hearing loss, whereas those with high-pitched tinnitus often have the least amount of hearing loss (Figure 5-1). The orderliness of this relationship is striking, and analysis of variance confirms that it is highly significant statistically ($p < .0001$).

The pitch of tinnitus also tends to correspond to the frequency region in which the audiogram exhibits a steep decline or the threshold has exceeded approximately 40 dB. These audiometric results might be evidence of a transition within the cochlea from normal or nearly normal lower-frequency regions to higher-frequency regions that have undergone damage. These findings provide support for the possibility that tinnitus might result from "edge effects."[8]

Tinnitus Localization

A second phenomenon related to audiometric findings is the perceived localization of tinnitus. Patients report a variety of different localizations,[9] which can be summarized in six groupings (Figure 5-2). There is a clear relationship between the localization of tinnitus and the hearing asymmetry between the two ears. In unilateral tinnitus (see Figure 5-2A) and in bilateral tinnitus that is louder on one side (see Figure 5-2B), the side on which tinnitus is heard corresponds to the ear with the poorer hearing. However, in patients with nonlateralized tinnitus (heard equally loudly on both sides or else heard "in the head"), the audiograms of the two ears tend to be quite symmetric (see Figure 5-2C).

These generalizations concerning audiometric correlates of tinnitus perceptions are based on group means, and it should be noted that there are individuals whose tinnitus perceptions differ from the general trends summarized here. Nevertheless, Figures 5-1 and 5-2 demonstrate that, in many people, there is a fairly precise dependence of tinnitus perceptions on peripheral hearing pathology. Thus, despite CNS mechanisms that may obscure such effects, we can conclude that the physiologic status of the cochlea exerts significant control over chronically sustained tinnitus perceptions.

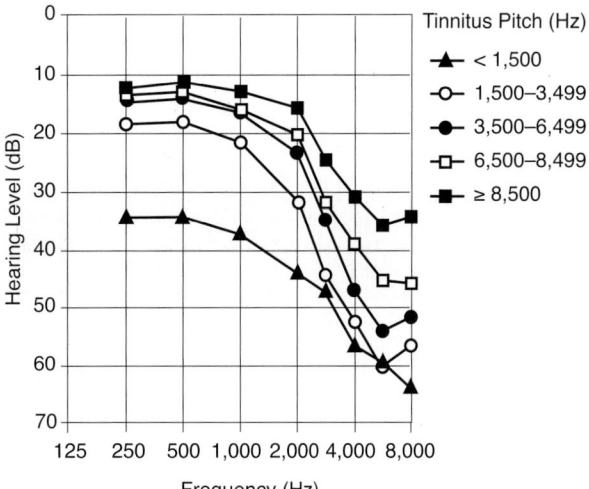

FIGURE 5-1. Relationship between tinnitus pitch and the audiogram. Mean thresholds for the right ear from a consecutive sample of 1,033 tinnitus clinic patients, of whom 803 were able to match the pitch of their tinnitus to a single frequency within one of the five frequency ranges indicated (excludes 230 patients with multiple tinnitus pitches). Pitch matches were obtained using a two-alternative forced-choice procedure with all tones matched in loudness to the patient's tinnitus (see Vernon and Meikle[6] for details). Adapted with permission from Meikle M.[9]

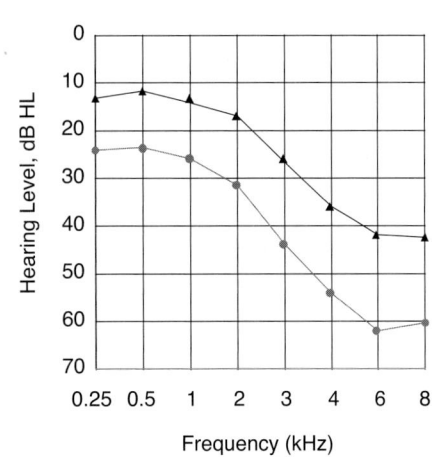
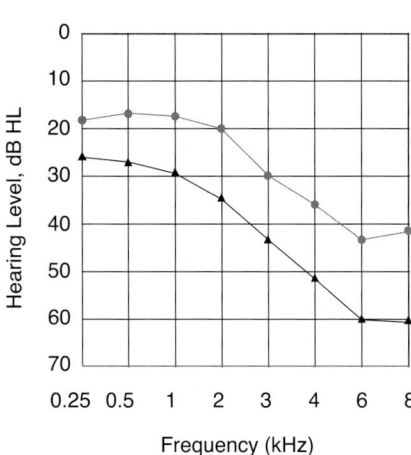
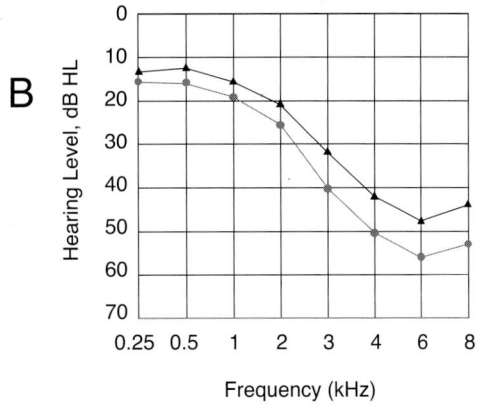
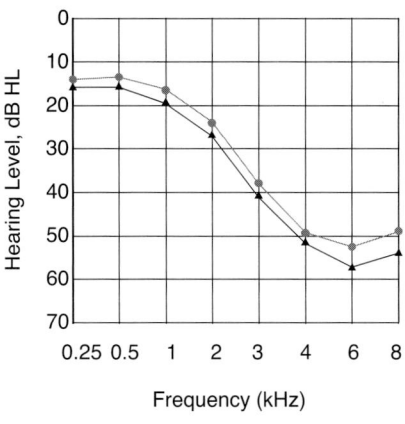
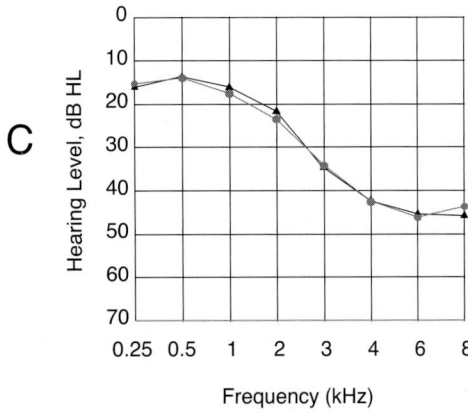
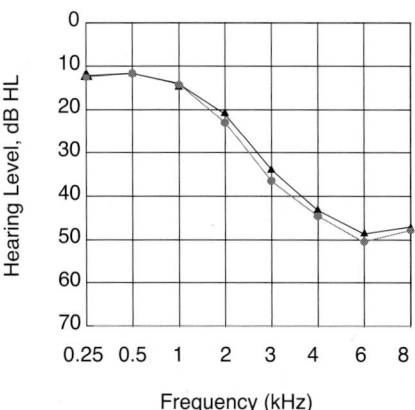

FIGURE 5-2. Relationship between tinnitus localization and the audiogram. Mean thresholds from the same sample of 1,033 patients, divided into six localization subgroups as indicated (omits a small percentage with mixed, uncertain, or variable location): *A*, unilateral (heard only on the left or only on the right); *B*, bilateral tinnitus, either louder on the left or louder on the right; *C*, nonlateralized tinnitus, heard either in the head or heard equally loudly on both sides. Triangles = right ear; circles = left ear.

EAR DISEASES AND RELATED CONDITIONS WITH ASSOCIATED TINNITUS

The close linkage between peripheral pathology and tinnitus is demonstrated in a variety of well-known clinical observations:

- Many individuals who experience gradually increasing hearing loss also report gradually increasing tinnitus with about the same time course.
- In cases of sudden-onset hearing loss, there is often a sudden onset of tinnitus or a dramatic increase of tinnitus if it was already present.
- Episodes of transient hearing loss (such as in Meniere's disease, temporary threshold shifts [TTSs] from noise trauma, and transient middle ear problems from otitis media) are typically accompanied by transient tinnitus.

Despite the fact that tinnitus is known to accompany nearly every form of hearing loss that has been studied, not all individuals with hearing loss experience tinnitus. It is not clear what genetic, environmental, or physiologic factors might predispose certain hearing-impaired individuals to develop tinnitus, whereas others with similar hearing losses do not.

In the large majority of individuals with hearing loss, the loss is peripheral in origin. Based on the model of the auditory nerve as the final common path for auditory input to the brain, any reduction in auditory nerve function has the potential to produce tinnitus. If this model is valid, then any auditory disorder or disease that ultimately compromises hearing (and auditory nerve activity) should commonly be accompanied by tinnitus. A survey of diseases of the peripheral auditory system confirms that expectation (Table 5-1).

STRIA VASCULARIS

The major role of the stria vascularis is to regulate the ionic concentrations within the endolymph. Along with the high potassium concentration of endolymph, it creates a +80 to 90 mV endolymphatic potential relative to perilymph. When this is coupled with the −80 mV intracellular potential of hair cells, it creates the approximately 160 mV potential that is necessary for inner ear sound transduction. The endothelial cells in the capillaries of the stria vascularis form the critical blood-labyrinth barrier that facilitates this control of ionic gradients and provides a protective barrier that prevents large molecules from entering the ear.[10–13] Any disease process that disrupts the stria vascularis will cause reduced perception of external sounds and potentially lead to tinnitus because of alterations in auditory processing.

There are certain auditory diseases that attack the stria specifically and in which tinnitus is an important symptom (see Table 5-1). The clinical classification of ear disease is somewhat confusing because some disorders are named for their pathologic processes (Meniere's disease), whereas others are named for their main symptom (sudden hearing loss), yet they can have similar laboratory findings (elevated immune complexes). Although some overlap is unavoidable, conventional terminology is followed to demonstrate which known hearing disorders have an important tinnitus component. Furthermore, the stria vascularis is capable of regeneration,[14] which may be a factor in the spontaneous recovery of some hearing disorders (sudden hearing loss) and the intermittent nature of others (Meniere's disease).

Meniere's Disease   Meniere's disease (etiology unknown) and Meniere's syndrome (etiology known) represent the combination of symptoms of hearing loss, vertigo, aural fullness, and tinnitus.[15,16] These symptoms are due to endolymphatic hydrops resulting from abnormal ionic control by the stria vascularis. The ability of the stria vascularis to recover presumably underlies the intermittent attacks and symptoms, particularly hearing loss and tinnitus. Meniere's disease can be confused with a number of other auditory system diseases, so differential diagnosis is critical,[17] particularly for effective treatment outcomes.[18,19]

Sudden and Rapidly Progressing Hearing Loss
Sudden and rapidly progressing hearing loss have a high incidence of tinnitus[20,21] (see Table 5-1). These hearing disorders are presented together because they are differentiated only by the time of hearing loss onset. Generally, if the hearing loss occurs in less than 24 hours, it is considered sudden hearing loss; any longer is rapidly progressing hearing loss. It may eventually be demonstrated that some of the same pathologic processes underlie both types, varying only in progression of damage to cause measurable hearing loss.

Both sudden and rapidly progressing hearing losses are symptoms of some type of cochlear pathology. Numerous causes of sudden hearing loss have been demonstrated, including immune disease, vascular disorders in the ear, inner ear infections (viral,

TABLE 5-1. Hearing Disorders with Associated Tinnitus

Lesion Location	Hearing Disorder	Reference
External ear	Cerumen in external canal, perforated or keratotic tympanic membrane	Roeser and Ballachanda,[34] Davidson and Morris,[35] Kartush,[36] Hallmo,[37] Soucek and Michaels[38]
Middle ear	Fluid, otitis media, cholesteatoma	van Cauwenberge et al,[43] Mills et al[42]
	Otosclerosis	Nager,[39] Lindsay[40]
	Ossicle disarticulation	Sperling and Kay[49]
	Temporomandibular joint disorders	Chole and Parker,[44] Rubenstein,[45] Ren and Isberg[46]
Inner ear Stria vascularis	Meniere's disease	Juhn et al,[11] Thai-Van et al,[16] Dickens and Graham,[15] Weber and Adkins[17]
	Immune-mediated inner ear disease	Hughes et al,[25] Sismanis et al,[19] Sperling et al,[27] Toubi et al,[114] Andonopoulos et al[26]
	Sudden and rapidly progressing hearing loss	Tomasi et al,[115] Byl,[21] Mattox and Simmons[20]
	Diuretics, antineoplastics	Seligmann et al,[31] Norris,[30] Meech et al[33]
	Labyrinthitis	Williams et al,[24] Veltri et al[22]
Hair cell	Noise trauma	Schleuning,[116] Reed[117]
	Antibiotics, salicylates, antineoplastics	Seligmann et al,[31] Norris[30]
Auditory nerve	Vestibular schwannoma (acoustic neuroma)	Magliulo et al,[50] Inoue et al,[51] Fahy et al,[53] Kentala and Pyykko,[52] Weber and Adkins,[17] Weissman and Hirsch[54]
	Vascular compression	Weissman and Hirsch,[54] Janetta[118]
	Acoustic nerve section	Coad et al[119]
	Multiple sclerosis and antibodies against Schwann cells	Weber and Adkins,[17] Fischer et al,[55] Cure et al,[56] Tomasi et al,[115] Yamawaki et al[120]

bacterial), acoustic neuroma, and endolymphatic hydrops.[20–24] Approximately 50 to 60% of sudden hearing loss cases will recover spontaneously,[20,21] suggesting that many of these pathologic processes affect the stria, which is capable of recovery.

Immune-Mediated Inner Ear Disease A large number of hearing loss patients have antibodies to a variety of inner ear proteins, although the role that these antibodies actually play in the hearing loss remains to be determined. Nevertheless, the clinical classification of immune-mediated inner ear disease is now used to describe hearing loss that has an antibody profile. Hearing disorders reported to have a potential immune basis and stria vascularis impact include Meniere's disease, autoimmune hearing loss, sudden hearing loss, and rapidly progressing hearing loss, all of which often have accompanying tinnitus (see Table 5-1).

Perhaps the best example of immune-mediated hearing loss is autoimmune inner ear disease. This type of hearing loss is seen in people with systemic autoimmune diseases, such as systemic lupus erythematosus, rheumatoid arthritis, and Cogan's syndrome.[25–27] The reversibility of autoimmune hearing loss with corticosteroid treatment[19,28] implies that it affects the vasculature and/or ionic control in the stria vascularis. Also, studies of hearing loss in autoimmune mice have shown that pathology is limited to the stria vascularis, leading to breakdown in the blood-labyrinth barrier and loss of the endocochlear potential (EP).[29]

Ototoxic Drugs Certain forms of drug therapy have a detrimental impact on the stria vascularis if given in high doses or for prolonged periods of time. Also, normal doses become ototoxic if the renal system of the patient is compromised. The ototoxicity of diuretics (ethacrynic acid, furosemide) is limited to the stria vascularis, and tinnitus often occurs in patients receiving these agents.[30,31] It also appears that blood vessels of the stria vascularis and spiral ligament are affected by diuretics.[32] Recovery of strial tissue occurs if treatment is terminated,[14] which explains the reversal of tinnitus with treatment cessation. Cisplatin, an antineoplastic drug, is also ototoxic and causes tinnitus.[30,31] Its impact on the ear is widespread, affecting both hair cells and stria vascularis.[33]

EXTERNAL AND MIDDLE EAR

Hearing loss occurs with any pathology of the external or middle ear that decreases the transmission of sound to the cochlea by interfering with the vibration of the tympanic membrane or the middle ear ossicles. This conductive hearing loss is often accompanied by tinnitus.

External Ear Canal Occlusion The overproduction of (or failure to clear) cerumen in the external auditory canal can sufficiently impede sound energy reaching the tympanic membrane or restrict membrane movement, and tinnitus can occur with the hearing loss.[34] The hearing loss begins in the high frequencies as cerumen occlusion occurs, gradually increasing impact on low frequencies as the canal becomes totally blocked. Resolution of the tinnitus is achieved with cerumen clearance.

Tympanic Membrane Perforation Similarly, any disruption of the tympanic membrane that decreases coupling of sound energy to ossicular movement will result in conductive hearing loss and often tinnitus. Tinnitus has been reported in cases of tympanic membrane perforation owing to trauma or otitis media,[35–37] as well as keratosis of the membrane.[38] In most cases, tinnitus subsides with restoration of the tympanic membrane and its mobility.

Any disease process that reduces ossicular vibration or stapes movement within the oval window will reduce sound perception. A number of such middle ear lesions have a tinnitus association.

Otosclerosis Otosclerosis results in fixation of the stapes footplate in the oval window, creating a conductive hearing loss. This reduction in cochlear stimulation causes tinnitus in a large number of patients.[39,40] Also, Paget's disease (osteitis deformans) can lead to conductive hearing loss and tinnitus if it occurs in the temporal bone.[41]

Otitis Media Otitis media is inflammation within the middle ear space, usually the result of bacterial infection. If fluid or purulent material accumulates and prevents tympanic membrane and ossicular movement, decreased hearing will occur. Otitis media can result in tinnitus,[42,43] presumably owing to a reduction in sound transmission.

Temporomandibular Joint Disorders Craniomandibular disorders or diseases of the joint between the skull and jaw can lead to tinnitus.[44–46] Often referred to as temporomandibular joint (TMJ) disorders, a large number of patients experience tinnitus with pain on movement of or application of pressure to this joint. Interestingly, most of the patients with tinnitus complain of the sensation of fullness or blockage of the middle ear,[46] suggesting some problem with middle ear pressure or increased impedance of the ossicular chain. Currently, the disease process underlying the tinnitus in TMJ disorders is unclear, but theories include blockage of the eustachian tube, clonus of tensor tympani muscle owing to its common innervation (trigeminal nerve) with muscles of the jaw, or a residual discomalleolar ligament that normally disappears in fetal development.[46–48] However, Chole and Parker argue against these mechanisms being able to produce the tinnitus described by patients.[44] Regardless of the cause, most of the symptoms, including tinnitus, decrease with surgery, suggesting that impaired sound conduction through the middle ear is the underlying cause of the tinnitus. This fits the final common path theory that suppressed sound transmission is responsible for tinnitus. The TMJ problems may not be causing the tinnitus directly but may initiate it through the hearing loss owing to impaired middle ear conduction.

Ossicular Disarticulation Reduced stimulation of the cochlea and tinnitus can result from disruption of the ossicular chain. For example, lateralization of a tympanic membrane graft (loss of its connection with the malleus) can cause tinnitus, which usually resolves when reparative surgery reconnects them.[49]

AUDITORY NERVE

Disorders that directly impact the auditory nerve also can be associated with tinnitus, even in the presence of a normal inner ear. Thus, tinnitus owing to a decrease in activity along the final common path is supported here as well.

Vestibular Schwannoma (Acoustic Neuroma or Neurinoma) Tumors of the vestibulocochlear nerve lead to tinnitus in the majority of patients.[50–53] Unfortunately, tumor removal does not necessarily relieve the patient of tinnitus and causes tinnitus in some patients who did not have it preoperatively.

Vascular Loops Tinnitus is also seen in some patients with vascular loops within the internal auditory canal that compress the auditory nerve.[17,54] This tinnitus may be pulsatile. Diagnosis is difficult because normally blood vessels lie against the auditory nerve without symptoms. Nevertheless, surgery to separate the vessel from the auditory nerve has been shown to relieve the tinnitus in some patients.

Multiple Sclerosis Demyelination of the auditory pathway in multiple sclerosis disrupts central auditory processing and causes hearing loss and tinnitus.[17,55,56] Although generally thought of as a CNS autoimmune disease, it can affect the auditory nerve directly,[55] possibly through antibodies to Schwann cells (see Table 5-1). Because the course of multiple sclerosis is variable and fluctuates, the auditory symptoms may occur only when the disease flares.[55] This waxing and waning of auditory symptoms sometimes makes the disease difficult to distinguish from Meniere's disease attacks.[17]

EXPERIMENTAL INSIGHTS INTO PERIPHERAL TINNITUS MECHANISMS

HAIR CELLS

Inner Hair Cells and Their Afferent Fibers Hair cell loss owing to noise trauma, presbycusis, or ototoxic drugs is generally accompanied by tinnitus (see Table 5-1). Numerous mechanisms are proposed to account for this. The concept of information flow to and from the cochlea was given the correct perspective with the publication of the landmark article by Spoendlin in the 1960s.[57] It was shown that 95% of afferent neurons exclusively contacted the inner hair cells (IHCs) and are called type I fibers. The smaller population of type II afferent fibers innervates groups of outer hair cells (OHCs). Efferent neurons also target hair cells in an unbalanced pattern. The fibers of the medial olivocochlear (MOC) bundle terminate on the soma of OHCs, whereas the axons of the lateral olivocochlear (LOC) system innervate the dendrites of the type I afferents. From the point of view of information leaving the cochlea, it is now known that IHCs and type I afferents are the main pathway. A single IHC feeds information to approximately 20 type I afferent fibers. This fact indicates that we should look carefully at the physiologic mechanisms of the IHC, its synapse with the type I afferent fiber, and the type I fibers themselves for a link to tinnitus. It is at these locations that the concept of the final common path mentioned earlier takes its physical meaning. The result can be an increase or a decrease in afferent fiber activity that the brain can interpret as sound.

The afferent fibers and IHC/type I afferent synapses are complex entities. It is possible that problems of ion channel function or regulation, or synaptic vesicle formation or release, may underlie some forms of tinnitus. For example, blockage of auditory neuron K^+ channels by quinine can result in distortion of the action potential waveform, leading to excessively long potentials.[58] As a stimulus mechanism, this excessively long action potential could lead to the release of excess neurotransmitter in the cochlear nucleus. Alternatively, faulty regulation of calcium homeostasis in IHCs could result in an excess, or deficient, IHC-released excitatory neurotransmitter (thought to be glutamate).[59]

The morphology of the IHC afferent synapse shows that the approximately 20 fibers are distributed in a unique radial pattern about the base of the IHC. The high spontaneous rate fibers, which also have high sensitivity, are located on the lateral sides of the cells.[60] Although there is no evidence to support the idea, such a partitioning of the fibers could mean that a subpopulation of the fibers at the IHC might be vulnerable to the effects of damage to nearby supporting cells or OHCs. Were this feasible, it would fit in the class of tinnitus mechanism hypotheses that propose rate change in a subpopulation of nerve fibers or the synchronization of their responses.

As far as is known, there is no synchronization of the spontaneous firing of one fiber on an IHC with another fiber from that cell or other IHCs.[61] Thus, the pattern of spontaneous activity across the neurons from a single IHC or among a population of IHCs is random and independent. The question is, "What happens under pathologic conditions?" Although Eggermont[62] and others have proposed increased synchrony as a tinnitus mechanism (see Chapter 13, "The Auditory Cortex and Tinnitus"), no one has published the direct test of this hypothesis from the simultaneous measurement of two afferent nerve fibers.

One way in which spontaneous activity is assessed is by measurement of the ensemble activity of the whole nerve using an electrode placed on the round window (RW).[63] An increase in the number of active fibers, or more synchrony among the active fibers, would lead to an increase in the magnitude of the Fourier transform of the RW time-dependent voltage signal. Consequently, salicylate (a known stimulus for human perception of tinnitus) has been tested to see if it alters the magnitude of the RW frequency spectrum. Cazals and colleagues found an increase in the RW noise provoked by chronic systemic salicylate administration in the guinea pig and proposed this as an increase in fiber synchrony and as an objective measure of tinnitus.[64] In addition, Searchfield and colleagues found an elevated peak around 200 Hz in the neural activity recorded from the RW in guinea pigs.[65] Their interpretation of the activity change as altered synchrony has been questioned.[66] It should be mentioned that others who gave salicylate as intravenous injections in acutely anesthetized guinea pigs did not observe an increase but rather a decrease in the peak magnitude of the RW noise spectrum following salicylate (also see the effects of salicylate on OHCs, below).[67]

Outer Hair Cells and Their Afferent Fibers The OHCs play a key role in the amplification of the acoustic energy that causes motion of the basilar membrane (BM). The synaptic processes of the type II afferent fibers that innervate OHCs and the information transferred to the brain are unknown. Attempts have been made to record the spike activity of type II fibers. Most recently, Robertson and colleagues reported that no spontaneous activity existed in type II fiber(s) and that sound did not evoke action potentials.[68] This result, which is consistent with previous reports, raises a problem for the type I or II fiber imbalance theory of tinnitus. Until sound-evoked nerve activity, pathology-altered activity, or spontaneous activity is proven, there is no physiologic basis for tinnitus owing to the imbalance of afferent activity mechanism.

Processes that Alter Afferent Output from the Organ of Corti

Endocochlear Potential Type I afferent fibers exhibit a varying but substantial spontaneous rate of firing. One of the earliest theories to account for tinnitus suggested that it results from an increase in the spontaneous activity of auditory nerve fibers. Theoretically, however, decreases in afferent fiber activity also could lead to perceptions of tinnitus. For example, if the normal average rate is the "setpoint" for the psychological percept of quiet, it is possible that the CNS could interpret downward modulation of the rate (relative to normal) as indicating the presence of sound. It is worthwhile, therefore, to consider what processes could increase or decrease the afferent fiber rate.

A variety of processes could alter afferent fiber rate initiated by the IHC. In addition to such hypothetical pathologic conditions as ion channel or calcium homeostatic malfunction, the main modulator of transmitter release is the IHC membrane potential. Figure 5-3 shows the main components in the process of determination of this potential. The essential elements are the electrochemical gradient across the cell that drives K^+ into and through the cell and the channels that regulate this current. Consideration is now given to the transduction channels of the OHC and the role of the EP in determining the IHC membrane potential.

The EP could have a paramount role in tinnitus because of the strict relationship of the intracellular resting potential to the EP. It has been shown that decreasing the EP level, which would result in decreasing the "standing current" passing into the IHC, will hyperpolarize the cell and decrease the spontaneous rate of afferent type I fibers.[69] Likewise, an increase in EP will depolarize the cells and increase the spontaneous activity of the fibers. Many mechanisms can affect the level of the EP. Some of these are "homeostatic" issues such as endolymphatic ionic concentrations and stria vascularis electrogenic activity (see above for more on strial mechanisms), whereas others directly involve the OHCs.

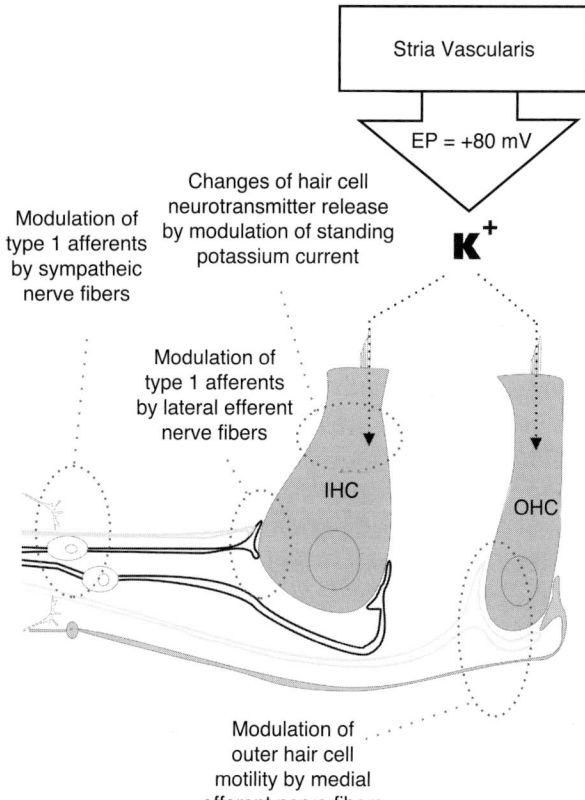

FIGURE 5-3. This schematic drawing of the organ of Corti and stria vascularis highlights the major mechanisms that modulate the "final common path," the neural discharge rate and pattern of the auditory afferent fibers. They are (1) changes of the endocochlear potential (EP), (2) modulation of the outer hair cells (OHCs) by the medial efferent nerve fibers, (3) modulation of the type I afferent nerve fibers by the lateral efferent nerve fibers, and (4) modulation of the type I afferent nerve fibers by sympathetic nerve fibers. IHC = inner hair cells.

It was shown by Fex in 1959 that the EP decreased when the medial olivocochlear bundle was stimulated.[70] The basis for this decrease is essentially an electrical impedance change of the OHCs that places more electrical load on the generating mechanism of the EP. With an increased electrical load, the voltage decreases slightly (about 3 mV).

Other examples of changes in electrical load are seen following loss of OHCs from toxic drug or loud sound exposure.[71] The manipulation of electrical load by the numbers of active OHCs, or by their ion channel properties, can place the OHCs in the domain of a regulator of EP.[72] In this scenario, for example, one can account for the tinnitus produced by salicylate by postulating that salicylate's known effect on prestin, the molecular motor protein of OHCs,[73] leads to a change in OHC somatic length (shortening), biasing the OHC stereocilia and closing transduction channels. As a result, the EP would increase, depolarize the IHCs, and cause release of neurotransmitter onto the dendrites of the type I afferents. The spontaneous rate of these fibers is thereby increased, even though the drug reduces the OHC-based amplification of the BM motion and reduces hearing thresholds. It should be apparent that any agent that causes the length of OHCs to change in a static or uncontrolled dynamic way will yield the same result. Prestin is one possible effector of the length change, but another OHC length-altering mechanism is the Ca^{2+}- and adenosine triphosphate–dependent slow motility of the OHC. Efferent neural input to the OHC is one activator of this slow motility, as discussed below.

A number of individuals experience tinnitus with no apparent change in audiometric threshold. Therefore, we also need to consider hair cell–based mechanisms that do not affect auditory sensitivity. One possibility is excessive activity of the OHC-based cochlear amplifier. This amplifier uses OHC electromotility as one component of a feedback system that enhances the physical power of the BM traveling wave that propagates as a result of sound stimulation. The BM has been observed to exhibit spontaneous motion evidenced with a wideband noise character, and this appears to be the result of random or thermal "noise."[74] If hyperactivity of the cochlear amplifier did occur, it could amplify IHC responses to the thermal "noise," possibly leading to tinnitus with either a tonal or a noise-like character. In such cases of excessive cochlear amplification, loudness perception also might be expected to be abnormal despite the apparent normality of auditory thresholds, and there is some evidence for decreased loudness tolerance in patients with tinnitus who have normal thresholds.[75]

Mechanical noise from BM motion could result from excessive cochlear amplification.[76,77] Instead, this concept of "cochlear motor tinnitus" was, in fact, put forth by Zenner and Ernst, who based their suggestions on the notion of distorted positive feedback control of organ of Corti motion.[78] Such distortions could occur, for example, by protein phosphorylation to alter the voltage-to-length transfer relation of the OHC motility apparatus (for similar ideas but related to efferent inhibition, see Frolenkov and colleagues[79] and Sziklai and Dallos[80]) or mechanical properties of the OHC (or even of organ of Corti–supporting cells).

It has been proposed that aberrations of positive feedback could result from degenerating OHCs and from missing OHCs.[81] One can ask, "What is the relationship of tinnitus and its pitch parameter to the type of cochlear lesion?" Above, we showed that clinical evaluation of patients with tinnitus does reveal a correlation between the shape of the audiogram and the tinnitus pitch.[9] From animal research, it is known that steeply sloping hearing losses are related to the edge of the cochlear region having relatively normal hair cells located next to abnormal or missing sensory cells, and a similar relationship probably exists in most humans with substantial high-frequency hearing loss. This strong evidence for the cochlear basis of some tinnitus also supports the concept that contrast in afferent fiber outputs over the transition region between cochlear lesions and the normally functioning hair cells could be responsible for generating phantom sounds. The concept of an "edge effect" in the generation of tinnitus originated with Kiang and colleagues[8] and has also been advocated by a number of others. As a hypothesis, it depends on the concept of a "comparator" or other central monitoring mechanism that is sensitive to differential inputs from the periphery; thus, it differs from hypotheses based simply on the presence or absence of input from OHCs. In at least one formulation, the "edge" or contrast hypothesis also involved hypothesizing that excessive efferent activity stimulates the OHCs adjacent to the lesion.

Loss of Sensory Cells The cochlear sensory cells (particularly the OHCs) have a well-known sensitivity to ototoxic agents. For example, loud sound can cause immediate, temporary deficits in auditory sensitivity, and there can be a corresponding tinnitus that is usually short-lived. Although it is parsimonious to assume that such tinnitus results from the same physiologic mechanism(s) as the TTS, that supposition is not necessarily true. A number of different physiologic mechanisms have been proposed to account for TTS, but other mechanisms may be responsible for the accompanying tinnitus (see the section on trigeminal innervation of the cochlea below). Regardless of the initial or "triggering" event, however, the end effect of TTS is now considered to be a temporary alteration in cochlear amplification. This alteration would be expected to produce a change in the sound-evoked pattern of activation of afferent fibers and their spontaneous rates. In this context, it is valuable to note that the pathologic effects of sound are not only on hair cells and supporting cells of the organ of Corti but also extend to involve the nerve fibers themselves. Puel and colleagues showed that a glutamate-induced excitotoxicity causes a temporary swelling and remodeling of afferent dendrites innervating the IHCs.[82]

In future studies using animal models of tinnitus, it would be useful to correlate the duration of sound-induced temporary tinnitus with the time courses of the various physiologic mechanisms of TTS, one of which (eg, EP change) might be the trigger for tinnitus. However, perhaps it is the degree of spontaneous activity decrease or the character of the fiber population involved that results in tinnitus. The so-called "edge effect" describes the dramatic decline in spontaneous discharge rate for type I afferent fibers on the basal side of a lesioned organ of Corti.[8] The edge is a transition from relatively normal morphology and function of hair cells in the organ of Corti on the apical (or low frequency) side of the lesion to missing or pathologic-appearing poorly functioning hair cells toward the basal side.

A permanent loss of OHCs occurs with prolonged loud sound exposure, certain ototoxic drugs, and aging (see Table 5-1). In most cases, such losses take a relatively long time. The tinnitus that results from such damage could be said to have been triggered by cochlear pathology, but with ample time for the CNS to modify the percept. As noted above, there is evidence from studying a large number of patients with chronic tinnitus that a high statistical association exists between the pitch of tinnitus and the pattern of cochlear lesions determined audiometrically. Thus, it seems reasonable to infer, when there has been permanent loss of OHCs, that cochlear processes continue to influence chronic, ongoing tinnitus perceptions or that cochlear processes have exerted a permanent cochleotopic effect on the CNS mechanisms subserving those percepts.

EFFERENT CONTROL OF AFFERENT ACTIVITY

In 1969, Spoendlin reported that most of the MOC efferent fibers terminating in the cochlea were on the cell bodies of OHCs.[83] A smaller portion, the LOC efferent fibers, primarily terminates on the dendritic processes of type I afferent fibers. Unfortunately, little is known about the physiology of the lateral efferent fibers. They contain a number of possible excitatory or inhibitory neurotransmitters and, because of their location, can theoretically control the excitability and spontaneous activity of type I afferents.[84]

The physiology of the medial efferent system is quite well known, although it is mainly in the context of the cholinergic neurotransmitters of the system. Acetylcholine is released from large efferent terminals and acts on a novel α_9 nicotinic receptor at the synaptic pole of the OHC. Efferent nerve activity leads to an OHC hyperpolarization, increased electrical conductance of the OHC soma, somatic elongation, and reduced mechanical stiffness of the OHC. A so-called MOC potential is seen in the scala media as a slight reduction in the EP caused by the conductivity change of the OHCs. This would lead to a decrease in spontaneous activity. The effect of the MOC fibers on OHC would change the mechanics of the organ of Corti, resulting in less cochlear amplification. Because tinnitus is not expected as a consequence of normal efferent activity (eg, sound evoked), this MOC potential could be taken as evidence that the expected decrease of type I fiber spontaneous activity is not the "trigger" for tinnitus.

MOC fibers also contain other neurotransmitters, such as γ-aminobutyric acid (GABA) and calcitonin gene-related peptide, and OHCs are known to have GABA receptors.[85] The physiology of this noncholinergic neurotransmission of the medial efferent fibers is unknown.

Adrenergic Innervation of the Cochlea

Not much has been written to attribute tinnitus to any malfunction of the adrenergic neural input to the cochlea. However, Meikle has pointed out the similarity of tinnitus to persistent pain states and the possible role of peripheral sympathetic nerve activity in maintaining tonic stimulation of sensitized neurons in the auditory CNS following peripheral damage.[9] Although many adrenergic fibers in the cochlea terminate on arteries and arterioles, it is valuable to realize that a portion of the fibers terminates as free endings in the vicinity of the auditory afferent fibers at the level of the spiral ganglion.[86] The functions of these fibers are unknown. It has been shown that they can affect afferent firing. For example, Hultcrantz and colleagues found that transection of the superior cervical ganglion produced a smaller dynamic range of afferent sound-evoked activity based on compound action potential measurements.[87] Transection also results in less permanent threshold shift[88] and TTS[89] following loud sound exposure. On the other hand, administration of noradrenaline reduces cochlear sensitivity based on measurements of the auditory nerve compound action potentials.[90,91] It is not clear how to separate the physiologic effects resulting from activity of the free sympathetic nerve endings from the possible effects on cochlear blood flow that would occur with activation or transection of the sympathetic fibers. Transection of the superior cervical ganglion does result in an increase in cochlear blood flow.[92] Although sympathetic ganglion block or removal has been claimed to relieve tinnitus,[93,94] the reports appear to be anecdotal, and the method is quite invasive. Certainly, one can conclude that any reduction of sympathetic input that reduces TTS would likely be accompanied by a reduction in the loudness of the tinnitus. Whether the reduced noradrenaline in the cochlea is responsible directly by action on nerve fibers or indirectly by effects on cochlear blood flow would be difficult to determine.

Hair Cell Mechanisms of Otoacoustic Emission Production and the Relationship to Tinnitus

Zwicker and later Zurek were among the first to note that there is little clinical evidence to link spontaneous otoacoustic emissions (SOAEs) to tinnitus,[95,96] although a few specific cases have been found in which the character of the emission has similarity to the tinnitus percepts.[97] The origin and generation of SOAEs in the cochlea are still controversial. The SOAEs are generally associated with normal cochlear sensitivity (ie, normal audiometric thresholds). SOAEs, following discovery, were immediately suspected of being responsible for perception of subjective tinnitus by Wilson and Kemp, and both reported that noise-induced tinnitus was correlated with enhanced SOAE activity.[81,98,99] One possible SOAE generator mechanism is "inhomogeneities" in the morphology of the organ of Corti, another type of edge effect. Studies in animals provide some basis for this idea.[100] Moreover, the concept of inhomogeneous mechanical impedance of the organ is a viable mechanism to generate and sustain SOAEs.[101] It is a curious fact that normal ears emit so much acoustic energy, but there is little perception of it. This seems to underscore the lack of association between SOAEs and tinnitus. Experimental research in humans has also indicated that the mechanisms for the two phenomena appear to be unrelated.[102] Tinnitus appears to reflect the altered information content carried by the type I afferent fibers, most commonly reflecting dysfunction or loss of the cochlear amplifier or other factors, whereas SOAEs appear to characterize a normal complement of OHCs and normal functioning of the cochlear amplification process.

COCHLEAR BLOOD FLOW AND ITS RELATIONSHIP TO TINNITUS

It is well known that turbulent flow in the carotid arteries of the neck can generate audible sounds and be a cause of objective tinnitus.[103] However, it is not known whether blood flow–related sounds generated within the cochlea itself can influence or cause tinnitus. This question was addressed by von Békésy, who speculated that the structure of the spiral capillary of the BM minimizes pulsatile motion of the vessel wall and does not impart any vibration to the BM itself.[104] Moreover, the arterioles more lateral to the spiral capillary will tend to dissipate the pressure wave caused by the cardiac pulse. Thus, the possible contribution of the spiral capillary to unwanted BM vibration may be minimal. Despite that conclusion, it has been found that the cardiac cycle does modulate the function of the organ of Corti.[105,106] The exact origin of the pressure variation is unclear, and evidence is lacking that could relate this modulation to any form of tinnitus. Nevertheless, approximately 6% of tinnitus clinic patients report experiencing tinnitus that has a pulsatile quality, usually experienced as a pulsation superimposed on other steady tinnitus sounds, such as ringing or hissing.[107]

It is generally agreed that the cochlea's use of potassium (rather than sodium) as the major contributor to mechanotransduction current into IHCs greatly reduces the energy needs of the hair cells. Ionic energy–expending pumps are not required to remove intracellular potassium because it moves down its concentration gradient and naturally exits the cell. Thus, the main energy-expending area of the cochlea is the stria vascularis, and the main capillary exchange area of the cochlea is located there. This anatomic configuration would be expected to reduce any effects of vascular vibrations in the vicinity of the sensory epithelium.

TRIGEMINAL INNERVATION OF THE COCHLEA

The analogy of tinnitus to pain has been discussed at least since 1981.[108,109] This literature will not be reviewed here, but the reader is referred to other reviews.[9,110] It is instructive to note that almost all tinnitus and pain analogies assume that the pain- or tinnitus-inducing event initially involves afferent fiber activity, which transmits information about cochlear damage to the CNS. Psychophysical interpretation of the signal then involves some type of plasticity of the CNS as an "adaptation" to the chronic and abnormal afferent activity.

However, there is a second or nonauditory type of afferent fiber that may convey pain from the cochlea. Vass and colleagues described a population of small-diameter neuropeptide-containing fibers on cochlear blood vessels that have cell bodies in the trigeminal ganglion.[111] That they also express transient receptor potential vanniloid type 1 (TRPV1) channels[112] puts these fibers in the category of type c primary sensory fibers. Such fibers usually trigger sensations of pain that are long lasting and slow to build up. TRPV1 channels are normally gated by temperature or pH. True pain from the ear is known to be associated with extremely loud sound stimulation, and it is possible that these fibers convey this pain information to the CNS. Activation of the small-diameter nonauditory fibers can also lead to substance P release and permeability changes of the blood vessels.[113] Regardless of whether there are direct pain sensations that may be initiated by activation of the cochlear c fibers, the resulting alteration of the fluid homeostasis of the inner ear could itself result in tinnitus from secondary mechanisms. Moreover, it is possible that the information carried by the cochlear c fibers is interpreted as sound by the CNS or modulates the percepts of tinnitus that are initiated by other, more conventional mechanisms. The latter possibility could have an anatomic basis in the trigeminal ganglion in analogy to somatosensory fibers, which are known to modulate tinnitus.

CONCLUSION

We have presented three different approaches to considering cochlear mechanisms involved in tinnitus by
- describing how several perceptual phenomena of tinnitus reveal a fairly precise dependence on the exact location and extent of peripheral pathology,

- citing otologic conditions that highlight the wide range of peripheral lesions giving rise to tinnitus, and
- reviewing physiologic mechanisms within the cochlea that have known or suspected potential for generating disordered auditory perceptions such as tinnitus.

The implication is not that all tinnitus is peripheral in origin. Although the most common forms of tinnitus are undoubtedly occasioned by peripheral insults that cause hearing impairment (exposure to damaging sound being the most prevalent), there are certainly clinical instances of tinnitus in which there is no discernible peripheral cause and systemic or central factors seem more likely.

It should be emphasized that tinnitus is a complex phenomenon, highly individual in nature, with many perceptual variants that may obscure relations to any related peripheral pathophysiology. At the same time, individuals may have developed tinnitus from more than one cause and may have multiple sounds, each with its own profile of characteristics. At this stage, our investigative tools are simply not adequate to analyze the various mechanisms that might account for multiple tinnitus sensations within a single individual.

Finally, what little evidence there currently is concerning cochlear mechanisms is circumstantial, meaning that, as yet, we cannot directly observe any of the potential tinnitus-generating mechanisms in human subjects who could verify the presence and nature of the resulting tinnitus. Until neural imaging methods in humans are more highly developed, or it becomes possible to document perceptual details of tinnitus in appropriate animal species in which cochlear physiology and anatomy can be evaluated, our ability to relate physiologic mechanisms to documented instances of tinnitus will remain conjectural.

ACKNOWLEDGMENTS

This work was supported by grants DC 00105, 00141, 03573, and 05593 from the National Institute on Deafness and Other Communication Disorders, National Institutes of Health; US Department of Education Special Project 10860006; and Department of Veterans Affairs Rehabilitation Research and Development Service (RCTR) 597-0160.

REFERENCES

1. Evered D, Lawrensen G. Tinnitus: facts, theories, mechanisms. Ciba Found Symp 1981;85:1–306.
2. McFadden D. Tinnitus facts, theories and treatments. Washington (DC): National Academy Press; 1982.
3. Vernon J, Møller AR. Mechanisms of tinnitus. Boston: Allyn and Bacon; 1995.
4. Axelsson A. Causes of tinnitus. In: Aran J-M, Dauman R, editors. Tinnitus 91. Proceedings of the Fourth International Tinnitus Seminar. Amsterdam: Kugler; 1992; p. 275–7.
5. Heller MF, Bergman M. Tinnitus aurium in normally hearing persons. Ann Otol Rhinol Laryngol 1953;62:73–83.
6. Vernon JA, Meikle MB. Tinnitus: clinical measurement. Otolaryngol Clin North Am 2003;36:293–305.
7. Meikle M, Griest SE, Press LS, Stewart BJ. Relationships between tinnitus and audiometric variables in a large sample of tinnitus clinic patients. In: Aran J-M, Dauman R, editors. Tinnitus 91. Proceedings of the Fourth International Tinnitus Seminar. Amsterdam: Kugler; 1992; p. 27–34.
8. Kiang NY, Moxon EC, Levine RA. Auditory-nerve activity in cats with normal and abnormal cochleas. Ciba Found Symp 1970;241–268.
9. Meikle M. The interaction of central and peripheral mechanisms in tinnitus. In: Vernon J, editor. Mechanisms of tinnitus. Boston: Allyn and Bacon, 1995. p. 181–206.
10. Wangemann P. Cochlear blood flow regulation. Adv Otorhinolaryngol 2002;59:51–7.
11. Juhn SK, Hunter BA, Odland RM. Blood-labyrinth barrier and fluid dynamics of the inner ear. Int Tinnitus J 2001;7:72–83.
12. Sterkers O, Bernard C, Ferrary E, et al. Possible role of Ca ions in the vestibular system. Acta Otolaryngol (Stockh) 1988;Suppl 460:28–32.
13. Weber PC, Cunningham CD, Schulte BA. Potassium recycling pathways in the human cochlea. Laryngoscope 2001;111:1156–65.
14. Roberson DW, Rubel EW. Cell division in the gerbil cochlea after acoustic trauma. Am J Otol 1994;15:28–34.
15. Dickens JRE, Graham SS. Meniere's disease—1983-1989. Am J Otol 1990;11:51–65.
16. Thai-Van H, Bounaix MJ, Fraysse B. Meniere's disease: pathophysiology and treatment. Drugs 2001;61:1089–102.

17. Weber PC, Adkins WY. The differential diagnosis of Meniere's disease. Otolaryngol Clin North Am 1997;30:977–85.
18. Hughes GB, Barna BP, Kinney SE, et al. Autoimmune endolymphatic hydrops: five-year review. Otolaryngol Head Neck Surg 1988;98:221–5.
19. Sismanis A, Wise CM, Johnson GD. Methotrexate management of immune-mediated cochleovestibular disorders. Otolaryngol Head Neck Surg 197;116:146–52.
20. Mattox DE, Simmons FB. Natural history of sudden sensorineural hearing loss. Ann Otol Rhinol Laryngol 1977;86:463–80.
21. Byl FM. Sudden hearing loss: eight years' experience and suggested prognostic table. Laryngoscope 1984;94:647–61.
22. Veltri RW, Wilson WR, Sprinkle PM, et al. The implication of viruses in idiopathic sudden hearing loss: primary infection or reactivation of latent viruses? Otolaryngol Head Neck Surg 1981;89:137–41.
23. Anderson RG, Meyerhoff WL. Sudden sensorineural hearing loss. Otolaryngol Clin North Am 1983;16:189–95.
24. Williams LL, Lowery HW, Shannon BT. Evidence of persistent viral infection in Meniere's disease. Arch Otolaryngol Head Neck Surg 1987;113:397–400.
25. Hughes G, Calabrese LH, Barna BP, et al. Immune inner ear disease: 1990 report. Trans Am Otol Soc 1990;78:86–91.
26. Andonopoulos AP, Naxakis S, Goumas P, Lygatsikas C. Sensorineural hearing disorders in systemic lupus erythematosus. A controlled study. Clin Exp Rheumatol 1995;13:137–41.
27. Sperling NM, Tehrani K, Liebling A, Ginzler E. Aural symptoms and hearing loss in patients with lupus. Otolaryngol Head Neck Surg 1998;118:762–5.
28. Alexiou C, Arnold W, Fauser C, et al. Sudden sensorineural hearing loss: does application of glucocorticoids make sense? Arch Otolaryngol Head Neck Surg 2001;127:253–8.
29. Trune D. Mouse models for immunologic diseases of the auditory system. In: Willott JF, editor. Handbook of mouse auditory research: from behavior to molecular biology. Boca Raton (FL): CRC Press; 2001. p. 505–31.
30. Norris CH. Drugs affecting the inner ear: a review of their clinical efficacy, mechanisms of action, toxicity and place in therapy. Drugs 1988;36:754–72.
31. Seligmann H, Podoshin L, BenDavid J, et al. Drug-induced tinnitus and other hearing disorders. Drug Saf 1996;14:198–212.
32. Ding D, McFadden SL, Woo JM, Salvi RJ. Ethacrynic acid rapidly and selectively abolishes blood flow in vessels supplying the lateral wall of the cochlea. Hear Res 2002;173:1–9.
33. Meech RP, Campbell KCM, Hughes LP, Rybak LP. A semiquantitative analysis of the effects of cisplatin on the rat stria vascularis. Hear Res 1998;124:44–59.
34. Roeser RJ, Ballachanda BB. Physiology, pathophysiology, and anthropology/epidemiology of human ear canal secretions. J Am Acad Audiol 1997;8:391–400.
35. Davidson BJ, Morris MS. The perforated tympanic membrane. Am Fam Physician 1992;45:1777–82.
36. Kartush JM. Tympanic membrane patcher: a new device to close tympanic membrane perforations in an office setting. Am J Otol 2000;21:615–20.
37. Hallmo P. Extended high-frequency audiometry in traumatic tympanic membrane perforations. Scand Audiol 1997;26:53–9.
38. Soucek S, Michaels L. Keratosis of the tympanic membrane and deep external auditory canal. A defect of auditory epithelial migration. Eur Arch Otorhinolaryngol 1993;250:140–2.
39. Nager GT. Histopathology of otosclerosis. Arch Otolaryngol 1969;89:157–79.
40. Lindsay JR. Otosclerosis. In: Paparella MM, Shumrick DA, editors. Otolaryngology. 2nd ed. Vol II. Philadelphia: WB Saunders Company; 1980. p. 1617–44.
41. Nager GT. Paget's disease of the temporal bone. Ann Otol Rhinol Laryngol 1975;84:1–32.
42. Mills RP, Albert DM, Brain CE. Tinnitus in children with chronic secretory otitis media. In: Lim DJ, Bluestone CD, Klein JO, Nelson JD, editors. Proceedings of the Fourth International Symposium on Otitis Media. Hamilton (ON): BC Decker Inc.; 1998. p. 420–2.
43. van Cauwenberge P, Watelet JB, Dhooge I. Uncommon and unusual complications of otitis media with effusion. Int J Pediatr Otorhinolaryngol 1999;49 Suppl 1:S119–25.
44. Chole R, Parker WS. Tinnitus and vertigo in patients with temporomandibular disorder. Arch Otolaryngol Head Neck Surg 1992;118:817–21.
45. Rubenstein B. Tinnitus and craniomandibular disorders—is there a link? Swed Dent J 1993;Suppl 95:1–46.
46. Ren YF, Isberg A. Tinnitus in patients with temporomandibular-joint internal derangement. Cranio 1995;13:75–80.
47. Ash CM, Pinto OF. The TMJ and the middle ear: structural and functional correlates for aural

symptoms associated with tempormandibular joint dysfunction. Int J Prosthodont 1991;4:51–7.
48. Eckerdal O. The petrotympanic fissure: a link connecting the tympanic cavity and the temporomandibular joint. Cranio 1991;9:15–22.
49. Sperling NM, Kay D. Diagnosis and management of the lateralized tympanic membrane. Laryngoscope 2000;110:1987–93.
50. Magliulo G, Zardo F, D'Amico R, et al. Acoustic neuroma: postoperative quality of life. J Otolaryngol 2000;29:344–7.
51. Inoue Y, Ogawa K, Kanzaki J. Quality of life of vestibular schwannoma patients after surgery. Acta Otolaryngol (Stockh) 2001;121:59–61.
52. Kentala E, Pyykko I. Clinical picture of vestibular schwannoma. Auris Nasus Larynx 1986;28:15–22.
53. Fahy C, Nikolopoulos TP, O'Donoghue GM. Acoustic neuroma surgery and tinnitus. Eur Arch Otorhinolaryngol 2002;259:299–301.
54. Weissman JL, Hirsch BE. Imaging of tinnitus: a review. Radiology 2000;216:342–9.
55. Fischer C, Mauguiere F, Ibanez V, et al. The acute deafness of definite multiple sclerosis: BAEP patterns. Electoencephalogr Clin Neurophysiol 1985;61:7–15.
56. Cure JK, Cromwell LD, Case JL, et al. Auditory dysfunction caused by multiple sclerosis: detection with MR imaging. AJNR Am J Neuroradiol 1990;11:817–20.
57. Spoendlin H. The innervation of the organ of Corti. J Laryngol Otol 1967;81:717–38.
58. Lin X, Chen S, Tee D. Effects of quinine on the excitability and voltage-dependent currents of isolated spiral ganglion neurons in culture. J Neurophysiol 1998;79:2503–12.
59. Nordang L, Cestreicher E, Arnold W, Anniko M. Glutamate is the afferent neurotransmitter in the human cochlea. Acta Otolaryngol (Stockh) 2000;120:359–62.
60. Merchan-Perez A, Liberman MC. Ultrastructural differences among afferent synapses on cochlear hair cells: correlations with spontaneous discharge rate. J Comp Neurol 1996;371:208–21.
61. Johnson DH, Kiang NY. Analysis of discharges recorded simultaneously from pairs of auditory nerve fibers. Biophys J 1976;16:719–34.
62. Eggermont JJ. Tinnitus: some thoughts about its origin. J Laryngol Otol 1983;Suppl 9:31–7.
63. Dolan DF, Nuttall AL, Avinash G. Asynchronous neural activity recorded from the round window. J Acoust Soc Am 1990;87:2621–7.
64. Cazals Y, Horner KC, Huang ZW. Alterations in average spectrum of cochleoneural activity by long-term salicylate treatment in the guinea pig: a plausible index of tinnitus. J Neurophysiol 1998;80:2113–20.
65. Searchfield G, Munoz DJB, Towns EC, Thorne PR. Ensemble spontaneous activity of the cochlear nerve: cochlear pathology and tinnitus. In: Patuzzi R, editor. Proceedings of the Seventh International Tinnitus Seminar, Perth, Australia. 2002. p. 53–5.
66. McMahon C, Patuzzi R. Spectral peaks in spontaneous and sound-evoked cochlear electrical activity and tinnitus. In: Patuzzi R, editor. Proceedings of the Seventh International Tinnitus Seminar, Perth, Australia. 2002. p. 34–8.
67. Meikle M, Charnell MG. Salicylate-induced changes in asynchronous neural activity recorded from the round window [abstract 394]. In: Abstracts of the Seventeenth Midwinter Research Meeting, Association for Research in Otolaryngology, St. Petersburg, FL, 1994. p. 99. Also available at www.aro.org.
68. Robertson D, Sellick PM, Patuzzi R. The continuing search for outer hair cell afferents in the guinea pig spiral ganglion. Hear Res 1999;136:151–8.
69. Sewell WF. The relation between the endocochlear potential and spontaneous activity in auditory nerve fibres of the cat. J Physiol 1984;347:685–96.
70. Fex J. Augmentation of cochlear microphonic by stimulation of efferent fibers to the cochlea. Acta Otolaryngol (Stockh) 1959;50:540–1.
71. Konishi T, Salt AN, Hamrick PE. Effects of exposure to noise on ion movement in guinea pig cochlea. Hear Res 1979;1:325–42.
72. Patuzzi R. Changes in guinea pig cochlea with salicylate perfusion and aspirin-induced tinnitus. In: Patuzzi R, editor. Proceedings of the Seventh International Tinnitus Seminar, Perth, Australia. 2002. p. 48–52.
73. Oliver D, He DZ, Klocker N, et al. Intracellular anions as the voltage sensor of prestin, the outer hair cell motor protein. Science 2001;292:2340–3.
74. Nuttall AL, Guo M, Ren T, Dolan DF. Basilar membrane velocity noise. Hear Res 1997;114:35–42.
75. Henry JA, Meikle MB. Pulsed versus continuous tones for evaluating the loudness of tinnitus. J Am Acad Audiol 1999;10:261–72.
76. Gold T. Hearing II. The physical basis of the action of the cochlea. Proc R Soc Lond B Biol Sci 1948;135:492–8.
77. Evans EF, Wilson JP, Borerwe TA. Animal models of tinnitus. Ciba Found Symp 1981;85:108–38.

78. Zenner HP, Ernst A. Cochlear motor tinnitus, transduction tinnitus, and signal transfer tinnitus: three models of cochlear tinnitus. In: Vernon J, Møller AR, editors. Mechanisms of tinnitus. Vol 1. Boston: Allyn and Bacon; 1995. p. 237–54.
79. Frolenkov GI, Mammano F, Belyantseva IA, et al. Two distinct Ca2+ dependent signaling pathways regulate the motor output of cochlear outer hair cells. J Neurosci 2000;20:5940–8.
80. Sziklai I, Dallos P. Acetylcholine controls the gain of the voltage-to-movement converter in isolated outer hair cells. Acta Otolaryngol (Stockh) 1993;113:326–9.
81. Kemp DT. Physiologically active cochlear micromechanics—one source of tinnitus. Ciba Found Symp 1981;85:54–81.
82. Puel JL, Ruel J, Gervais d'Aldin C, Pujol R. Excitotoxicity and repair of cochlear synapses after noise-trauma induced hearing loss. Neuroreport 1998;9:2109–14.
83. Spoendlin H. Innervation patterns in the organ of Corti of the cat. Acta Otolaryngol (Stockh) 1969;67:239–54.
84. Puel JL, Ruel J, Guitton MJ, et al. The inner hair cell synaptic complex: physiology, pharmacology and new therapeutic strategies. Audiol Neurootol 2002;7:49–54.
85. Plinkert PK, Gitter AH, Mohler H, Zenner HP. Structure, pharmacology and function of GABA-A receptors in cochlear outer hair cells. Eur Arch Otorhinolaryngol 1993;250:351–7.
86. Spoendlin H, Lichtensteiger W. The adrenergic innervation of the labyrinth. Acta Otolaryngol (Stockh) 1966;61:423–34.
87. Hultcrantz E, Nuttall AL, Brown MC, Lawrence M. The effect of cervical sympathectomy on cochlear electrophysiology. Acta Otolaryngol (Stockh) 1982;94:439–44.
88. Hildesheimer M, Henkin Y, Pye A, et al. Bilateral superior cervical sympathectomy and noise-induced, permanent threshold shift in guinea pigs. Hear Res 2002;163:46–52.
89. Giraudet F, Horner KC, Cazals Y. Similar half-octave TTS protection of the cochlea by xylazine/ketamine or sympathectomy. Hear Res 2002;174:239–48.
90. Juhn SK, Li W, Kim JY, et al. Effect of stress-related hormones on inner ear fluid homeostasis and function. Am J Otol 1999;20:800–6.
91. Muchnik C, Hildesheimer M, Nebel L, Rubinstein M. Influence of catecholamines on cochlear action potentials. Arch Otolaryngol 1983;109:530–2.
92. Laurikainen EA, Ren T, Miller JM, et al. The tonic sympathetic input to the cochlear vasculature in guinea pig. Hear Res 1997;105:141–5.
93. Atkinson M. Tinnitus aurium: observations on its nature and control. Ann Otol Rhinol Laryngol 1944;53:742–51.
94. Passe ERG. Surgery of the sympathetic for Meniere's disease, tinnitus and nerve deafness. Arch Otolaryngol 1953;57:257–66.
95. Zwicker E. A model describing nonlinearities in hearing by active processes with saturation at 40 dB. Biol Cybern 1979;35:243–50.
96. Zurek PM. Spontaneous narrowband acoustic signals emitted by human ears. J Acoust Soc Am 1981;69:514–23.
97. Plinkert PK, Gitter AH, Zenner HP. Tinnitus associated spontaneous otoacoustic emissions. Active outer hair cell movements as common origin? Acta Otolaryngol (Stockh) 1990;110:342–7.
98. Wilson JP, Sutton GJ. Acoustic correlates of tonal tinnitus. Ciba Found Symp 1981;85:82–107.
99. Kemp DT. Otoacoustic emissions, travelling waves and cochlear mechanisms. Hear Res 1986;22:95–104.
100. Lonsbury-Martin BL, Martin GK, Probst R, Coats AC. Spontaneous otoacoustic emissions in a nonhuman primate. II. Cochlear anatomy. Hear Res 1988;33:69–93.
101. Zweig G, Shera CA. The origin of periodicity in the spectrum of evoked otoacoustic emissions. J Acoust Soc Am 1995;98:2018–47.
102. Penner MJ, Burns EM. The dissociation of SOAEs and tinnitus. J Speech Hear Res 1987;30:396–403.
103. Sismanis A. Pulsatile tinnitus. Int Tinnitus J 1997;3:39–40.
104. von Békésy G. Experiments in hearing. New York: McGraw-Hill; 1960.
105. Long GR, Talmadge CL. Spontaneous otoacoustic emission frequency is modulated by heartbeat. J Acoust Soc Am 1997;102:2831–48.
106. Ren T, Nuttall AL. Acoustical modulation of electrically evoked otoacoustic emission in intact gerbil cochlea. Hear Res 1998;120:7–16.
107. Meikle MB, Johnson RM, Griest SE, et al. 1995. Oregon tinnitus data archives 95-01. Available at: http://www.ohsu.edu/ohrc-otda or http://www.tinnitusArchive.org (accessed 03/05/2004).
108. Aran J-M, Cazals Y. Electrical suppression of tinnitus. Ciba Found Symp 1981;85:217–71.
109. House JW, Brackmann DE. Tinnitus: surgical treatment. Ciba Found Symp 1981;85:204–16.

110. Moller AR. Similarites between severe tinnitus and chronic pain. J Am Acad Audiol 2000;11:115–24.
111. Vass Z, Shore SE, Nuttall AL, et al. Trigeminal ganglion innervation of the cochlea—a retrograde transport study. Neuroscience 1997;79:605–15.
112. Vass Z, Steyger P, Trune D, Nuttall AL. Co-localization of the vanilloid TRPV1 and TrkA Substance P in the trigeminal sensory neurons that mediate vascular permeability in cochlear and vertebro-basilar arteries. Neuroscience 2004;124:919–27.
113. Vass Z, Steyger PS, Hordichok AJ, et al. Capsaicin stimulation of the cochlea and electric stimulation of the trigeminal ganglion mediate vascular permeability in cochlear and vertebro-basilar arteries: a potential cause of inner ear dysfunction in headache. Neuroscience 2001;103:189–201.
114. Toubi E, Ben-David J, Kessel A, et al. Autoimmune aberration in sudden sensorineural hearing loss: association with anti-cardiolipin antibodies. Lupus 1997;6:540–2.
115. Tomasi JP, Lona A, Deggouj N, Gersdorff M. Autoimmune sensorineural hearing loss in young patients. Laryngoscope 2001;111:2050–3.
116. Schleuning AJ. Neurotologic evaluation of subjective idiopathic tinnitus. J Laryngol Otol 1981;Suppl 4:99–101.
117. Reed GF. An audiometric study of two hundred cases of subjective tinnitus. Arch Otolaryngol 1960;71:94–104.
118. Janetta PJ. Microvascular decompression surgery for tinnitus. In: Vernon J, editor. Tinnitus: treatment and relief. Vol 1. Boston: Allyn and Bacon; 1998. p. 218–22.
119. Coad ML, Lockwood A, Salvi R, Burkard R. Characteristics of patients with gaze-evoked tinnitus. Otol Neurotol 2001;22:650–4.
120. Yamawaki M, Ariga T, Gao Y, et al. Sulfoglucuronosyl glycolipids as putative antigens for autoimmune inner ear disease. J Neuroimmunol 1998;84:111–6.

CHAPTER 6

Otoacoustic Emissions and Tinnitus

Brenda L. Lonsbury-Martin, PhD, Glen K. Martin, PhD

Otoacoustic emissions (OAEs), which were discovered by Kemp over 25 years ago,[1] are small acoustic signals presumed to be generated by the electromotile activity of the outer hair cells (OHCs) of the cochlea[2] and propagated into the external auditory canal via the middle ear ossicles and tympanic membrane. The two general classes of emissions, evoked and spontaneous (SOAEs), are detected in the sound pressure of the ear canal by a sensitive microphone assembly contained in an acoustic probe that is positioned snugly in the canal. Levels of both SOAEs and evoked OAEs vary but, on average, are relatively minute in that they are around 0 and 10 dB sound pressure level (SPL), respectively, for adults. In infants and young children, however, it is not uncommon for both types of OAEs to be approximately 10 dB greater in magnitude. When measured conventionally in a quiet environment, that is, in the absence of the synchronizing clicks used by some commercial systems, SOAEs are most commonly measured between approximately 0.8 and 4 kHz, with the majority being detected between 1 and 2 kHz. Alternatively, evoked OAEs are typically measured from approximately 0.5 to 6, 8, or 16 kHz, depending on the OAE class and equipment manufacturer. Experimentally, distortion-product otoacoustic emissions (DPOAEs) have been determined as high as 20 kHz.[3] The presence of OAEs, in general, over this wide range of frequencies is consistent with the typical extent of normal hearing sensitivity for humans.

The OAEs are of special interest with respect to tinnitus for several reasons. First, when OAEs were initially discovered, there was great hope that SOAEs, that is, emissions occurring in the absence of deliberate external acoustic stimulation, were an objective indicator of the beginning stages of tinnitus.[4,5] Certainly, that the ear can naturally emit narrowband acoustic signals logically suggests that SOAEs may be the physical counterpart to tinnitus, that is, the perception of sound without an external acoustic stimulus. Thus, there is an early history between SOAEs and tinnitus, in particular, that is of historical importance, and this past includes research involving both animal models and humans. Second, the evoked OAEs, and specifically the subclasses of transient evoked otoacoustic emissions (TEOAEs) and DPOAEs, have been evaluated for their usefulness as a diagnostic index of tinnitus by a number of investigators.

The following discussion reviews the roles of SOAEs and evoked OAEs in research on tinnitus. This discourse initially addresses SOAEs in more detail and then focuses on the relationship of this specific emission type to tinnitus. Similarly, some relevant details on evoked OAEs and, in particular, TEOAEs and DPOAEs are presented before discussing how these particular emissions have been used to provide some insight into the fundamental cochlear mechanisms underlying tinnitus. Finally, the role of the cochlear efferent system in tinnitus is addressed by reviewing the findings of several investigators who studied the effects of tinnitus on the efferent-induced suppression of emitted activity using the contralateral acoustic stimulation (CAS) paradigm.

SPONTANEOUS OTOACOUSTIC EMISSIONS

SOAEs, as noted above, are narrowband acoustic signals generated within the cochlea in the absence of deliberate sound stimulation. This class of OAE was discovered by Kemp shortly after he originally described the TEOAE subtype of evoked emissions.[1,4] Figure 6-1A illustrates a number of SOAEs (arrowheads) measured in a normal human ear as sharp peaks above the noise floor (NF) in the spectral analysis of the average output of the ear-canal microphone. SOAEs are detected at one or more discrete frequencies in approximately 72% of humans with normal hearing and approximately 56% of the ears of such individuals,[6] with this emission type being more prevalent in both female and right ears. Interestingly, using sensitive research equipment that is capable of more sophisticated data analysis than typical commercial devices, SOAEs can be measured in up to 80 to 85% of normal-hearing humans,[7] thus inferring that all normal ears likely exhibit SOAEs. Also, like the other types of emissions, SOAEs are very stable in the absence of ear pathology in that they vary by only a few hertz and/or decibels, even when measured over periods of many years. These frequency or magnitude features, which are unique to each emitting ear, in particular, make SOAEs less useful as a diagnostic clinical test because it is difficult to index such idiosyncratic properties in terms of their being normal or abnormal. It is also noteworthy that SOAEs are usually measured in ears with normal hearing and that they systematically decrease in incidence as hearing levels increase over approximately 20 dB HL.[8]

Spontaneous OAEs are thought to be generated primarily by the same reflection process(es) as TEOAEs and the stimulus-frequency OAE subtype of evoked emission,[9] that is, as a result of continual feedback of the output of the emission generator into its input. At frequencies at which this feedback is positive, if the loop gain is sufficient, self-sustaining oscillation will result, which is observed in the ear canal as an SOAE.[5] Thus, SOAEs can be thought of as continuously self-eliciting evoked OAEs. Consistent with this notion is the observation that SOAEs are typically detected in regions of strong evoked emissions[5,10] and rarely exceed 20 dB SPL, presumably owing to the compressive nonlinearity of the OAE generator.

Although it is not unusual for normal human ears to emit SOAEs, detecting SOAEs in the normal ears of laboratory animal species is much rarer. For example, although monkeys have SOAEs, their prevalence of approximately 20% is somewhat lower than that in humans.[11,12] Otherwise, however, the frequency or magnitude properties of monkey SOAEs are essentially identical to the typical SOAEs observed for normal-hearing humans.[13]

The nonprimate laboratory mammals, in contrast, rarely have SOAEs. In systematic surveys of a number of mammalian species typically used in hearing research, only the Hartley strain of albino guinea pig exhibited SOAEs in approximately 21% of the ears examined.[14] Again, like monkey emissions, these guinea pig SOAEs demonstrated properties similar to the typical, low-level SOAEs observed for normal-hearing humans.

Although SOAEs were initially thought to be an objective indicator of a developing tinnitus condition, common sense suggested that this notion was flawed. That is, SOAEs are typically detected in very normal ears, whereas tinnitus is commonly linked to abnormal hearing. In fact, SOAEs disappear once hearing levels deteriorate to approximately 30 to 35 dB HL.[8] However, despite the disassociation of tinnitus and SOAEs, there are a few situations in which SOAEs do cause tinnitus. For example, a common approach to classifying tinnitus is to label it as being either subjective or objective. That is, subjective tinnitus is audible only to the patient, whereas objective tinnitus is also audible to the examiner.

In general, SOAEs are inaudible to the patient. However, several early investigators observed a rare subtype of SOAE that differs in a number of respects from the SOAEs routinely observed in normal human ears.[15–17] Specifically, these rare atypical SOAEs, being audible and up to 60 dB SPL, were much larger than normal SOAEs, occurred in a higher frequency range than the majority of SOAEs, and tended to be associated with regions of audiometric abnormality. Another feature that differentiates these abnormally large from the more typical low-level SOAEs is that they often exhibited considerable short-term instability of frequency and level. Finally, when they are suppressed, that is, reduced in magnitude by externally applied tones, the resulting contours or tuning curves, rather than displaying sharp, single-lobed isosuppression tuning, had broad, multilobed shapes. One interpretation of this latter observation is that such abnormal SOAEs, rather than originating from a discrete set of localized OHCs, are generated by a much broader region of aberrant OHCs. Thus, these audible SOAEs appear to cause objective tinnitus.

There have been reports in nonprimate mammals of audible SOAEs that display properties resembling those of the high-level, atypical SOAEs observed in some pathologic ears rather than the low-level SOAEs common to normal human ears.[18–21] In particular, these SOAEs, like their human counterparts, had large magnitudes (up to 59 dB SPL), and most of them were unstable in frequency and level and/or demonstrated broad or multilobed isosuppression contours. It is noteworthy that in the nonprimate laboratory mammals, such as the chinchilla, some of the particularly large SOAEs were associated with regionally re-

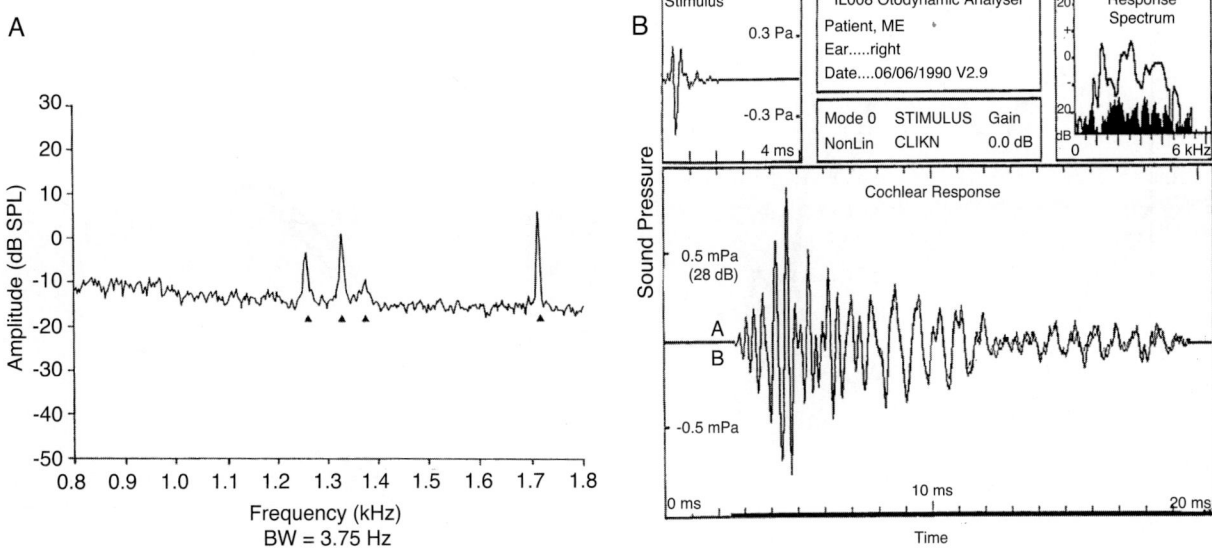

FIGURE 6-1. Examples of three types of otoacoustic emissions. *A,* Four spontaneous otoacoustic emissions (SOAEs) (*arrowheads*) recorded from the left ear (L) of a normal-hearing female subject. Thirty samples were taken of the ear canal activity in the absence of external stimulation and were averaged to reveal the spectrum illustrated here. SOAEs were detected from approximately 1.2 to 1.7 kHz. Note the low-level (< 10 dB SPL) features of these emissions and, in general, their sharp peaks. *B,* An example of a transient evoked otoacoustic emission (TEOAE) elicited by clicks administered by a common commercial device (see text). The patient was a 45-year-old female with normal hearing. The upper left panel illustrates the acoustic waveform of the click, the upper middle panel provides routine information about the subject and test parameters, and the upper right panel displays the amplitude spectrum of the averaged TEOAE. The lower portion of the plot shows the temporal waveform features of the mean response. Note that the rapid high-frequency components occurred early over the 20 ms monitoring period followed systematically by the middle- and low-frequency elements. Also note from the spectral response pattern that the TEOAE was present for this subject from about 0.7 to 5 kHz. (*Figure continues on next page.*)

stricted cochlear lesions[18,20] or, in the dog, apparent audiometric abnormalities.[21]

Thus, both humans and some nonprimate mammals demonstrate both the typical low-level and atypical high-level SOAEs. However, it appears that in the nonprimates, the typical SOAEs are less prevalent than in humans, whereas the atypical type, although rare, may be more common in nonprimates than in humans. The very different properties of the uncommon SOAEs and their apparent association with cochlear pathology suggest that the mechanism of generation of these SOAEs in both humans and laboratory mammals may be different from that of the more typical SOAEs.

Penner was the first investigator to examine in detail the association of tinnitus and the conventional low-level SOAEs in humans,[22,23] although other researchers also were intrigued with this potential relationship.[24] In fact, Penner and Burns identified several lines of evidence that can be used empirically to support SOAE-induced tinnitus.[25] First, when SOAEs are suppressed, tinnitus should be inaudible. Second, pitch matches to the tinnitus should correspond approximately to an SOAE frequency. Third, more intense SOAEs should be associated with louder tinnitus sensations. Fourth, suppression tuning curves for an SOAE should correspond to the isomasking contour for the related tinnitus, that is, be frequency specific. In a subsequent report, Penner further proposed that, in contrast to the stable SOAEs typically determined for normal-hearing individuals, unstable SOAEs, that is, those that can be present or absent during different measurement sessions and/or change frequency values, might be audible to the patient and thus cause bothersome tinnitus.[22]

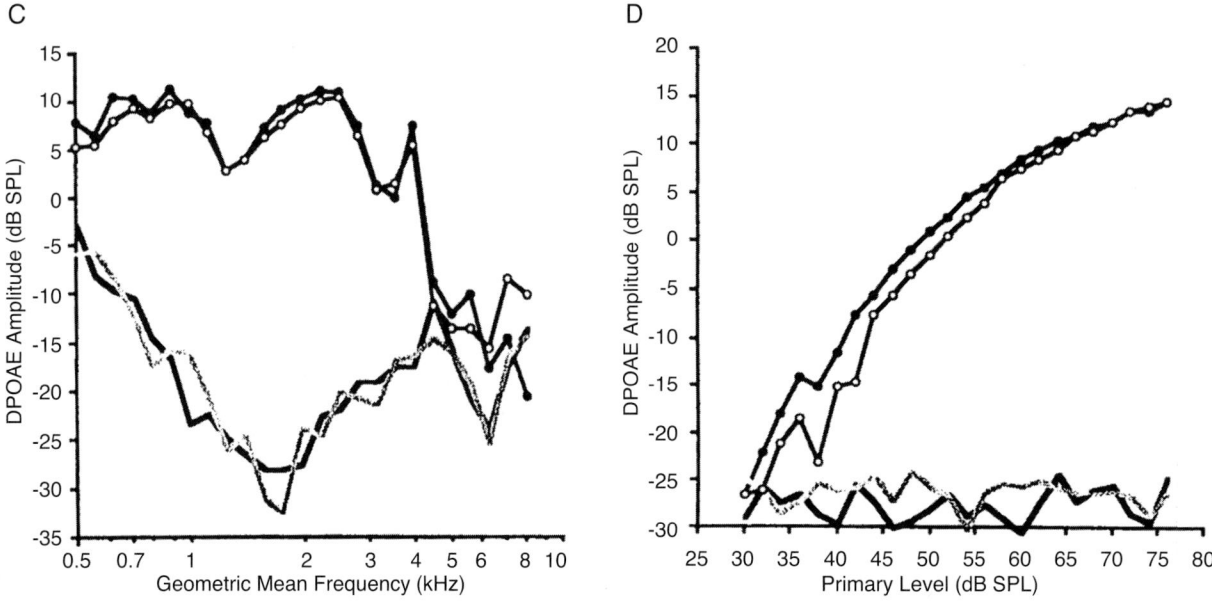

FIGURE 6-1 CONTINUED. *C*, DP-gram showing distortion-product otoacoustic emission (DPOAE) levels as a function of the geometric mean of f_1 and f_2 primary tones (see text) elicited from the left ear of a 27-year-old male, who also displayed a high-frequency hearing loss for frequencies above approximately 4 kHz (not shown). The DPOAEs were measured at 10 points per octave in response to f_1 and f_2 primary tone levels of the level of f_1 (L_1) = 65 dB and the level of f_2 (L_2) = 55 dB SPL (f_2/f_1 = 1.22). In this case, the solid-circle function of the top set of curves represents responses elicited in the absence of contralateral acoustic stimulation (CAS), whereas the open-circle curve shows the slight suppression, particularly at the lower frequencies, induced by CAS, which is attributed to activation of the suppressive activity of the cochlear efferent system. The lower set of curves represents the noise floor of the measurement system in the absence (*dark solid line*) and presence (*stippled line*) of the CAS. *D*, Response/growth or input/output (I/O) function at the geometric mean frequency of 2 kHz illustrating DPOAE level in response to systematic increases of the primary tone in 2 dB steps from 30 to 76 dB SPL. Again, the solid-circle function represents DPOAE levels in the absence of CAS, whereas the open-circle curve indicates the suppressing effects of the CAS, particularly at the lower-intensity values of the primary tones.

In most cases, however, there is little correspondence between SOAEs and tinnitus. For example, although suppressing an SOAE typically leads to a frequency-specific tuning curve, characteristically, tones of any frequency are equally effective in masking tinnitus. Although, as noted above, most patients complaining of tinnitus have abnormal hearing that is not usually associated with SOAEs, Penner estimated that between 1 and 9% of patients with tinnitus do have SOAEs that are at least partially responsible for generating tinnitus, with the most likely percentage being about 3%.[26] Clearly, such patients have normal to near-normal hearing, at least, in the frequency region of the SOAE.[25] As an example of such a patient, Penner and Glotzbach reported on a female subject who was discovered to have as many as 21 bilateral SOAEs that were associated with her problematic tinnitus, that is, tinnitus that kept her awake at night and interfered with her concentration during the day.[27] One practical consequence of Penner's research is that patients with distressing tinnitus and normal to near-normal hearing should be tested for SOAEs to confirm if such emissions produce the abnormal perception.

Based on an earlier observation that SOAEs can be abolished by aspirin,[28] Penner and associates investigated whether this pharmacologic agent would make an effective treatment for tinnitus caused by SOAEs. For example, Penner and Coles reported on a patient for whom SOAEs caused tinnitus and who was taking two 300 mg tablets of aspirin four times per day.[29] The results proved provocative in that an SOAE in one ear was abolished and the tinnitus in that ear became inaudible after the patient had ingested 2.4 g of aspirin. Thus, aspirin may be an acceptable palliative for SOAE-caused tinnitus.

More recent studies of the relationship between SOAEs and tinnitus have focused more on the stability of these emissions in the ears of patients with tinnitus. For example, Prasher and colleagues showed unexpectedly that the incidence of SOAEs was greater in noise-exposed mill workers than previously observed, that is, SOAEs were present in 73% of tinnitus subjects, whereas only 50% of the nontinnitus but noise-exposed control subjects exhibited these emissions.[30] Most interestingly, as observed earlier by Penner,[22] for the tinnitus sufferers, the stability of SOAEs from week to week, that is, their presence and frequency values, was significantly more variable in the workers with subjective tinnitus than in their control counterparts. Thus, it is likely that such noise-induced instability within the cochleas of these patients with tinnitus directly altered the properties of their SOAEs in the form of shifted frequencies and poor intersession reproducibility.

EVOKED OTOACOUSTIC EMISSIONS

The TEOAE and DPOAE subclasses of evoked OAEs have contributed substantially to our basic knowledge about how the normal peripheral ear processes sound, as well as to clinical practice. For example, in basic studies of cochlear function, evoked emissions have been used extensively to investigate the active processes underlying the function of the cochlear amplifier, which uses the OHCs' electromechanical feedback mechanisms to counter the problematic damping characteristics of the cochlea. Clinically, the evoked OAEs have also been used widely for both neonatal hearing screening and site-of-lesion testing, that is, for determining the cochlear versus retrocochlear basis of a complaint about hearing problems. Other clinical uses include serial monitoring for progressive disorders such as ototoxicity in patients receiving potentially damaging drugs and ruling out pseudohypacusis in medicolegal cases involving monetary compensation.

The average TEOAE illustrated in Figure 6-1B is most commonly elicited by several hundred acoustic clicks, which, in this case, were generated by one of the most widely used diagnostic TEOAE commercial devices, the ILO88 (Otodynamics Ltd, Hatsfield, Herts, UK). Although TEOAEs can be displayed in their temporal (lower portion of Figure 6-1B) or spectral (upper right plot in Figure 6-1B) form, the latter measure is mainly used. Currently, these emissions are thought to be the most clinically useful OAE with respect to newborn hearing screening and are conventionally scored as being either present or absent over several 1,000 Hz frequency bands extending from approximately 1 to 5 kHz. As with all of the evoked OAEs, TEOAEs are detectable in about 98% of individuals with normal hearing, regardless of gender or age, and the two ears of any subject produce essentially identical emissions.

The DPOAEs are elicited by two simultaneous, long-lasting (~ 90 ms) tonebursts related in frequency in that the higher-frequency primary tone at f_2 is ideally 1.22 times the frequency of the lower-frequency primary tone at f_1, that is, $f_2/f_1 = 1.22$, to produce, on average, the largest emissions. This class of evoked OAE is typically measured in terms of either a plot of DPOAE levels elicited by constant-level primary tones as a function of stimulus frequency (DP-gram) or a response/growth or input/output (I/O) function. Figure 6-1, C and D, illustrates each of these DPOAE measures obtained with (open circles) and without (solid circles) contralateral acoustic stimulation, which affected mainly the low-frequency (see Figure 6-1C) and lower-level (see Figure 6-1D) aspects of the DP-gram and 2 kHz I/O function, respectively.

As shown in Figure 6-1C, the DP-gram describes DPOAE level as a function of stimulus frequency, which, in this case, is the geometric or logarithmic mean of f_1 and f_2, that is, $(f_1 \times f_2)^{0.5}$. In obtaining a DP-gram, stimulus frequency is usually changed in regular ascending steps of a third to a tenth of an octave (ie, either 3 or 10 frequency points per octave, respectively), whereas primary-tone levels (L_1) and (L_2), whether equilevel (eg, $L_1 = L_2 = 65$ dB SPL) or offset in level (eg, $L_1 - L_2 = 10$ dB), are constant across the frequency range examined. Figure 6-1D illustrates a typical I/O function for a midgeometric mean frequency of 2 kHz. In obtaining I/O measures, the primary tones are kept constant in frequency, whereas their levels are systematically increased in, typically, 2 or 5 dB steps. From the resulting function, certain features, such as detection threshold, growth slope, level that elicits the largest magnitude response, and the shape of the curve (eg, nonmonotonic or compressive, monotonic or linear), can be determined. In clinical testing, DPOAEs are considered to be particularly useful in establishing a differential diagnosis through intentionally assessing functional status over a specific frequency region of the cochlea.

One common experimental approach for relating evoked OAEs to tinnitus has been, as with the SOAE studies reviewed above, to use emissions as an objective correlate of tinnitus. Toward this end, many investigators have made comparisons of the common properties of evoked OAEs, usually magnitude, between groups of subjects with normal hearing and patients with tinnitus who have typically been matched for age and gender, along with hearing level. Again, the assumption here is that if a common anomaly associated with the tinnitus condition is identified, an objective test of tinnitus using evoked OAEs would be useful as a tool for determining the origin of this abnormal perception and for assessing the effectiveness of subsequent treatments.

For example, Shiomi and colleagues found that the average DP-gram of a normal-hearing tinnitus group was significantly smaller than that of a group of normal-

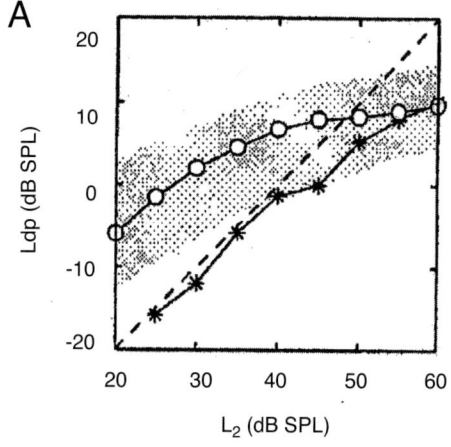

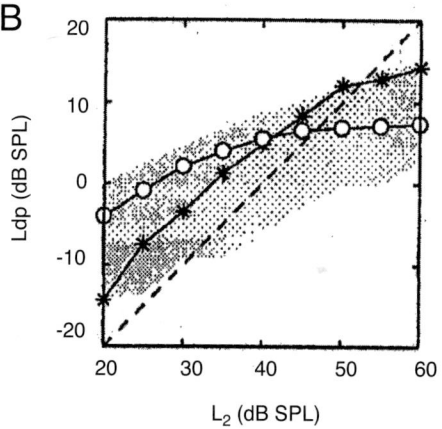

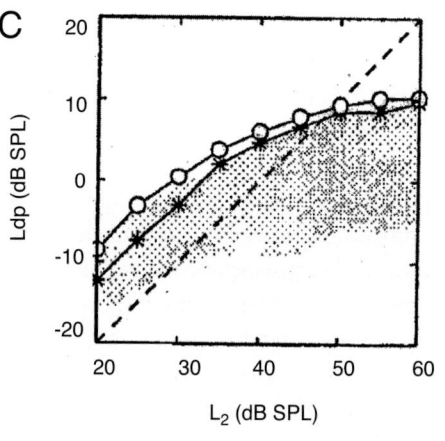

FIGURE 6-2. Input/output (I/O) functions plotting distortion-product otoacoustic emission (DPOAE) growth against the level of the upper-frequency primary tone, L_2, obtained from a 21-year-old female during an episode of acute acoustic trauma and tinnitus (*star symbols*) associated with visiting a discotheque and following the subsequent recovery period (*open circles*). The shaded area on each plot indicates the range of ±1 SD of the DPOAE levels for a normal-hearing control group at the corresponding frequencies. *A*, I/O at 4,492 Hz, which was associated with a 4 kHz notch (30 dB HL) in the audiogram (not shown). Note that the DPOAE losses during trauma occurred predominantly at the lowest stimulus levels showing almost a 25 dB decrement at $L_2 = 25$ dB SPL, with little change at the highest stimulus level of $L_2 = 60$ dB SPL. *B*, I/O at 6,055 Hz in the tinnitus region. Note that above $L_2 = 40$ dB SPL, the DPOAE level was higher during trauma by about 10 dB, even though the corresponding audiometric hearing loss around 6 kHz was about 20 dB (not shown). *C*, I/O at 7,666 Hz in a region of normal hearing showing similar DPOAE growth during both the trauma and recovery states. Note the steep slope up to 1 dB/dB in the lower primary-tone level region and a flat slope, as low as 0.1 dB/dB, in the upper compressive region that is characteristic of normal hearing. Diagonal dashed line on each plot indicates slope = 1 dB/dB.

hearing subjects in that DPOAE levels for tinnitus subjects were associated with very low-level emissions.[31] This finding infers that even in the presence of normal hearing sensitivity, some subtle cochlear pathology may be developing. These findings are also in agreement with the results of a number of other studies performed in patients with various forms of sensorineural hearing loss and tinnitus. Thus, as expected, the level of evoked OAEs is typically related to hearing threshold in that, as hearing threshold increases, the corresponding emission level tends to decrease.

In contrast, Janssen and colleagues discovered that for a number of individuals with tinnitus, that is, 44% of their patient sample of 39 chronic tinnitus ears, DPOAE I/O levels actually increased as hearing threshold increased.[32] That is, these investigators observed that an abnormal pattern of increased DPOAEs as a function of the increasing stimulus level was related to tinnitus. The panels of Figure 6-2 illustrate these findings in some detail for another subject, that is, for a 21-year-old female, who suffered from acoustic trauma and tinnitus following a visit to a discotheque. In this work, DPOAE I/Os were obtained within a few days of the trauma (star symbols) and after the subsequent recovery (open circles) for several frequencies surrounding both the noise-induced 4 kHz notch (see Figure 6-2A) in the patient's audiogram (not shown) and the tinnitus frequency (see Figure 6-2B). In addition, the I/O of Figure 6-2C illustrates normal DPOAE response/growth within a normal-hearing frequency region, that is, the steep trajectory of DPOAE growth (eg, slope = 1 dB/dB) in response to the lower-level primary tones followed by compressive growth (eg, slope = 0.1 dB/dB) in response to higher-level primaries. The I/Os were measured using a variable L_1, L_2 protocol (ie, $L_1 = 0.4L_2 + 39$), which accounts for the nonlinear interaction of the two primary tones at the DPOAE generation site at f_2 as a function of stimulation level.[33]

Basically, Janssen and colleagues observed a linearization of the I/O that was associated with the hearing loss (see Figure 6-2A) and the tinnitus frequency (see Figure 6-2B) regions, which was in contrast to the typical compressive growth curve observed for regions associated with normal hearing (see Figure 6-2C).[32] Interestingly, for the tinnitus I/O function (see Figure 6-2B), the linear trajectory continued to the high-level portion of the I/O curve so that DPOAE levels in response

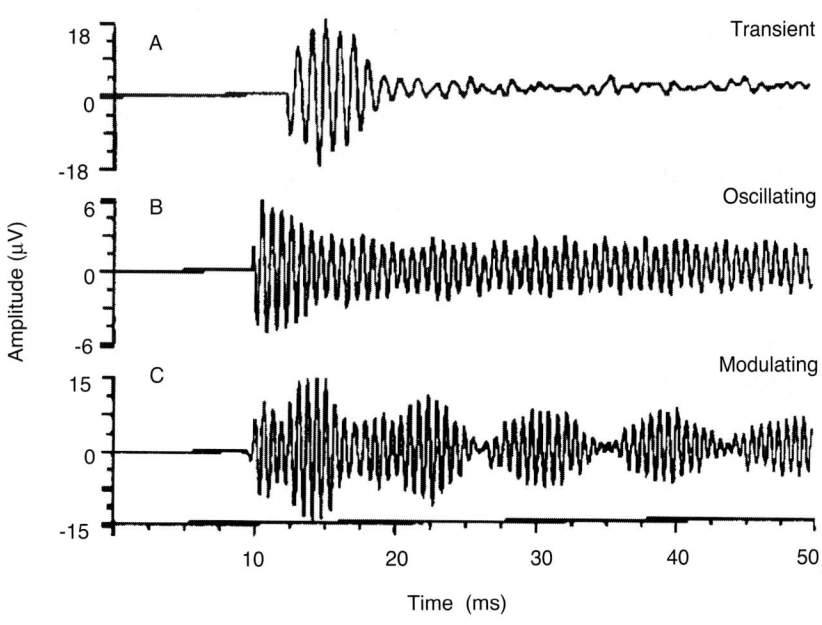

FIGURE 6-3. Three types of temporal patterns of transient evoked otoacoustic emissions (TEOAEs) recorded from ears with chronic tinnitus. *A,* A transient response elicited by 1 kHz tone-pips that occurs succinctly within the initial measurement interval for one patient with tinnitus; *B,* an oscillating response elicited by 1.5 kHz tone-pips and showing a continual response presence throughout the ~ 50 ms recording period; and *C,* a modulating TEOAE elicited by 1.5 kHz tone-pips showing a waxing and waning response pattern that also persisted throughout the monitoring interval. Adapted from Norton SJ et al.[34]

to $L_2s > 45$ dB SPL were greater by as much as 10 dB than in the subsequent recovery period. Thus, the presence of abnormal linear rather than more normal compressive I/Os, particularly over the mid- to high-level portion of the curve, may be a useful indicator of an underlying cochlear pathology associated with the tinnitus state.

In another study, Norton and colleagues used TEOAEs in an attempt to develop an objective test for identifying tinnitus of peripheral origin.[34] These investigators reasoned that the presence of a prolonged, "ringing" tonal emission in response to transient stimuli such as tone-pips would be consistent with a cochlear mechanical origin of tinnitus. In their study of six patients with chronic tinnitus and two control subjects with no tinnitus, five of the six patients with tinnitus showed oscillating or modulating TEOAEs. In contrast, one patient with tinnitus and the two nontinnitus subjects exhibited no "ringing"-type emissions.

The panels of Figure 6-3 illustrate the various TEOAE patterns evoked by tone-pip stimuli from 1 to 2 kHz. Such patterns consist of, in Figure 6-3A, the transient ($n = 3$) prototype typically shown by the latter nonringing subjects, along with, in Figure 6-3B, the oscillating ($n = 4$) and, in Figure 6-3C, the modulating ($n = 1$) TEOAE patterns exhibited by the remaining five patients with tinnitus. Note that although the transient TEOAE is brief and occurs within the initial portion of the approximately 50-millisecond recording period, the oscillating and modulating emissions persisted throughout the measurement interval. Thus, for these specific patients with tinnitus, the majority, according to Norton and colleagues, exhibited a type of tinnitus that was consistent with pathologic cochlear micromechanics.[34]

EVOKED OTOACOUSTIC EMISSIONS, THE AUDITORY EFFERENT PATHWAY, AND TINNITUS

Some investigators have proposed that the central auditory efferent pathway may play an important role in the generation of tinnitus.[35–37] In this theory, tinnitus is thought of as an extracochlear phenomenon in which a reduction in the central efferent-induced suppression of cochlear micromechanics leads to an increase in the gain of the cochlear amplifier, which results in an overactivity-related symptom such as tinnitus. A simple method for assessing the global effectiveness of the cochlear efferent pathway is to compare the levels of OAEs with and without mild contralateral acoustic stimulation using a broadband noise of about 30 dB SL, with the expectation being that such contralateral stimulation reduces the magnitude of the emissions. This mechanism is thought to be mediated, at least in part, through the medial olivocochlear efferent pathway innervating the OHCs of the ipsilateral test ear. For certain, some investigators have found a significant difference in either the amount of OAE suppression or the varying extent of suppression values, with the tinnitus group exhibiting less suppression[36] and more variability[38] than their normal group counterparts. However, like the similar correlational studies of spontaneous and evoked emissions, such findings are not overpowering. Certainly, no general principles concerning tinnitus can be drawn from the global testing of the functional status of the cochlear efferent pathway. Perhaps some of the newer efferent pathway testing protocols that use long-lasting primaries of 1 second or more administered binaurally to study the efferent-mediated fast adaptation response[39] will make more effective assessors of the role of cochlear efferents in the generation of certain classes of tinnitus.

SUMMARY

OAEs are a sensitive and frequency-specific tool for assessing cochlear damage. Since their discovery, many investigators have thought that emissions might provide a unique method of objectively evaluating both the origin of the tinnitus and the efficacy of subsequent tinnitus treatments. However, as hearing loss progresses, the probability of detecting either SOAEs or evoked OAEs decreases, so that these objective measures of cochlear function cannot be used as a tinnitus tool when the degree of hearing loss is > 35 to 45 dB. Moreover, given the multiple mechanisms associated with tinnitus, it is unlikely that cochlear mechanisms contribute appreciably to more than only a few types of tinnitus. However, even though, for example, SOAEs are associated with tinnitus in only a few patients, it may be beneficial for the clinician and the patient to screen for SOAE-induced tinnitus, particularly in individuals with normal to near-normal hearing. Thus, in such cases, details about the cochlear origin of this auditory pathology may be uncovered in a small percentage of the patient population with tinnitus, which, hopefully, would lead to the most efficacious treatment.

ACKNOWLEDGMENT

This work was supported in part by funds from the National Institutes of Health (DC00613, DC03114, DC03086).

REFERENCES

1. Kemp DT. Stimulated acoustic emissions from within the human auditory system. J Acoust Soc Am 1978;64:1386–91.
2. Brownell WE. Outer hair cell electromotility and otoacoustic emissions. Ear Hear 1990;11:82–92.
3. Dreisbach LE, Siegel JH. Distortion-product otoacoustic emissions measured at high frequencies in humans. J Acoust Soc Am 2001;110:2456–69.
4. Kemp DT. Evidence of mechanical nonlinearity and frequency selective wave amplification in the cochlea. Arch Otorhinolaryngol 1979;224:37–45.
5. Kemp DT. Physiologically active cochlear micromechanics—one source of tinnitus. Ciba Found Symp 1981;85:54–81.
6. Talmadge CL, Long GR, Murphy WJ, Tubis A. New off-line method for detecting spontaneous emissions in human subjects. Hear Res 1993:71:170–82.
7. Zhang T, Penner MJ. A new method for the automated detection of spontaneous otoacoustic emissions embedded in noisy data. Hear Res 1998;117:107–13.
8. Probst R, Lonsbury-Martin BL, Martin GK, Coats AC. Otoacoustic emissions in ears with hearing loss. Am J Otolaryngol 1987;8:73–81.
9. Shera CA, Guinan JJ Jr. Evoked otoacoustic emissions arise by two fundamentally different mechanisms: a taxonomy for mammalian OAEs. J Acoust Soc Am 1999;105:782–98.
10. Zwicker E, Schloth E. Interrelation of different otoacoustic emissions. J Acoust Soc Am 1984;75:1148–54.
11. Martin GK, Lonsbury-Martin BL, Probst R, Coats AC. Spontaneous otoacoustic emissions in the nonhuman primate: a survey. Hear Res 1985;20:91–5.
12. Lonsbury-Martin BL, Martin GK. Incidence of spontaneous otoacoustic emissions in macaque monkeys: a replication. Hear Res 1988;34:313–7.
13. Martin GK, Lonsbury-Martin BL, Probst R, Coats AC. Spontaneous otoacoustic emissions in a nonhuman primate. I. Basic features and relations to other emissions. Hear Res 1988;33:49–68.
14. Ohyama K, Wada H, Kobayashi T, Takasaka T. Spontaneous otoacoustic emissions in guinea pig. Hear Res 1991;56:111–21.
15. Wilson JP, Sutton GJ. A family with high-tonal objective tinnitus—an update. In: Klinke R, Hartmann R, editors. Hearing—physiological bases and psychophysics. Berlin: Springer-Verlag; 1983. p. 97–103.
16. Yamamoto E, Takagi A, Hirono Y, Yagi N. A case of "spontaneous otoacoustic emission." Arch Otolaryngol Head Neck Surg 1987;113:1316–8.
17. Mathis A, Probst R, De Min N, Hauser R. A child with unusually high-level spontaneous otoacoustic emission. Arch Otolaryngol Head Neck Surg 1991;117:674–6.
18. Zurek PM, Clark WW. Narrow-band acoustic signals emitted by chinchilla ears after noise exposure. J Acoust Soc Am 1981;70:446–50.
19. Decker TN, Fritsch JH. Objective tinnitus in the dog. J Am Vet Med Assoc 1982;180:74.
20. Clark WW, Kim DO, Zurek PM, Bohne BA. Spontaneous otoacoustic emissions in chinchilla ear canals: correlation with histopathology and suppression by external tones. Hear Res 1984;16:299–314.
21. Ruggero MA, Kramek B, Rich NC. Spontaneous otoacoustic emissions in a dog. Hear Res 1984;13:293–6.
22. Penner MJ. Audible and annoying spontaneous otoacoustic emissions. A case study. Arch Otolaryngol Head Neck Surg 1988;114:150–3.
23. Penner MJ. Linking spontaneous otoacoustic emissions and tinnitus. Br J Audiol 1992;26:115–23.
24. Plinkert PK, Gitter AH, Zenner HP. Tinnitus associated spontaneous otoacoustic emissions. Active outer hair cell movements as common origin? Acta Otolaryngol (Stockh) 1990;110:342–7.
25. Penner MJ, Burns EM. The dissociation of SOAEs and tinnitus. J Speech Hear Res 1987;30:396–403.
26. Penner MJ. An estimate of the prevalence of tinnitus caused by spontaneous otoacoustic emissions. Arch Otolaryngol Head Neck Surg 1990;116:418–23.
27. Penner MJ, Glotzbach L. Covariation of tinnitus pitch and the associated emission: a case study. Otolaryngol Head Neck Surg 1994;110:304–9.
28. Wier CC, Pasanen EB, McFadden D. Partial dissociation of spontaneous otoacoustic emissions and distortion products during aspirin use in humans. J Acoust Soc Am 1988;84:230–7.
29. Penner MJ, Coles RR. Indications for aspirin as a palliative for tinnitus caused by SOAEs: a study. Br J Audiol 1992;26:91–6.
30. Prasher D, Ceranic B, Sulkowski W, Buzek W. Objective evidence for tinnitus from spontaneous emission variability. Noise Health 2001;3:61–73.

31. Shiomi Y, Tsuji J, Naito Y, et al. Characteristics of DPOAE audiogram in tinnitus patients. Hear Res 1997;108:83–8.
32. Janssen T, Kummer P, Arnold W. Growth behavior of the 2 f1-f2 distortion product otoacoustic emission in tinnitus. J Acoust Soc Am 1998;103:3418–30.
33. Kummer P, Janssen T, Arnold W. The level and growth behavior of the 2 f1-f2 distortion product otoacoustic emission and its relationship to auditory sensitivity in normal hearing and cochlear hearing loss. J Acoust Soc Am 1998;103:3431–44.
34. Norton SJ, Schmidt AR, Stover LJ. Tinnitus and otoacoustic emissions: is there a link? Ear Hear 1990;11:159–66.
35. Chery-Croze S, Truy E, Morgon A. Contralateral suppression of transiently evoked otoacoustic emissions and tinnitus. Br J Audiol 1994;28:255–66.
36. Attias J, Bresloff I, Furman V. The influence of the efferent auditory system on otoacoustic emissions in noise induced tinnitus: clinical relevance. Acta Otolaryngol (Stockh) 1996;116:534–9.
37. Castello E. Distortion products in normal hearing patients with tinnitus. Boll Soc Ital Biol Sper 1997;73:93–100.
38. Graham RL, Hazell JW. Contralateral suppression of transient evoked otoacoustic emissions: intra-individual variability in tinnitus and normal subjects. Br J Audiol 1994;28:235–45.
39. Kim DO, Dorn PA, Neely ST, Gorga MP. Adaptation of distortion product otoacoustic emission in humans. J Assoc Res Otolaryngol 2001;2:31–40.

EDITORIAL COMMENTARY

Ryan and Mullen point to the roles of ion transport and channel genes in ionic and fluid balance of the inner ear as possible sources of tinnitus arising in the inner ear. These mechanisms might include leakage of potassium ions from the endolymph into the extracellular fluid of the dendrites of the auditory nerve or excessive or deficient endolymphic volume causing deformation of the basilar membrane, increasing the spontaneous impulse rate in auditory neurons. Because mice with a deletion of a glutamate transporter gene are more susceptible to noise-induced hearing loss, it is possible that decreased glutamate clearance from the hair cell afferent dendrite synapse could also lead to increased neuronal discharge. Of perhaps greater general importance, they articulate that because most tinnitus appears to be the result of plasticity in the central nervous system, the genes involved in neuronal changes may provide clues to the molecular mechanisms of tinnitus.

Of particular interest in neural plasticity in memory is the calcium response element binding protein (CREB). The expression of CREB is up-regulated in the central auditory pathway for months after noise-induced cochlear trauma. Also of interest in plasticity is the 65 kDa isoform of the glutamate decarboxylase (*GAD65*) gene involved in the synthesis of γ-aminobutyric acid, a major inhibitory transmitter in the central auditory pathway. Reduction of the *GAD65* gene occurs in learning and might participate in the neuroplasticity associated with tinnitus.

Ryan and Mullen point out that because there have been no reports of tinnitus that is inherited without hearing loss, it is unlikely that tinnitus can be linked to a single gene. It is more likely that changes in the expression of genes that participate in the mechanisms underlying the generation of tinnitus will be found. They also call attention to the possibility that benefit to the patient with tinnitus may more likely come from advances in the molecular therapy of depression and anxiety.

Nuttall and colleagues emphasize that most tinnitus occurs in response to auditory system pathology, the majority of which is in the cochlea. In that sense, the auditory nerve can be thought of as the final common path in tinnitus. The absence of normal activity and the presence of abnormal activity in the auditory nerve may be perceived as sound.

Based on the linkage between the psychoacoustic parameters of tinnitus, particularly pitch and localization, and the extent of the cochlear damage, they posit that there is an ongoing dynamic interaction between the cochlea and brain centers in tinnitus. Drawing on examples of ear disease, tinnitus tends to mirror the natural history of the associated hearing loss temporally and in severity. They point out the critical role of the stria vascularis in the recovery from or the intermittency of Meniere's disease, sudden idiopathic sensorineural hearing loss, autoimmune inner ear disease, and diuretic ototoxicity through regulation of ionic gradients and maintenance of the endolymphatic potential and the blood-labyrinth barrier.

Nuttall and colleagues draw attention to a possible mechanism in the generation of tinnitus caused by the edge effect of relatively normal hair cells on the low-frequency side and missing or poorly functioning hair cells on the high-frequency side of the lesion. They discuss other intriguing peripheral mechanisms, including excessive release of neurotransmitter at the inner hair cell–type I afferent synapse, increased cochlear amplification leading to mechanical noise from basilar membrane motion, and decreased cochlear amplification reducing the spontaneous rate in the afferent auditory neurons.

Lonsbury-Martin and Martin note the usual disassociation of spontaneous otoacoustic emissions and tinnitus and the fact that, in general, spontaneous otoacoustic emissions are inaudible by the subject. However, they point out that a rare type of spontaneous otoacoustic emissions is audible, much larger, and at a higher frequency range than the usual spontaneous otoacoustic emissions associated with regions of audiometric abnormality and attributable to a broad region of aberrant outer hair cells. Based on Penner's work with individuals with unstable low-level spontaneous otoacoustic emissions, Lonsbury-Martin and Martin recommend that patients with distressing tinnitus and normal or nearly normal hearing should be tested for spontaneous otoacoustic emissions to confirm if such emissions are responsible for their tinnitus. Furthermore, they point out that aspirin is an acceptable means of relieving this kind of tinnitus.

Lonsbury-Martin and Martin emphasize that evoked otoacoustic emissions tend to be smaller in individuals with tinnitus even when the hearing appears to be normal and suggest that this finding infers that, even in the presence of normal hearing sensitivity, some subtle cochlear lesions may be developing.

James B. Snow Jr

CHAPTER 7

Animal Models of Tinnitus

David B. Moody, PhD

The laboratory study of tinnitus using animal models presents unique problems, primarily because there are no simple objective means of determining when tinnitus is present. Although there have been demonstrations of physiologic correlates of tinnitus, those measures may not always correspond on a one-to-one basis with the perceptions being experienced by the subject. In other words, tinnitus is a very private experience. Humans, of course, can tell us when they have tinnitus and, in many cases, seem to be able to provide accurate descriptions of what it sounds like. But humans are not ideal subjects for invasive experimentation, so we resort instead to using an animal model and forgo the luxury of verbal reports. To do so, we must develop other ways to determine when a subject is experiencing tinnitus. The goal of this chapter is to review some of the behavioral methods that have been developed for detecting tinnitus in an animal model and to discuss some of the advantages and disadvantages of each. The chapter is not intended to be a "cookbook" that will enable the reader to carry out behavioral measures of tinnitus; rather, it is a starting point to understand the issues involved and the approaches that have been tried.

When the phenomenon we wish to study is highly variable, as is tinnitus, it would seem to be desirable to specify something of its quality and magnitude as well. To that end, this chapter also describes some of the ways in which procedures have been adapted to look at the perceived quality of the tinnitus. Because the manifestation of tinnitus may vary significantly from subject to subject, it becomes useful to be able to obtain meaningful data from a single subject so that individual differences can be studied. The chapter also touches on the extent to which it has been possible to do so with the methods described.

The chapters in this volume describe what is known about the phenomenon of tinnitus. To appreciate the problems associated with developing a behavioral animal model of tinnitus, it is also necessary to delve into matters concerned with getting animals to behave in ways that provide us with information on what they hear. There are two major problems associated with training an animal to tell us when tinnitus is present. The first is that we do not know when the animal is experiencing tinnitus; thus, we cannot reward correct behavior and punish or extinguish incorrect behavior. The second major problem is that we do not have control of when the stimulus is present; we cannot gate the tinnitus on for test trials and off for "catch trials," as we do with electronically produced acoustic stimuli. Both of these problems present difficult challenges for behaviorally training subjects to report what they hear, but the first, knowing when the subject is correctly reporting tinnitus, is perhaps the greater of the two problems. Methods have been developed to overcome this challenge to some extent, but those methods require that the experimenter have the ability to control when test stimuli are being presented. For example, in our laboratory, we wanted to know whether a monkey perceived a novel vocalization as a member of one communication class or another; in other words, we wanted to find out what the vocalization "meant" to the monkey. Although we did not know the answer to that question a priori, we could train the animal to respond differently to known members of the two communication classes, and once that task was learned, we could present the novel vocalization, and, from the responses of the monkey, we could determine the communication class to which the stimulus belonged.[1] An important aspect of these experiments was that it was never possible to reward (or punish) the subjects when the novel vocalization was presented. Instead, we assumed that, as a result of prior training, the subject would respond appropriately in the absence of any feedback.

However, because the novel stimuli were controlled by the experimenter and were presented on only a small number of trials in a testing session, rewards could still be given for correct responses when the original training stimuli were presented.

Now consider the case of tinnitus. As in the experiment just described, subjects could be trained to respond in one way when various sounds were presented to simulate tinnitus and in a different way when no sound was presented. Then, without reinforcing either type of response, tinnitus could be experimentally induced, and behavioral testing could be carried out. However, because the tinnitus could not be gated on and off, reward must be discontinued for the duration of the testing session. In the absence of reward, the trained behavior would be expected to deteriorate. Thus, inability to reward correct behavior and inability to control presentation of the test stimuli (the perceived tinnitus) greatly complicate efforts to determine when tinnitus is occurring and what it sounds like to the subject.

The sounds heard by tinnitus sufferers are described variously as ringing, whistling, buzzing, or humming. They may be heard in one ear, both ears, or the middle of the head, or it may be difficult to pinpoint their exact location. They may be low, medium, or high pitched. There may be a single noise or two or more components. The noise may be continuous, or it may come and go. These descriptions, adapted from the Web site of the British Tinnitus Association, emphasize the point that tinnitus is highly variable in its manifestations but also make it clear that, whatever tinnitus sounds like, the one thing it does not sound like is silence.[2]

JASTREBOFF PROCEDURE

In the mid- to late-1980s, Jastreboff and colleagues realized that animals trained to respond in a particular way in silence would fail to do so if tinnitus was present.[3,4] Whatever it was they were hearing, it was not silence. Jastreboff and colleagues' contribution was a major breakthrough, one that has served as a basis for a number of the procedures that have followed. It did not, however, lead to an overwhelming number of other laboratories "jumping on the bandwagon" of tinnitus research in animal models, at least until the interest in (and support for) tinnitus research increased in the past decade.

The Jastreboff procedure is based on a behavioral effect known as conditioned suppression. Basically, that means that if a stimulus warns an animal that something aversive is about to happen, the animal will cease whatever it was doing while the warning stimulus is present. In the following discussion, I use the term *conditioned stimulus* (CS) to indicate the warning stimulus and the term *unconditioned stimulus* (US) to represent the aversive stimulus. In the Jastreboff procedure, the CS was silence, the US was a brief electric shock, the behavior that was measured was licking a water spout, and the subjects were rats. The procedure consisted of three main stages: acclimation, training, and extinction. In the early experiments, subjects were maintained in a sound field, even in their home cages. The only time they experienced silence was during the warning stimulus periods. Because silence was a novel stimulus, it was first necessary to verify that animals did not suppress licking to silence itself. To do so, an acclimation session was carried out in which several periods of silence were presented without any pairing with the US. During the subsequent training session, the silent CS period was paired with a brief shock presented at the end of the CS, and subjects learned to suppress responding during the silent interval. After training, testing sessions were carried out in extinction, that is, without any shock. For each trial, a suppression ratio was calculated as the number of licks during the CS (X) divided by the number of licks in an equal period before the stimulus (Y) plus the number of licks during the CS, that is, $X/(X + Y)$. This metric equals 0.5 if the animal continues responding at the same rate in the silent interval and equals 0 if the animal totally suppresses responding. Smaller ratios mean more suppression. Therefore, the prediction would be that an animal trained to suppress responding during a silent interval would fail to do so if sound was perceived.

Figure 7-1 presents data that Jastreboff and colleagues obtained using acoustic stimuli to simulate the presence of tinnitus.[3] The triangles connected by the lighter line illustrate what happened in the control condition, that is, when silence (ie, cessation of a background noise) was the warning stimulus. There was no suppression to the CS during the acclimation session, but during the training session, the animal learned to suppress licking, and this suppression continued well into the extinction sessions (E1–5). This is the pattern of behavior that would be expected if the warning stimulus during extinction was the same as

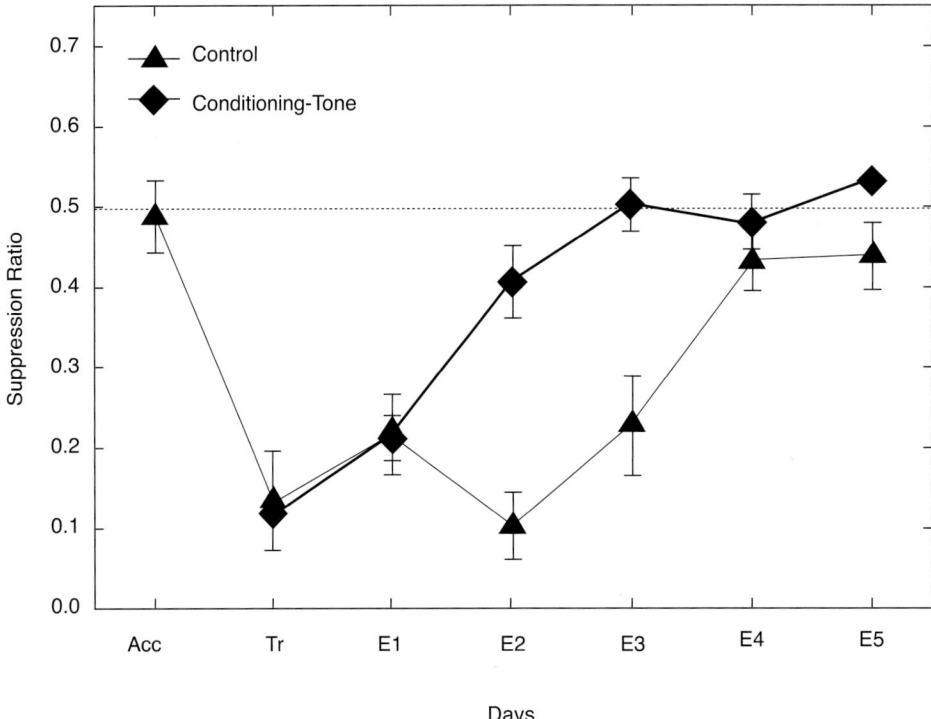

FIGURE 7-1. Behavioral suppression ratios (see text) obtained with the Jastreboff procedure when an external acoustic stimulus was presented to simulate tinnitus. For both the Control and Conditioning-Tone groups, the conditioned stimulus was the offset of a background noise. For the Conditioning-Tone group, the acoustic stimulus was introduced after training and was continuously present during testing sessions, resulting in different conditioned stimulus conditions during training and testing. Therefore, recovery from suppression was more rapid relative to the control group. Adapted from Jastreboff PJ et al.[3] Acc = acclimation session; Tr = training session.

that during training. However, if the warning stimulus during extinction was different from that during training, then the licking response rate should recover more rapidly. The function plotted with the diamonds (Conditioning-Tone) was obtained with silence as the CS during training and with a constant tone present at all times subsequent to training, including during the testing sessions in extinction. Thus, for the Conditioning-Tone group, the CS during training was termination of the noise background, and the CS during extinction testing was termination of the noise background but with the tone still present. This group simulated what would be expected if the tinnitus was induced following training and maintained during extinction testing. Although there was still some suppression during the extinction sessions, licking recovered much more rapidly than when the CS was silence during both training and extinction tests. In data not shown in Figure 7-1, Jastreboff and colleagues also demonstrated that when the tonal background was introduced prior to the training session and maintained during extinction, then the pattern of suppression again continued well into extinction, as it did with silence as the CS during both training and extinction. These data were from one of Jastreboff and colleagues' control conditions and demonstrated what behavior should look like if the animal perceived a sound during training and/or extinction.

The demonstration that the procedure worked as expected with acoustic stimuli was important, but the critical question was what happened when something was done that was assumed to produce tinnitus—in these experiments, administration of large doses of salicylate (300 mg/kg of salicylate acid). Figure 7-2 shows the results from this manipulation. The control data shown by the triangles are the same data set shown in Figure 7-1. The data shown by the squares (Conditioning-Salicylate) were obtained when salicylate was administered starting after training; in other words, the animals were trained to suppress to silence and were then tested when it was assumed that tinnitus might be present—the same situation present in

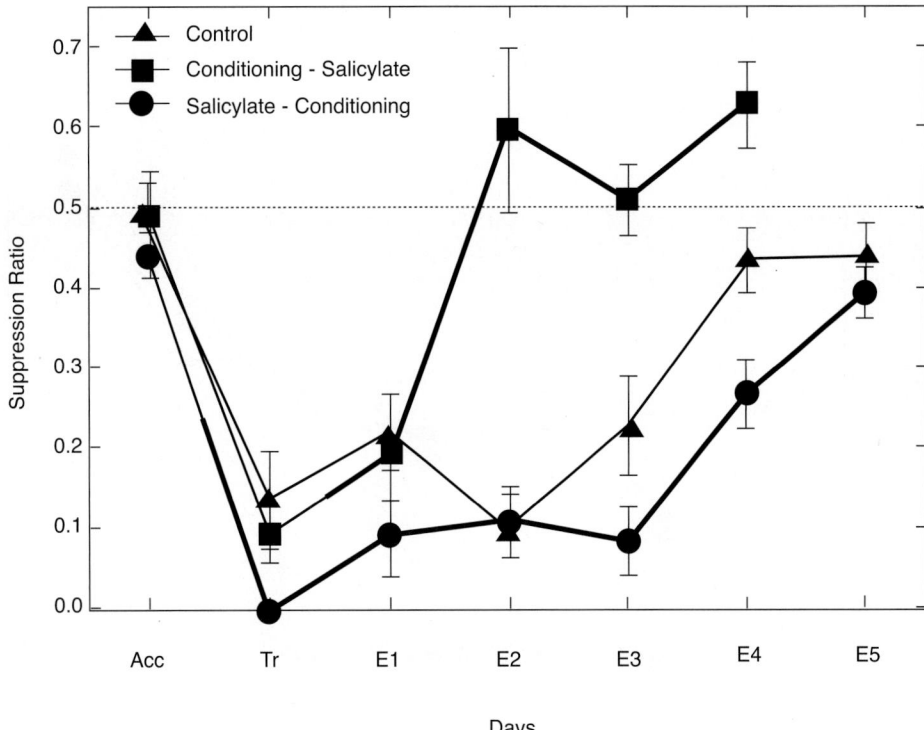

FIGURE 7-2. Behavioral suppression ratios obtained with the Jastreboff procedure when salicylate was administered to produce tinnitus. The salicylate administration began either before (Salicylate-Conditioning) or after (Conditioning-Salicylate) training. The *thicker lines* in the figure indicate the salicylate administration periods. When the conditioned stimulus conditions were different in training and testing (Conditioning-Salicylate), recovery from suppression was more rapid than when they were the same (Control and Salicylate-Conditioning groups). Adapted from Jastreboff PJ et al.[3] Acc = acclimation session; Tr = training session.

the Conditioning-Tone data shown in Figure 7-1. Figure 7-2 shows that the suppression disappeared fairly rapidly, just as it did when an acoustic stimulus was used as the CS during extinction. When salicylate was administered before training and continued during the extinction sessions, the suppression was prolonged. In other words, if the subject experienced a different CS during extinction from that experienced during training, the licking response rate recovered more rapidly during extinction testing. Thus, Jastreboff and colleagues' data supported the assumption that the behavior observed following salicylate administration indicated the perception of an auditory sensation that was different from silence.

An important control in these experiments was the demonstration that the effect was related to an auditory sensation rather than to some effect of salicylate. To do so, the experiment was repeated using light offset as the CS instead of sound offset.[3] The assumption was that the visual stimulus would not be compromised as a cue to whether additional auditory sensations were present. As seen in Figure 7-3, that was exactly what happened. Lick suppression extinguished almost identically under all conditions. It appears, therefore, that this procedure seems to detect tinnitus when it is likely that tinnitus would be present. A number of additional control experiments that were reported in the original article support this interpretation. For example, Jastreboff and colleagues showed that when the CS was a tone during both training and extinction testing, the suppression data were almost identical to those obtained when the CS was silence. Also, the authors showed that under reduced levels of motivation, which would be expected to reduce the amount of licking, a pattern of results similar to that shown in Figure 7-2 was observed.[3]

The Jastreboff procedure appears to be fairly efficient in terms of training but somewhat inefficient

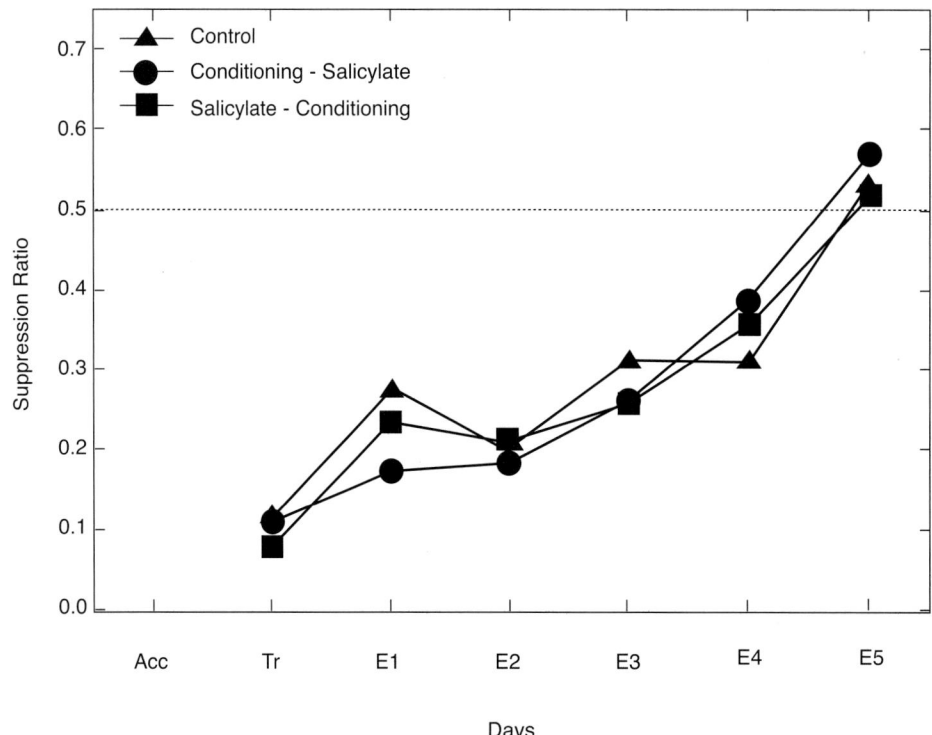

FIGURE 7-3. Behavioral suppression ratios obtained with the Jastreboff procedure when a visual stimulus was used as the conditioned stimulus. The salicylate administration began either before (Salicylate-Conditioning) or after (Conditioning-Salicylate) training. The lack of a difference between treatment groups demonstrates that there was no generalized effect of the salicylate administration. Adapted from Jastreboff PJ et al.[3] Acc = acclimation session; Tr = training session.

in terms of the amount of data derived per animal. In the early reports, each session contained only four CS intervals. The data were group averages from six animals in each group, but the standard errors indicated that the effect may have been strong enough to be seen in individual subjects, although comparison between subjects receiving different treatments would still have been required. As presented, however, the data tell us nothing about the nature of the tinnitus that was observed—only that it was something other than silence.

In subsequent studies, attempts were made to quantify the magnitude of the perceived tinnitus. For example, Jastreboff and Brennan looked at the behavioral measure (suppression ratio) as a function of salicylate dose and produced the results shown in the inset in Figure 7-4.[5] The inset contains two functions: one for a 300 mg/kg dose of salicylate before training and one for salicylate after training. Similar functions were obtained for doses ranging from 75 to 300 mg/kg. If one assumes that the amount of tinnitus is related to the salicylate dose, then it is possible to use a measure based on the area between the salicylate-before and salicylate-after functions, as shown by the shaded portion in the inset in Figure 7-4. The assumption, presumably, was that the primary difference between the salicylate-before and salicylate-after groups was that tinnitus was present during training for the salicylate-before group and therefore that the differences observed between groups reflected the effect of that tinnitus rather than any effect of salicylate on the behavioral performance. The area measure is shown in the main part of Figure 7-4 as a function of salicylate dose, and a linear relationship between the behavioral measure and salicylate dose is demonstrated.

It was then necessary to determine if the behavioral measure was also related to the level of an acoustic stimulus substituted for the presumed tinnitus. Those

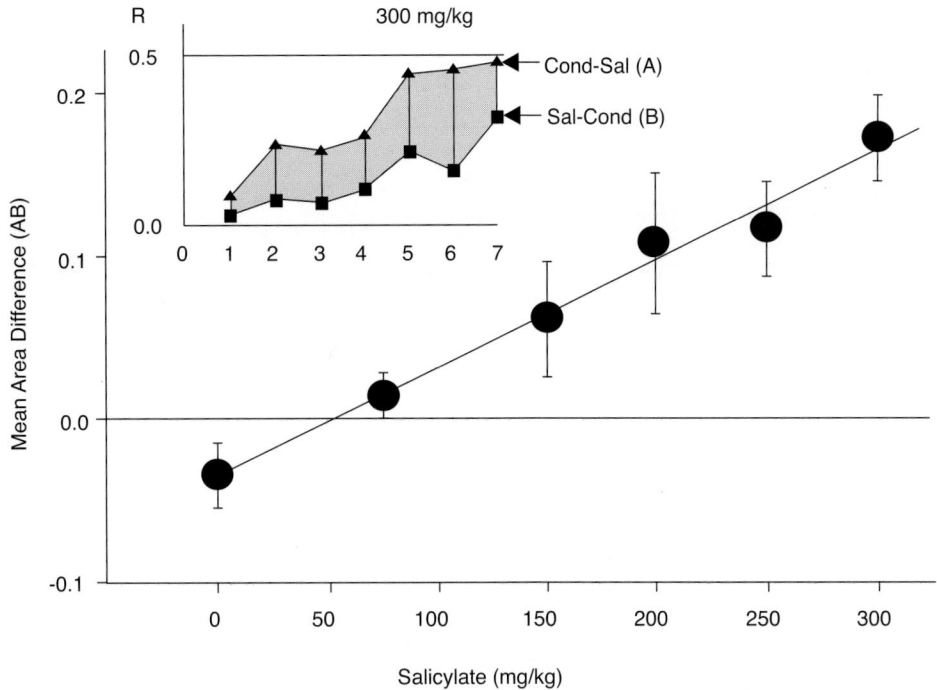

FIGURE 7-4. The *inset* shows suppression ratios (R) obtained during seven extinction testing sessions with a salicylate dose of 300 mg/kg. The *triangles* present data obtained from Conditioning-Salicylate sessions, and the *squares* present data from Salicylate-Conditioning sessions. The area between the two functions shown by the *shaded area* in the inset was used as a metric to indicate the level of the perceived tinnitus. The main portion of the figure plots this metric as a function of salicylate dose and suggests a relationship between salicylate dose and amount of perceived tinnitus. Adapted from Jastreboff PJ and Brennan JF.[5]

results are shown in Figure 7-5, which demonstrates that the area measure also resulted in a linear relationship to acoustic stimulus level over a 30 dB range. The inset in Figure 7-5 shows the data points from the main graph but with the results for 72 and 82 dB SPL stimuli included. For those levels, the linear relationship broke down, and, in fact, the salicylate-before group extinguished more rapidly than the salicylate-after group. Jastreboff and Brennan suggested that this breakdown in the linear relationship may have been the result of masking of the tonal stimuli below 72 dB SPL by the noise background, which, in this study, was at a level of 62 dB SPL.[5] At 72 and 82 dB SPL tone levels, the tone would have been audible throughout the session, and a reversal of the tone-before and tone-after effects might be expected.

Although the method has not been adopted in its original form by other laboratories, it has been used by Jastreboff and colleagues to demonstrate the experimental induction of tinnitus by quinine and the amelioration of tinnitus by ginkgo biloba extract.[6,7] Thus, the method seems to have applicability in several areas of the study of tinnitus.

In summary, the Jastreboff procedure seems to produce behavioral results that are consistent with the presence of tinnitus following treatments that would be expected to produce tinnitus. The magnitude of the behavioral measure corresponds to the dose of the salicylate used to induce tinnitus, suggesting that it might be an index of the amount of tinnitus being perceived. The procedure is relatively efficient in terms of the time required for training and testing but is relatively inefficient in terms of the amount of data that can be obtained from each subject because of the necessity of testing in extinction. The method yields results based on group averages and on comparison between groups rather than from individual subjects and allows for statistical validation of the results. However, it may not be useful in determining individual differences in perceived tinnitus.

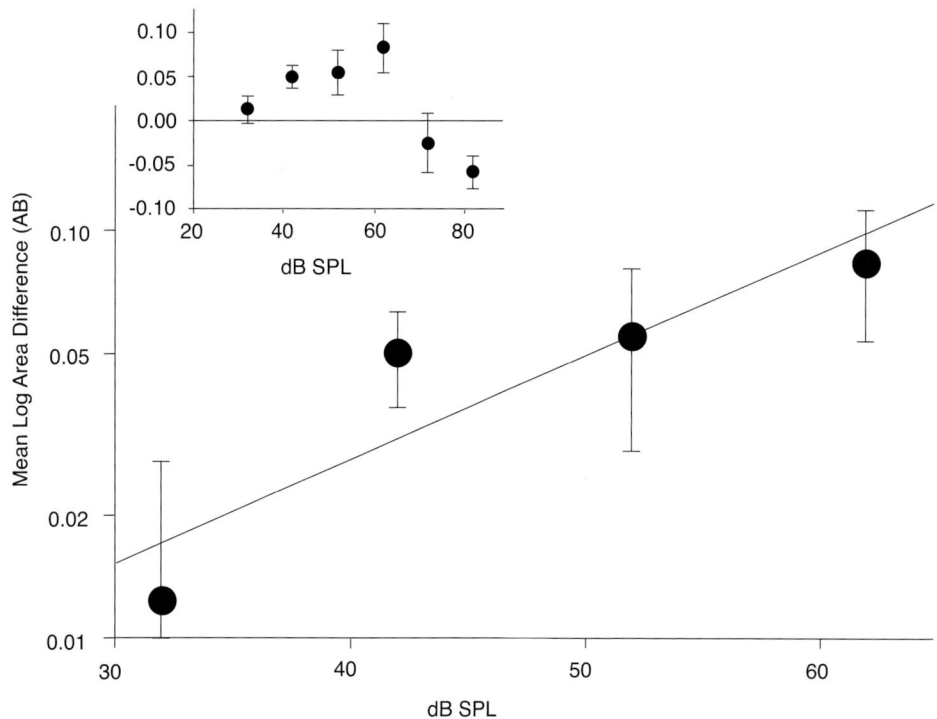

FIGURE 7-5. Area between the conditioning-tone and tone-conditioning suppression ratio functions in the Jastreboff procedure, calculated as shown in Figure 7-4, as a function of level of an external tone used to simulate tinnitus. The *inset* includes the data from the main graph with the addition of the 72 and 82 dB SPL levels. Comparison of this function with Figure 7-4 allows estimation of the level of the perceived tinnitus. Reproduced with permission from Jastreboff PJ and Brennan JF.[5]

BAUER PROCEDURE

The procedures that have been developed since the original Jastreboff and colleagues' publications have largely been efforts to improve on the approach that Jastreboff introduced. For example, Bauer and colleagues developed a procedure that allowed evaluation of tinnitus over extended periods of time and gathered more data from each subject.[8,9] As in the Jastreboff procedure, during both training and testing, there was a CS period (offset of a broadband noise) that terminated in a US (mild foot shock). The behavior measured was pressing a response lever, responses were reinforced with food, and the subjects were rats. A significant difference between the Jastreboff and Bauer studies is that, in the Bauer procedure, the US was presented only if the suppression ratio was greater than or equal to 0.2, that is, the animal received a foot shock only if it failed to suppress to the silent CS intervals. Technically, this procedure should be referred to as a passive avoidance procedure. The animal avoided an aversive event by ceasing to press the lever during the silent CS interval. In the Bauer procedure, not all of the CS intervals were silent; some intervals contained a tonal stimulus of one of several levels and frequencies. When the CS interval contained a tone, shock was never delivered at the end of the interval.

In a recent study by Bauer and Brozoski, tinnitus was induced by unilateral exposure to 16 kHz octave-band noise at 105 dB SPL.[9] Three groups of animals were tested: no exposure (controls), 1-hour exposure, and 2-hour exposure. Data from this study are shown in Figure 7-6, which plots the suppression ratio as a function of the level of a 20 kHz tone presented during the CS interval. These data were obtained 12 months after the noise trauma. The results indicate less suppression (larger ratios) for the unexposed control group than for the noise trauma group. Bauer and Brozoski's interpretation of these results is as follows. First, both groups suppressed to

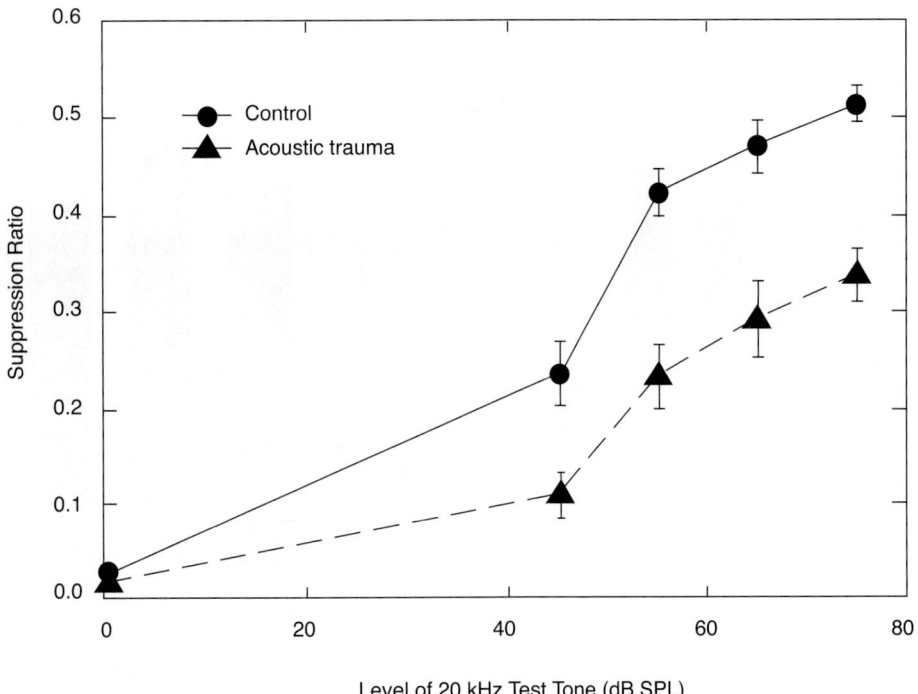

FIGURE 7-6. Results from the Bauer procedure showing suppression ratio as a function of the level of a 20 kHz test tone presented during the conditioned stimulus interval. The authors suggested that the acoustic trauma group showed greater suppression than the controls because they were "perceptually more challenged" by the similarity of the test tone to their perceived tinnitus. Adapted from Bauer CA and Brozoski TJ.[9]

the no-tone condition (which the authors refer to as 0 dB). That result is not surprising because training occurred after noise exposure. Presumably, the exposure groups were trained to suppress to a CS of whatever tinnitus they were experiencing; in other words, for the control group, the CS was silence, but for the exposed groups, the CS was the sound of tinnitus. What this procedure does is train animals in the control group to discriminate between silence and various sounds and animals in the exposed group, assuming that they were experiencing tinnitus, to discriminate between tinnitus and tinnitus plus various sounds. What Bauer and Brozoski suggested was that if tinnitus was present, then the animals were (in their words) "perceptually more challenged with test stimuli that were qualitatively more similar to their tinnitus."[9] Another way of stating that would be that the more similar the test stimuli were to the tinnitus, the more difficult was the discrimination, so the animals showed greater suppression of responding.

This explanation of the suppression effect seems feasible but is brought into question by an earlier study by Bauer and colleagues using a very similar procedure but in which tinnitus was produced by salicylate presented in the drinking water after initial training.[8] In that study, the animals presumed to have tinnitus showed less suppression than did controls; the opposite effect was seen in the noise exposure study.[9] In the salicylate study, the authors interpreted the lesser suppression shown by the experimental group as possibly being the result of the animals hearing the combination of the test tones plus the perceived tinnitus as sounding louder than the test tones alone. It is difficult to resolve these opposite results from experiments using a similar behavioral method but different procedures for inducing tinnitus.

Any interpretation of the data that involves an interaction between tinnitus and tonal stimuli suggests that tonal tinnitus should result in greater frequency specificity of the suppression effect than would noisy tinnitus. Examples of both outcomes are shown in Figure 7-7, which plots cumulative difference in suppression ratio between control and exposed groups as a function of test tone frequency.[9] This is a measure

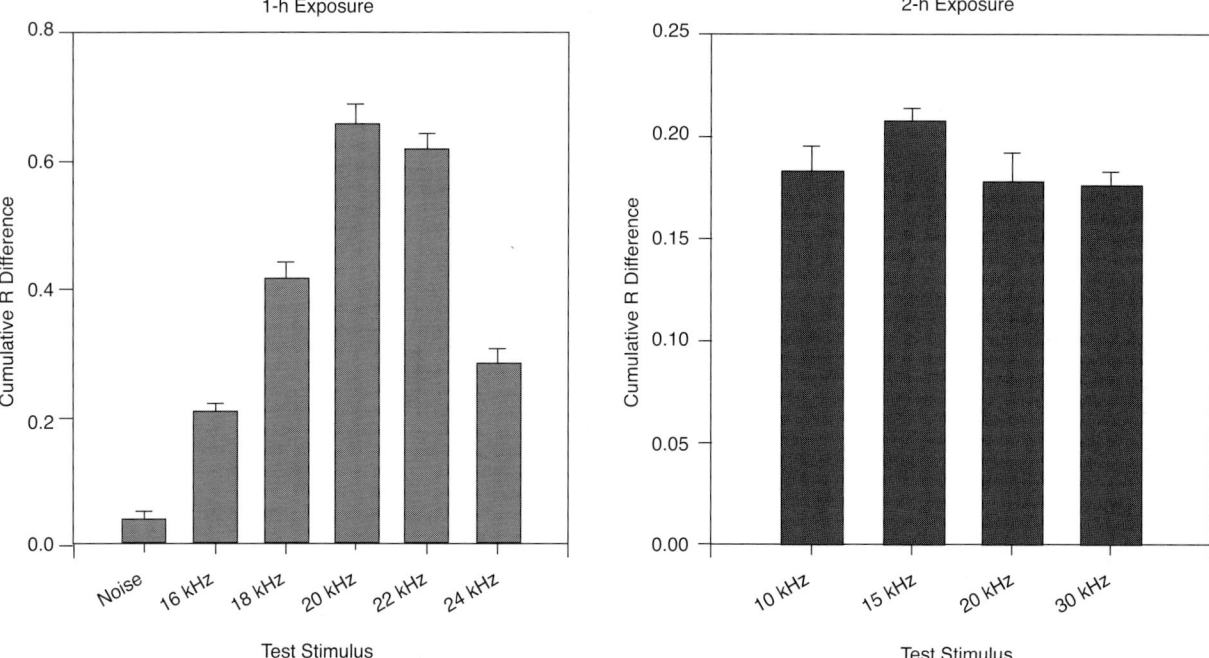

FIGURE 7-7. Cumulative difference in suppression ratio values between control and noise trauma groups for different test stimulus frequencies and noise and for the 1- and 2-hour exposure groups. Tonal stimuli were predicted to have a greater effect on tonal tinnitus that was most similar to the test frequency. Such an outcome is seen for the 1-hour group around 20 kHz but not for the 2-hour group. Adapted from Bauer CA and Brozoski TJ.[9]

similar to what Jastreboff and Brennan used to measure the magnitude of perceived tinnitus.[5] The left half of the figure shows data from the 1-hour exposure group, and the right half is from the 2-hour exposure group. In the 1-hour exposure group, the maximum effect was seen at 20 kHz, suggesting a tonal tinnitus, whereas in the 2-hour exposure group, there was almost no difference in the effect across a broad frequency range, suggesting a noisy tinnitus. In the study using salicylate-induced tinnitus, a frequency-specific suppression was also shown at 15 kHz.[8] Unfortunately, there is no independent means of determining whether these data accurately represent differences in what the animals perceived. Based on the representative histology that is presented by Bauer and Brozoski, there appeared to be little difference in the cochlear damage between the two noise exposure conditions. Both examples showed almost complete loss of both outer and inner hair cells in the basal-most 60% of the cochlea, suggesting that these animals had a significant high- to midfrequency hearing loss in the exposed ear.[9] In fact, auditory brainstem responses (ABRs) obtained 90 days postexposure using both click and pure-tone stimuli showed thresholds in the exposed ear of approximately 100 dB SPL but thresholds in the unexposed ear of between 20 and 40 dB SPL.

In summarizing the Bauer procedure, it should be noted that it is also a group design, that is, comparison of two groups is required to demonstrate the effect. The procedure offers the apparent advantage of being able to obtain data over longer periods of time than does the Jastreboff procedure. In the study of noise-induced tinnitus, Bauer and Brozoski used this feature to demonstrate the therapeutic effectiveness of a γ-aminobutyric acid agonist to reversibly attenuate tinnitus.[9] Another positive contribution of that article was the use of monaural noise exposure to produce the tinnitus. One of the problems encountered with most studies of experimentally produced tinnitus is that the means used to induce the tinnitus will usually also produce hearing loss, so the behavioral procedure needs to be able to distinguish between those two outcomes. The use of monaural noise exposure may be one way around that problem. In such a preparation, one might expect that subjects could detect sounds normally with the unexposed ear but would experience tinnitus in the exposed ear even though the ear was essentially insensitive to acoustic stimulation.

HEFFNER PROCEDURES

Another behavioral method to detect and assess tinnitus was recently reported by Heffner and Harrington.[10] The basic idea will, by now, sound familiar. Golden hamsters were trained to lick from a drinking spout in the presence of noise and/or tone and to stop drinking in silence to avoid a mild electric shock. The duration of each test trial was 15 seconds, and the shock was delivered only if the animal licked the spout during the last half of silent test trials. Tinnitus was induced by monaural exposure to a 10 kHz tone at 124 dB SPL for four different periods from 30 minutes to 4 hours. During tinnitus testing, no shocks were delivered. Because the animals were unilaterally exposed, the authors were concerned that the resulting monaural tinnitus might provide a differential cue relative to acoustic stimuli heard in the normal ear. Therefore, test stimuli were presented from several locations to reduce the likelihood that animals with a unilateral hearing loss would respond based on the apparent source of sound. As in the other procedures, the assumption was that animals experiencing tinnitus should behave during silent trials as if a tone was present and continue to lick. The dependent variable used in these studies was the average percent time that the subject was in contact with the drinking spout during noise trials and was not in contact with the spout during silent trials—in other words, the average percent time the animal was behaving in a manner appropriate to the stimulus being presented. Using this metric, the presence of tinnitus would be indicated by a lower percent correct score.

Some results from this study are shown in Figure 7-8 and are consistent with the presence of tinnitus. In the test sessions, obtained starting 5 days after exposure

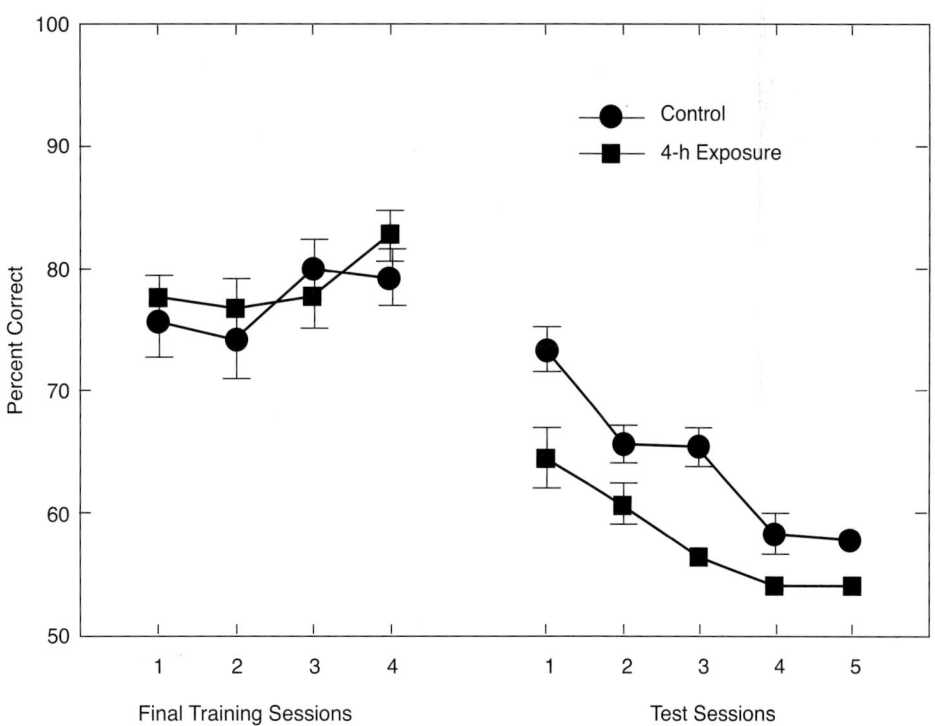

FIGURE 7-8. Percent correct responses during final training and testing in the Heffner procedure. Percent correct is defined as the average percent time during the last half of test trials that the animal was in contact with a drinking spout during noise trials and not in contact during silent trials. Lower percent correct following exposure was taken as an indication that the animal was experiencing tinnitus during silent trials. Adapted from Heffner HE and Harrington IA.[10]

and shown in the right-hand set of functions, the exposed groups showed lower percent correct scores. For both groups, percent correct decreased over time, presumably because shocks had been discontinued; thus, the trained behavior was extinguished. By taking the difference between the exposed and unexposed groups, an index of the magnitude of the tinnitus could be derived.

What about examining the nature of the perceived tinnitus with this procedure? In other words, is the reduction in percent correct an indication of the magnitude of the perceived tinnitus? Without an independent measure of the tinnitus, that question cannot be answered directly, but it is possible to examine differences in the behavioral measure as a function of exposure parameters. The results of such comparisons are shown in Figure 7-9, which depicts, for individual subjects, the behavioral measures obtained at four different exposure durations from 0.5 to 4 hours. In this figure, the shaded area represents the entire range of data obtained from unexposed controls. It will come as no surprise to anyone who has worked with noise damage that there is quite a bit of variability among individuals. However, it is apparent that longer exposures tend to produce behavioral results consistent with more tinnitus, although the effect may be nonmonotonic, as indicated by the greater number of individual functions within the normal range for the 4-hour exposure relative to the 2-hour exposure. Although the behavioral results were variable, it is important to note that Kaltenbach has shown, in measures on animals from which Heffner had obtained behavioral measures, that this variability was correlated with differences in neural activity measured in the dorsal cochlear nucleus (see Chapter 11, "Neural Correlates of Tinnitus"). Thus, the observed variability in the behavioral results may, in fact, have been indicative of differences in the perceived tinnitus being experienced by the subjects.

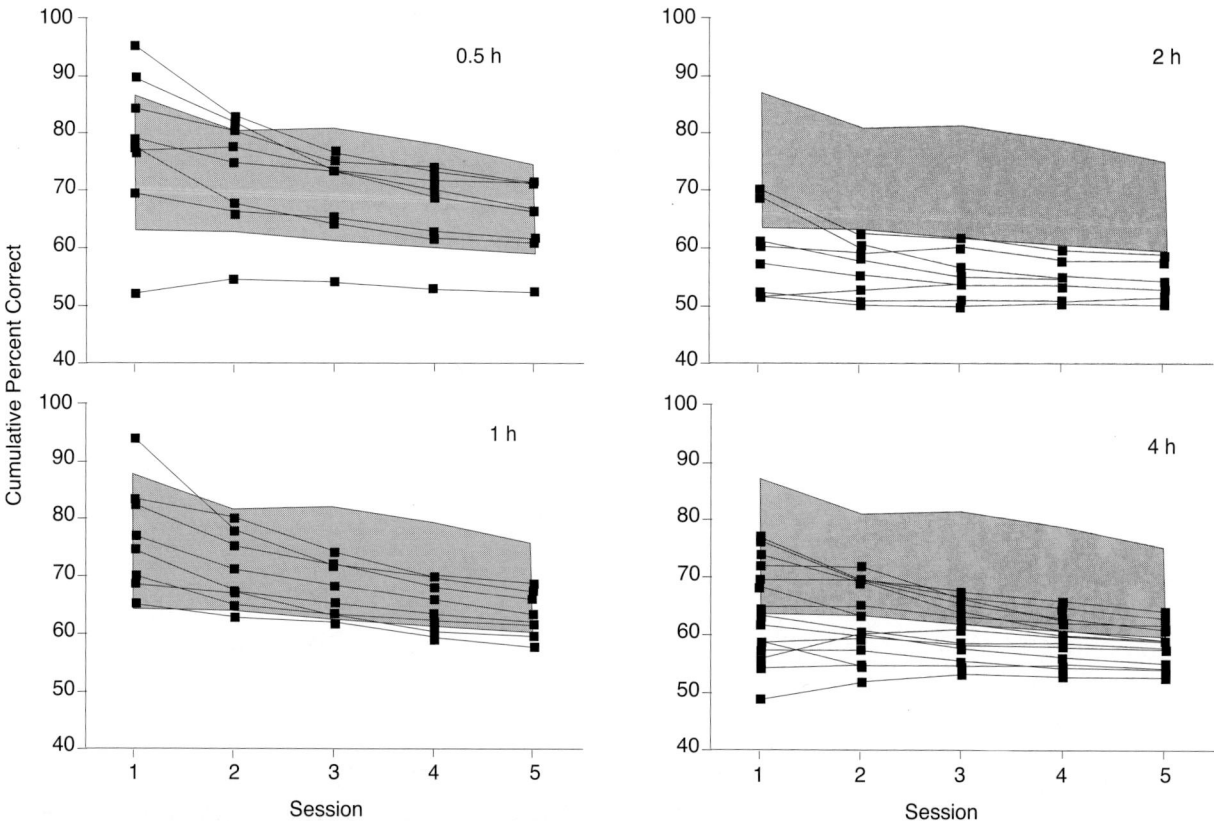

FIGURE 7-9. Individual percent correct functions for four exposure durations. The percent correct measure is as described for Figure 7-8. The *shaded areas* represent the range of values obtained from unexposed controls. Generally greater suppression is seen for longer exposure durations. Adapted from Heffner HE and Harrington IA.[10]

The possibility that the hearing loss and resulting tinnitus produced by unilateral noise exposure resulted in lateralized perception has recently been explored by Heffner in an ingenious procedure in which animals are initially trained to make one of two different responses depending on the location from which sound was presented.[11] Following this initial training, subjects were tested in the absence of sound to determine any response preference. Then the ear on the opposite side from that of any preferred response direction was exposed to intense sound to induce tinnitus. Following exposure, in the absence of acoustic stimulation, animals tended to make the response appropriate to sound presented from the side that was exposed, suggesting that they were hearing lateralized tinnitus in that ear. The number of sessions on which this response tendency was observed was significantly correlated with the amount of hearing loss as determined by ABR estimates of threshold. That is, the greater the hearing loss, the longer the animals demonstrated tinnitus. An important contribution of this procedure is that subjects were trained to make a specific response when they heard a sound rather than respond in some way when there was no sound. It is also notable because it seems appropriate for use with individual subjects and because it does not seem to be influenced by the hearing loss produced by the sound exposure. However, both of the procedures developed by Heffner require that testing be carried out in extinction, so the amount of testing possible following the induction of tinnitus is limited. Nonetheless, both of these procedures have succeeded in relating the behavioral measure of tinnitus from individual subjects to other measures from the same subjects: activity in the nervous system or amount of hearing loss.

GUITTON PROCEDURE

Recently, yet another procedure for detecting tinnitus was reported by Guitton and colleagues in which rats were trained to avoid shock by climbing a pole when they heard a 10 kHz tone presented at a level of 50 dB SPL.[12] Training was carried out until subjects responded correctly on 80% of the training trials by climbing the pole within 1 second of the tone onset. During testing sessions, animals were shocked if they failed to respond to sound. Two measures of behavior were recorded: "score" (correct responses to tone presentation) and "false alarms" (positive responses in the absence of the 10 kHz tone). Salicylate (300 mg/kg) was administered 2 hours prior to testing sessions. Animals treated with salicylate made fewer correct responses and more false-positive responses. Both of these metrics suggested that the presence of tinnitus made the auditory warning stimulus less distinctive, that is, the perceived tinnitus during the silent intervals between trials was interpreted as a warning stimulus, so animals made more false-positive responses, whereas the tone presentations may have become less effective as a warning stimulus because of the hearing loss produced by the salicylate. In this study, the choice of 10 kHz as the warning stimulus frequency was based on the assumption that the perceived tinnitus might be at about that frequency. Based on that assumption, it was predicted that a 4 kHz acoustic warning stimulus would not be similar to the perceived tinnitus and would yield different behavioral results on postsalicylate test trials. In this condition, no increase was seen in false-positive responses, but a decrease was seen in the percent correct score. One interpretation of these results is that the two behavioral measures of tinnitus may reflect different underlying processes: the decrease in percent correct may reflect a loss in hearing sensitivity, whereas the increase in false-positive rate may reflect the presence of tinnitus. This interpretation was strengthened by results obtained following administration of mefenamate, which, like salicylate, is a cyclooxygenase inhibitor. Those results showed no change in the percent correct score but an increase in false-positive responses.

MOODY PROCEDURE

Finally, in our laboratory, we have been working on developing procedures that are aimed at evaluating tinnitus in single subjects. The most promising of these procedures is one that we borrowed from behavioral pharmacologists, who use it to determine the perceived effects of drugs in animal models.[13,14] Pharmacologists face one of the same problems with drugs that we face when we try to study tinnitus: namely, that once the effect is initiated, it cannot be gated on and off at the will of the experimenter; rather, the effect is present for extended periods of time. The pharmacologists' procedure is remarkably straightforward. Subjects were trained for food reward to press one response lever on sessions in which they received one drug and a second response lever on sessions in which they received another drug (or an inactive injection). Then, in sessions in which no reward was given, a novel drug was administered, and the distribution of lever presses between the two levers was used as an indication of the perceived effect of the drug. The transfer of this concept to the study of tinnitus was, we assumed, quite straightforward. Guinea pigs were trained to respond on one lever in the presence of various sounds and on a second lever in silence. An advantage of this procedure is that the subject made a positive response to indicate the perception of sound and another response to indicate silence. In adapting the procedure to the study of tinnitus, we had to make several modifications to the pharmacologists' procedure. In their version of the procedure, for example, animals were rewarded during training after they made a fixed number of responses on the correct lever. We, however, determined that subjects would press one lever a number of times, and if no reward occurred, they would switch to the other lever. In other words, reward, rather than auditory cues, was determining behavior. In the current tinnitus procedure, the amount of time between reward availability was randomly varied, and the first lever press after the random time produced the reward. In studies of drug discrimination, a drug effect was present for the entire training session, whereas with tinnitus, sound and silent periods could be randomly alternated within training sessions. The change in the schedule of reward and the random alternation of sound and silent periods during training served to improve the control of behavior by acoustic stimuli (either real or the perceptions from tinnitus). Once subjects were trained so that most responding occurred on the stimulus-appropriate lever, probe sessions were carried out in which auditory stimuli were present (tone probes) or absent (quiet probes) during the entire session, and no responses were rewarded.

We found that the best way to look at the data from these probe sessions is in the form of what is known as a cumulative record—a means of data presentation that is probably familiar to anyone who ever took a Skinnerian "rat lab" course. Such a record is shown in Figure 7-10, which presents the results of three different testing conditions for a single subject. In this figure, time is shown on the abscissa. Every time the animal responded on one lever or the other, the y value of the appropriate function was incremented by a fixed amount. In this figure, the thicker lines represent responses on the "sound" lever, and the thinner lines represent responses on the "quiet" lever.

The upper panel of Figure 7-10 presents data from a "sound probe" session, that is, a session in

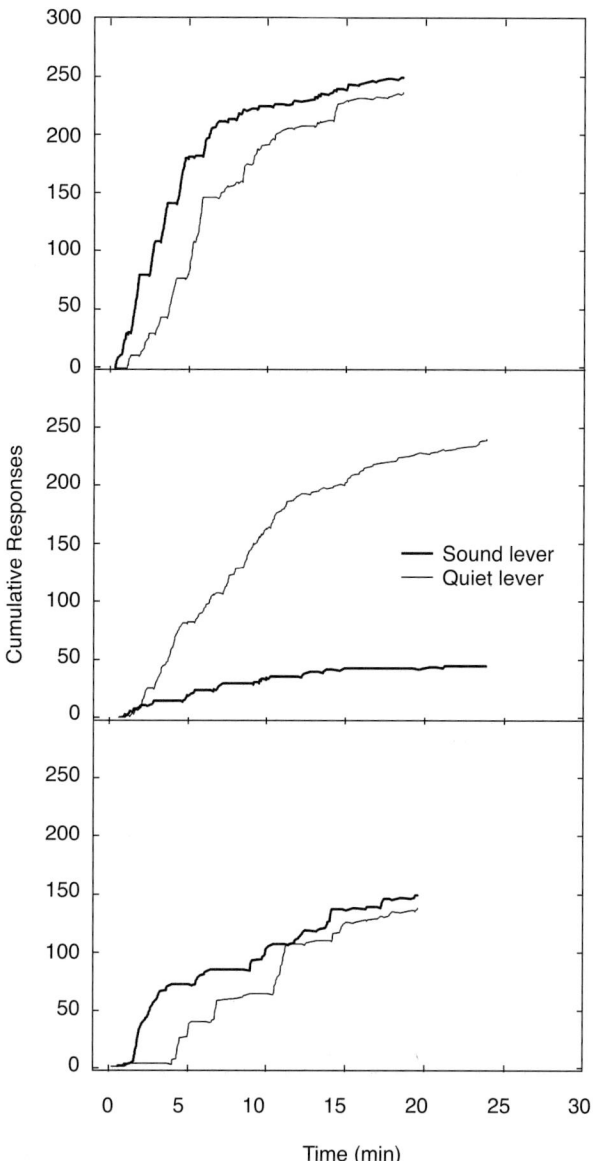

FIGURE 7-10. Patterns of responding observed during tone-probe (*top panel*), quiet-probe (*middle panel*), and 2 days postsalicylate (*bottom panel*) sessions in the Moody procedure. In the functions, time is plotted on the x-axis, and each time a response occurs on one of the levers, the y value for that function is incremented. The greater responding on the sound lever following salicylate administration indicates that the animal was experiencing tinnitus.

which a continuous background tone was present to simulate tinnitus. In the top panel, more responding is seen to occur on the sound lever, although significant responses also occurred on the quiet lever. The middle panel in Figure 7-10 shows the response patterns from a "quiet" probe session in which no external acoustic stimulus was present. During this session, most responding occurred on the quiet lever, as it should, with relatively little responding on the sound lever. The bottom panel of the figure shows the pattern of behavior obtained in a probe session carried out after 2 days of salicylate administration (300 mg/kg). No external acoustic stimuli were presented during this session, but the animal responded primarily on the sound lever. This pattern of behavior was taken as indicating that the animal was hearing a sound—tinnitus—even though no external sound was present.

The pattern of responding on the sound and quiet probe sessions was fairly typical for this subject, but response patterns varied among subjects. For example, some subjects responded on the stimulus-appropriate lever only during the early parts of the probe sessions and then began to respond on both levers. The same pattern of behavior is often seen when the procedure is used to evaluate drugs. The reason for this apparent lack of control by the acoustic stimulus during probe sessions is quite clear. During training, animals were reinforced for correct responding. They learned which lever was correct by attending to what they heard but also by which lever produced a reward. It is not surprising, therefore, that when the "correct" lever no longer produced food, the animals responded on the other lever. It seems likely, therefore, that it will be necessary to determine the pattern of responding on sound and quiet probe sessions for each subject and then to compare the results obtained following induction of tinnitus with those patterns to determine if tinnitus is being reported.

A major advantage of this procedure is that it was designed to obtain results from individual subjects. In fact, it appears that it may be necessary to evaluate the data from each subject on an individual basis. At this point, however, it seems unlikely to provide much information about the nature of the perceived tinnitus.

We also tried to develop a procedure that was based on the assumption that the presence of tinnitus would interfere with the detection of acoustic signals that resembled the tinnitus—in other words, that perceived tinnitus would mask external stimuli.

Although this procedure showed a reduction in sensitivity following salicylate administration, the sensitivity shift did not seem to be frequency specific, as would be expected with the tonal tinnitus typically produced by salicylate. Instead, I believe that the reduction in sensitivity was the result of hearing loss that resulted from the salicylate. Many clinicians believe that all loss of sensitivity with tinnitus is the direct result of the underlying hearing loss and that there is no masking effect of the perceived tinnitus on external acoustic stimuli.

THE IDEAL PROCEDURE: IS THERE SUCH A THING?

So far, this chapter has covered a number of different approaches that have been used to detect tinnitus in an animal model. Each technique demonstrated a behavioral effect that was consistent with the presence of tinnitus, and most of the techniques were able to offer something about the nature of the tinnitus that was perceived, its magnitude or its quality. Several of the methods required comparison with data from control groups to demonstrate the presence of tinnitus, but the variability of the results from those methods suggested that data from individual subjects might be meaningful.

At this point, it is reasonable to consider which method is the best for detecting tinnitus in an animal model. The answer is that no method is the best one; each has some advantages and some disadvantages. Instead, we can consider what features an ideal method should possess and then measure the procedures that we have discussed against that list of features. If one ignores concerns about what might actually be possible, a set of criteria for the ideal behavioral procedure for evaluating tinnitus might include the following:

- The model should reliably detect the presence of tinnitus from a variety of causes, including spontaneous tinnitus.
- It should yield interpretable results from individual subjects.
- It should allow statistical validation of the results.
- It should provide results that can be interpreted as the perceived level and quality of the tinnitus.
- It should readily discriminate between the presence of tinnitus and the hearing loss that results from agents that produce tinnitus.

- It should be efficient in terms of the time required for training.
- It should allow for collection of data over extended time periods without loss of behavioral performance.

Although it might be reasonable to assume that the ideal procedure in a well-trained subject might be able to detect spontaneous tinnitus if, for example, the subject suddenly started responding as if sound were present when there was none, it would probably always remain a question as to whether tinnitus was actually present or whether behavioral performance had deteriorated. The remaining points, however, have been achieved to some extent by one or more of the procedures described in this chapter.

The original Jastreboff procedure is relatively efficient in terms of time required for training and testing, but like any of the procedures that require testing to be conducted in extinction, it is not suited to the collection of data over extended time periods.[3,4] The procedure is not well suited to interpretation of data from individual subjects, but the group design is better suited to statistical validation of the results. The relationship shown between salicylate dose and the behavioral measure suggests that the method may have the possibility of specifying the level of the perceived tinnitus.

The Bauer procedure, on the other hand, seems suited to the collection of data over longer time periods, and training time is relatively short.[8,9] Like the Jastreboff procedure, its group design allows statistical validation at the cost of interpretable data from individual subjects. The procedure seems to be able to specify the perceived quality of the tinnitus. The use of unilateral sound exposure to produce tinnitus should result in a preparation in which a normal-hearing ear is available to detect stimuli, whereas the exposed ear experiences tinnitus. However, the apparently conflicting direction of behavioral change in the two Bauer studies is troublesome.

The Heffner procedure is relatively efficient in terms of training, but because testing must take place in extinction, it is not suited to the collection of data over longer time periods.[10] Although it is a group design, individual differences in the behavioral measure have been shown to reflect differences in neural activity at higher levels of the auditory system. Thus, this method has demonstrated the usefulness and potential advantages of evaluating data from individual subjects. The procedure also demonstrates a relationship between the behavioral measure and the exposure duration, suggesting a correlation with the level of the perceived tinnitus. Like the Bauer method, unilateral sound exposure leaves one normal-hearing ear and one ear with presumed tinnitus, so that inability to detect acoustic stimuli should not be an issue. The Heffner procedure, in fact, considers the possibility that the lateralized changes in auditory function might confound the results and attempts to test and control for that possibility. The more recent Heffner procedure uses the lateralization of the perceived tinnitus as the indication that tinnitus is present.[11]

The Guitton procedure is also a group design, thus minimizing the possibility of meaningful data from individual subjects but allowing statistical validation of the results.[12] Training time was relatively short. The avoidance contingencies were continued during tinnitus testing, allowing evaluation of changes in the behavioral measures over time but with the risk of biasing responding. The use of two separate behavioral metrics may have allowed differentiation between evaluation of tinnitus and effects of hearing loss. No data are available from this method to determine directly its usefulness in evaluation of the quality or level of the perceived tinnitus, although the differences seen between different test tone frequencies suggest that such evaluation may be possible.

The Moody procedure, based on techniques from behavioral pharmacology, was specifically designed to obtain data from individual subjects, but to do so required extensive training and determination of patterns of responding during probe sessions with and without the presence of simulated tinnitus. Thus, it was not particularly efficient. Because comparison of complex patterns of response is needed to evaluate the outcome of testing, it was not readily amenable to statistical validation. However, when used with an agent such as salicylate that produced a reversible effect, it was possible to carry out repeated testing with intervening retraining. It was not a technique ideally suited to evaluation of the quality or level of the perceived tinnitus. Because subjects made separate responses to perceived sound and silence, the method was probably not susceptible to biases resulting from hearing loss produced by the tinnitus-inducing agent.

To summarize, then, there are behavioral procedures that can detect when an animal model is experiencing tinnitus. From the published reports, it is sometimes difficult to evaluate the problems and pitfalls of the various techniques and to compare their effectiveness. Although several reports have attempted to specify the nature of the perceived tinnitus, that goal remains elusive. In particular, an important unanswered question is whether different behavioral techniques would give comparable estimates of the nature of the perceived tinnitus following identical treatments. Nonetheless, it is encouraging that there has been a recent increase in the number of laboratories working on developing an optimal animal model in which to evaluate the nature and physiologic basis of this common but elusive problem.

ACKNOWLEDGMENTS

The preparation of this chapter and a portion of the research presented were supported by a grant from the Tinnitus Research Consortium and by the University of Michigan Hearing Research Core Center grant from the National Institute on Deafness and Other Communication Disorders (P30 DC-005188). Dr. Colleen G. Le Prell is thanked for her comments on an earlier version of this chapter and Ms. Beth Hand and Ms. Laura Grant for their help in carrying out the experiments described as "the Moody procedure."

REFERENCES

1. Le Prell CG, Moody DB. Perceptual salience of acoustic features of Japanese monkey coo calls. J Comp Psychol 1997;111:261–74.
2. British Tinnitus Association. What is Tinnitus? Available at: http://www.tinnitus.org.uk/information/what_is_tinnitus.htm (accessed July 18, 2003).
3. Jastreboff PJ, Brennan JF, Coleman JK, et al. Phantom auditory sensation in rats: an animal model for tinnitus. Behav Neurosci 1988;102:811–22.
4. Jastreboff PJ, Brennan JF, Sasaki CT. An animal model for tinnitus. Laryngoscope 1988;98:280–6.
5. Jastreboff PJ, Brennan JF. Evaluating the loudness of phantom auditory perception (tinnitus) in rats. Audiology 1994;33:202–17.
6. Jastreboff PJ, Zhou S, Jastreboff MM, et al. Attenuation of salicylate-induced tinnitus by ginkgo biloba extract in rats. Audiol Neurootol 1997;2:197–212.
7. Jastreboff PJ, Brennan JF, Sasaki CT. Quinine-induced tinnitus in rats. Arch Otolaryngol Head Neck Surg 1991;117:1162–6.
8. Bauer CA, Brozoski TJ, Rojas R, et al. Behavioral model of chronic tinnitus in rats. Otolaryngol Head Neck Surg 1999;121:457–62.
9. Bauer CA, Brozoski TJ. Assessing tinnitus and prospective tinnitus therapeutics using a psychophysical animal model. J Assoc Res Otolaryngol 2001;2:54–64.
10. Heffner HE, Harrington IA. Tinnitus in hamsters following exposure to intense sound. Hear Res 2002;170:83–95.
11. Heffner HE. Relationship between hearing loss and tinnitus in hamsters exposed to intense sound [abstract]. In: Santi PA, editor. Abstracts of the Twenty-Sixth Annual Mid Winter Research Meeting of the Association for Research in Otolaryngology. Mt. Royal (NJ): Association for Research in Otolaryngology; 2003. p. 192.
12. Guitton MJ, Caston J, Ruel J, et al. Salicylate induces tinnitus through activation of cochlear NMDA receptors. J Neurosci 2003;23:3944–52.
13. Colpaert FC, Rosecrans JA. Stimulus properties of drugs: ten years of progress. New York: Elsevier/North Holland Biomedical Press; 1978.
14. Woods JH, Bertalmio AJ, Young AM, et al. Receptor mechanisms of opioid drug discrimination. In: Colpaert FC, Balsters RL, editors. Transduction mechanisms of drug stimuli. New York: Springer-Verlag; 1988. p. 95–106.

CHAPTER 8

The Neurophysiological Model of Tinnitus

Pawel J. Jastreboff, PhD, ScD

The neurophysiological model of tinnitus postulates that many systems in the brain are involved in tinnitus and decreased sound tolerance, with the auditory system playing a secondary role. Stress is on the role of the limbic and autonomic nervous systems, subconscious processing of information, subconscious learning, and creation and extinction of conditioned reflexes. The model is based on general neurophysiology and behavioral neuroscience. A clear distinction is made between tinnitus perception and tinnitus-evoked reactions (eg, annoyance, anxiety, depression, difficulty concentrating). Tinnitus as a problem arises from sustained activation of the limbic and autonomic nervous systems, particularly of the sympathetic part of the autonomic nervous system.

Tinnitus is defined as a phantom auditory perception,[1] that is, perception of the sound without corresponding acoustic or mechanical correlates in the cochlea. In other words, tinnitus results exclusively from perception of an activity within the nervous system (the tinnitus-related neuronal activity) and is not related to any external or internal auditory stimulus.

As presented in this chapter, the model is sufficiently general to encompass the perception of and reaction to tinnitus and external sounds. Issues related to decreased tolerance to external sounds are discussed in Chapter 2, "Decreased Sound Tolerance," and are only briefly alluded to in this chapter. The description of the model focuses on the functional interactions of the various systems in the brain rather than on their anatomic components. The model, however, remains the same as described previously.[1-4]

POTENTIAL MECHANISMS RESPONSIBLE FOR EMERGENCE OF TINNITUS PERCEPTION

Although the specific mechanisms responsible for emergence of tinnitus-related neuronal activity are irrelevant for the model, it is customary and convenient to delineate the potential mechanisms generating the tinnitus-related neuronal activity and tinnitus perception while discussing tinnitus. Therefore, the discordant dysfunction theory[1,4] is briefly outlined here. The discordant dysfunction theory postulates that tinnitus-related neuronal activity is generated in the dorsal cochlear nucleus as a result of disinhibition caused by the decreased or absent signal from type II auditory nerve fibers resulting from damaged or dysfunctional outer hair cells (OHCs), whereas inner hair cells (IHCs) are still functioning reasonably well. Each part of the cochlear basilar membrane with local damage to the OHCs will serve as a source for tinnitus-related neuronal activity, with the strength of the signal depending on the difference in functional properties between OHCs and IHCs located on this particular part of the basilar membrane. If there is only one area with discordant dysfunction of OHCs and IHCs, the individual will perceive tonal tinnitus. In typical cases of complex tinnitus sound perception, the final tinnitus signal is composed of signals created at many locations.

This signal is further enhanced in the subconscious part of the auditory pathways and is finally perceived at a high cortical level. Recent experimental data support the discordant dysfunction theory by showing that tinnitus is related to damage to OHCs but not IHCs or hearing loss.[5]

This theory explains many tinnitus puzzles, for example, why approximately 20% of individuals with tinnitus have normal hearing (local, partial damage to OHCs might not affect the audiogram but be sufficient to create unbalanced stimulation of cells in the dorsal cochlear nucleus); why tinnitus is absent in 27% of deaf individuals (if damage to OHCs and IHCs is complete, imbalance is not present or small, and tinnitus, when present, would emerge owing to increased gain within central auditory pathways); why the pitch of tinnitus typically corresponds to the bottom of the threshold slope or the dip in the threshold curve on the audiogram (this is the frequency area where larger differences exist between the damage of OHCs and IHCs); why it might be impossible to suppress tinnitus even with a high level of sound (the tinnitus-related neuronal activity results from disinhibition of neurons in the dorsal cochlear nucleus and takes the form of bursting, epileptic-like activity[6,7]; this type of activity is very powerful and difficult to suppress by sound-induced activity); why salicylate, quinine, and sound exposure are the most powerful methods of inducing tinnitus in animals (all of these methods, although acting through different mechanisms, have one feature in common, that is, damage or dysfunction of OHCs); and why it is not possible to document tinnitus-related neuronal activity by recording the activity of type I auditory fibers (tinnitus-related neuronal activity first appears at the level of the dorsal cochlear nucleus, and the only change that could be observed within the auditory nerve is decreased activity in type II fibers innervating the OHCs, without any change in activity of type I fibers innervating the IHCs).[1,4]

MECHANISMS CONTRIBUTING TO AND MODULATING THE STRENGTH OF THE TINNITUS SIGNAL

AUTOMATIC GAIN CONTROL

Several mechanisms can modify the strength of the tinnitus signal and its perception. First, all sensory systems work in an "automatic gain control" manner; that is, when an average level of incoming signals is low, then various mechanisms are activated to increase amplification of incoming signals. This is well recognized in the visual system (gradually increased perception of a low-light signal when the subject is in darkness), and automatic gain control is present in the auditory system as well. At the peripheral level, activation of the efferent system increases mechanical amplification by the OHC system. At the central level, studies have shown increased sensitivity of the neurons at various subconscious levels of the auditory pathways.[8–12]

STRENGTH OF A STIMULUS DEPENDS ON THE DIFFERENCE RELATIVE TO THE BACKGROUND

Second, the strength of signals within the nervous system and the perception of sensory stimuli depend on the prominence of the signal relative to the background. For example, sound-induced neuronal activity of 50 spikes per second will have a different relative strength and effect on the next neuron, depending on whether the prestimulus spontaneous activity was 5 versus 45 spikes per second. At the perceptual level, the same intensity of sound would be louder when presented in silence versus a noisy environment.

These two mechanisms can explain the Heller and Bergman experiment, which showed that 94% of people develop tinnitus after a few minutes in an anechoic chamber,[13] as well as the commonly reported increase of tinnitus in a quiet environment. When subjects are in silence for a few minutes, the gain within the auditory pathways increases, whereas background neuronal activity decreases. Under a typical situation, with some environmental sounds present, even a high level of random spontaneous activity recorded from the auditory pathways is filtered out and not perceived. When a subject is in a quiet environment, the gain within the auditory pathways increases, and fluctuations of spontaneous activity are detected and perceived as tinnitus.

In individuals with preexisting tinnitus, both phenomena will enhance the strength and perception of the intensity of the tinnitus. This is particularly relevant for sleep because people tend to select a quiet environment for sleeping. However, because tinnitus is enhanced in silence and induces stronger autonomic and behavioral reactions, an individual with tinnitus may experience problems falling asleep and with continuing sleep throughout the night. This last aspect is related to the fact that sleep occurs in cycles of about 90 minutes, and in every cycle, there is a period when sleep is very shallow. During the shallow period, one may wake up for a short time only to fall asleep again without realizing that this has happened.

During this period, an individual's tinnitus will be enhanced by the silence. This will activate the autonomic nervous system, waking the individual and preventing him or her from falling back to sleep.

PERCEPTION OF A SIGNAL DEPENDS ON THE STATUS OF THE LIMBIC AND AUTONOMIC NERVOUS SYSTEMS

A third factor contributing to the enhancement of the tinnitus signal relates to the involvement of the limbic and autonomic nervous systems in assessing the strength of sensory signals. The activation of these systems yields increased arousal and awareness and promotes the tuning of neuronal networks in the auditory pathways, enhancing perception of the tinnitus signal. Many individuals exhibit strong and cyclic modulation of perceived tinnitus loudness. However, when an audiometric loudness match is performed, the intensity of the tinnitus is the same or may even move in the direction opposite to the perception, that is, the loudness match can be lower when the tinnitus is perceived to be very loud and higher when the tinnitus is perceived as softer. The modulation of perceived loudness can be related to stress, anxiety, and emotional status.

MECHANISM AND THE BRAIN SYSTEMS GOVERNING EMERGENCE OF TINNITUS AS A PROBLEM

As long as the tinnitus-related neuronal activity is constrained to the auditory pathways, individuals "experience" tinnitus but do not "suffer" because of it, that is, the presence of tinnitus will not result in negative behavioral reactions (eg, anxiety, annoyance). This is actually the situation for over 80% of people with tinnitus.[14,15] Notably, there is no difference in psychoacoustic characterization of tinnitus (pitch and loudness matching, maskability) between the group that just experiences tinnitus and the group that suffers because of it, proving that the auditory system is secondary in tinnitus-induced problems.

The distinction is made between perceiving tinnitus and having a problem because of it. The proposed term, *clinically significant tinnitus*, is defined as tinnitus that bothers people, affects their life, and causes them frequently to seek professional help and become patients (thus the descriptor "clinically significant"). According to surveys performed in various countries, approximately 4% of the population has clinically significant tinnitus (approximately 10 to 12 million people in the United States).[14,16,17]

Analysis of tinnitus-related problems shows that they are associated with a high level of activation of the sympathetic part of the autonomic nervous system and the limbic system. Patients exhibit anxiety, annoyance, problems with sleep, decreased ability to enjoy life activities, and other symptoms when the sympathetic part of the autonomic nervous system is at a high level of activity. In the remaining text, for brevity, the term *autonomic nervous system* denotes the sympathetic part of the autonomic nervous system. Patients show strong emotional responses to tinnitus, which necessitate involvement of the limbic system. The tinnitus signal becomes highly significant, as indicated by difficulty (or even inability) to shift attention from it to other subjects. Therefore, brain centers involved in attention are involved as well. Other centers, such as the prefrontal cortex (tendency to perseveration, problems with task switching) and the cerebellum (eg, multisensory integration, interaction with somatosensory system) must be considered in clinically significant tinnitus.[1]

The crucial question is why these systems are activated in some people with tinnitus but not in others, keeping in mind that there is no difference in the psychoacoustic characterization of tinnitus in patients with clinically significant tinnitus and in people just experiencing it. What are the mechanisms of this activation? Why is it, in the majority of patients, that the trigger for clinically significant tinnitus is not related to the auditory system? Why does the same tinnitus signal create a high level of anxiety during the day while promoting (contrary to a typical situation) sleep at night?[1] Why is it difficult to modify tinnitus, and why can it persist for decades without improvement?

The answers come from an analysis of the mechanisms governing development and modification of conditioned reflexes, mechanisms of subconscious processing of information, and reflexes working at the subconscious level.

PRINCIPLES OF CREATING CONDITIONED REFLEXES

Conditioned reflexes allow any physical stimulus to be linked to reinforcement and then to induce a reaction, the specifics of which are determined by the reinforcement. Consequently, the reaction and its strength depend primarily on reinforcement and not on the stimulus; for example, tinnitus and external sound, in a case of misophonia (strong dislike of sound), can share the same reactions, although the stimuli are different.

Adequacy of Temporal Association of Stimulus and Reinforcement to Create a Reflex

A particular feature of conditioned reflexes provides an explanation as to why only some individuals with tinnitus have a problem with it, whereas over 80% just experience it. Specifically, to create a conditioned reflex, it is not necessary to have a causal relation between the stimulus and reinforcement; temporal association is sufficient for the so-called "superstitious conditioned reflexes" (Jerzy Konorski, personal communication, 1971). Indeed, while training animals to perform a specific task, care should be taken to prevent creation of "superstitious reflexes," for example, animals turning around before pressing a bar or performing other additional, irrelevant tasks, because they slow the process of training and increase the latency of the required response.

Therefore, the conditioned reflex arc is created when the tinnitus-related neuronal activity temporarily coexists with (1) cognitively induced activation of the limbic and autonomic nervous systems (eg, the patient is told that the tinnitus might be related to a brain tumor or other medical condition and might reach the conclusion that the tinnitus is something bad) or (2) "by chance" temporal coexistence of stimulus and activation of the limbic and autonomic nervous systems (eg, high level of stress and anxiety related to retirement, problem at work, divorce, a health problem, such as a broken leg or cancer).

These mechanisms provide the initial negative reinforcement, which is sufficient to create a conditioned reflex arc linking the tinnitus-related neuronal activity present in the auditory pathways with the limbic and autonomic nervous systems (Figure 8-1). Consequently, the tinnitus signal starts to activate the limbic and autonomic nervous systems on its own. Reactions evoked by this activation act, in turn, as negative reinforcement, further enhancing this reflex. This process can be described as a feedback loop or "vicious circle." In essence, it enhances and sustains the reflex, preventing its spontaneous extinction, that would occur when a stimulus is present, but the reinforcement is absent.

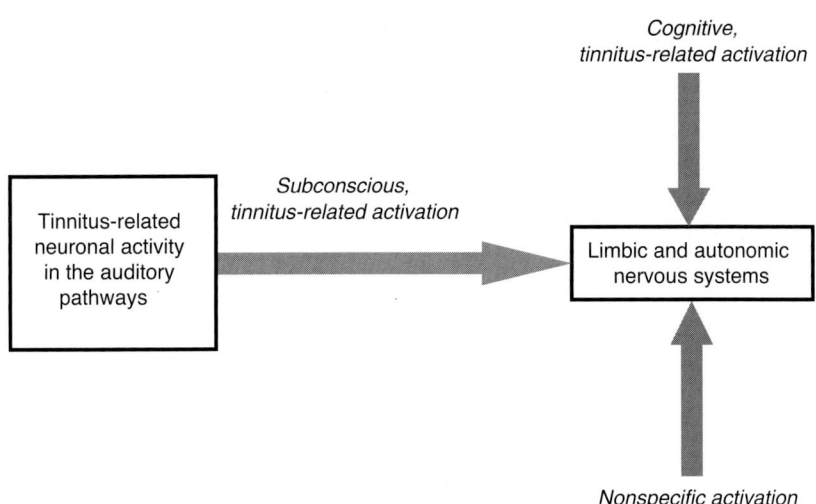

FIGURE 8-1. Creation of a conditioned reflex arc. Note that nonspecific, coincidental but concurrent with the presence of a sensory stimulus activation of the limbic and autonomic nervous systems is sufficient to initiate development of a conditioned reflex arc.

IMPORTANCE OF CLASSIFICATION OF STIMULI FOR DEVELOPMENT OF CONDITIONED REFLEXES

Stimuli to which people are exposed are classified on a continuous scale from completely insignificant (irrelevant) to highly (extremely) important and on an independent scale as having a positive or a negative connotation. The brain attends the most important signal to which the subject is exposed at a given moment. Thus, the same signal of moderate significance in a general sense may become dominant when there are no other competing stimuli, for example, tinnitus during the night, when there is a limited number of other stimuli and tasks to attend.

The negative reinforcements, particularly evoking survival reflexes or reactions, are the strongest. Positive stimuli do not evoke survival reactions (except reproduction-linked ones). On the other hand, anything that can potentially affect health and the ability to work and provide means for living could induce survival reactions. This principle is true for stimuli that are linked with just discomfort, even though the significance of these stimuli and the reaction evoked by them are weaker than stimuli related to survival. Tinnitus evokes all varieties of negative reactions, starting from mild annoyance up to preventing people from working and participating in everyday activities. Typically, concern about health and the repercussions of losing good health are common but coexisting factors providing a high level of activation of the autonomic nervous system; for example, retirement, divorce, and other health problems can be a sufficient stimulant of the limbic and autonomic nervous systems to initiate a conditioned reflex arc.

Classification of stimuli can be conscious or subconscious, and the subject may not necessarily be aware which particular element of the stimulus determines the classification, for example, trust or mistrust evoked by seeing a face. Individuals may not be aware even of the presence of a stimulus and may still have negative reactions. There is growing awareness that training, developing reflexes, and learning can occur at subconscious levels[18–25] or that subconscious learning can be a significant element in training. Note that there is a direct subconscious connection between the auditory (medial geniculate body) and the limbic (lateral nucleus of amygdala) systems.

It is important to realize that for any stimulus, conscious or subconscious, activation of the limbic and autonomic nervous systems at the same time there is some activity within the auditory system (the tinnitus-related neuronal activity or sound-evoked activity in the case of misophonia) can create a conditioned reflex arc.

CONDITIONING TO COMPLEX STIMULI

In a situation in which tinnitus acquires some cognitively recognized negative significance, it is classified as important, and activation of the limbic and autonomic nervous systems is aimed at preparing the subject for a defensive action. Typically, there is no action that would improve tinnitus, and these systems remain on an increased level of activity for a prolonged time, even many years. Consequently, as long as the tinnitus signal is classified as significant (important), the activation persists, sustaining and enhancing (owing to dynamic balance scenario) the conditioned reflex arc.

Another important aspect of conditioned reflexes is that the stimulus, although assessed and classified as an individual entity, may be physically complex and consists of a number of independent stimuli, even from various sensory modalities. The final reaction depends on this complex stimulus, detected as a pattern, and can be completely different from reactions evoked by individual components.[26] This property can explain a case in which a patient was highly annoyed by his tinnitus during the day, but, paradoxically, the tinnitus was facilitating sleep.[1] It turned out that during his happy childhood, he slept in a room with heating pipes in the walls that produced a hissing sound close to the perception of his tinnitus. The complex stimulus consisting of the sound of the tinnitus, darkness, and a comfortable bed acted as a relaxing stimulus. Notably, this patient had had problems with sleep before he started to experience tinnitus. When other components of this complex signal were removed during the day, the tinnitus signal induced the opposite reaction of a high level of anxiety.

CONSOLIDATION OF TINNITUS-CONDITIONED REFLEX ARCS

The creation of the reflex does not ensure its persistence. Neural networks require some time to establish functional connections; therefore, there is a need for tinnitus and reinforcement (stimulation of the limbic and autonomic nervous systems) to be concurrently present for the same time so that connections needed for clinically significant tinnitus can solidify. In the case of transient tinnitus, even if stimulation of the limbic and autonomic nervous systems is strong, the conditioned reflex is not developed because there is only an intermittent sensory signal. This is the physiologic basis of the explanation as to why transient tinnitus is practically never clinically significant.

However, once the arc has reached a sufficient strength, it can be sustained and enhanced (and enhanced activity within the limbic and autonomic nervous systems can be preserved), even when the stimulant that provided the initial negative reinforcement is no longer present. This happens because reactions induced by the autonomic nervous system will provide the negative reinforcement needed for sustaining this conditioned reflex. Figure 8-2 presents a situation for classical conditioning with the use of external sound and external reinforcement (Figure 8-2A) versus conditioning involving tinnitus (Figure 8-2B). The main difference is that in the case of tinnitus, the signal (the tinnitus-related neuronal activity) is continuously present, and reactions of the limbic and autonomic nervous systems act as internal self-reinforcement. Both factors prevent the extinction of the reflex. This scenario could explain why spontaneous remission of tinnitus is low.[27] Of course, if the stimulant providing reinforcement is still present, the arc is strengthened faster.

If tinnitus is associated with pleasure (positive reinforcement), as in the case of "disco tinnitus," or the belief that tinnitus represents the voice of God, the functional connections are typically weaker and can be easily extinguished. Reactions associated with a positive reinforcement are positive as well. Consequently, subjects do not have problems with them and with tinnitus, which, consequently, is not classified as clinically significant.

ROLE AND FUNCTION OF THE CLASSIFICATION CENTER

In the scenario described above, classification of each stimulus is the determining factor for developing the reflex. Higher significance translates into stronger reaction and higher probability of establishing the reflex, whereas the type of reinforcement (positive or negative) determines the type of reaction. Classification occurs at

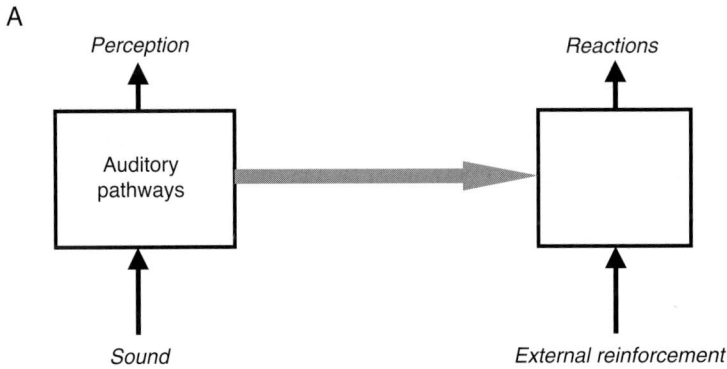

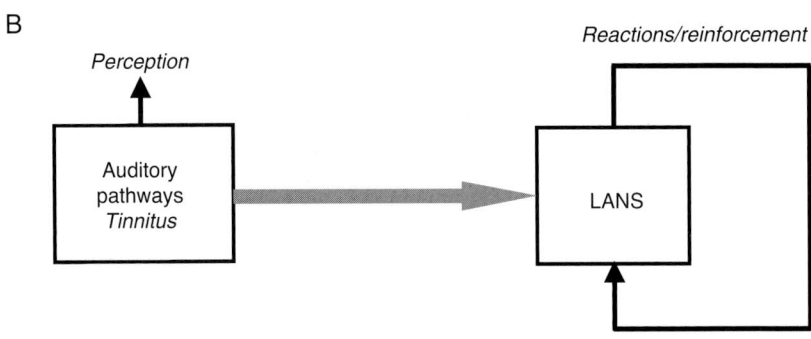

FIGURE 8-2. Similarities and differences in (A) conditioning involving external sound and external reinforcement versus (B) conditioning occurring in the case of tinnitus. LANS = the limbic and autonomic nervous systems.

a relatively high level of the nervous system because it requires integration of various sensory systems and information stored in memory. However, classification has to occur at both conscious and subconscious levels because blocking of a stimulus from reaching awareness (habituation of perception) has to be carried out at a subconscious level. Moreover, evaluation has to occur simultaneously for a number of stimuli, a task that cannot be performed at the cognitive level. Cortical areas involved in task switching[28] have to be engaged, as well as the brain's system, which takes part in integrating information from various sensory modalities, attention, memory, and emotions. Recent literature supports previously proposed involvement of the limbic and autonomic nervous systems, prefrontal cortex, and cerebellum.[1] Notably, an increasing number of articles show the important role of the cerebellum in autonomic functions, cognition, attention, sensory and cognitive integration, conditioning, language development and cognitive development.[29–34] Finally, there are data showing direct modulation of cerebellar activity in relation to tinnitus.[35] Therefore, it seems likely that the cerebellum plays an important role in networks processing tinnitus-related neuronal activity.

It is proposed that sensory stimuli are continuously evaluated at the subconscious level on the basis of past experiences. Note that although one can perform only one task requiring full attention at a given time (including focusing attention on one stimulus), more than one stimulus can be evaluated and processed at the subconscious level. The stimuli are ranked in order of importance. The stimulus that is most important is passed to higher cognitive centers when it is consciously perceived. At the same time, if any physical or mental action is expected or the stimulus has a high level of significance or strong emotional connotations, then the limbic and autonomic nervous systems are activated as well. It is possible to switch attention consciously from one stimulus to another, but this task requires a conscious decision. If a stimulus has strong negative associations, particularly if it belongs to a category evoking survival reflexes, then shifting attention from it might be difficult, and the person will be forced to recheck the status of this particular stimulus all of the time.

Clinically significant tinnitus acquires classification as a significant, negative signal. Consequently, it is ranked highly in the order of importance and has a tendency to dominate perception (patients frequently report that they perceive tinnitus close to 100% of the time) and through this mechanism affects attention, which can be committed to other stimuli and tasks. Tinnitus induces a strong negative reaction of the limbic and autonomic nervous systems, resulting at the behavioral level in anxiety, annoyance, panic, and, notably, a decrease in or suppression of the ability to enjoy life activities.

The classification center receives input from sensory systems, integrating this information, comparing it with memory, and providing relative assessment of the significance of a given stimulus and its positive or negative connotation. Outputs of this center perform several functions: First, gate the access to awareness so that the person is fully aware of the most important stimulus at a given time and ensure that only the dominant task requiring attention is to be carried on. The system is involved in task switching and opening and closing sensory inputs for stimuli required for voluntary selected tasks. Second, modulate sensory input to the limbic and autonomic nervous systems. Third, modulate the general level of the activation of the limbic and autonomic nervous systems.

In the case of tinnitus, once it achieves a high level of significance, the classification center will open its access to awareness, enhance this signal on its passage from the auditory system to the limbic and autonomic nervous systems, and enhance the general level of activation of these systems. All of these changes will result in a higher level of activation of the limbic and autonomic nervous systems evoked by the same tinnitus-related neuronal activity in the auditory pathways. The functional centers and their connections discussed above are presented in Figure 8-3, whereas Figure 8-4 shows the same neurophysiological model of tinnitus but with a focus on anatomic sites, as has been presented previously.[2]

ENHANCING FUNCTIONAL CONNECTIONS WITHIN THE NEUROPHYSIOLOGICAL MODEL OF TINNITUS

All connections in the brain are subject to continuous changes dependent on the existing activations of interactive neuronal pathways (the dynamic balance scenario).[36,37] Once initial functional connections are created, owing to naturally existing excitatory feedback loops, they undergo enhancement until a physiologically determined metastable state is achieved. The decisive factor determining the extent of reactions

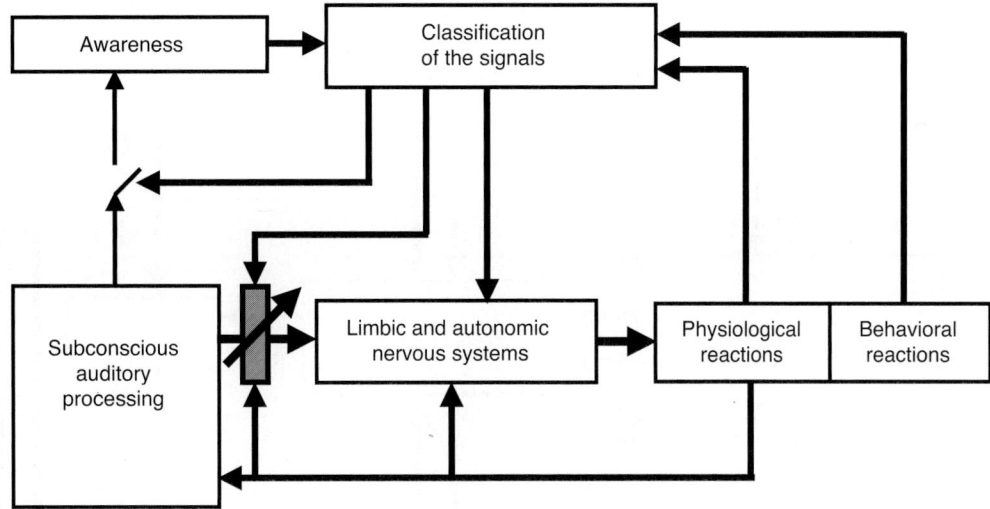

FIGURE 8-3. Functional centers and their connections involved in tinnitus and misophonia.

to tinnitus is the strength of connection between the auditory system and the limbic and autonomic nervous systems and not the strength of the tinnitus-related neuronal activity.

Some level of stress and activation of the limbic and sympathetic parts of the autonomic nervous system is needed for optimal performance of a subject in learning or performing any type of activity. Both too low and too high levels of activation cause a decrease in performance. One of the postulated functions of the classification center is adjusting the general level of activation of the limbic and autonomic nervous systems to optimize performance, resulting in enhancing the strength of connections between auditory and other systems.

At the cognitive level, increased awareness of tinnitus will further enhance its importance, which, in turn, further increases the proportion of time in which patients are aware of tinnitus. At the subconscious level, feedback influence of the limbic and autonomic nervous systems on the auditory system (physiologic reactions) enhances tuning of neuronal networks to a specific pattern of neuronal activity related to tinnitus. In the case of misophonia, similar tuning will occur to patterns evoked by specific categories of sound.

SUSTAINING OR REVERSING FUNCTIONAL CONNECTIONS

The strength of connections in the brain is governed by the principle of dynamic balance, changes continuously, and requires a specific action to be preserved and not extinguished. As argued above, owing to the continuous presence of the tinnitus signal and the fact that reactions evoked by this signal act as self-reinforcement for the conditioned reflex arc (see Figure 8-2), the strength of this particular arc is continuously promoted. Consequently, once this arc is established, it is very stable and does not undergo extinction. Two systems are involved in sustaining this reflex (see Figure 8-3): the classification system and the self-reinforcement provided by reactions. Although both systems involve conscious and subconscious processes, physiological reactions act, however, at the purely subconscious level, for example, changes in levels of stress-related hormones and neuromodulators.

EXTINCTION (RETRAINING) OF THE TINNITUS-RELATED CONDITIONED REFLEX ARCS

Note that both systems must be modified to remove the enhancement action of the tinnitus signal on the reflex arc to be able to decrease or even remove functional connections between the sensory (auditory) system and the limbic and autonomic nervous systems. Preserved activity in one of these systems would be sufficient in sustaining the reflex arc connecting the auditory with the autonomic nervous system. Physiological reactions are prewired and cannot be changed, or, at least, it is very difficult to modify them. As long as the classification system facilitates and enhances connections between the auditory system and the limbic and autonomic nervous systems, the arc

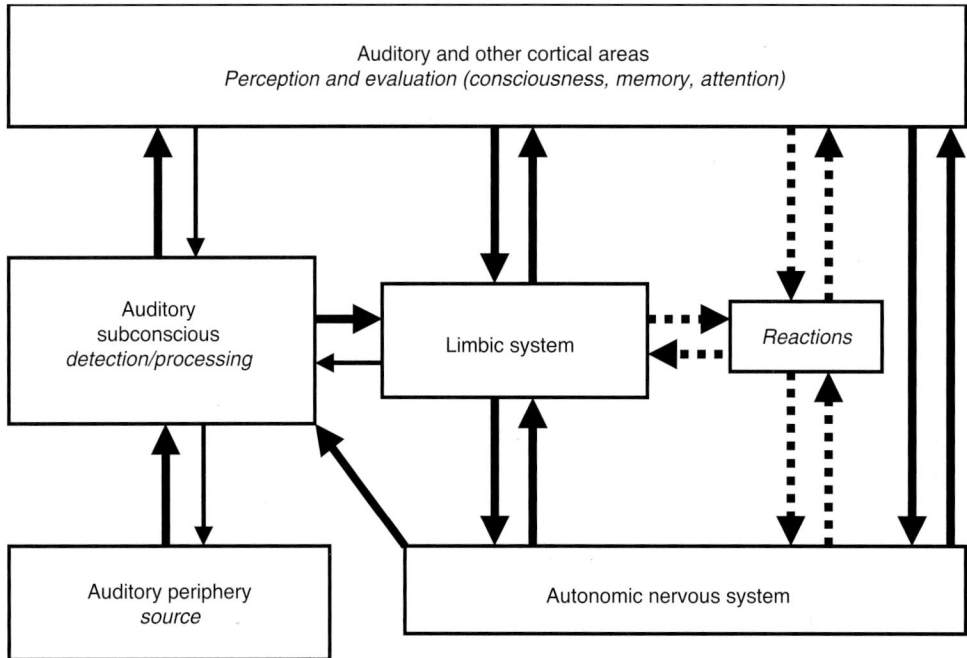

FIGURE 8-4. The neurophysiological model of tinnitus, as presented previously, with focus on anatomic sites. Dashed arrows indicate the interactions between various systems in the nervous system and reactions.

will remain active and stable. Thus, the first crucial step in the process yielding removal of this functional connection is to reclassify the tinnitus signal, aiming at decreasing its importance.

However, it is not necessary to make the signal totally neutral to initiate the process of weakening connections of the auditory system with other systems. At the same time, even if the importance of the signal decreases to neutral, the connections of the auditory system with other systems will remain active owing to the sustaining action of physiological reactions. However, it is also possible to weaken connections between reactions and the classification system.

Successful reclassification of the tinnitus signal to a neutral category will initially result in a decrease in the activation of the limbic and autonomic nervous systems and in a decrease in the strength of the connection between the auditory system and other systems, creating the basis for the gradual extinction of this connection. In the case of mild tinnitus, this might be sufficient for initiating a further decrease in the strength of the connections and the final extinction of the conditioned reflex arc. Typically, it is not sufficient because the tinnitus signal is unchanged and the physiological reactions remain and are adequate to sustain the reflex arc. Therefore, in a majority of cases, it is beneficial to add another factor: decrease the strength of the tinnitus-related neuronal activity.

Simultaneous decrease of the output from the classification system (achieved by reclassification of the tinnitus) and decrease of the strength of the tinnitus signal create the optimal condition for breaking connections of the auditory system with the limbic and autonomic nervous systems by a concurrent decrease of the signal, of the negative reinforcement, and of awareness. This, in turn, results in a further decrease in the reactions induced by the tinnitus signal. Finally, disappearance of the tinnitus-evoked reactions occurs as a result of the repeated presence of the weakened tinnitus signal while the reinforcement is decreased.

HABITUATION (PASSIVE EXTINCTION) OF TINNITUS-RELATED CONDITIONED REFLEXES

If it would be possible to remove the reinforcement totally while preserving the same strength of the conditioned stimulus, this process would fit exactly the definition of passive extinction of conditioned reflexes,[26] which is also called habituation.[38] In the case of tinnitus, owing to the self-reinforcing nature of the reflex arc, extinction is achieved with decreasing strength of the signal and the reinforcement. Owing to the inability to remove the reinforcement totally, the process of extinction happens more gradually but, in turn, is facilitated by a decrease in the signal strength. Note that a decrease in the tinnitus-related neuronal activity will reduce the input to the classification system, further limiting its output (see Figure 8-3) and further facilitating extinction of the reflex arc.

Once the tinnitus signal is classified as more neutral, awareness will decrease because of the ongoing process of habituation to all neutral signals. As long as the tinnitus signal retains some importance, the proportion of time that a patient is aware of tinnitus will depend on the level of the significance of the tinnitus versus the significance of other stimuli to which the subject is exposed and on the importance of other tasks in which the patient is involved.

CERTAIN RAMIFICATIONS OF THE NEUROPHYSIOLOGICAL MODEL OF TINNITUS

A specific method of treatment implementing the described model into clinical practice is known as tinnitus retraining therapy (TRT) (see Chapter 21, "Tinnitus Retraining Therapy"). TRT uses teaching or counseling sessions to reclassify the tinnitus signal and sound to decrease the strength of the tinnitus-related neuronal activity. The same general principles described above are used in the model for decreased sound tolerance (presented in Chapter 2) and in its treatment (see Chapter 21).

Note that total blockage of the tinnitus-related neuronal activity by suppression ("masking") will, by definition, prevent retraining because it is impossible to retrain neuronal networks to a signal that cannot be detected by the brain. Partially suppressed tinnitus can still be habituated, but the effectiveness of habituation will decrease because retraining will occur not to the original but to the modified signal.

There are some further ramifications of the model. The method aimed at habituation of signal works outside the auditory system (specifically at connections between the auditory system and the limbic and autonomic nervous systems) or at the highest level of the auditory system (gating mechanism of perception). Therefore, the source of the signal within the auditory system is irrelevant, and the method can be used for any type or cause of tinnitus and for physical sound, for example, somatosounds and misophonia.

The model and approach are aimed at habituation of reactions induced by a sensory signal and its perception and can be used for other sensory modalities, for example, pain, somatosensory perception, and smell.

REFERENCES

1. Jastreboff PJ. Phantom auditory perception (tinnitus): mechanisms of generation and perception. Neurosci Res 1990;8:221–54.
2. Jastreboff PJ, Jastreboff MM. Tinnitus and hyperacusis. In: Snow JB, Ballenger JJ, editors. Ballenger's otorhinolaryngology head and neck surgery. 16th ed. Hamilton (ON): BC Decker; 2003. p. 456–75.
3. Jastreboff PJ, Jastreboff MM. The neurophysiological model of tinnitus and its practical implementation: current status. In: Myers EN, Bluestone CD, Brackman DE, et al, editors. Advances in otolaryngology-head and neck surgery. Vol 15. St. Louis: Mosby; 2001. p. 135–47.
4. Jastreboff PJ. Tinnitus as a phantom perception: theories and clinical implications. In: Vernon J, Møller AR, editors. Mechanisms of tinnitus. Boston: Allyn & Bacon; 1995. p. 73–94.
5. Kaltenbach JA, Rachel JD, Mathog TA, et al. Cisplatin-induced hyperactivity in the dorsal cochlear nucleus and its relation to outer hair cell loss: relevance to tinnitus. J Neurophysiol 2002;88:699–714.
6. Chen G-D, Jastreboff PJ. Salicylate-induced abnormal activity in the inferior colliculus of rats. Hear Res 1995;82:158-178.
7. Kwon O, Jastreboff MM, Hu S, et al. Modification of single-unit activity related to noise-induced tinnitus in rats. In: Hazell J, editor. Proceedings of the Sixth International Tinnitus Seminar, Cambridge, UK. London: The Tinnitus and Hyperacusis Centre; 1999. p. 459–62.
8. Boettcher FA, Salvi RJ. Functional changes in the ventral cochlear nucleus following acute acoustic overstimulation. J Acoust Soc Am 1993;94:2123–34.
9. Gerken GM, Saunders SS, Paul RE. Hypersensitivity to electrical stimulation of auditory nuclei follows hearing loss in cats. Hear Res 1984;13:249–59.
10. Gerken GM, Simhadri-Sumithra R, Bhat KHV. Increase in central auditory responsiveness during continuous tone stimulation or following hearing loss. In: Salvi RJ, Henderson D, Hamernik RP, Colletti V, editors.

Basic and applied aspects of noise-induced hearing loss. New York: Plenum Publishing Corporation; 1986. p. 195–211.
11. Salvi R, Saunders S, Powers N, Gratton MA. Acoustic trauma can "enhance" evoked response amplitudes in chinchillas. In: Berglund B, Berglund U, Karlsson J, Lindvall T, editors. Noise as a public health problem. Vol 2. Hearing, communication, sleep and nonauditory physiological effects. Stockholm: Swedish Council for Building Research; 1988. p. 347–52.
12. Salvi RJ, Saunders SS, Gratton MA, et al. Enhanced evoked response amplitudes in the inferior colliculus of the chinchilla following acoustic trauma. Hear Res 1990;50:245–58.
13. Heller MF, Bergman M. Tinnitus in normally hearing persons. Ann Otol Rhinol Laryngol 1953;62:73–93.
14. Davis A, El Refaie A. Epidemiology of tinnitus. In: Tyler RS, editor. Tinnitus handbook. San Diego (CA): Singular, Thomson Learning; 2000. p. 1–23.
15. Coles RR. Epidemiology of tinnitus: (1) prevalence. J Laryngol Otol Suppl 1984;9:7–15.
16. Sindhusake D, Mitchell P, Newall P, et al. Prevalence and characteristics of tinnitus in older adults: the Blue Mountains Hearing Study. Int J Audiol 2003;42:289–94.
17. Axelsson A, Ringdahl A. Tinnitus—a study of its prevalence and characteristics. Br J Audiol 1989;23:53–62.
18. Hoshiyama M, Kakigi R, Watanabe S, et al. Brain responses for the subconscious recognition of faces. Neurosci Res 2003;46:435–42.
19. David D, Brown RJ. The impact of different directed forgetting instructions on implicit and explicit memory: new evidence from a modified process dissociation procedure. Q J Exp Psychol A 2003;56:211–31.
20. Snodgrass M. Disambiguating conscious and unconscious influences: do exclusion paradigms demonstrate unconscious perception? Am J Psychol 2002;115:545–79.
21. Klapp ST, Hinkley LB. The negative compatibility effect: unconscious inhibition influences reaction time and response selection. J Exp Psychol Gen 2002;131:255–69.
22. Salidis J. Nonconscious temporal cognition: learning rhythms implicitly. Mem Cognit 2001;29:1111–9.
23. Bargh JA, Gollwitzer PM, Lee-Chai A, et al. The automated will: nonconscious activation and pursuit of behavioral goals. J Pers Soc Psychol 2001;81:1014–27.
24. Caldwell JI, Masson ME. Conscious and unconscious influences of memory for object location. Mem Cognit 2001;29:285–95.
25. Esteves F, Para C, Dimberg U, Ohman A. Nonconscious associative learning: pavlovian conditioning of skin conductance responses to masked fear-relevant facial stimuli. Psychophysiology 1994;31:375–85.
26. Konorski J. Conditioned reflexes and neuronal organization. Cambridge (UK): Cambridge University Press; 1948.
27. McFadden D. Tinnitus: facts, theories, and treatments. Washington (DC): National Academy Press; 1982.
28. Kimberg DY, Aguirre GK, D'Esposito M. Modulation of task-related neural activity in task-switching: an fMRI study. Brain Res Cogn Brain Res 2000;10:189–96.
29. Schmahmann JD, Sherman JC. The cerebellar cognitive affective syndrome. Brain 1998;121(Pt 4):561–79.
30. Schmahmann JD, Sherman JC. Cerebellar cognitive affective syndrome. Int Rev Neurobiol 1997;41:433–40.
31. Gottwald B, Mihajlovic Z, Wilde B, Mehdorn HM. Does the cerebellum contribute to specific aspects of attention? Neuropsychologia 2003;41:1452–60.
32. Miller MJ, Chen NK, Li L, et al. fMRI of the conscious rabbit during unilateral classical eyeblink conditioning reveals bilateral cerebellar activation. J Neurosci 2003;23:11753–8.
33. Marien P, Engelborghs S, Fabbro F, De Deyn PP. The lateralized linguistic cerebellum: a review and a new hypothesis. Brain Lang 2001;79:580–600.
34. Marien P, Engelborghs S, De Deyn PP. Cerebellar neurocognition: a new avenue. Acta Neurol Belg 2001;101:96–109.
35. Reyes SA, Salvi RJ, Burkard RF, et al. Brain imaging of the effects of lidocaine on tinnitus. Hear Res 2002;171:43–50.
36. Albus JS. A theory of cerebellar function. Math Biosci 1971;10:25–61.
37. Pribram KH. Languages of the brain—experimental paradoxes and principles in neurophysiology. Englewood Cliffs (NJ): Prentice Hall; 1971.
38. The American heritage dictionary. 3rd ed. Boston: SoftKey International; 1994.

EDITORIAL COMMENTARY

Moody evaluates several existing and developing animal models of tinnitus and concludes that they are useful approaches to detect the experiencing of tinnitus by animals. Jastreboff's seminal contribution provides a means for specifying the intensity of tinnitus that a group of animals is experiencing. The procedure of Bauer and associates allows longer-term experiments. Heffner's procedures allow study of individual animals for correlation with hearing parameters and neural activity in the central auditory centers.

Moody's efforts toward the ideal model capable of evaluating tinnitus in individual subjects is based on the behavioral pharmacologists' study of drug effects in animals. In addition, the ideal animal model should provide measures of the intensity, frequency, and spectrum of the tinnitus and allow discrimination between the presence of tinnitus and the effects of the associated hearing loss. The increased scientific effort in this endeavor is encouraging.

Jastreboff emphasizes that in individuals who suffer with tinnitus as opposed to those who only experience tinnitus, the auditory system plays a secondary role. He stresses the role of the sustained activation of the limbic and autonomic nervous systems, particularly the sympathetic part of the autonomic nervous system. According to his neurophysiological model of tinnitus, when tinnitus-related neuronal activity is temporally associated with cognitively induced or high stress–induced activation of the limbic and autonomic nervous systems, a conditioned reflex is established. Initially, these mechanisms provide negative reinforcement for the reflex. Subsequently, the tinnitus signal activates the limbic and autonomic nervous systems without adverse cognition or stress. Physiological and behavioral reactions evoked by the activation of the limbic and autonomic nervous systems provide negative reinforcement of the reflex, and a vicious circle ensues.

Jastreboff points out that tinnitus is classified by the individual as to its importance and its positive or negative connotation. Reinforcement becomes stronger with greater importance of the stimulus, and the type of reaction is determined by the type of connotation. The continuous tinnitus-related neuronal activity and the reactions caused by the activation of the limbic and autonomic nervous systems prevent the extinction of the reflex.

Jastreboff makes the compelling case for the need for the patient to reclassify tinnitus to decrease activation of the limbic and autonomic nervous systems, to weaken the connection between the auditory system and the limbic and autonomic nervous systems, and to decrease the strength of the tinnitus-related neuronal activity aimed at weakening the reflex arc. In tinnitus retraining therapy, counseling helps the patient reclassify the tinnitus signal, and sound therapy is used to decrease the strength of the tinnitus-related neuronal activity.

James B. Snow Jr

CHAPTER 9

Somatic Tinnitus

Robert A. Levine, MD

When the quality of tinnitus is nonspecific (such as buzzing, tonal, hissing, humming, ringing, roaring, rushing, whistling and whooshing, crickets), establishing a cause for the tinnitus is a challenging problem. An experienced clinician has observed, "If the probability is assessed as being over 50% that a particular condition is causing the tinnitus, ...most cases of tinnitus would have to be classified as 'unknown'" (ie, idiopathic).[1]

Among the reasons why establishing the cause for nonspecific tinnitus is so difficult is the fact that tinnitus is common in the general population presumably because it can be a normal physiologic phenomenon. At one extreme is the study by Heller and Bergman, who found that 94% of people they studied had tinnitus.[2] A more recent study found that although 19% of adults, when questioned, reported tinnitus, when the same individuals were then taken to a quiet room, another 28% described some tinnitus, so that a total of 47% described nonspecific tinnitus.[3]

Another reason contributing to the difficulty in establishing a cause for nonspecific tinnitus is that for any pathologic process associated with tinnitus, not all subjects with this diagnosis will, in fact, develop tinnitus. An extreme case is individuals who are deaf; 80% have tinnitus, but 20% have no tinnitus.[4] Hence, the presence of tinnitus and the existence of a pathologic process by themselves do not imply that the two are related.

Another consideration in attempting to establish a diagnosis to account for a patient's tinnitus is that the cause of the tinnitus may be multifactorial. A closely related idea is that tinnitus can be considered a threshold phenomenon,[5] such that whereas any one factor, such as chronic progressive hearing loss, may not be sufficient to elicit a tinnitus complaint, two or more factors may synergistically lead to the tinnitus becoming symptomatic. For example, it is well established that the prevalence of tinnitus increases with increasing hearing loss for any type of chronic progressive sensorineural hearing loss, such as presbycusis, chronic acoustic trauma, or a hereditary hearing loss. The recent onset of tinnitus in a patient with a known chronic progressive sensorineural hearing loss suggests that some other factor might be combining with the sensorineural hearing loss to lead to the tinnitus. Along a similar vein, several authors have put forth the concept of "triggering factors" that can lead to symptomatic chronic tinnitus.[1,6]

What might be some of these triggering factors? First, any pathologic process associated with tinnitus can be a triggering factor. Some classes of medications probably can be triggering factors, although this has not been well established for any medication. From our clinical experience, α_1-selective adrenoreceptor blocking agents, benzimidazole inhibitors of gastric acid secretion, and angiotensin-converting enzyme inhibitors appear to be triggering factors in some cases. Finally, any factor that has been associated with changes in tinnitus loudness would also qualify as a triggering factor. At least three factors often are associated with changes in the loudness of tinnitus, namely psychosocial stress, high-intensity sound exposure, and head and neck "somatic" factors. People with clinical tinnitus commonly describe one or more of these three factors as altering their perception of their tinnitus.

If a patient reports that his or her tinnitus is intermittent or has wide fluctuations in loudness or other qualities, and there is neither exposure to intense sound nor evidence of stress, then somatic modulation must be suspected. Consider the following case: *Case 1.* A 77-year-old woman, who had two major thyroid operations at age 23 and 26 years, reported 5 months of non-lateralized intermittent tinnitus. The tinnitus was always present upon awakening but at times would disappear during the day. Pure-tone thresholds were normal for both ears except at 8 kHz where both ears had thresholds of 60 dB HL and at 4 kHz for the left ear where the threshold was 30 dB HL. Brief firm pressure at the insertion of her right sternocleidomastoid (SCM) muscle onto the mastoid process abolished her right ear tinnitus for more than 8 minutes and reduced her left ear tinnitus loudness from 5/10 to 3/10 on a 0 to 10 loudness scale for less than a minute.

A history of variations in tinnitus loudness raises the suspicion of a somatic factor modulating the percept's loudness (Table 9-1). At an extreme are patients who describe that they have periods when their tinnitus cannot be heard, even in the quiet. Others report wide variations in the loudness of their tinnitus. For still others, their tinnitus is unilateral when it is relatively quiet but becomes nonlateralized when the tinnitus is louder (see case 6 below). Such phenomena suggest that there are ongoing somatically mediated factors modulating the tinnitus percept.

Diurnal fluctuations in the tinnitus percept also suggest that somatic modulation is operative. Patients who describe their tinnitus as louder on awakening raise the possibility that somatic factors such as bruxism (grinding of the teeth) are active during sleep and are causing an increase in tinnitus loudness. Others report that their tinnitus has usually vanished by the time they awaken and then returns a few hours into the day; this scenario suggests that, during the day, they are reactivating their tinnitus through somatic mechanisms, such as the tonic muscle contractions required to support the head in an upright position or clenching the jaws related to the stress of daily activities. Finally, others report that their tinnitus is louder after awakening from a nap in a chair; this may relate to somatic factors such as stretching of the neck muscles when their head passively falls forward while dozing in a sitting position.

In this chapter, I explore further this "somatic" factor. I review the effects of muscle contractions and other closely related somatic factors on auditory perception in general and tinnitus in particular. The evidence is reviewed for (1) how somatic factors are commonly responsible for fluctuations in tinnitus perception, (2) how somatic factors can act as a trigger factor and thereby lead to the somatic tinnitus syndrome, and (3) how somatic factors can combine with other conditions to cause tinnitus on a multifactorial basis. Finally, I provide a hypothesis that can serve as a conceptual framework to account for the interactions between hearing and a variety of nonotic factors, including the somatic factor.

SOMATIC FACTORS ARE COMMONLY RESPONSIBLE FOR FLUCTUATIONS IN TINNITUS PERCEPTION

It has long been known, almost as a curiosity, that some people can modulate their tinnitus somatically. Møller and colleagues showed that median nerve stimulation could modulate tinnitus in close to 40% of subjects.[7] Rubinstein found that approximately one-third of her subjects could influence their tinnitus with jaw movements or pressure on the temporomandibular joint (TMJ).[8] When interviewed, approximately 20% of patients in our tinnitus clinic reported that they can somatically modulate the acoustic properties of their tinnitus by head and neck movements or muscle contractions such as clenching the teeth together.[9] In a systematic study of 70 consecutive patients in my tinnitus clinic, my colleagues and I found that 68% could somatically modulate their tinnitus with head or neck maneuvers.[10] With the same maneuvers, Sanchez and colleagues reported almost identical results (65%).[11] When we added jaw maneuvers to our test battery (Table 9-2), the percentage of those who could somatically modulate their tinnitus rose to 80%.[3] Thus, somatic modulation of tinnitus is very common in clinical tinnitus subjects. A typical pattern of somatic modulation is illustrated by the following case.

Case 2. A 50-year-old man had nonlateralized high-pitched tinnitus that had begun with an upper respiratory infection 9 months earlier. Prior to his visit, he had noticed that jaw protrusion increased the loudness of his tinnitus, and he suspected that his tinnitus was louder on awakening when he had consumed modest quantities of wine the previous night. His audiogram was symmetric, and all pure-tone thresholds were 25 dB HL or better. His pattern of modulation is the most common type (Table 9-3): his tinnitus only became louder, and the change in loudness did not persist following the release of a forceful contraction. Also typical is the pattern of tinnitus mod-

TABLE 9-1. Tinnitus Properties Suggesting a Somatic Component

Intermittency
Large fluctuations in loudness
Variability of location
Diurnal pattern
No hearing loss but head, neck, or dental insult

TABLE 9-2. Maneuvers Currently Being Used to Test for Somatic Modulation (All Use Maximal Force)

Jaw Contractions

1. Clench teeth together
2, 3. Open mouth, with and without restorative pressure
4, 5. Protrude jaw, with and without restorative pressure
6, 7. Slide jaw to left, with and without restorative pressure
8, 9. Slide jaw to right, with and without restorative pressure
10. Retract jaw

Head and Neck Contractions

With the head in the neutral position, contractions are made to resist pressure applied by the examiner to

11. The forehead
12. The occiput
13. The vertex
14. The left temple
15. The right temple
16. The left zygoma, with the head turned fully to the left
17. The right zygoma, with the head turned fully to the right
18. The left temple, with the head turned to the right and tilted to the left (left sternocleidomastoid muscle)
19. The right temple, with the head turned to the left and tilted to the right (right sternocleidomastoid muscle)

Extremity Contractions

20. Pulling apart the locked fingers of the two hands

Resisting pressure to

21. Left hip flexion
22. Right hip flexion
23. Left shoulder abduction
24. Right shoulder abduction

---

ulation that occurred with the maneuvers that can be attributed to the contraction of a single muscle; namely, lateral deviation of the jaw (subserved by the contralateral medial pterygoid muscle) is usually associated with changes in the contralateral ear only, whereas SCM muscle contractions usually affect only the ipsilateral ear.

To assess whether somatic modulation is a general phenonenon and not restricted to clinical tinnitus subjects, my colleagues and I tested somatic modulation in 62 nonclinical subjects (friends and relatives).[3] Our only exclusion criterion was that they had never sought any medical care for tinnitus. Twelve (19%) knew that they had tinnitus, but it was not a problem, and 17 (27%) were unaware that they had tinnitus until we brought them into a low–ambient noise room and asked them what they heard. In this group of 29 nonclinical subjects with tinnitus, 23 (again about 80%) could modulate their tinnitus. Hence, somatic modulation of tinnitus is not restricted to the clinical population; its incidence (80% with our test battery) is the same for all populations with tinnitus and probably all causes of tinnitus. This implies that the ability to modulate tinnitus somatically is not what makes tinnitus a clinical problem.

Finally, when we tested the other 33 nonclinical subjects who in the quiet had no tinnitus whatsoever, even when pointedly questioned, somatic testing elicited an acoustic perception ("tinnitus") in 19, or almost 60%. Thus, somatic modulation of auditory perception is a fundamental property of the auditory system that happens to be most obvious in tinnitus subjects because they have spontaneous ongoing auditory perception. In fact, it has been shown that the perception of external sounds can also be somatically modulated. Møller and Rollins reported that the perception of ex-

TABLE 9-3. Somatic Testing for Case 2

Maneuver*	Right Ear Tinnitus Loudness	Left Ear Tinnitus Loudness
Baseline (0–10 scale)	7	7
2. Open mouth	8.5	8.5
3. Open mouth, against resistance	9	9
4. Protrude jaw	9	9
5. Protrude jaw, against resistance	9	9
9. Slide jaw to right, against resistance	7	9
11. Forehead	7.5	7.5
18. Sternocleidomastoid muscle, left	7	7.5
19. Sternocleidomastoid muscle, right	8	7

*Only maneuvers that modulated the patient's tinnitus are shown.

ternally generated sounds can be modulated by a nonphysiologic type of somatosensory stimulation, namely median nerve stimulation at the wrist.[12] Of those who could modulate, 83% perceived the external sound as louder and 17% as softer. Although they found that 60% of subjects could modulate their perception of the external sound, they did not use a physiologic stimulus and did not stimulate the most sensitive region for somatic modulation of tinnitus, the head and upper neck (see below). It is likely that even more subjects would modulate their perception of an external sound with other types of somatosensory stimuli.

Now that it has been established that subjects without tinnitus can somatically modulate their auditory perception, the lower incidence of change in auditory perception with somatic testing in subjects with no tinnitus than in subjects with tinnitus is readily explained. From our observations of clinical and nonclinical tinnitus subjects, it is clear that somatic testing can increase and/or decrease tinnitus loudness and pitch (see below). If such changes in auditory perception are happening equally for all groups of subjects, one would expect the incidence of a change in auditory perception to be less in people without tinnitus than in those who have an ongoing auditory perception (tinnitus) for at least two reasons: (1) if somatic modulation decreases the loudness of auditory perception, then this would not be detected in the nontinnitus subjects, similarly for any change of pitch, and (2) if somatic testing causes only a small degree of change in the level of activity in the auditory system, such as might be perceived in tinnitus subjects as a small change in their tinnitus loudness, subjects without tinnitus might raise the overall activity in their auditory pathways but not enough to cross the threshold of auditory perception. Thus, for these two reasons, the incidence of change in auditory perception will be lower in the nontinnitus groups than in the tinnitus groups.

A similar result was obtained for the effect of loud sounds on tinnitus. We asked all 62 nonclinical subjects whether they had ever experienced tinnitus after a loud sound; 32% of those without tinnitus in the quiet reported affirmatively compared with 63% of those experiencing tinnitus at the time.[5] This highly significant difference ($p < .01$) can be explained in a similar way using the threshold idea. If loud sounds cause only a small degree of change in the level of activity in the auditory system, such as might be perceived in tinnitus subjects as a small change in their tinnitus loudness, subjects without tinnitus might raise the overall activity in their auditory pathways but not enough to cross the threshold of auditory perception.

Alterations in tinnitus perception that occurred with somatic testing of the clinical and nonclinical tinnitus subjects were similar and included changes in loudness, pitch, or location. By far, most common were changes in tinnitus loudness that could be either louder or softer or louder for some maneuvers and quieter for others in the same subject. Of these, increased loudness alone was the most frequent, as shown in Table 9-4 for nonclinical subjects. Five of the subjects with ongoing tinnitus at the time of testing could increase their tinnitus loudness with some contractions and decrease it with others; in four of these five, their tinnitus was not perceptible with at least one of the maneuvers. Pitch changes were described by 13 of the subjects; in all except 1 subject, loudness changes also occurred. Four of the subjects described the pitch change as a new sound in addition to their baseline tinnitus percept, which continued to be present unchanged.

TABLE 9-4. Loudness Changes with Somatic Testing Reported by Subjects with Ongoing Tinnitus Using the 0 to 10 Loudness Scale

Direction of Change	Number of Subjects	Range		Mean
		Minimum	Maximum	
Increase in loudness	20	0.5	5	2.2
Decrease in loudness	7	0.1	3	1.0

Sometimes the effects of somatic testing were prolonged. In 21% of subjects who could change or induce tinnitus with a somatic manipulation, the effect persisted after the contraction was released. This effect could be for a few seconds or up to 10 minutes. The two longest ones (5 and 10 minutes) occurred in subjects who had had no tinnitus before the somatic modulation testing. The maneuvers that altered a subject's tinnitus varied from subject to subject. On average, seven different maneuvers altered a subject's auditory perception (range 1–20). This average and range were about the same whether or not a subject had tinnitus at the time of testing.

Head and neck contractions changed tinnitus more effectively than extremity contractions. Without exception, whenever extremity maneuvers modulated or elicited tinnitus, head and neck maneuvers also did so, but the reverse was not always true. In fact, twice as many subjects could modify or elicit tinnitus with head and neck contractions as with extremity contractions. Whichever the direction of the loudness changes, those elicited by head and neck maneuvers in any subject were always equal to or larger than those from extremity maneuvers of the same subject. Although Cullington reported a single subject who could somatically modulate his left ear tinnitus with active movement of his left long finger, the report does not describe the effect of head and neck movements, so it is unclear what head and neck movements would have done for this subject.[13] In any case, we have never encountered such a subject.

We have probed further into our understanding of somatic modulation of tinnitus by testing individuals who are deaf (cochlear implant subjects with their implant disconnected). At present, 13 deaf subjects have been tested in the standard manner ("somatic testing"). At the time of testing, 10 subjects had ongoing tinnitus and 3 did not. Five of the 10 (50%) with ongoing tinnitus could modulate their tinnitus with somatic testing, whereas 2 of the 3 (67%) without tinnitus could elicit an auditory percept with somatic testing. As with hearing subjects, loudness changes were the most common type of somatic modulation. Of the five with ongoing tinnitus, three increased and two decreased their tinnitus loudness with somatic testing. No subjects of this group did both. Likewise, the effects of somatic testing could persist; the longest was for a subject whose tinnitus disappeared for 4 minutes. Pitch changes also occurred but only in one subject. For this subject, loudness increased for some maneuvers, whereas pitch increased for others. In all of these subjects, head and neck maneuvers were more effective in altering auditory perception than extremity maneuvers.

Consider the following two examples. In case 3 somatic testing elicited tinnitus in a deaf subject who had no ongoing tinnitus. In case 4 somatic testing modulated tinnitus in a deaf subject who had ongoing tinnitus.

Case 3. This 52-year-old woman had received a left cochlear implant 12 years earlier. She had no tinnitus with her processor connected or disconnected. Three months prior to testing, she experienced 45 minutes of left ear tinnitus three times over a week but not subsequently. The effects of somatic testing are shown in Table 9-5.

Case 4. This 52-year-old man had received a right cochlear implant 16 years earlier. He had no tinnitus with his processor connected but heard "wind" in his right ear with the processor disconnected. His tinnitus persisted louder for up to 2 minutes with forehead pressure and 1 minute with right temple pressure (Table 9-6).

Our findings in the cochlear implant subjects with and without tinnitus, who describe changes in their auditory perceptions with somatic testing, clearly indicate that acoustic sounds are not responsible for their results because these subjects are deaf and their implant was not activated at the time of somatic testing. Furthermore, the similarities in the characteristics of the changes in auditory perception that occur for all groups suggest that the mechanism operating in individuals who are deaf is likewise operating for most, if not all, of the other groups. Thus, I

TABLE 9-5. Somatic Testing for Case 3

Maneuver*	Right Ear Tinnitus Loudness	Left Ear Tinnitus Loudness
Baseline (0–10 scale)	0	0
2. Open jaw	0	1
5. Protrude jaw against resistance	0	0.5
10. Retract jaw	0	0.5

*Only maneuvers that elicited the patient's tinnitus are shown.

conclude that somatosensory-auditory neural interactions within the central nervous system account for most, if not all, somatic modulations of tinnitus and the development of auditory percepts with somatic testing.

Some of our observations provide insights into the neural system responsible for somatic modulation of auditory perception (somatic modulation of tinnitus). The cutaneous sensory system is unlikely. Never in our clinical experience or from clinical reports have intact patients reported that light touch can modify auditory perception. The only report of cutaneous stimulation causing modulation of auditory perception is in two patients who had been deafened by posterior fossa surgery.[14] On the other hand, the motor system is likely because the actions that elicit modulations of auditory perception are almost exclusively non-noxious but forceful muscle contractions. Such contractions involve (1) the entire voluntary efferent motor system (motor cortex, corticospinal or corticobulbar tracts, and primary motoneurons) and (2) the motor afferent system, which begins with the deep muscle receptors such as the muscle spindles and tendon organs.

One fortuitous occurrence has shown that muscle fatigue can abolish somatic modulation of auditory perception.

Case 5. A 57-year-old man with lifelong nonlateralized tinnitus could increase the loudness of his tinnitus with jaw protrusion from an estimated loudness of 4 of 10 to 6 of 10. After being a subject of a functional magnetic resonance imaging (fMRI) experiment in which he repeatedly modulated his tinnitus with jaw protrusion for approximately an hour, for the next 3 to 4 days, he could not modulate his tinnitus, following which his ability to modulate with jaw protrusion gradually returned over about a day.

Muscle fatigue is principally due to fatigue (weakening) of the muscle fibers per se and not the motor efferent system. Unlike the efferent system, the motor afferent system requires contraction of the muscle fibers to be activated. Therefore, muscle fatigue inactivates the motor afferent system but not the motor efferent system. Hence, the motor afferent system (from muscle spindles and Golgi tendon organs) is responsible for at least some, if not all, somatic modulation of auditory perception.

The Golgi tendon organ senses muscle tension, and the muscle spindle senses muscle length. Because somatic testing is done principally with isometric muscle contractions (ie, little change in muscle length), our results favor the Golgi tendon organ as the source for somatic modulation of auditory perception.

TABLE 9-6. Somatic Testing for Case 4

Maneuver*	Right Ear Tinnitus Loudness	Left Ear Tinnitus Loudness
Baseline (0–10 scale)	4	0
3. Open jaw against resistance	5	0
5. Protrude jaw against resistance	5	0
11. Forehead pressure	5	0
15. Right temple pressure	6	0
16. Left turn	5	0
18. Left sternocleidomastoid muscle	5	0

*Only maneuvers that modulated the patient's tinnitus are shown.

On the other hand, another observation favors the muscle spindle.

Case 6. A 69-year-old woman with tinnitus for about 2½ years described her hissing tinnitus as varying in location and intensity. When soft, it was heard in the right ear and when loud throughout the head. It was never heard in the left ear only. At the time of one of her visits, her tinnitus was very loud and perceived throughout the head. She rated its loudness as 8 on a 0 to 10 scale. On examination, her left SCM muscle was taut and tender; her right SCM muscle was normal. Vibration with a handheld massager applied to her right SCM muscle did not alter her tinnitus. However, when applied to her left SCM muscle, she noticed that the tinnitus gradually became quieter (4 of 10) over about 5 minutes and shifted its location from throughout the head to the right ear only. It remained quieter and in the right ear for about 30 minutes.

Because vibration is known to be a potent activator of muscle spindles, this result provides support for the hypothesis that muscle spindle activation is a mediator of somatic modulation.

Hence, our observations support the hypothesis that both the muscle spindles and the Golgi tendon organs of the motor afferent system may be responsible for somatic modulation of auditory perception. This conclusion is consistent with Kanold and Young's findings, which implicate activation of the cat's pinna muscle spindles and/or Golgi tendon organs as the likely source of neural activity ultimately affecting the dorsal cochlear nucleus (DCN).[15]

Possible sites of neural somatosensory-auditory interactions include the inferior colliculus because it is known to exhibit tinnitus-related abnormalities and it receives somatosensory inputs.[16] Experimentally, the firing of all units in the cat central nucleus of the inferior colliculus can be somatically modulated.[17] The DCN appears to be critical when tinnitus is due to ear disorders and is an established site of somatosensory-auditory interaction.[15,18]

If the change in auditory perception is unilateral, the DCN becomes a highly likely site for somatic-auditory interaction. Nonlateralized tinnitus suggests either the bilateral cochlear nucleus or some higher center, such as the inferior colliculus.

SOMATIC FACTORS CAN TRIGGER THE SOMATIC TINNITUS SYNDROME

Our finding that people without tinnitus (even when specifically questioned in a very low–ambient noise environment) can develop tinnitus from forceful head and neck contractions suggests that it is likely that some cases of clinical tinnitus may be due to activation of latent somatic-auditory interactions. One such example follows.

Case 7. A 29-year-old woman with normal audiometry had highly distressing right ear tinnitus for 7 months, which had resolved approximately 2 months prior to her visit to our tinnitus clinic. On physical examination, she had increased muscle tension and tenderness in her right SCM muscle compared with the left. At the time of somatic testing, she was hearing slight constant ringing of both ears (1 of 10), which was much fainter than her prior right ear tinnitus. With somatic testing, each time that her right SCM muscle was forcefully contracted, she reported hearing right ear tinnitus identical to her prior distressing tinnitus (Table 9-7). The right ear tinnitus did not persist after her somatic testing.

In some of our clinical cases, a well-described event occurred that precipitated the tinnitus. Many of these people had normal audiograms as well. We refer to such cases as examples of the somatic tinnitus syndrome.

Case 8. A 52-year-old woman underwent a right interscalene block to have manipulation of her frozen shoulder performed. With the injection, anesthesia of the shoulder did not occur; rather, she developed anesthesia of her right ear, right postauricular region,

TABLE 9-7. Somatic Testing for Case 7

Maneuver*	Right Ear Tinnitus Loudness	Left Ear Tinnitus Loudness
Baseline (0–10 scale)	1	1
Forehead pressure	4	1
Mandibular pressure	4	1
Right sternocleidomastoid muscle	4	1

*Only maneuvers that modulated the patient's tinnitus are shown.

and slightly right side of the face, with a dull ache in the same distribution. There was no facial weakness or dizziness. The numbness resolved within 14 hours. But immediately on injection of the local anesthetic (15 mL of 1.5% mepivacaine), she developed right ear tinnitus that has persisted unchanged for more than 10 years. She described her tinnitus as a high-pitched ringing in the right ear that sounds "like the brakes of a bus." An otolaryngologic evaluation 2 weeks later noted right occipital spasm. The audiograms for both ears were normal at the six standard audiometric frequencies. Her tinnitus was matched to a 3 kHz tone. Tympanograms and the stapedial reflexes were normal. Two subsequent audiograms in the next month remained similar but unlike the first audiogram; in these later audiograms, 6 kHz was also tested, and her thresholds for 6 kHz were 25 dB HL for both ears. All other frequencies tested were approximately 10 dB HL. On two of these occasions, her tinnitus was matched to a 6 kHz tone at 10 and 5 dB SL. Spontaneous otoacoustic emissions were not detected. A bolus of intravenous lidocaine abolished the tinnitus for 10 minutes. Oral mexiletine provided marginal benefit. Contrast magnetic resonance imaging (MRI) a year following the onset showed in the posterior part of the right cerebellar hemisphere two small regions of chronic infarction estimated to be more than 6 months old. A magnetic resonance angiogram of the neck arteries was normal. Her neurologic examinations have always been normal.

Case 9. A 45-year-old, right-handed man developed left dental pain and left-sided high-pitched tinnitus at about the same time. Treatment of an abscessed left upper molar with analgesics and antibiotics followed by a root canal procedure resolved his dental pain in a few days, whereas his tinnitus remained unchanged. An audiogram 3 months following the onset of the tinnitus was normal. Over the next several months, his tinnitus slowly became quieter but never totally resolved. Its pitch was matched to a 10 kHz tone. After 8 years, the tinnitus is still heard only in the left ear but is generally barely perceptible except for episodes of abrupt growth in loudness followed by a gradual return to its baseline loudness over the ensuing few days to weeks. Sleeping with the left ear down may precipitate such an episode. He described a vague strange feeling in the left periauricular region since the onset of his tinnitus.

Case 10. A 34-year-old, right-handed man presented to an otolaryngologist complaining of 5 days of high-pitched, left ear tinnitus and a history of 3 to 4 months of left-sided facial pain, which, more recently, had been associated with left facial swelling and mild pain. An abscessed left upper molar had been surgically treated 1 day previously. His examination and audiometry were unremarkable. The facial pain and swelling resolved, and the tinnitus improved for approximately a week following the dental surgery but then worsened again. When evaluated 2 months later, his tinnitus was present about 80% of the time. His left posterior cervical muscles were under increased tension compared with the right but were nontender. Clenching of the teeth on the left or pressure on the left mastoid abolished his tinnitus. After another 3 months of nearly continuous tinnitus, the tinnitus stopped. At no time did he have any vestibular complaints.

Case 11. A 6-year-old girl fell off her bicycle, fracturing the left mandibular ramus and dislocating the left TMJ. Within 4 months, the fracture and dislocation healed without surgery, but she had some persistent discomfort in the left preauricular and infra-auricular regions. She never complained of tinnitus or hearing loss after the accident, but 2 years later, she failed a routine school hearing test and did poorly on some subsequent audiograms because of the left ear. Otoacoustic emissions were normal. Temporal bone computed tomographic scans and contrast MRIs were normal. Once it was realized that she had left ear tinnitus, she was taught the difference between her tinnitus and the audiometer tones. Subsequent audiograms have been normal. Her left ear tinnitus was described as buzzing like a dial tone. She had noticed that her tinnitus became quieter with tilting her head to the left and louder with tilting to the right. When examined 3 years after the accident, she had full range of motion of her neck, but her left SCM muscle was rope-like in consistency and tender. Her baseline tinnitus was 8 of 10 in the left ear; by tilting to the right, it became 9 of 10, and by tilting to the left, it became 5 of 10. With somatic testing, contracting the left SCM muscle, such as with forehead pressure, left temple pressure, or left SCM muscle testing, her tinnitus became much louder, as high as "13 of 10." Other maneuvers caused pain but did not change the loudness of her tinnitus.

Case 12. A 39-year-old, right-handed woman described hearing a high-pitched ringing principally in the right ear since at least her teens. Her tinnitus has been unchanged over the years, with the exception of becoming louder during the last months of her two pregnancies, and returned to baseline within 3 months of parturition, despite nursing both infants for a year. On one of these occasions, she was treated with physical therapy for "stiffness" of her neck, but her tinnitus was unchanged. Head position has always modulated her tinnitus loudness. On a 0 to 10 loudness scale, she rates her tinnitus as 3 of 10. With turning the head to either side or tilting to the left, loudness increases to 5 of 10, whereas with tilting to the right, the loudness was barely perceptible (1 of 10). Clenching her teeth increased the loudness only slightly (4 of 10). On examination, two regions of increased muscle tension and tenderness were noted in the right neck compared with the corresponding regions on the left, namely the upper part of the SCM muscle and the medial part of the suprascapular region. Otherwise, her otoneurologic examination was unremarkable. An audiogram was normal. Her tinnitus matched to an 11 kHz tone at 10 dB SL.

Case 13. As a 50-year-old man was swallowing some sleeping pills, he sneezed and developed acute right ear pain. The next day he noticed right ear tinnitus. An otolaryngologic evaluation 2 days later detected an abrasion of his right side of his nasopharynx, which resolved uneventfully. His audiogram was normal. He matched his tinnitus to a 10 kHz tone. His right ear tinnitus has persisted for more than 2 years. With somatic testing, his tinnitus went from a baseline of 3 of 10 up to 4 of 10 with forceful contraction of his right SCM muscle.

CLINICAL FEATURES OF SOMATIC TINNITUS SYNDROME

These seven cases illustrate the characteristic features of the somatic tinnitus syndrome. First, the tinnitus is closely associated temporally with factors relating to the head or upper neck. We have never encountered patients with tinnitus similarly associated with the upper extremities, torso, or lower extremities, nor have others reported such findings. There appears to be a predilection for the periauricular region and particularly the upper part of the SCM muscle in many cases. Second, the tinnitus is always described as coming from the ear ipsilateral to the somatic event. The tinnitus is usually described as a high-pitched constant ringing. Third, there are no other associated hearing or vestibular complaints and no abnormalities on the neurologic examination. The syndrome can occur in people with no hearing loss. Pure-tone and speech audiometry of the two ears is symmetric and often within normal limits. Hyperacusis is not a feature of any of these cases. Note that successful treatment of the associated disorder may resolve the tinnitus in some cases but not in others.

REVIEW OF PRIOR REPORTS

There has been little description in the literature of the clinical features of nonotic somatic tinnitus. The association between whiplash and tinnitus has been well described, particularly in the German literature, and has been attributed to "functional disturbances of the upper cervical spine."[19,20] Beside being frequently associated with other elements of the whiplash syndrome (dizziness, pain, and nausea) and unrelated to hearing loss, rarely is any detail about the tinnitus provided. Wyant described intermittent unilateral tinnitus in a presumably normal-hearing man that was associated with neck pain radiating to the ipsilateral side of the face and eye.[21]

Many articles describe an association between tinnitus and pain in the region of the ear or TMJ. Some authors emphasize the joint's role and refer to the syndrome as TMJ syndrome, Costen's syndrome, or craniomandibular disorder. Others stress muscle tension as the key to the syndrome and describe it as myofascial pain-dysfunction syndrome. A recent report of tinnitus and TMJ syndrome associated the tinnitus with muscle dysfunction and not joint dysfunction.[22] The fact that somatic tinnitus would appear to have been previously described as part of TMJ syndrome suggests that somatic tinnitus not only is limited to the craniocervical regions but may more likely be from the lateral craniocervical regions, the periauricular regions.

Although virtually all reports include tinnitus as part of TMJ syndrome, detailed characteristics of the location of the tinnitus are few. Three reports describe some features of tinnitus consistent with our cases of somatic tinnitus. Curtis reported the tinnitus as lateralized to the side with the pain in 14 of the 17 patients in whom the pain was unilateral, whereas the three other patients reported bilateral tinnitus.[23] Of the 28 patients with bilateral but asymmetric pain, the tinnitus was lateralized to the side of greater pain in 13 and was bilateral in the other 15 patients. Ten other patients had symmetric otalgia, and all had bilateral tinnitus. Travell and Simons described a patient who had tinnitus ipsilateral to a trigger point in the upper posterior part of the masseter muscle.[24]

A controlled study of tinnitus and TMJ syndrome defined the syndrome as "both clicking in the joint and pain in the region of the ear (joint)."[25] Based on questionnaire data, the authors found that tinnitus was significantly more prevalent in the patients with TMJ syndrome than in two control groups.

MULTIFACTORIAL TINNITUS: SOMATIC FACTORS AND HEARING LOSS INTERACT

Three cases illustrate that factors predisposing individuals toward otic tinnitus can interact with factors predisposing individuals toward somatic tinnitus.

Case 14. A 50-year-old woman carried the diagnosis of unilateral otosclerosis manifested by a left, predominantly sensorineural, hearing loss. Her hearing loss predated her intermittent left ear tinnitus by more than 5 years. She reported that her tinnitus had begun following neck manipulation a few months prior to being seen in our clinic. When initially examined, she was not having tinnitus. Her left suboccipital muscles, however, were noted to be tender and under increased muscle tension compared with the corresponding muscles on the right side. Within an estimated 5 minutes of examining the cervical musculature, she reported that her left-sided tinnitus had started. On reexamination, her left suboccipital muscle tension had become much more pronounced. Within another 5 minutes, her tinnitus abated, and her suboccipital muscles were again more relaxed.

Case 15. A 50-year-old man reported that he had noticed very faint tinnitus in his left ear for many years. On a 0 to 10 loudness scale, he rated it as 1 of 10. An audiogram at age 41 revealed normal thresholds bilaterally except 25 dB HL at 4 kHz for the left ear. At age 45, 5 to 6 days after placement of a permanent crown on a left lower molar, his left ear tinnitus became much louder (4 to 5 of 10). At about the same time, he had also attended a loud concert. His tinnitus then remained unchanged until age 48, when it vanished (0 of 10) following placement of a temporary inlay on the tooth that occludes with the left lower molar crown. Two weeks later, while leaving the dentist's office after the placement of the permanent gold inlay, his tinnitus suddenly became very loud (10 of 10) and remained that way for the next 6 months. A repeat audiogram revealed normal thresholds except again at 4 kHz in the left ear, in which the threshold was now 40 dB HL. Over the last 2 years, his tinnitus loudness has gradually decreased to the 6 to 7 of 10 range.

Case 16. A 62-year-old man had been doing "facial exercises" for about 20 years to improve his scowl. One evening, while vigorously contracting his facial muscles, he developed right face and lateral neck discomfort associated with right ear tinnitus. He had had an upper respiratory infection at the time. He was evaluated at our clinic 8 months later. The tinnitus and facial discomfort persisted. Facial massage could temporarily resolve the facial pain and lower the intensity of the tinnitus. On examination, his right SCM muscle was tender. An audiogram revealed normal thresholds bilaterally except for his right ear at 4 kHz (35 dB HL) and 8 kHz (25 dB HL). He matched his tinnitus to a 15 dB SL narrowband noise centered at 8 kHz. His auditory brainstem responses were normal. His right ear tinnitus has persisted for more than 10 years.

These observations are dramatic examples of how tinnitus of presumably otic origin can interact with craniocervical somatic factors. Although these cases, like the cases of purely somatic tinnitus, are all restricted to the head or upper cervical region, somatic modulation of tinnitus is likewise predominantly a head and neck phenomenon. With the possible exception of the Cullington case report, there have been no reports of somatic modulation outside the head and upper neck in physiologically intact individuals using physiologic stimuli.[13] Somatic modulation of tinnitus can easily be accounted for by central nervous system interactions between the auditory and somatic systems, such as is proposed by our neurologic model (presented below). Otic-somatic interactions may account for (1) why some patients with a hearing disorder develop tinnitus and others with an otherwise identical hearing disorder do not, (2) why some patients with chronic progressive hearing loss develop tinnitus at some point in time, and (3) why patients with symmetric hearing loss can develop tinnitus in only one ear.

NEUROLOGIC MODEL OF SOMATIC TINNITUS AND AUDITORY INTERACTIONS

Because somatic tinnitus syndrome is closely related to somatic modulation of auditory perception, and I have shown that somatic modulation occurs because of central nervous system interaction, I propose a neurologic model of somatic tinnitus that will account for all features of somatic modulation of auditory perception (Figure 9-1). This model follows directly from the clinical characteristics of somatic tinnitus.

In the afferent auditory pathway, although binaural interaction can occur at the cochlear nucleus, it is probably at the level of the superior olivary complex, where the binaural interaction necessary for sound lateralization first occurs.[26,27] At these higher levels of the auditory pathway, all degrees of lateralization are probably represented. Accordingly, activation of these regions would not likely result in lateralization of the percept to one ear exclusively. On the other hand, at lower levels such as the cochlear nucleus, auditory nerve, or inner ear, lateralization of the percept exclusively to one ear would be expected. In fact, clinically, it is known to be the case that tinnitus is lateralized exclusively to the ipsilateral ear for disorders of the auditory nerve and cochlea. The unilateral characteristic of somatic tinnitus suggests that nonauditory interaction with the auditory system for somatic tinnitus occurs at the level of the cochlear nucleus because it is the only part of the afferent central auditory pathway before the trapezoid body, where the first auditory decussation important for sound lateralization is located.[28] The fact that our defining cases of somatic tinnitus always report their tinnitus as coming from one ear suggests that the cochlear nucleus is the site on the auditory pathway where the nonauditory inputs interact with the auditory system to initiate the neural discharge patterns that are ultimately interpreted as tinnitus.

That the defining cases of somatic tinnitus are associated only with processes that involve the ipsilateral head and upper neck also must be accounted

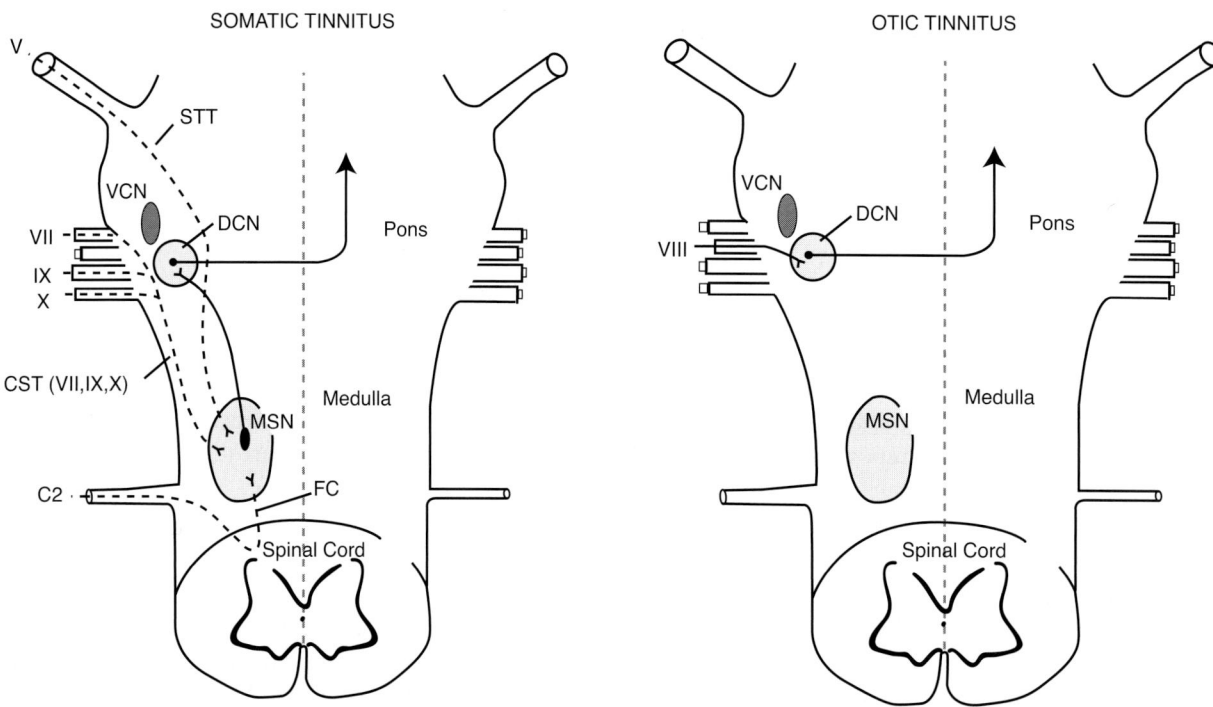

FIGURE 9-1. Schematic diagram of the brainstem and upper cervical part of the spinal cord, depicting the anatomic basis for the dorsal cochlear nucleus (DCN) hypothesis: both somatic and otic tinnitus occur owing to disinhibition of the DCN. In both cases, tinnitus is due to increased activity in the output of the DCN (*curved arrow*), which projects to the other centers and eventually leads to activation of the auditory perceptual machinery responsible for tinnitus. For somatic tinnitus (*left panel*), sensory inputs (*long dashed lines*) from (1) the face via the trigeminal (V) nerve in the spinal trigeminal tract (STT); (2) the external and middle ears via the common spinal tract of the facial, glossopharyngeal, and vagus nerves [CST (VII, IX, X)]; and (3) the neck via the C2 dorsal root and the fasciculus cuneatus (FC) converge to a common region of the lower part of the medulla, the medullary somatosensory nuclei (MSN), from which fibers project to the ipsilateral DCN (*solid line*). Modulation of activity in the MSN-DCN pathway results in disinhibition of the DCN. For otic tinnitus (*right panel*), loss of input (spontaneous activity) from the auditory (VIII) nerve leads to disinhibition of the DCN. VCN = ventral cochlear nucleus.

for by any hypothesis regarding the neuroanatomic basis of this type of tinnitus. If we assume that all cases of somatic tinnitus have a similar neuroanatomic substrate, the possible neuroanatomic regions involved are limited. Sensation of the face is subserved principally by the trigeminal nerve, but the second cervical root also contributes to the sensation of the auricle and, to some extent, the nearby face. Parts of the auricle, ear canal, and tympanic membrane are innervated by branches of the facial, glossopharyngeal, and vagus nerves. Sensation of the upper neck is via the upper cervical roots, namely C2 and C3. The branches of cranial nerves VII, IX, and X that innervate the ear join the spinal tract of cranial nerve V most medially (Figure 9-2), where they come to assume a position adjacent to the most lateral fibers of the fasciculus cuneatus.[29] Kunc suggests that this distinct bundle should be called the "common spinal tract of the facial, glossopharyngeal, and vagus nerves" [CST(VII, IX, X)].[29] In awake patients, according to Kunc, mechanical stimulation of CST(VII, IX, X) elicits pain in the "auditory passage, the pharynx and the tonsil. Stimulation of the lateral portion of this small tract evokes pain in the area served by the third division of the trigeminal nerve. Stimulation of the medial portion causes pain over the area innervated by the second cervical spinal root."[29] Thus, despite the fact that somatic nonotic tinnitus is associated with the upper cervical dorsal roots and four cranial nerves (V, VII, IX, and X), these primary sensory pathways associated with somatic tinnitus all converge to the region of the CST (VII, IX, X), namely the ipsilateral dorsolateral lower medulla and upper cervical spinal cord. This region has been referred to as the "medullary somatosensory nuclei" (MSN).[30] I hypothesize that this region of anatomic convergence is involved in somatic tinnitus.

For this hypothesis to be reasonable, there must be a connection between MSN and the primary auditory pathway. In fact, both experimental anatomic and electrophysiologic studies provide support for such a pathway between this location and the ipsilateral cochlear nucleus, principally the DCN. Anatomic and physiologic studies of the cat and rat demonstrate a direct projection between MSN and the ipsilateral DCN.[31,32] Although the initial effect of activation of this pathway may be to excite the DCN granule cells, the overall effect appears to be inhibition of the DCN projection neurons, the pyramidal cells, through a multisynaptic system within the DCN. There is evidence that stimulation of the granule cells excites the cartwheel cells, which, in turn, inhibits the pyramidal cells. These authors go on to argue that this pathway may be important in sound localization because pinna position can modify the activity within the ipsilateral DCN via this pathway. I hypothesize that somatic tinnitus occurs because of inappropriate excitation of the auditory pathway, which is due to pathology within a somatic pathway that is normally present and innervates the DCN.

Another line of reasoning based on our somatic modulation observations also implicates the DCN. The fact that somatic modulation appears to originate from the proprioceptive muscle receptors (Golgi tendon organs and muscle spindles) suggests interaction with the part of the auditory system requiring proprioceptive information, that is, for sound localization. Furthermore, because somatic modulation can affect only one ear, then the auditory structure involved must be involved with the mode of sound localization requiring only one ear,

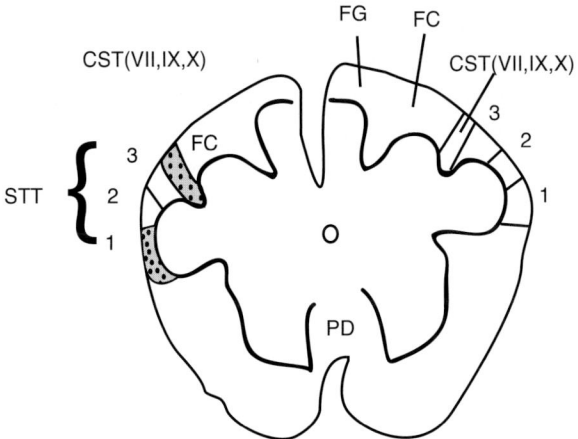

FIGURE 9-2. Cross-section of the lower part of the medulla at the level of the decussation of the pyramidal tract (PD). *Stippled* on the left is the position of the fibers from the facial (nervus intermedius), glossopharyngeal, and vagus nerves making up the common spinal tract [CST(VII, IX, X)], as shown in relationship to (1) the positions of the fibers of the first, second, and third divisions (1, 2, 3) of the trigeminal nerve in the spinal trigeminal tract (STT) and (2) the fasciculus cuneatus (FC). FG = fasciculus gracilis. Adapted from Kunc Z.[29]

that is, vertical and front-back sound localization. Finally, animal ablation experiments have implicated the DCN as being involved in vertical and front-back sound localization.[33] Thus, our somatic modulation results also converge on the DCN as the locus of somatic-auditory interactions related to tinnitus.

In summary, consideration of the clinical features of somatic tinnitus syndrome and the properties of somatic modulation of tinnitus, along with experimental neuroanatomy and electrophysiology, leads to the hypothesis that somatic modulation of tinnitus and the somatic tinnitus syndrome occur through modulation of the pathway from the MSN to the ipsilateral DCN. If increased activity in the primary output cells of the DCN is associated with tinnitus, as has been suggested for noise-induced tinnitus, our speculation can be taken a step farther to suggest that inhibition of the MSN to DCN pathway could lead to tinnitus through disinhibition of the DCN fusiform cells.[34] The findings in case 8 are consistent with this hypothesis because her tinnitus began with an injection of a local anesthetic to her upper neck, which, presumably, reduced activation of the lateral part of the fasciculus cuneatus, which, in turn, might result in less DCN inhibition. As will be shown, cases of otic tinnitus also give us reason to think that disinhibition in the DCN is involved in the origin of otic tinnitus.

Relationship to Otic Tinnitus

Multiple theories have been put forward to account for tinnitus related to disturbances of the peripheral part of the auditory system, auditory nerve, and cochlea. Based on the observation that aminoglycoside-induced hair cell loss was associated with loss of spontaneous activity of auditory nerve fibers innervating the region of hair cell loss, one proposal was that tinnitus was a consequence of decreased neural input to the cochlear nucleus.[35] It was hypothesized that the absence of active neural input from the auditory nerve to the central nervous system resulted in increased neural activity within the auditory pathways, leading to perception of sound (tinnitus).

Support for this theory also comes from patients who have received auditory nerve electrical stimulation. Although reports vary in the degree of tinnitus improvement with cochlear implants, in our experience, about 80% of these deaf subjects report tinnitus just prior to receiving their cochlear implants. Following a multichannel cochlear implant, the tinnitus associated with the ear that received the implant improved in 88% (M. A. Jalaludin, D. K. Eddington, R. A. Levine, M. Whearty, unpublished data). Rubinstein and colleagues also reported that, in about half of subjects with high-frequency sensorineural hearing loss of varying degrees, high-rate pulse trains applied to the cochlea suppressed tinnitus, with no perception of the stimulus.[36] These observations are consistent with the theory that tinnitus in individuals who are deaf owing to a cochlear disorder is due to the absence of neural input from the auditory nerve because reestablishment of auditory nerve activity with electrical stimulation abolishes or decreases the tinnitus.

Further support for this theory has come from reports of the effect of inner ear lesions on DCN spontaneous activity. In experimental animals with cochlear hearing losses (acoustic trauma or ototoxic drugs), which are known to be associated with loss of type I auditory nerve fiber spontaneous activity, increased spontaneous activity was found in the regions of the DCN tonotopically corresponding to the regions of cochlear injury (particularly outer hair cells) and the associated loss of auditory nerve fiber spontaneous activity.[37] The original suggestion that a decrease in spontaneous activity in auditory nerve fibers can lead to increased spontaneous activity from higher levels of the auditory pathway (and thereby tinnitus) is supported by multiple DCN studies.[18,34,37] In fact, these studies support the idea that the DCN may play an important role in otic tinnitus, possibly through its projections to the inferior colliculus, ventral cochlear nucleus, or medial geniculate body.[38]

Our model (see Figure 9-1) now generalizes this theory for otic tinnitus to somatic tinnitus by proposing that tinnitus can also occur from a somatic source of DCN disinhibition via a pathway originating from the MSN.

More recent anatomic studies of the DCN have shown that not only do the auditory nerve and MSN provide inputs to the DCN, but multiple other regions of the central nervous system likewise project to the DCN (Figure 9-3).[39] Thus, our hypothesis can be further generalized to include the vestibular system, pontine nuclei (including the medial olivocochlear efferent system), and inferior olive. Such inputs, many of which are not readily measured or observed, could account for (1) the high incidence of idiopathic tinnitus and (2) the fact that tinnitus is multifactorial.

OTHER CASES

Although I selected for presentation some of our most clear-cut cases with somatic tinnitus, other cases that, at first, might appear to be obvious cases of otic tinnitus, viewed from this new perspective, may actually be cases of somatic tinnitus. The following case is an example.

Case 17. A 25-year-old, left-handed woman developed an upper respiratory infection with ear discomfort, particularly on the right. As her physician irrigated her right ear canal, she developed excruciating ear pain, hearing loss, and bleeding from the external auditory meatus. By the next day, she was aware of right ear tinnitus as well. A 20% central perforation of the posterior part of the right tympanic membrane was identified, and audiometry revealed a 10 to 20 dB conductive hearing loss. Within 2 weeks, her perforation had healed, and her audiogram returned to normal. However, the right ear tinnitus has remained unchanged for over 2 years. It is described as a high-pitched ring and was matched to a 7 kHz tone at 5 dB SL. She had no other hearing complaints.

Considering that at no time did this patient have any auditory or vestibular complaints attributable to the inner ear, another possible mechanism that would account for her tinnitus is somatic, namely originating from the somatic innervation of the tympanic membrane in a manner analogous to cases of facial or dental pain (cases 9, 10, and 13). Coles described several cases of tinnitus following ear canal cleaning that could be on a similar basis.[1]

INDIVIDUAL DIFFERENCES IN SUSCEPTIBILITY TO TINNITUS

The fact that for the same otic or somatic insult some individuals will develop tinnitus but others will not suggests that there are differences among individuals in their susceptibility to tinnitus. For example, tooth abscesses are very common, but the development of tinnitus with a tooth abscess is rare (cases 9 and 10). We must conclude that there is something different about the neuroanatomy and/or physiology of individuals who develop tinnitus compared with those who do not develop tinnitus. What these differences may be will require further study but may relate to the wide variety of influences on the DCN. That the cerebellum, which projects to the pontine nuclei, could be involved is suggested by case 8, whose MRI showed small cerebellar infarcts. However, a similar situation obtains for otic tinnitus. Patients with similar diseases of the auditory periphery and indistinguishable audiometry may or may not have tinnitus. Given apparently similar insults to hearing, some people will develop tinnitus, whereas others will not. Nothing about the changes in hearing that occur from an insult have revealed which human subjects have tinnitus and which do not. However, animal models of tinnitus suggest that outer hair cell rather than inner hair cell dysfunction is more likely to cause tinnitus.[37] Furthermore, transection of the auditory nerve in patients with otic tinnitus does not reliably diminish the tinnitus.[40,41]

TINNITUS TREATMENT

From our experience and those of others, it is not clear whether somatic tinnitus can generally be treated successfully by addressing what appears to be the associated condition, such as TMJ syndrome or myofascial pain syndrome involving the craniocervical region. At least two possible explanations can be offered for this experience. First, as can be seen from cases 9, 10, and 13, as well as case 8, there would appear to be a general principle regarding all types of subjective tinnitus that removal of what would appear to be the initial source for the tinnitus does not guarantee that the tinnitus will resolve. Second, in general, treatment for

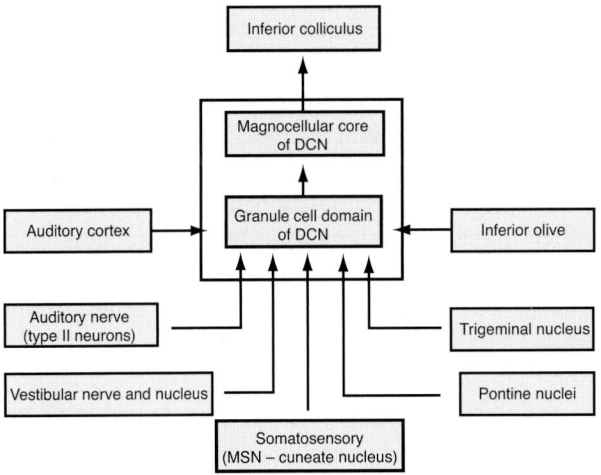

FIGURE 9-3. Block diagram that summarizes the multiple inputs to the granule cell domain of the dorsal cochlear nucleus (DCN). Such organization is consistent with the multifactorial nature of tinnitus. Adapted from Ryugo DK, et al.[39]

TMJ syndrome or cervical myofascial pain syndrome has mixed results.

On the other hand, our hypothesis suggests that restoration of DCN inhibition through either the auditory or the somatic inputs to the DCN could suppress some types of unilateral tinnitus (Table 9-8). In fact, there is ample evidence that increasing the inhibition from the ear-DCN pathway through electrical stimulation of the auditory nerve or DCN can suppress tinnitus, for example, with (1) cochlear implants (M. A. Jalaludin, D. K. Eddington, R. A. Levine, M. Whearty, unpublished data), (2) auditory brainstem implants, or (3) high-rate pulse trains applied to the cochlea.[36,42] Likewise, there are reports suggesting that somatic stimulation of the head or upper neck can suppress tinnitus through this somatic pathway. For example, placebo-controlled studies have shown that mastoid to mastoid electrical stimulation can suppress tinnitus in some patients.[43,44] Chouard and colleagues suggested that such effects were due to "direct action on sensitive cutaneous fibres, rather than direct action on the cochlea."[45] Likewise, reports of acupuncture suppressing tinnitus could be mediated by activation of this somatic pathway.[46]

An altogether different approach to treating this type of tinnitus, namely reduction of DCN output, also follows from our hypothesis. If tinnitus is due to increased neural activity projecting from the DCN to higher centers, interruption of this pathway might abolish the tinnitus. Such a procedure (ablating the DCN or transecting the dorsal acoustic stria) is likely to have little effect on hearing because the behavioral evidence from chronic ablation of DCN outflow pathways in experimental animals suggests that, beside orienting to an elevated sound source, loss of the DCN has no detectable effect on hearing.[33] Patients who would have elected to have their auditory nerve sectioned for control of their unilateral tinnitus may have derived more benefit from a DCN procedure because sectioning of the auditory nerve guarantees deafness and, in general, has about as much likelihood to worsen as to improve tinnitus; on the other hand, for patients with strictly lateralized otic or somatic tinnitus, our hypothesis suggests a more promising tinnitus treatment with little impact on hearing.

Alternative Hypotheses

The proposed model for somatic tinnitus is based on combining our clinical observations and known anatomy and physiology. Undoubtedly, there are other possible models that would be consistent with our current state of knowledge. For example, the inferior colliculus receives somatic inputs, and all units of the central nucleus of the inferior colliculus of the cat can be somatically modulated.[17] So the inferior colliculus is another possible site of auditory-somatic interaction. Because the inferior colliculus occurs after the auditory chiasm, activation from this center might not be expected to result in a perception that is consistently fully lateralized. It is for this reason that the inferior colliculus was felt to be a less likely site in the auditory pathway for the initial somatic-auditory interaction.

Another reservation about this model pertains to the DCN. Not only have there been no human studies regarding a pathway from the cuneate or spinal tract of cranial nerve V to the ipsilateral DCN, but the architecture of the human DCN differs from that of many other mammals.[47,48] The two most superficial layers (granular and molecular layers) are said to be vestigial in adult humans. Nonetheless, some report that, although the relative numbers may differ, in humans, all classes of DCN neurons are found as in other mammals.[49] Further advances, such as with fMRI, may provide more insights into the neurology of somatic tinnitus that will allow refinement of this model and, ultimately, effective treatment.

TABLE 9-8. Treatments Suggested by the Dorsal Cochlear Nucleus Disinhibition Hypothesis

Restoration of DCN Inhibition	Reduction of DCN Output
Electrical stimulation of auditory nerve	Transect the output tracts of the DCN
Electrical or mechanical stimulation of somatic pathway	Lesion the DCN

DCN = dorsal cochlear nucleus.

CONCLUSION

In this chapter, I reviewed the evidence that the somatosensory system plays a major role in clinical tinnitus. Not only can somatic events cause tinnitus (somatic tinnitus syndrome), but changes in the somatosensory system can account for changes in ongoing tinnitus loudness, pitch, and location (somatic modulation of tinnitus). These somatic-auditory interactions occur within the central nervous system and are not limited to tinnitus but are a fundamental property of the auditory system. The somatosensory inputs appear to originate from motor afferents (Golgi tendon organs and muscle spindles) and almost exclusively from the upper cervical and head regions. Among the principal muscles involved are the SCM and the pterygoids. When somatic-auditory interactions are restricted to one ear, the DCN appears to be the site of interaction. The somatosensory system is probably only one of several nonauditory neural systems that modulate the DCN activity.

These multiple influences on the DCN, many of which are not readily measured or observed, may account for much of the difficulties in determining the cause of and devising effective treatments for tinnitus. The challenge for the future is to understand these relationships so that improved tinnitus treatments can be developed.

REFERENCES

1. Coles RRA. Tinnitus. In: Stephens D, editor. Adult audiology. Guilford (UK): Butterworth Heinemann; 1996. 2/18/10.
2. Heller MF, Bergman M. Tinnitus aurium in normally hearing persons. Ann Otol Rhinol Laryngol 1953;62:73–83.
3. Levine RA, Abel M, Cheng H. CNS somatosensory-auditory interactions elicit or modulate tinnitus. Exp Brain Res 2003;153:643–8.
4. Levine RA. Somatic (craniocervical) tinnitus and the dorsal cochlear nucleus hypothesis. Am J Otolaryngol 1999;20:351–62.
5. Abel M, Levine RA. Muscle contractions and auditory perception in tinnitus patients and non-clinical subjects. Cranio. [In press]
6. Fowler EP. Control of head noises: their illusions of loudness and timbre. Arch Otolaryngol 1943; 37:391–8.
7. Møller AR, Møller MB, Yokota M. Some forms of tinnitus may involve the extralemniscal auditory pathway. Laryngoscope 1992;102:1165–71.
8. Rubinstein B. Tinnitus and craniomandibular disorders—is there a link? Swed Dent J Suppl 1993;95:1–46.
9. Levine RA, Kiang NYS. A conversation about tinnitus. In: Vernon JA, Møller AR, editors. Mechanisms of tinnitus. Boston: Allyn and Bacon; 1995. p. 149–62.
10. Levine RA. Somatic modulation appears to be a fundamental attribute of tinnitus. In: Hazell J, editor. Proceedings of the Sixth International Tinnitus Seminar. London: The Tinnitus and Hyperacusis Centre; 1999. p. 193–7.
11. Sanchez TG, Guerra GC, Lorenzi MC, et al. The influence of voluntary muscle contractions upon the onset and modulation of tinnitus. Audiol Neurootol 2002;7:370–5.
12. Møller AR, Rollins PR. The non-classical auditory pathways are involved in hearing in children but not in adults. Neurosci Lett 2002;319:41–4.
13. Cullington H. Tinnitus evoked by finger movement: brain plasticity after peripheral deafferentation. Neurology 2001;56:978.
14. Cacace AT, Cousins JP, Parnes SM, et al. Cutaneous-evoked tinnitus. I. Phenomenology, psychophysics and functional imaging. Audiol Neurootol 1999;4:247–57.
15. Kanold PO, Young ED. Proprioceptive information from the pinna provides somatosensory input to cat dorsal cochlear nucleus. J Neurosci 2001;21:7848–58.
16. Melcher JR, Sigalovsky IS, Guinan JJ Jr, Levine RA. Lateralized tinnitus studied with functional magnetic resonance imaging: abnormal inferior colliculus activation. J Neurophysiol 2000;83:1058–72.
17. Davis KA. Effects of somatosensory stimulation on neurons in the inferior colliculus [abstract]. In: Popelka GR, editor. Abstracts of the Twenty-Second Annual Midwinter Research Meeting of the Association for Research in Otolaryngology. Mt. Royal (NJ): Association for Research in Otolaryngology; 1999. p. 215–6.
18. Kaltenbach JA, McCaslin DL. Increases in spontaneous activity in the dorsal cochlear nucleus following exposure to high intensity sound: a possible neural correlate of tinnitus. Audit Neurosci 1996;3:57–78.
19. Becker R, Meyer ED. Cervical syndrome due to trauma. In: Claussen C-F, Kirtane MV, editors. Vertigo, nausea, tinnitus, and hypoacusia due to head and neck trauma: proceedings of the XVIIth Scientific Meeting of the

Neurootological and Equilibriometric Society. Amsterdam: Excerpta Medica; 1991. p. 259–63.
20. Tjell C, Tenenbaum A, Rosenhall U. Auditory function in whiplash-associated disorders. Scand Audiol 1999;28:203–9.
21. Wyant GM. Chronic pain syndromes and their treatment. II. Trigger points. Can Anaesth Soc J 1979;26:216–9.
22. Peroz I. [Dysfunctions of the stomatognathic system in tinnitus patients compared to controls]. HNO 2003;51:544–9.
23. Curtis AW. Myofascial pain-dysfunction syndrome: the role of nonmasticatory muscles in 91 patients. Otolaryngol Head Neck Surg 1980;88:361–7.
24. Travell JG, Simons DG. Myofascial pain and dysfunction: the trigger point manual. Baltimore (MD): Williams & Wilkins; 1983. p. 223.
25. Chole RA, Parker WS. Tinnitus and vertigo in patients with temporomandibular disorder. Arch Otolaryngol Head Neck Surg 1992;118:817–21.
26. Mast TE. Binaural interaction and contralateral inhibition in dorsal cochlear nucleus of the chinchilla. J Neurophysiol 1970;33:108–15.
27. Young ED, Brownell WE. Responses to tones and noise of single cells in dorsal cochlear nucleus of unanesthetized cats. J Neurophysiol 1976;39:282–300.
28. Glendenning KK, Masterton RB. Acoustic chiasm: efferent projections of the lateral superior olive. J Neurosci 1983;3:1521–37.
29. Kunc Z. Treatment of essential neuralgia of the 9th nerve by selective tractotomy. J Neurosurg 1965;23:494–500.
30. Young ED, Nelken I, Conley RA. Somatosensory effects on neurons in dorsal cochlear nucleus. J Neurophysiol 1995;73:743–65.
31. Wright DD, Ryugo DK. Mossy fiber projections from the cuneate nucleus to the cochlear nucleus in the rat. J Comp Neurol 1996;365:159–72.
32. Nelken I, Young ED. Why do cats need a dorsal cochlear nucleus? J Basic Clin Physiol Pharmacol 1996;7:199–220.
33. Sutherland DP, Glendenning KK, Masterton RB. Role of acoustic striae in hearing: discrimination of sound-source elevation. Hear Res 1998;120:86–108.
34. Brozoski TJ, Bauer CA, Caspary DM. Elevated fusiform cell activity in the dorsal cochlear nucleus of chinchillas with psychophysical evidence of tinnitus. J Neurosci 2002;22:2383–90.
35. Kiang NYS, Moxon EC, Levine RA. Auditory-nerve activity in cats with normal and abnormal cochleas. In: Wolstenholme GEW, Knight J, editors. Sensorineural hearing loss: a Ciba Foundation symposium. London: Churchill; 1970. p. 241–73.
36. Rubinstein JT, Tyler RS, Johnson A, Brown CJ. Electrical suppression of tinnitus with high-rate pulse trains. Otol Neurotol 2003;24:478–85.
37. Kaltenbach JA, Rachel JD, Mathog TA, et al. Cisplatin-induced hyperactivity in the dorsal cochlear nucleus and its relation to outer hair cell loss: relevance to tinnitus. J Neurophysiol 2002;88:699–714.
38. Malmierca MS, Merchan MA, Henkel CK, Oliver DL. Direct projections from cochlear nuclear complex to auditory thalamus in the rat. J Neurosci 2002;22:10891–7.
39. Ryugo DK, Haenggeli CA, Doucet JR. Multimodal inputs to the granule cell domain of the cochlear nucleus. Exp Brain Res 2003;153:477–85.
40. Pulec JL. Cochlear nerve section for intractable tinnitus. Ear Nose Throat J 1995;74:468, 470–6.
41. Jackson P. A comparison of the effects of eighth nerve section with lidocaine on tinnitus. J Laryngol Otol 1985;99:663–6.
42. Soussi T, Otto SR. Effects of electrical brainstem stimulation on tinnitus. Acta Otolaryngol (Stockh) 1994;114:135–40.
43. Lyttkens L, Lindberg P, Scott B, Melin L. Treatment of tinnitus by external electrical stimulation. Scand Audiol 1986;15:157–64.
44. Dobie RA, Hoberg KE, Rees TS. Electrical tinnitus suppression: a double-blind crossover study. Otolaryngol Head Neck Surg 1986;95:319–23.
45. Chouard CH, Meyer B, Maridat D. Transcutaneous electrotherapy for severe tinnitus. Acta Otolaryngol (Stockh) 1981;91:415–22.
46. Marks NJ, Emery P, Onisiphorou C. A controlled trial of acupuncture in tinnitus. J Laryngol Otol 1984;98:1103–9.
47. Moore JK. The human auditory brain stem: a comparative view. Hear Res 1987;29:1–32.
48. Adams JC. Neuronal morphology in the human cochlear nucleus. Arch Otolaryngol Head Neck Surg 1986;112:1253–61.
49. Moore JK, Osen KK. The cochlear nuclei in man. Am J Anat 1979;154:393–418.

CHAPTER 10

Sensory Nuclei in Tinnitus

Susan E. Shore, PhD

Tinnitus has long been considered an exclusive disorder of the auditory system. Accumulating evidence, however, suggests that tinnitus is an expression of neural plasticity encompassing diverse reactions of multisensory neurons to changes in their external environment. Tinnitus, according to this view, is not a passive consequence of interrupted peripheral input to a central location but rather an active process generated partly in the periphery and partly by complex plastic changes across central sensory modalities.

Tinnitus is often associated with hearing loss, a reduction of auditory input to the brain, but changes in somatosensory input can likewise lead to the sensation of tinnitus. As many as two-thirds of patients who have hearing losses accompanied by tinnitus are able to modulate their tinnitus by clenching the jaw or touching the skin on the face, regions innervated by the trigeminal nerve.[1,2] Positron emission tomographic studies correlating increased blood flow to the medial geniculate body with changes in tinnitus substantiate verbal reports of such alterations. Many of these patients can attribute their onset of tinnitus to a somatic insult in the head and neck region ("somatic tinnitus").[2] There have been reports in the literature of tinnitus following tooth abscesses and neck injuries, which can resolve following recovery.[2] Additionally, changing the direction of gaze, which involves trigeminal pathways, can evoke tinnitus, especially after deafening.[3,4] Finally, the findings that median nerve stimulation can result in modulating the perception of tinnitus in some patients has led Møller and colleagues to propose that tinnitus can occur through reactivation of "non-classical," extralemniscal pathways that have connections with somatosensory systems.[5–7] (For additional information on the crossmodal effects on tinnitus, see Cacace[4] and Chapter 12, "The Limbic System and Tinnitus.")

The present chapter reviews the neuroanatomic connections of the somatosensory system with the auditory portion of the brainstem and touches on connections with the auditory portion of the midbrain.[8] The focus is on the neuroanatomy of somatosensory connections with the cochlear nucleus (CN) and the physiologic effects of electrically stimulating somatosensory centers that project to this region. The role of the somatosensory system in the generation of the perception of tinnitus is discussed.

BACKGROUND

SOMATOSENSORY INNERVATION OF THE AUDITORY PORTION OF THE BRAINSTEM

Neuroanatomy Regions of the auditory portion of the brainstem and midbrain receiving somatosensory innervation are depicted in Figure 10-1. Also included in this diagram are somatosensory projections to the blood vessels and perhaps spiral ganglion cells of the cochlea. Projections to the CN, the superior olivary complex (SOC), and the inferior colliculus (IC) arise primarily in the trigeminal ganglion, dorsal column, and trigeminal nuclei, as well as neurons of the reticular formation, which themselves receive trigeminal input. These neuroanatomic connections form the basis of any theories incorporating multisensory integration into a comprehensive theory of tinnitus.

COCHLEAR NUCLEUS. The CN, in addition to receiving afferent connections from the auditory nerve and efferent information from higher auditory centers,[9] is innervated by somatosensory neurons, which subserve tactile and kinesthetic sensations. Somatosensory innervation can originate in as peripheral a location as the trigeminal ganglion. Both the ophthalmic and mandibular divisions of the trigeminal ganglion innervate

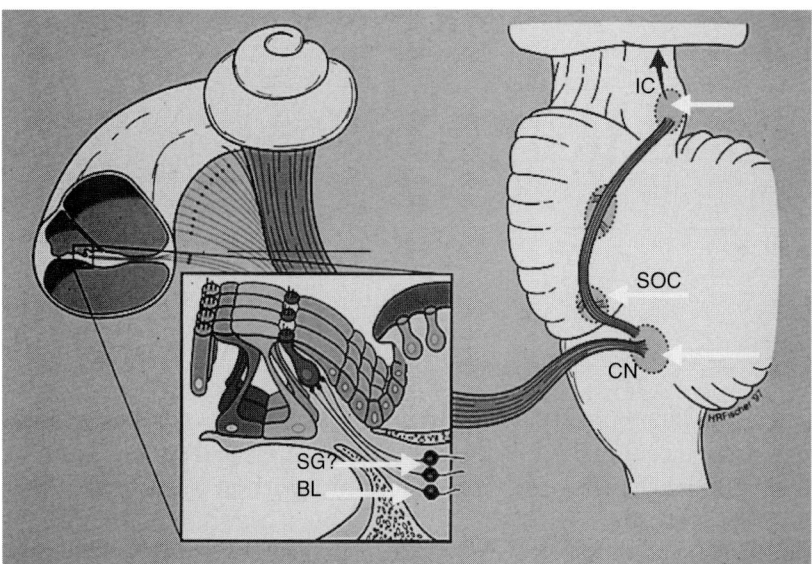

FIGURE 10-1. Schematic view of the cochlea and auditory parts of the brainstem and midbrain. *Inset* shows amplified view of the sensory hair cells and spiral ganglion cells. *Arrows pointing left* indicate regions of the auditory parts of the brainstem and midbrain receiving innervation from somatosensory ganglia or brainstem nuclei. These pathways originate primarily in dorsal column nuclei, trigeminal nuclei, and the trigeminal ganglion. *Arrows pointing right* indicate somatosensory projections to the blood vessels and perhaps spiral ganglion cells of the cochlea. BL = blood vessels of the cochlea; CN = cochlear nucleus; IC = inferior colliculus; SG = spiral ganglion; SOC = superior olivary complex.

the magnocellular and granule regions of the ventral cochlear nucleus (VCN).[10] The marginal cell region, especially, is innervated by axodendritic terminals containing small spherical vesicles indicative of excitatory neurotransmission (Figure 10-2). Larger cells, within the body of the VCN, are also innervated by the trigeminal ganglion (Figure 10-3). The same divisions of the trigeminal ganglion that project to the CN, that is, the ophthalmic and mandibular divisions, project to the cochlea and middle ear, respectively.[11] The observation

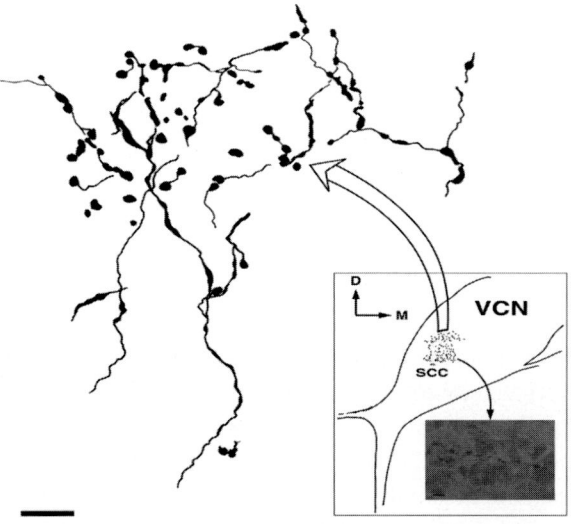

FIGURE 10-2. Biotinylated-dextran-amine (BDA) injection into the trigeminal ganglion produced BDA-labeled terminals from thin axons of the trigeminal ganglion in the small cell cap (SCC) region of the anteroventral cochlear nucleus. A transverse section (*inset*) of the ventral cochlear nucleus (VCN) is shown, indicating the location of terminals. The *large arrow* points to an expanded drawing of some of these terminals at upper left. The *small arrow* points to the photomicrograph at the lower right, showing an expanded view of some of the terminals. The axons typically form boutons de passage. Large scale bar = 5 μm; small scale bar = 10 μm. These axodendritic terminals containing small spherical vesicles are likely to be excitatory. Reproduced with permission from Shore SE et al.[10]

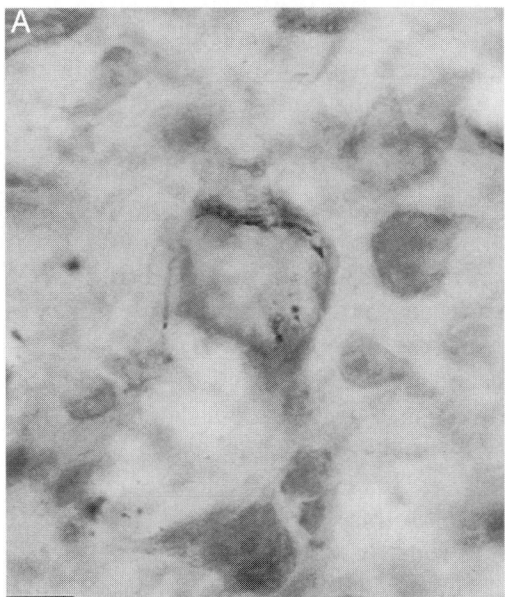
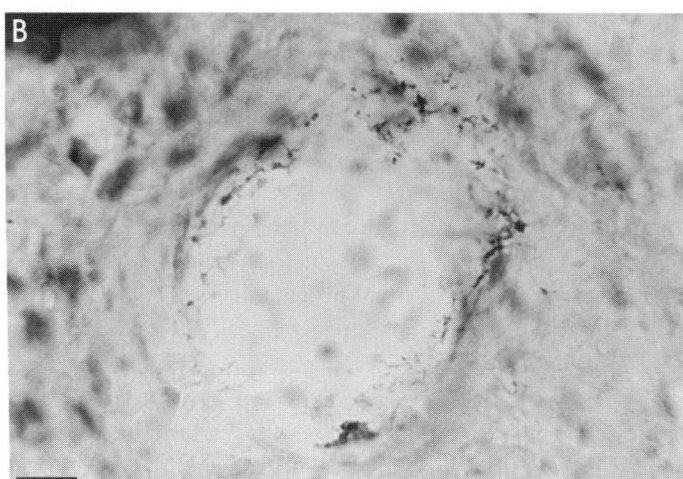

FIGURE 10-3. *A*, A multipolar cell in the anteroventral cochlear nucleus with biotinylated-dextran-amine (BDA)-labeled puncta surrounding the soma after a BDA injection into the ipsilateral trigeminal ganglion. Scale bar = 10 μm. Reproduced with permission from Shore SE et al.[10] *B*, A blood vessel in the ventral cochlear nucleus surrounded with BDA-labeled puncta after a BDA injection into the ipsilateral trigeminal ganglion. Scale bar = 20 μm (BDA was visualized with diaminobenzidene [DAB]; stain was neutral red). Reproduced with permission from Shore SE et al.[10]

that the ophthalmic portion of the trigeminal ganglion innervates extraocular muscles[12] raises the interesting possibility that this connection might be involved in the vestibulo-ocular reflexes. Direct connections from the vestibular end-organs to the CN have, indeed, been demonstrated.[13]

The regions of the trigeminal ganglion that innervate the CN overlap the regions that innervate both the cochlea and the middle ear.[10] The ophthalmic division innervates the cochlea, and the mandibular division innervates the middle ear.[11] The intriguing possibility, therefore, exists of a role for the trigeminal ganglion in the middle ear reflex. Support for this hypothesis is suggested by the finding that cutaneous stimulation of the periorbital and external ear regions can evoke the middle ear reflex.[14] The form of this reflex arc could include an ascending limb involving the trigeminal input from the external auditory meatus. The first central relay station of the middle ear reflex is the VCN, which sends a projection bilaterally to the motoneurons of the tensor tympani and stapedius muscles located in the trigeminal and facial nuclei, respectively.[15] Thus, it is possible that the trigeminal ganglion, activated by cutaneous stimulation in the region of the external ear, directly modulates the activity of neurons in the VCN, which, in turn, project to motoneurons of the tensor tympani and stapedius. Because my colleagues and I have shown that the trigeminal ganglion projects to the middle ear, the cochlea, and the VCN,[10,11] modulation of the middle ear reflex could occur through direct trigeminal ganglion projections to the VCN and middle ear muscles.

Biocytin injections into the trigeminal ganglion resulted in labeled puncta in the VCN that were located not only on neurons but also around the lumina of blood vessels.[10] This suggests an involvement of this pathway in the regulation of blood flow or metabolism in the CN and SOC. Stimulating the trigeminal ganglion results in changes in cochlear and cerebral blood flow.[16] Additionally, in peripheral and central blood vessels, low-dose administration of capsaicin, which stimulates release of substance P, produces sustained vasodilatation, increased vascular permeability, and an increase in cochlear blood flow.[17,18] In cerebral circulation, substance P–containing neurons may be associated with headache pain or reactions to trauma such as breakdown of the blood-brain barrier.[18] In the cochlea, the trigeminal ganglion may play a role in the pathophysiology of Meniere's disease.[19]

The granule cell region of the VCN is also innervated by the interpolar and caudal spinal trigeminal nuclei and the cuneate nucleus. The projection from the cuneate nucleus gives rise to mossy fiber terminals that synapse in both the dorsal cochlear nucleus (DCN) and granule cell region of the VCN.[20]

LATERAL SUPERIOR OLIVARY COMPLEX. The trigeminal ganglion innervates both neurons and blood vessels in the "shell" regions of the lateral superior olivary complex, which are known to send projections to cochlear hair cells and type I auditory nerve fibers.[10,21,22] The small cell cap region of the CN, which is innervated by the trigeminal ganglion, is also innervated by type II spiral ganglion cells and by collaterals of the olivocochlear system. Because the trigeminal ganglion innervates both the auditory and vestibular portions of the labyrinth,[23] olivocochlear neurons, and the small cell cap region, which has a reciprocal connection with olivocochlear neurons, it is primed to form part of the olivocochlear feedback system.[24]

INFERIOR COLLICULUS. The task of determining the orientation of sound in space was originally attributed solely to centers such as the superior colliculus, where convergence of auditory and somatosensory inputs was first described. Somatosensory innervation from the dorsal column nuclei and spinal trigeminal complex, as well as reticular formation to the IC, was subsequently described[25] and was shown to be, at least partially, glutamatergic.[26] The projections from somatosensory nuclei terminate primarily in the external nucleus of the inferior colliculus (ICx). Interestingly, some cells of the spinal trigeminal and dorsal column nuclei project both to the CN and ICx by way of axon collaterals.[27] Thus, neurons of both the central nucleus of the inferior colliculus (ICc), which receive input from the CN, and those neurons in the ICx receiving direct trigeminal input would be expected to be influenced by the somatosensory system.

Functional Aspects Electrical stimulation of somatosensory brainstem regions has been shown to primarily inhibit but can also excite cells in the superficial and deep layers of the DCN and VCN.[28,29] Inhibition of DCN neurons is produced through excitation of cells in the granular regions, which, in turn, modify (inhibit) the activity of principal cells in the DCN through interneurons (cartwheel cells). Tactile stimulation of the pinna, likewise, can inhibit DCN neurons, suggesting that some of the cells stimulated electrically are those that represent the pinna and back of the head.[28] Thus, brainstem somatosensory input concerning pinna position may provide sound localization information to DCN cells. Somatosensory input from the trigeminal ganglion to the CN or SOC (see below) might be involved in olivocochlear feedback and mechanisms related to neck movements that play a role in orientation to acoustic stimuli. Because the vocal apparatus is also strongly innervated by the trigeminal system, trigeminal input to auditory structures may form part of a vocal structure feedback system necessary for speech production and perception. Support for this hypothesis is given by studies that demonstrate that some neurons in the spinal trigeminal complex and adjacent reticular formation do, indeed, respond to vocalizations.[30]

Trigeminal input directly from the trigeminal ganglion or from brainstem somatosensory nuclei to the CN and other auditory brainstem neurons could have a significant impact on the response characteristics of CN neurons if it targets both the neurons and their vascular supply. Because changes in peripheral hearing structures occurring with deafness may affect the structure of central auditory neurons, pathologic changes in innervation from peripheral somatosensory structures could also profoundly affect auditory functions requiring multisensory input, such as the localization of sound in space or vocal structure feedback for the purposes of speech. Thus, the perception of tinnitus in patients who receive somatic insults could similarly be a result of disrupted somatosensory input to the CN.

HOW DOES TRIGEMINAL INPUT AFFECT ACTIVITY OF CN NEURONS?

To assess the effects of somatosensory pathways connecting to the CN, my colleagues and I have electrically stimulated regions where the somatosensory inputs originate. Tract tracing studies have demonstrated that neurons in the trigeminal ganglion, trigeminal nucleus, and reticular formation project to the VCN of guinea pigs. Accordingly, we have positioned bipolar, concentric stimulating electrodes in each of these regions and passed current while recording unit activity in the VCN. Electrical stimuli consisted of bipolar pulses, 100 or 200 μs/phase. Single-shank, 16-channel silicon recording probes, manufactured by the University of Michigan Bioengineering Department, were placed in the CN to determine unit responses to the electrical stimulation. Each recording site was separated by 100 μm. These electrodes provide high spatial resolution in a dorsal-ventral direction. Off-line sorters were used to isolate multiunit clusters into single units using principal component analysis. Sound stimuli were presented to classify neurons according to previously described types. In some cases, sound and trigeminal stimuli were presented simultaneously to determine whether multisensory integration was occurring in CN neurons.

ELECTRICAL STIMULATION OF THE TRIGEMINAL GANGLION

Electrical stimulation of the trigeminal ganglion produces single- or multipeaked excitation of VCN neurons.[29] The excitation can be long lasting, up to 60 milliseconds, and is often followed by even longer-lasting inhibition. In some cases, units are inhibited by electrical stimulation of the trigeminal ganglion. Thresholds among VCN units vary between 20 and 50 μA.[29] Figure 10-4 shows responses from 4 channels of a 16-channel electrode to stimulation of the trigeminal ganglion at 60 μA. Three of the four units shown in this figure are vigorously excited by electrical stimulation and show suppression of activity below the spontaneous rate following the excitation. One unit is totally inhibited by the stimulation. The excitatory responses last approximately 60 milliseconds, whereas recovery from inhibition can take up to 100 milliseconds.

What Type of VCN Units Are Affected by Trigeminal Ganglion Stimulation? All unit types in the VCN, that is, primary-like, onset, and chopper units, are affected by trigeminal ganglion stimulation. There is no particular response pattern elicited by electrical stimulation that is specific to a unit type group. Figure 10-5 shows the typical response of a primary-like unit to a best-frequency toneburst. A high firing rate is observed at the onset of the sound that tapers off to a steady-state rate. The response of this unit to trigeminal ganglion stimulation showed a multipeaked response, which could also be seen in other types. Similarly, the onset unit in Figure 10-6 shows a typi-

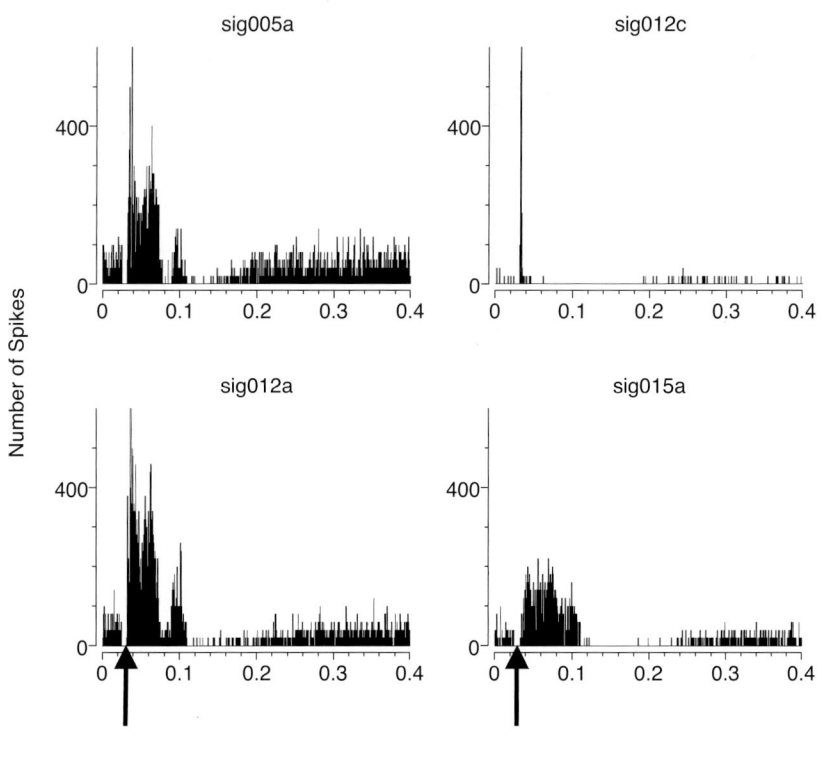

FIGURE 10-4. Poststimulus time histograms of unit responses from 4 channels of a 16-channel University of Michigan probe. Three of the units are initially excited and then inhibited by bipolar current pulses (200 μs/phase) applied to the ipsilateral trigeminal ganglion. One unit is inhibited by trigeminal ganglion stimulation. Reproduced with permission from Shore SE et al.[29]

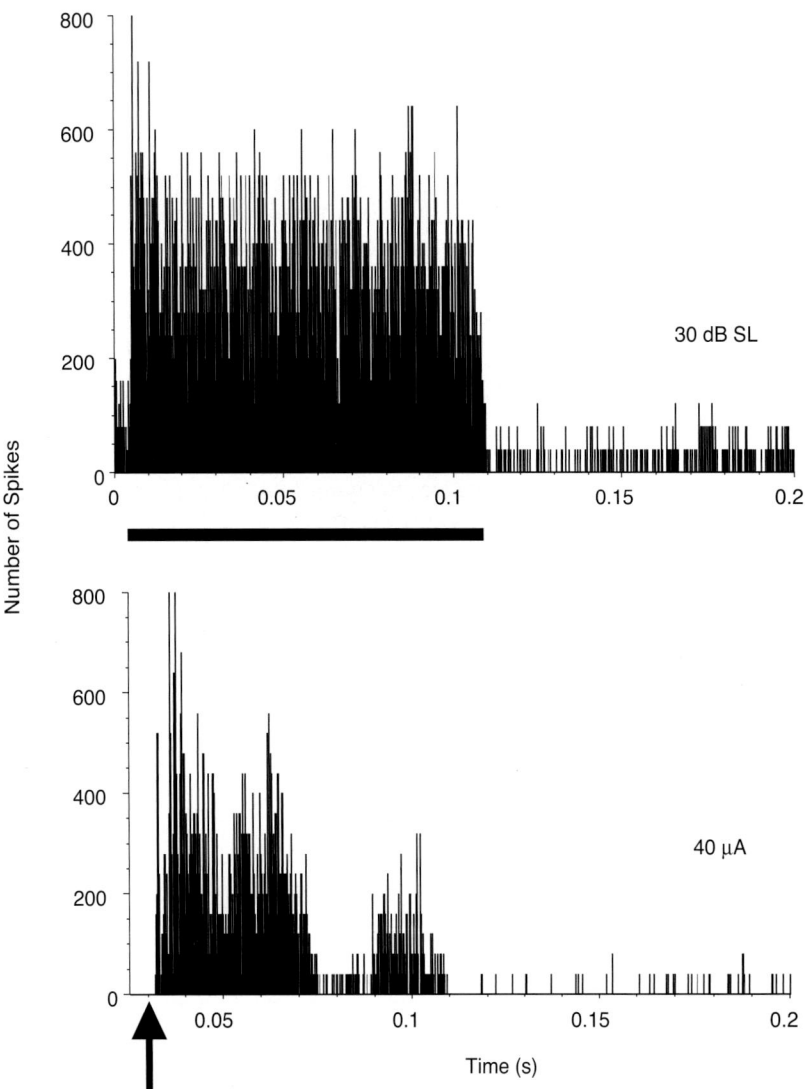

FIGURE 10-5. Poststimulus time histograms of unit responses from a ventral cochlear nucleus primary-like unit in response to best-frequency tonebursts (*top*) and trigeminal ganglion stimulation (*bottom*). The response to the best-frequency toneburst, together with a coefficient of variation value greater than 0.3, defines this unit as a primary-like unit. *Bar* indicates onset and duration of toneburst; *arrow* indicates onset of trigeminal stimulation. Reproduced with permission from Shore SE et al.[29]

cal high firing rate at the onset of the best-frequency toneburst, with little response to the rest of the sound. The response to trigeminal stimulation is a biphasic excitatory response. Both response types shown in Figures 10-5 and 10-6 are observed in primary-like, onset, and chopper units.

There is a tendency for more inhibitory responses to trigeminal ganglion stimulation to be observed in the posteroventral cochlear nucleus (PVCN), close to the DCN border, as well as units within the DCN. Figure 10-7A shows the change in firing rate (from spontaneous) elicited by 80 μA electrical stimulation of the trigeminal ganglion in units at the PVCN-DCN border and within the DCN.

Depression of firing rate is seen more frequently than elevation, in contrast to the primarily excitatory responses observed in the VCN. An example of the response from one DCN unit to trigeminal ganglion stimulation is shown in Figure 10-7B. Some DCN units can take up to 150 milliseconds to recover from inhibition from trigeminal ganglion stimulation.

Integration by CN Units of Auditory and Somatosensory Information Integration of auditory, somatosensory, and visual information has been well demonstrated for multimodal neurons in the superior colliculus, amygdala, and primary and secondary sensory cortices.[31] My laboratory studies provide

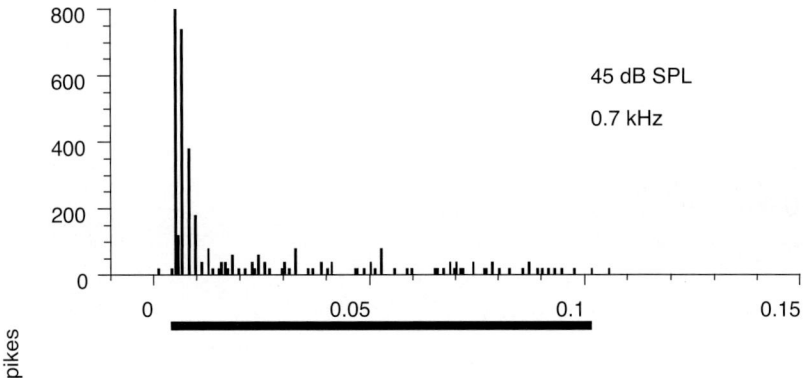
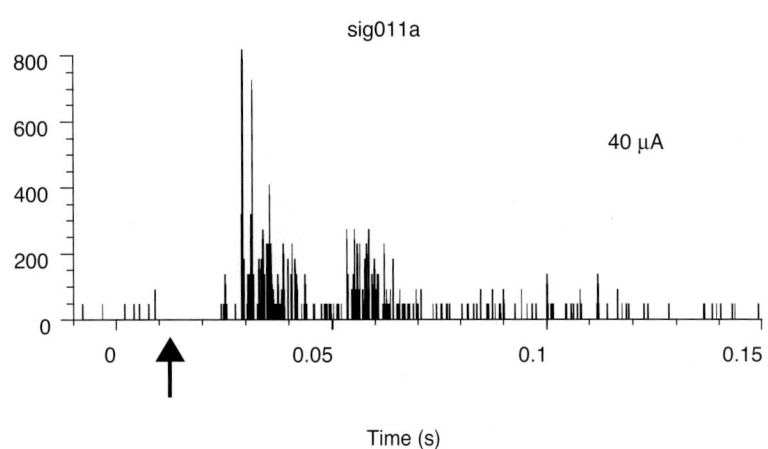

FIGURE 10-6. Poststimulus time histograms of unit responses from the ventral cochlear nucleus onset unit in response to best-frequency tonebursts (*top*) and trigeminal ganglion stimulation (*bottom*). The response pattern to the best-frequency toneburst showing an onset-to-average ratio of > 10:1, together with an interval histogram showing strong phase locking, defines this unit as an onset unit (see Godfrey DA et al.[50]). *Bar* indicates onset and duration of toneburst; *arrow* indicates onset of trigeminal stimulation. Reproduced with permission from Shore SE et al.[29]

evidence that trigeminal and acoustic stimuli can be integrated by VCN units. This means that responses to both stimuli, when presented simultaneously, are greater than (or less than) the sum of the responses to each stimulus alone. An example of such integration is shown in Figure 10-8. Responses of this VCN unit to sound show a primary-like response with a maximum firing rate around 200 spikes/s at the onset of the stimulus, which levels out to a steady-state firing rate below 100 spikes/s. The response to trigeminal stimulation shows a maximum spike count around 100 spikes. In contrast, when both signals are presented together, the firing rate increases dramatically over the duration of the sound, eliminating the reduced-rate steady-state level. The multisensory integration demonstrated here is not unique to the CN but has been demonstrated in higher auditory, somatosensory, and visual centers.[31] This enhancement of CN and IC (see below) responses to sound by somatosensory stimulation could give us clues as to how multisensory integration may play a role in somatic tinnitus.

ELECTRICAL STIMULATION OF BRAINSTEM SOMATOSENSORY NUCLEI

Responses of CN Neurons The large distribution of response latencies to trigeminal ganglion stimulation among VCN units indicates that many of these units are being activated through multiple synapses (Figure 10-9). This would be expected because, in addition to direct projections from the trigeminal ganglion, the CN receives projections from brainstem somatosensory nuclei. In my laboratory studies, stimulation of the trigeminal nuclei in the brainstem can produce responses similar to those observed with trigeminal ganglion stimulation (Figure 10-10). The right panel

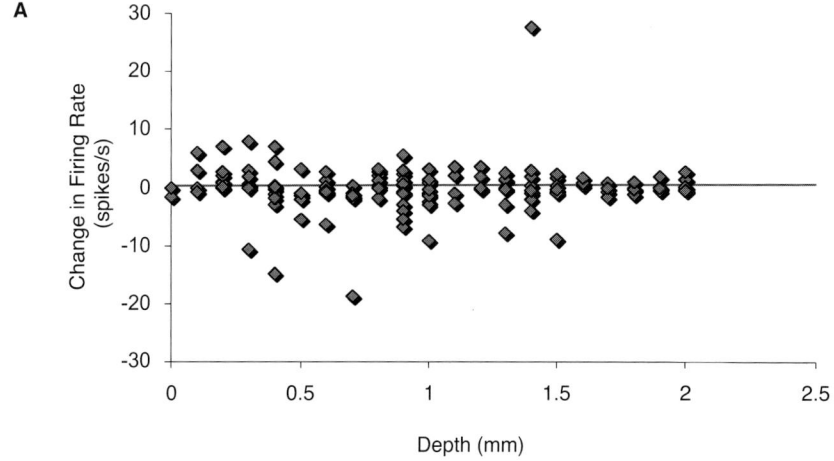

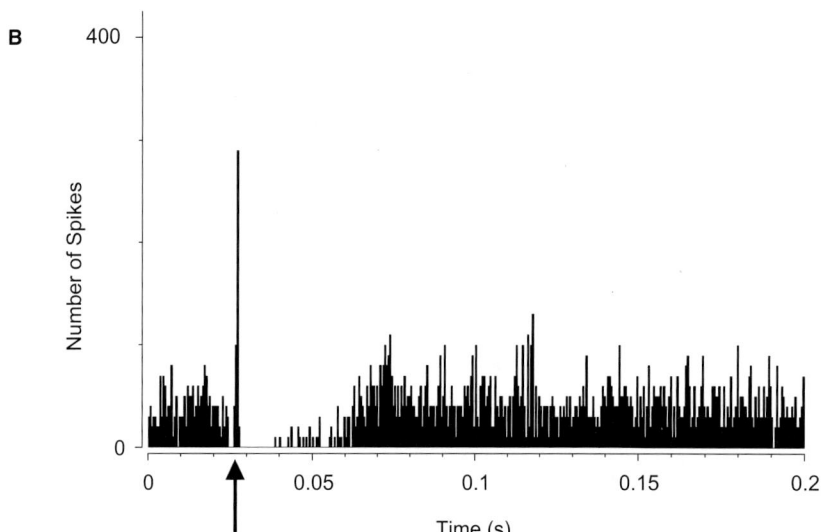

FIGURE 10-7. *A*, Change in firing rate of units at the posteroventral cochlear nucleus—dorsal cochlear nucleus (DCN) border and units within the DCN produced by stimulating the trigeminal ganglion with biphasic pulses at a current level of 80 μA. Zero represents spontaneous rate. Each symbol represents one single unit or a multiunit cluster. Inhibition of spontaneous rate is observed more frequently than excitation. *B*, Poststimulus time histograms of unit responses from one DCN unit in response to trigeminal ganglion stimulation (50 μA). *Arrow* indicates onset of trigeminal ganglion stimulation. Inhibition subsides slowly. Recovery to previous spontaneous rate takes approximately 100 milliseconds.

of Figure 10-10 demonstrates the responses of three units recorded on a 16-channel recording probe placed in the VCN. The top unit shows a long-duration response to the short-duration electrical pulse (the arrow shows the onset of electrical stimulus). The units in the middle and lower panels show short-duration excitation followed by inhibition. Responses to electrical stimulation of the trigeminal nuclei were often of longer duration than those observed with trigeminal ganglion stimulation. The latencies of responses obtained from trigeminal nucleus stimulation ranged from 3 to 12 milliseconds, largely excluding the possibility of monosynaptic activation and suggesting activation through the granule cell circuit or synaptic nests.[32,33] Similarly, stimulation of the lateral paragiganticular region of the reticular formation, which itself receives trigeminal input, can produce excitation of VCN units. Conventional tract tracing methods were used to establish the locations of neurons in the trigeminal nucleus and reticular formation that project to the cochlear nucleus. The left panel of Figure 10-10 shows the results of such an experiment in which the tracer fluorgold (Fluorochrome, LLC, Denver, CO) was injected into the lateral PVCN and produced labeled cells in the spinal trigeminal nucleus and the lateral paragiganticular reticular formation. The location of these labeled cells guided the placement of stimulating electrodes.

Responses of IC Neurons Because somatosensory nuclei innervate the ICx and the CN, it is not surprising that stimulation of trigeminal nuclei can directly and indirectly (through the CN) alter the responsiveness of neurons in the IC. Unit responses were recorded

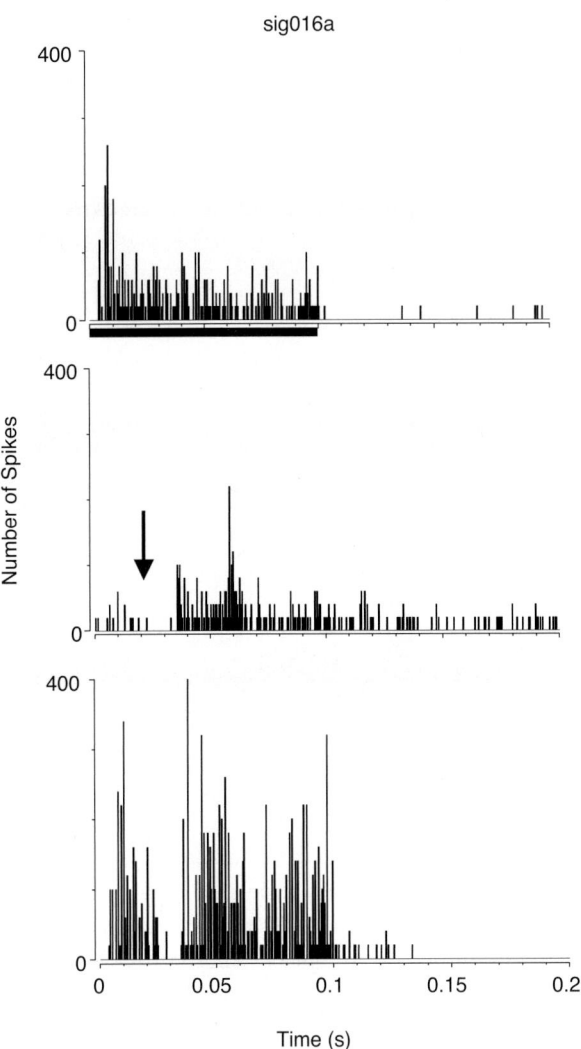

FIGURE 10-8. Responses of a primary-like unit to a best-frequency toneburst (100 milliseconds, 30 dB SPL) in the top panel; a 60 μA pulse delivered to the trigeminal ganglion beginning at 25 milliseconds (*arrow*) in the middle panel; and both signals together in the lower panel. The *bar* below the histogram in the top panel indicates the duration of the toneburst. The response to electrical stimulation of the trigeminal ganglion dramatically enhances the response to the toneburst over its duration.

from the ICx and ICc in response to trigeminal nucleus and reticular formation stimulation and showed that such stimulation can increase or decrease the firing rate of these neurons, especially in the presence of sound stimulation. In one example (Figure 10-11), the stimulating electrode was located in the spinal trigeminal nucleus and the recording electrode in the ICc. Figure 10-11A shows rate-level functions to broadband noise with and without a 200 μs/phase electrical pulse applied to the trigeminal nucleus. Several current levels

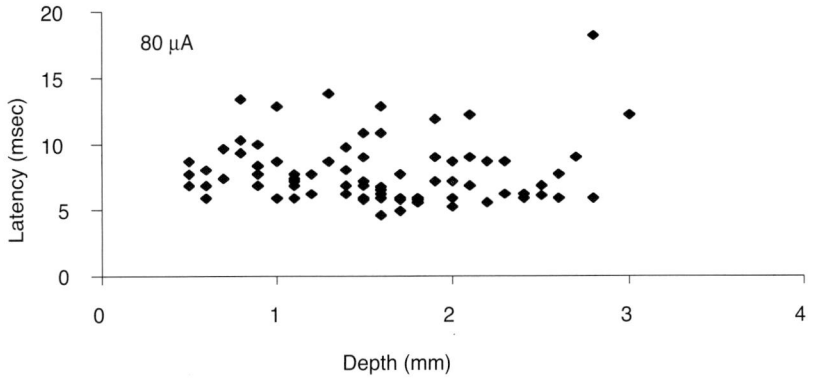

FIGURE 10-9. The latencies of ventral cochlear nucleus (VCN) unit responses elicited by trigeminal ganglion stimulation are shown as a function of the depth of the recording site within the VCN. Depth is indicated as millimeters from the surface of the dorsal cochlear nucleus. Reproduced with permission from Shore SE et al.[29]

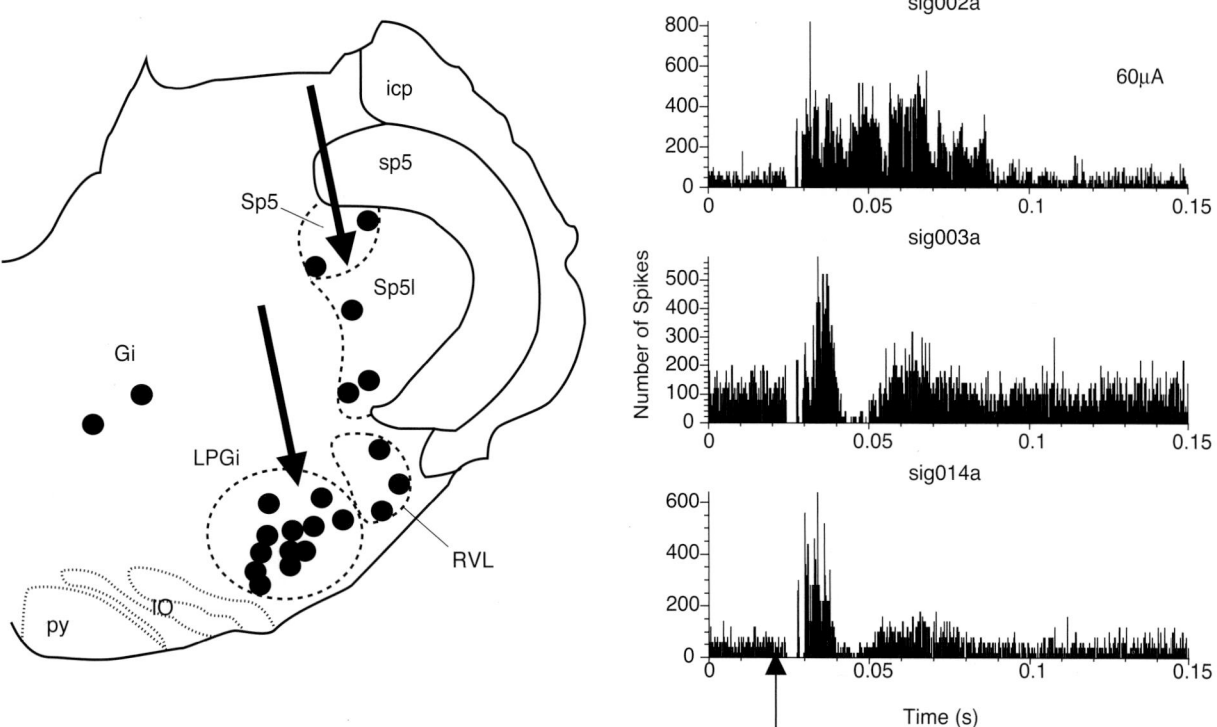

FIGURE 10-10. Left, Transverse section of the brainstem caudal to the cochlear nucleus. *Filled circles* indicate locations of fluorgold (FG)-labeled cells following an injection of FG into the posteroventral cochlear nucleus. icp = inferior cerebellar peduncle; IO = inferior olive; LPGi = ipsilateral lateral paragiganticular reticular formation; py = pyramidal tract; RVL = lateroventral reticular formation; sp5 = spinal tract of cranial nerve V; Sp5l = spinal nucleus of cranial nerve V. *Arrows* indicate locations of stimulating electrodes that produced the type of responses shown at right. *Right,* Poststimulus time histograms of responses obtained in three different ventral cochlear nucleus units to electrical stimulation of the Sp5, indicated by the *top arrow in the left panel.*

are shown. The suppressive effects of electrical stimulation peak around sound levels of 20 dB SPL, and the responses decline above 40 dB SPL. This is true whether the sound is excitatory, as shown in Figure 10-11A, or inhibitory (see Figure 10-11B) to the IC neuron. The finding that electrical stimulation of the trigeminal nuclei has more pronounced effects when combined with sound stimulation suggests the occurrence of multisensory integration, as shown in other sensory systems and described above for VCN neurons. If the combined response to the two stimuli is different from the algebraic sum of responses to each stimulus alone, integration is occurring. Figure 10-11C shows such integration for the unit shown in Figure 10-11A unit 2 (U2) and unit 12 (U12). In these examples, the algebraic sum (E + S) of responses to each stimulus is much larger than the combined response (ES), indicating the occurrence of integration that is inhibitory in nature. The surprising aspect of these findings is the inhibitory nature of the stimulation because projections to the IC from trigeminal regions have been shown to be glutamatergic. However, most of the projections are to ICx, and our recordings in this case were in ICc, suggesting a multisynaptic connection or indirect activation through projections from the CN.

CROSSMODAL PLASTICITY AND TINNITUS

Just as amputation of an arm can lead to perceptions of pain in the absent limb ("phantom pain"),[34] so can absence of auditory input to the central nervous system lead to the perceptions of "phantom" sounds, or tinnitus. Clinical reports showing that tinnitus often persists after surgical resection of the auditory nerve stress the importance of tinnitus having central components.[35] Several investigators have proposed

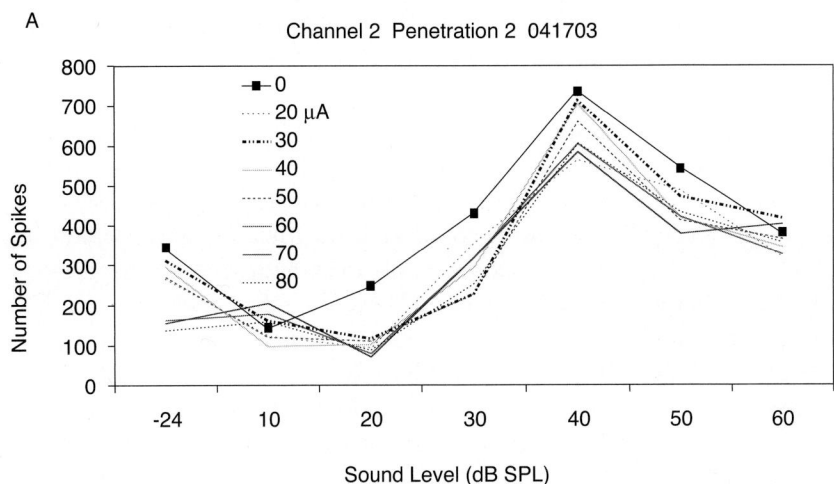

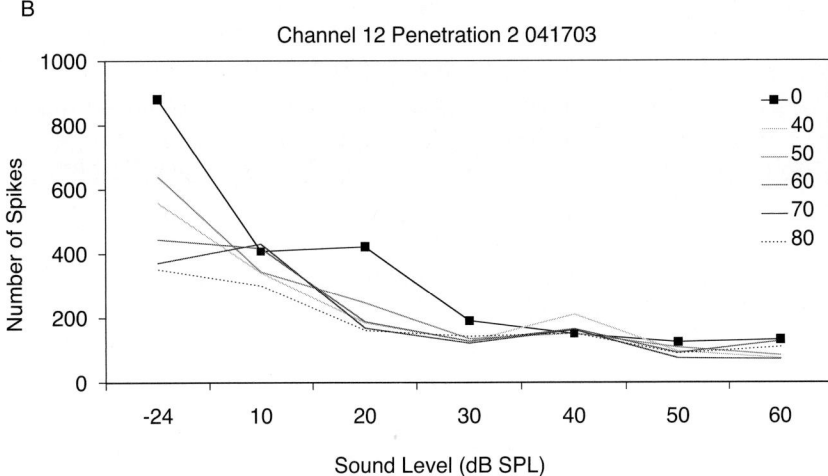

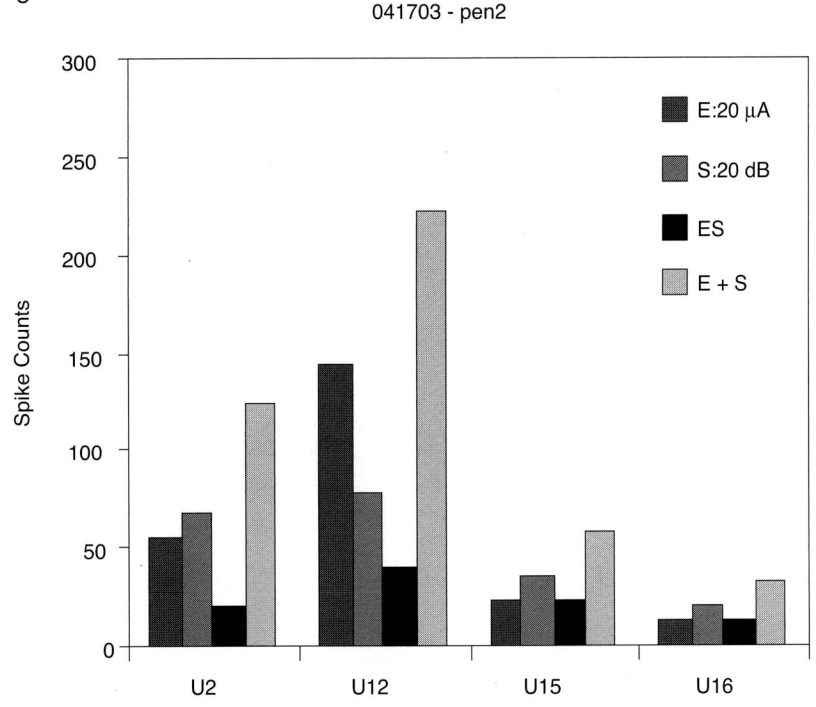

FIGURE 10-11. A, The number of spikes elicited from one inferior colliculus (IC) unit in response to noise bursts is shown as a function of the noise level. Electrical stimulation is applied at the trigeminal nucleus at several different current levels, as shown. Depression of the responses to the noise is especially evident at low sound levels. This depression occurs for a range of current levels from 20 to 80 μA. *B*, The number of spikes elicited from a different IC unit in response to noise bursts is shown as a function of the noise level. Electrical stimulation is applied at the trigeminal nucleus at several different current levels, as shown. Depression of the responses to the noise, even in a unit inhibited by sound, is especially evident at low sound levels. This depression occurs for a range of current levels from 20 to 80 μA. *C*, The number of spikes elicited by sound stimulation (S), electrical stimulation (E), and sound plus electrical stimulation (ES) is compared with the number of spikes obtained by the algebraic summation of E and S. Units 2 and 12 show multisensory integration because their response to electrical and sound stimulation is dramatically smaller than the responses obtained by algebraic summation of their responses to each signal alone.

that tinnitus involves disturbances of spontaneous activity at central levels of the auditory pathway.[36,37] This notion is supported by studies showing that sodium salicylate treatment and noise exposure result in altered spontaneous activity in the central auditory system, including the CN.[36–38] Those animals treated with sodium salicylate or noise exposure also experience tinnitus-like percepts.[39,40]

How does this increase in spontaneous discharge occur? One possibility is that inhibitory pathways are downgraded,[41–44] whereas another is that unmasking of silent, glutamatergic synapses occurs.[45–47] How might auditory-somatosensory interactions contribute to these alterations, especially at the brainstem level? It is intriguing that loss of outer hair cells may be a necessary ingredient for the increased excitation that occurs in the central auditory system after damage to the cochlea.[37] Outer hair cells are innervated by type II auditory nerve fibers, which centrally innervate the granule cell region of the CN.[21,48] The granule cell region, in turn, receives input from many areas of the brain, including somatosensory systems.[10,20,21] Thus, the decreased innervation of the granule cell region resulting from outer hair cell loss might be a signal for compensatory crossmodal reinnervation of this area, resulting in changes in the balance of excitation and inhibition. Decreased peripheral auditory input to central structures may, in some cases, lead to pathologic plastic changes or overcompensation for decreased auditory input and thus to the perception of tinnitus. It is well established that crossmodal reafferentation of denervated cortical regions occurs after blindness and deafness.[49]

What happens when we stimulate the locations of trigeminal connections to the CN in animals that have been deafened? Figure 10-12A shows responses of three VCN units to trigeminal ganglion stimulation before and after one guinea pig was deafened by cochlear ablation. Compound action potentials were recorded before and after the procedure to demonstrate the presence of total deafness. The unit responses shown here have diminished amplitudes after cochlear ablation. Most units showed this pattern after cochlear ablation.[29] Most units also showed decreased spontaneous rate after cochlear ablation. The reduced responsiveness to trigeminal stimulation could then be a result of descending inhibitory influences dominating the unit responses because auditory nerve drive is reduced. Some units, however, show an increased responsiveness to trigeminal stimulation after cochlear ablation (see Figure 10-12B, right panel, lower histogram). In such a case, increased responses to trigeminal input could account for a perceived phantom sound, most notably in somatic tinnitus. Studies are under way that will examine the effects of trigeminal stimulation on VCN responses in animals deafened for longer periods of time. In cases with longer-duration deafness, we would expect not a decrease but an increase in the spontaneous rate of CN neurons,[38] which could, in turn, facilitate the responses of CN neurons to trigeminal input. Alternatively, given time for plastic changes such as reinnervation of the sensory-deprived region (CN), there could be increased somatosensory innervation of the CN, an alternative substrate mechanism for certain forms of tinnitus.

Just as the areas that show cortical reorganization after sensory deprivation are predominantly those that mediate multisensory integration in normal individuals, so might more peripheral sites that integrate multimodal stimuli, such as in the CN or IC, be more susceptible to plastic changes. Changes in brainstem regions after deprivation have been shown to contribute to reorganization at the level of the thalamus and cortex. Therefore, discovering which brainstem areas mediate multisensory integration might give us cues as to where to expect plastic reorganization after sensory deprivation. Understanding the mechanisms that mediate such reorganization will contribute to our understanding of the differentiation of sensory systems and how they might go awry after deprivation, producing by-products such as phantom pain and tinnitus.

ACKNOWLEDGMENTS

The author would like to thank the following people who have contributed to this chapter with their hard work and talents, and without whom this chapter would not have been possible: Helena Bissinger, Roshini Jain, Jianzhong Lu, Christian Sumner, Seth Koehler, and Jianxun Zhou. This work was supported by grants from the National Institutes of Health (ROI DC 004825), the Tinnitus Research Consortium, and the American Tinnitus Association.

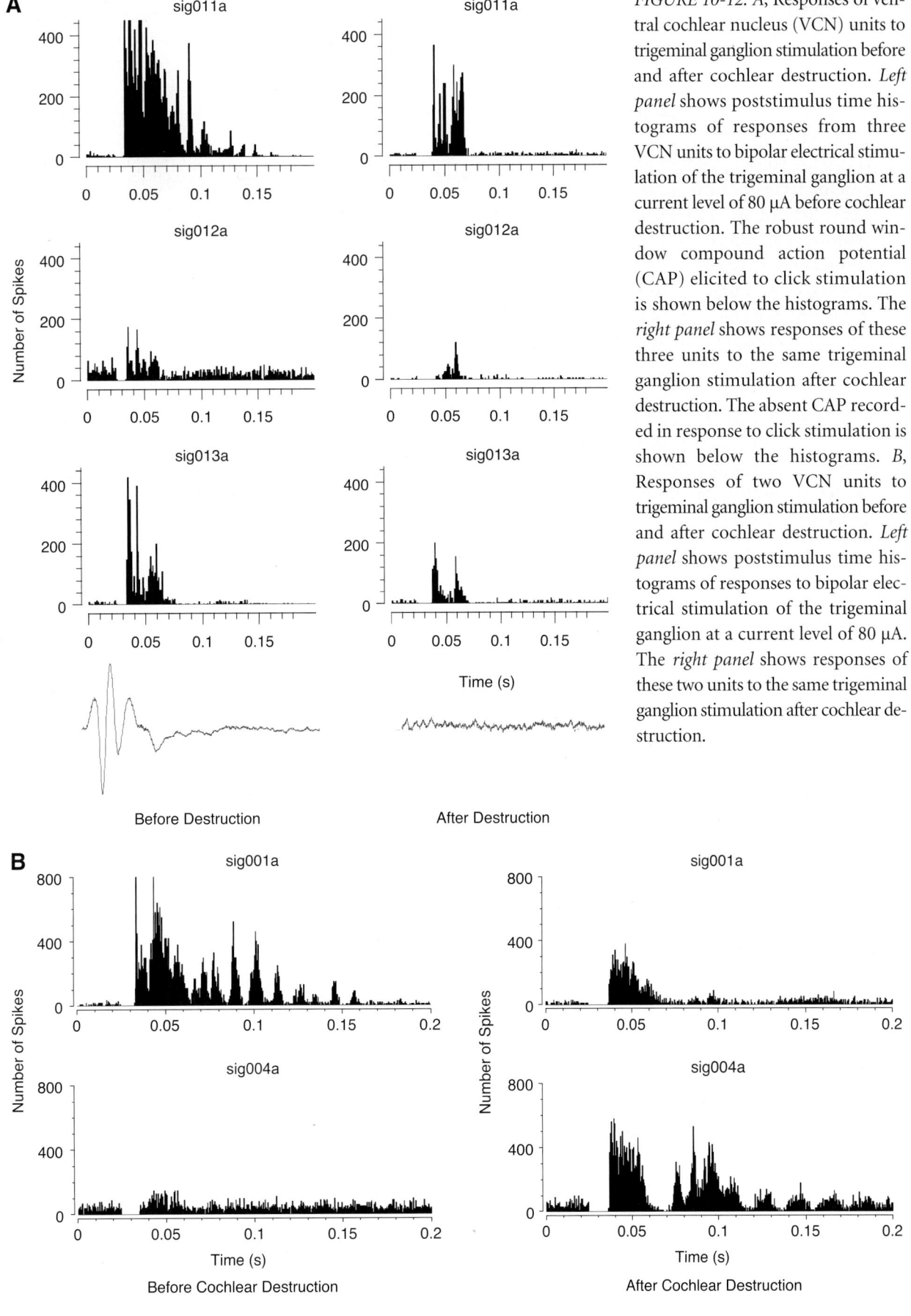

FIGURE 10-12. *A*, Responses of ventral cochlear nucleus (VCN) units to trigeminal ganglion stimulation before and after cochlear destruction. *Left panel* shows poststimulus time histograms of responses from three VCN units to bipolar electrical stimulation of the trigeminal ganglion at a current level of 80 μA before cochlear destruction. The robust round window compound action potential (CAP) elicited to click stimulation is shown below the histograms. The *right panel* shows responses of these three units to the same trigeminal ganglion stimulation after cochlear destruction. The absent CAP recorded in response to click stimulation is shown below the histograms. *B*, Responses of two VCN units to trigeminal ganglion stimulation before and after cochlear destruction. *Left panel* shows poststimulus time histograms of responses to bipolar electrical stimulation of the trigeminal ganglion at a current level of 80 μA. The *right panel* shows responses of these two units to the same trigeminal ganglion stimulation after cochlear destruction.

REFERENCES

1. Lockwood AH, Salvi RJ, Coad ML, et al. The functional neuroanatomy of tinnitus: evidence for limbic system links and neural plasticity. Neurology 1998;50:114–20.
2. Levine RA. Somatic modulation of tinnitus appears to be a fundamental attribute of tinnitus. In: Hazell J, editor. Proceedings of the Sixth International Tinnitus Seminar. London: The Tinnitus and Hyperacusis Centre; 1999. p. 193–7.
3. Whittaker CK. Intriguing change in tinnitus with eye movement. Am J Otol 1983;4:273.
4. Cacace AT. Expanding the biological basis of tinnitus: crossmodal origins and the role of neuroplasticity. Hear Res 2003;175:112–32.
5. Møller AR, Møller MB, Yokota M. Some forms of tinnitus may involve the extralemniscal auditory pathway. Laryngoscope 1992;102:1165–71.
6. Møller AR, Rollins PR. The non-classical auditory pathways are involved in hearing in children but not in adults. Neurosci Lett 2002;319:41–4.
7. Møller AR. Sensory systems: anatomy and physiology. San Diego (CA): Academic Press; 2003. p. 69.
8. Malmierca M, Merchan MA, Henkel CK, et al. Direct projections from cochlear nuclear complex to auditory thalamus in the rat. J Neurosci 2002;22:11091–7.
9. Shore SE, Helfert RH, Bledsoe SC, et al. Descending projections to the dorsal and ventral divisions of the cochlear nucleus in guinea pig. Hear Res 1991;52:255–68.
10. Shore SE, Vass Z, Wys NL, et al. The trigeminal ganglion innervates the auditory brainstem. J Comp Neurol 2000;419:271–85.
11. Vass Z, Shore SE, Nuttall AL, et al. Trigeminal ganglion innervation of the cochlea—a retrograde transport study. Neuroscience 1997;79:605–15.
12. Aigner M, Lukas JR, Denk M, et al. Sensory innervation of the guinea pig extraocular muscles: a 1,1′-dioctadecyl-3,3,3′3′-tetramethylindocarbocyanine perchlorate tracing and calcitonin gene-related peptide immunohistochemical study. J Comp Neurol 1997;380:16–22.
13. Kevetter GA, Perachio AA. Projections from the sacculus to the cochlear nuclei in the Mongolian gerbil. Brain Behav Evol 1989;34:193–200.
14. Moller AR. The acoustic middle ear reflex. In: Keidel WD, Neff WD, editors. Handbook of sensory physiology: auditory system. Vol V/2. Berlin: Springer-Verlag; 1975. p. 519–48.
15. Rouiller EM, Capt M, Dolivo M, et al. Neuronal organization of the stapedius reflex pathways in the rat: a retrograde HRP and viral transneuronal tracing study. Brain Res 1989;476:21–8.
16. Vass Z, Nuttall AL, Coleman JK, et al. Capsaicin-induced release of substance P increases cochlear blood flow in the guinea pig. Hear Res 1995;89:86–92.
17. Vass Z, Steyger PS, Hordichok AJ, et al. Capsaicin stimulation of the cochlea and electric stimulation of the trigeminal ganglion mediate vascular permeability in cochlear and vertebro-basilar arteries: a potential cause of inner ear dysfunction in headache. Neuroscience 2001;103:189–201.
18. Duckles SP, Buck SH. Substance P in the cerebral vasculature: depletion by capsaicin suggests a sensory role. Brain Res 1982;245:171–4.
19. Vass Z, Shore SE, Nuttall AL, et al. Endolymphatic hydrops reduces retrograde labeling of trigeminal innervation to the cochlea. Exp Neurol 1998;151:241–8.
20. Ryugo DK, Haenggeli C, Doucet JR. Multimodal inputs to the granule cell domain of the cochlear nucleus. Exp Brain Res 2003;153:477–86.
21. Shore SE, Moore JK. Sources of input to the cochlear granule cell region in the guinea pig. Hear Res 1998;116:33–42.
22. Warr W, Beck Boche JE, Ye Y, et al. Organization of olivocochlear neurons in the cat studied with the retrograde tracer cholera toxin-B. J Assoc Res Otolaryngol 2002;3:457–78.
23. Vass Z, Shore SE, Nuttall AL, et al. Direct evidence of trigeminal innervation of the cochlear blood vessels. Neuroscience 1998;84:559–67.
24. Benson TE, Berglund AM, Brown MC. Synaptic input to cochlear nucleus dendrites that receive medial olivocochlear synapses. J Comp Neurol 1996;365:27–41.
25. Willard FH, Martin GF. Collateral innervation of the inferior colliculus in the North American opossum: a study using fluorescent markers in a double-labeling paradigm. Brain Res 1984;303:171–82.
26. Saint Marie RL. Glutamatergic connections of the auditory midbrain: selective uptake and axonal transport of D-[3H]aspartate. J Comp Neurol 1996;373:255–70.
27. Li H, Mizuno N. Single neurons in the spinal trigeminal and dorsal column nuclei project to both the cochlear nucleus and the inferior colliculus by way of axon collaterals: a fluorescent retrograde double-

labeling study in the rat. Neurosci Res 1997; 29:135–42.
28. Young ED, Nelken I, Conley RA. Somatosensory effects on neurons in dorsal cochlear nucleus. J Neurophysiol 1995;73:743–65.
29. Shore SE, El-Kashlan HK, Lu J. Effects of trigeminal ganglion stimulation on unit activity of ventral cochlear nucleus neurons. Neuroscience 2003;119:1085–101.
30. Kirzinger A, Jurgens U. Vocalization-correlated single-unit activity in the brain stem of the squirrel monkey. Exp Brain Res 1991;84:545–60.
31. Wallace MT, Stein BE. Sensory and multisensory responses in the newborn monkey superior colliculus. J Neurosci 2001;21:8886–94.
32. Wright DD, Ryugo DK. Mossy fiber projections from the cuneate nucleus to the cochlear nucleus in the rat. J Comp Neurol 1996;365:159–72.
33. Hutson KA, Morest DK. Fine structure of the cell clusters in the cochlear nerve root: stellate, granule, and mitt cells offer insights into the synaptic organization of local circuit neurons. J Comp Neurol 1996;371:397–414.
34. Møller AR. Similarities between severe tinnitus and chronic pain. J Am Acad Audiol 2000;11:115–24.
35. Soussi T, Otto SR. Effects of electrical brainstem stimulation on tinnitus. Acta Otolaryngol (Stockh) 1994;114:135–40.
36. Jastreboff PJ, Sasaki CT. Salicylate-induced changes in spontaneous activity of single units in the inferior colliculus of the guinea pig. J Acoust Soc Am 1986;80:1384–91.
37. Kaltenbach JA, Rachel JD, Mathog TA, et al. Cisplatin-induced hyperactivity in the dorsal cochlear nucleus and its relation to outer hair cell loss: relevance to tinnitus. J Neurophysiol 2002;88:699–714.
38. Kaltenbach JA, Afman CE. Hyperactivity in the dorsal cochlear nucleus after intense sound exposure and its resemblance to tone-evoked activity: a physiological model for tinnitus. Hear Res 2000;140:165–72.
39. Jastreboff PJ, Brennan JF, Sasaki CT. Quinine-induced tinnitus in rats. Arch Otolaryngol Head Neck Surg 1991;117:1162–6.
40. Heffner HE, Harrington IA. Tinnitus in hamsters following exposure to intense sound. Hear Res 2002;170:83–95.
41. Syka J. Plastic changes in the central auditory system after hearing loss, restoration of function, and during learning. Physiol Rev 2002;82:601–36.
42. Mossop JE, Wilson MJ, Caspary DM, et al. Down-regulation of inhibition following unilateral deafening. Hear Res 2000;147:183–7.
43. Wang J, Caspary D, Salvi RJ. GABA-A antagonist causes dramatic expansion of tuning in primary auditory cortex. Neuroreport 2000;11:1137–40.
44. Szczepaniak WS, Møller AR. Evidence of decreased GABAergic influence on temporal integration in the inferior colliculus following acute noise exposure: a study of evoked potentials in the rat. Neurosci Lett 1995;196:77–80.
45. Baba H, Doubell TP, Moore KA, et al. Silent NMDA receptor-mediated synapses are developmentally regulated in the dorsal horn of the rat spinal cord. J Neurophysiol 2000;83:955–62.
46. Atwood HL, Wojtowicz JM. Silent synapses in neural plasticity: current evidence. Learn Mem 1999; 6:542–71.
47. Li P, Zhuo M. Silent glutamatergic synapses and nociception in mammalian spinal cord. Nature 1998;393:695–8.
48. Brown MC, Berglund AM, Kiang NY, et al. Central trajectories of type II spiral ganglion neurons. J Comp Neurol 1988;278:581–90.
49. Ryugo DK, Ryugo R, Globus A, et al. Increased spine density in auditory cortex following visual or somatic deafferentation. Brain Res 1975;90:143–6.
50. Godfrey DA, Kiang NY, Norris BE. Single unit activity in the posteroventral cochlear nucleus of the cat. J Comp Neurol 1975;162:269–84.

EDITORIAL COMMENTARY

Levine argues that somatic modulation of perception is a fundamental property of the auditory system and that somatic modulation of tinnitus loudness, pitch, and location is a common phenomenon. Head and neck maneuvers are more frequently effective in modulating tinnitus than are extremity contractions. Levine reasons that sensory afferent input from muscle spindle and Golgi tendon organ activation ultimately to the dorsal cochlear nucleus or inferior colliculus is responsible for the change in tinnitus.

Somatic tinnitus is temporally associated with injury or disease of the musculoskeletal system, particularly of the head and neck and most especially the preauricular area and the upper part of the sternocleidomastoid muscle. Levine points out that somatic tinnitus is characteristically unilateral and ipsilateral to the somatic lesion.

Levine's neurologic model of somatic tinnitus states that the origin of the somatic tinnitus most frequently results from input from the upper cervical dorsal roots, trigeminal nerve in the spinal trigeminal tract, or the common spinal tract of the facial, glossopharyngeal, and vagus nerves to the medullary somatosensory nuclei located dorsolaterally in the lower part of the medulla and upper cervical part of the spinal cord and then to the ipsilateral dorsal cochlear nucleus, resulting in inappropriate excitation (disinhibition) of the auditory pathway. Levine also presents convincing histories and findings of patients in whom somatic factors interact with tinnitus of otic origin.

The somatosensory innervation of the cochlear nucleus, superior olivary complex, and inferior colliculus provides the bases for somatic tinnitus. Shore has delineated the anatomic details and perhaps, in part, the physiologic mechanisms underlying somatic tinnitus.

Stimulation of the trigeminal ganglion or nuclei results in both excitation and inhibition of the cochlear nucleus and inferior colliculus neurons. Shore has demonstrated integration of acoustic and somatosensory stimuli in the cochlear nucleus and inferior colliculus resulting in an enhanced or diminished response that is greater or less than the sum of the parts. This integration could play a role in the generation of somatic tinnitus.

James B. Snow Jr

CHAPTER 11

Neural Correlates of Tinnitus

James A. Kaltenbach, PhD, Jinsheng Zhang, PhD, Mark A. Zacharek, MD

The identification of the neural correlates of tinnitus has been a major research objective for many years. Knowledge of these correlates is of fundamental importance for an understanding of the structures and mechanisms involved in tinnitus. Although progress in achieving this objective has been slow, this field of investigation has recently gained considerable momentum. There has been a rapid increase in the number of studies describing physiologically relevant changes in the auditory systems of animals that were treated with tinnitus-inducing agents. In parallel with these efforts, a number of laboratories have developed behavioral methods for the psychophysical assessment of tinnitus in animals. This has opened up new possibilities for testing the relationship between changes in neural function recorded electrophysiologically and the presence of tinnitus demonstrated behaviorally.

At the same time, the clinical literature has matured to new levels, providing fresh insights and perspectives. Modern imaging technologies have made possible the identification of regions of abnormal activity in the brains of human subjects with tinnitus. These studies have revealed that tinnitus is associated with hyperactivity at the cortical and subcortical levels of the auditory system and some nonauditory areas. They further show that the central part of the auditory system is an important and, sometimes, the exclusive source of tinnitus-associated signals. It has recently been discovered that modulation of tinnitus by certain somatic manipulations is more common than previously realized. Maneuvers, such as clenching of the jaws, applying pressure to the shoulder or neck, or movement of the eyes, cause a change in the percepts of tinnitus in the majority of individuals (see Chapter 9, "Somatic Tinnitus"). This suggests that neural correlates of tinnitus should be sought in structures of the brain that integrate information from the auditory and nonauditory systems. Also, new information has been published on the psychophysical characteristics of tinnitus. These results suggest that as many as 75% of patients with tinnitus match their tinnitus to frequencies above 4 kHz, and the median pitch is 6 kHz.[1] These characteristics help define the types of stimuli that most resemble the percepts of tinnitus and bring the search for tinnitus correlates into a narrower focus.

In this chapter, we review the progress that has been made in the search for neural correlates of tinnitus in various animal models. The chapter is divided into three sections. The first section reviews the psychophysical aspects of tinnitus, describing the principal attributes of these percepts that are most revealing of its underlying neural basis. The second section reviews the history of the search for its neurophysiological correlates, examining the neural responses to acoustic stimuli that resemble tinnitus and summarizing the effects of tinnitus-inducing agents on resting activity in the auditory system. The third section focuses on the results of studies implicating hyperactivity of the dorsal cochlear nucleus (DCN) as a possible site of tinnitus generation. We summarize what is known about the relationship between altered activity in the DCN and tinnitus and then discuss experimental findings that have helped uncover some of the mechanisms by which these alterations are induced.

PSYCHOPHYSICAL CHARACTERISTICS OF TINNITUS

An appreciation of the perceptual features of tinnitus is essential if an understanding of the underlying correlates is to be obtained. This seems especially true given that the attributes will vary depending on the underlying lesions, which, in turn, will depend on the inducing agent, and, for a given inducing agent, the correlates will depend on the severity of its effects. Unfortunately, tinnitus is difficult to study systematically as a function of the cause and degree of exposure because many inducers of tinnitus carry a risk of permanent injury. For this reason, most of our knowledge about the psychophysics of tinnitus has come from studies using agents of induction with relatively low risk levels. These include salicylate and brief exposures to moderate or high levels of sound. These agents have been found to be very effective inducers of the reversible (acute) form of tinnitus. In addition, several studies have examined the characteristics of tinnitus induced by more prolonged exposures to sound that have caused the chronic form of tinnitus. The acute and chronic forms of tinnitus induced by these agents are described here.

SALICYLATE-INDUCED TINNITUS

Salicylate induces the acute form of tinnitus, which is usually reversible and has an onset that is clearly correlated with the ingestion of the drug. This form usually becomes noticeable within a few hours to a few days following ingestion of high-dose salicylate. The dose that seems necessary for tinnitus induction generally ranges between 100 and 500 mg/kg of body weight, although a dose of 200 mg/kg is the most commonly reported threshold. Increases in dose result in corresponding increases in tinnitus loudness.[2] The induced tinnitus is characterized as a continuous high-pitched tone, hum, or noise. The pitch is typically matched to frequencies above 7 kHz,[3] although matches to lower frequencies have been reported.[2] Usually, salicylate-induced tinnitus is associated with hearing loss, although some studies suggest that the threshold and time course of the induced hearing loss and tinnitus differ somewhat.[4] For example, the onset of tinnitus is sometimes reported as preceding that of the hearing loss. The hearing loss and the tinnitus generally disappear within a few days following cessation of treatment.

ACUTE NOISE-INDUCED TINNITUS

It is important to distinguish between the various severities of noise-induced tinnitus because they likely involve different mechanisms. Depending on the exposure conditions and the susceptibility of the individual, noise-induced tinnitus can be acute or chronic. Acute tinnitus can last from a few minutes to a few weeks after the exposure. The duration of chronic tinnitus ranges from months to years. The psychophysical characteristics of acute noise-induced tinnitus in humans have been described in several reports.[5–8] In these investigations, humans were exposed for 5 minutes to tones (500–3,000 Hz), white noise, or narrowband noise with center frequencies of 2 to 6 kHz. The levels varied between 90 and 120 dB sound pressure level (SPL). Each of these exposure conditions induced tinnitus immediately after exposure. The tinnitus was most commonly perceived as being tonal and short in duration (15–50 minutes). For tonal and narrowband noise exposures, the frequency matching the pitch of the induced tinnitus was generally shifted upward with increases in exposure frequency and was usually higher than the frequency of the exposure sound (Figure 11-1A). The size of the octave interval between the frequency of the tinnitus pitch match and the frequency of the exposure stimulus was dependent on the frequency of the exposure stimulus.[6] In most cases, the tinnitus was associated with hearing loss, although the interval between the frequency at which hearing loss was greatest and the frequency of the tinnitus pitch match varied. However, one consistent feature was that when tinnitus was induced by pure-tone exposure, the pitch match was usually higher in frequency than the frequency of maximal hearing loss (Figure 11-1B, upper curve); when the inducing sound was narrowband noise, the pitch match was usually lower in frequency than the frequency of maximum hearing loss (Figure 11-1B, lower curve). In the majority of cases, the tinnitus was lateralized to the side of the exposed ear, although some subjects perceived the tinnitus on the side opposite the exposed ear.[7,8] Noise-induced tinnitus was also found to be maskable by presenting noise to the unexposed ear. These latter two observations suggest that this form of tinnitus might have an important central component.

CHRONIC NOISE-INDUCED TINNITUS

Almost all of what is known about this form of tinnitus comes from retrospective clinical evaluations of patients with histories of noise exposure or noise-induced hearing loss. This is a potential weakness of the literature because an association of tinnitus with a history of noise exposure does not necessarily establish noise as the causative agent. However, it is apparent

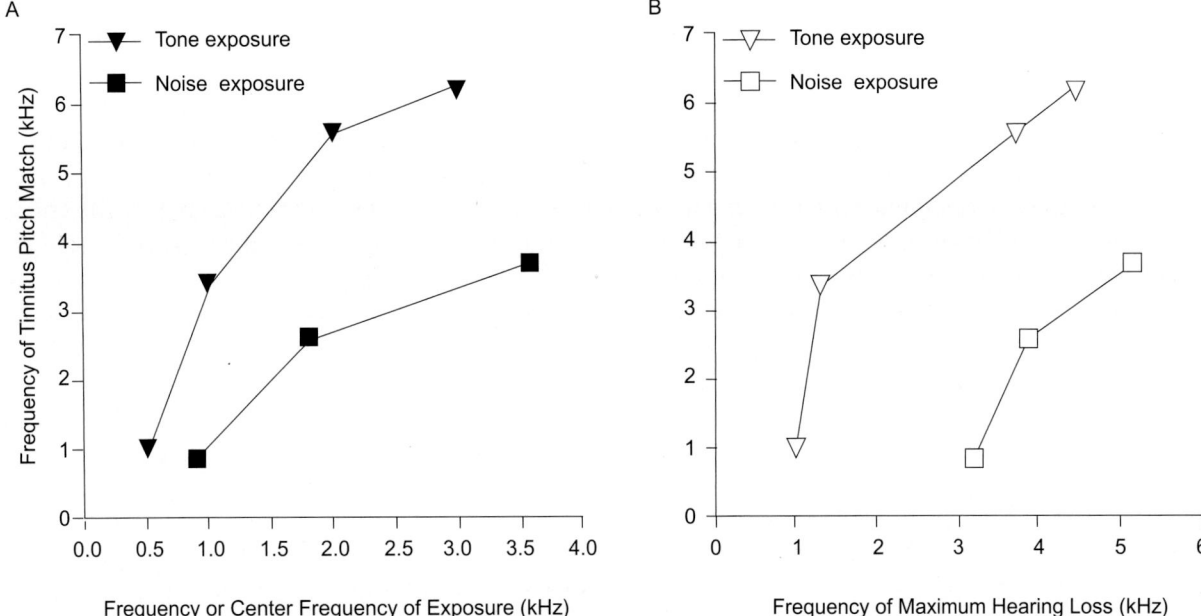

FIGURE 11-1. The relationships between pitch of intense sound-induced tinnitus and frequency of exposure tone or center frequency of noise (*A*) and between pitch of tinnitus and frequency of maximal hearing loss (*B*). Note in *A* that for both tonal and noise exposures, the frequency to which the pitch is matched shifts upward with exposure tone frequency. However, the pitch matches for tone exposures are generally higher than those of narrow bands of noise of equivalent center frequency.[6] *B* shows that the pitch match occurs at frequencies that are higher than the frequency of maximal hearing loss when the tinnitus-inducing sound was a tone but lower than the frequency of maximal hearing loss when the inducing sound was a narrow band of noise. Based on data from Loeb M and Smith RP.[6]

in these studies that considerable efforts have been made to rule out other possible causes. Axelsson and Barrenas briefly reviewed this topic,[9] and a summary of the principal findings follows. An important aspect of chronic noise-induced tinnitus, which seems to distinguish it from acute noise-induced tinnitus, is its time course. Acute noise-induced tinnitus is usually noticeable immediately after the acoustic exposure, whereas the chronic form is seldom remembered as developing immediately following an exposure. Although immediate onsets are sometimes reported, these have usually been associated with exposures to high-level, explosive noises such as firecrackers, cap guns, and gunshots. Subjects with permanent noise-induced tinnitus usually do not recall the onset time, and the impression conveyed in patient interviews is that their tinnitus developed gradually over many years. The reported incidences of tinnitus in subjects with noise-induced hearing loss vary widely across studies, spanning a range of 5 to 80%. This variation may be related to differences in exposure histories of the selected patient populations or could reflect differences in methods across studies. In any case, the lack of a consistent association between chronic noise-induced hearing loss and tinnitus indicates that the mechanisms underlying these two hearing disorders are probably to some degree independent. Chronic noise-induced tinnitus has usually been reported as being tonal or like a narrow band of noise. The loudness is usually matched to sounds within 10 dB of hearing thresholds. Its pitch is most commonly matched to frequencies between 3 and 8 kHz, with 4 kHz being the average for tonal noise-induced tinnitus and 6 kHz for noise-induced tinnitus resembling narrowband noise. Axelsson and Sandh found that the relationship between the tinnitus pitch and the frequency at which hearing loss was greatest depended on the pitch of the tinnitus.[10] When the pitch match was below 4 kHz, the frequency of greatest hearing loss was usually slightly higher than the frequency of the tinnitus pitch match; when the pitch match was above 4 kHz, the frequency of the pitch match corresponded well with the frequency of maximum hearing loss.[10] Slightly different results were reported by Man and Naggan, who found little correlation between the frequency of the pitch match and the frequency of maximum hearing loss.[11] As with temporary noise-induced tinnitus, the chronic form of tinnitus is most commonly lateralized to the ear with the greater hearing loss. Surprisingly, chronic noise-induced tinnitus, like the acute form, is sometimes reported on the side opposite the ear with the greater hearing loss.[9] This is an additional finding suggesting that hearing loss and tinnitus involve separate mechanisms.

OTHER FORMS OF TINNITUS

Although tinnitus induced by noise and tinnitus induced by salicylate are the best characterized forms of tinnitus, there are numerous other causes. Acute tinnitus and chronic tinnitus are common symptoms among those treated with certain ototoxic drugs, particularly the aminoglycosides (eg, tobramycin, gentamicin, streptomycin), certain antineoplastic agents (cisplatin and carboplatin), antimalarial agents (quinine, chloroquine), and loop diuretics (ethacrynic acid, furosemide).[12] Unfortunately, little is known about the psychophysical characteristics of tinnitus caused by these agents. Aminoglycosides and platin drugs have been shown to cause high-frequency hearing loss, and the pathology underlying this loss usually involves damage to the hair cells in the basal end of the cochlea. This would predict that the induced tinnitus is probably high in pitch, which is consistent with the fact that patients treated with these agents often describe their tinnitus as a ringing sound. This is contrasted to the type of tinnitus that is associated with Meniere's disease, which is commonly described as a low-pitched, roaring sound.

NEUROPHYSIOLOGICAL CORRELATES OF TINNITUS

Current views on the neural correlates of tinnitus have been influenced by two separate but complementary lines of inquiry. First, insights have been obtained from studies examining how the auditory system responds to sound. Although the precise nature of the neural code that leads to sound percepts is not yet known, much has been learned about how neurons behave when they are responding to sounds, particularly the simple dimensions of sound such as pitch and loudness, features that are also characteristic of most forms of tinnitus. This information provides important suggestions of what we should expect a neural "code" of tinnitus to look like. Additional insights have been provided by studies examining the effects of tinnitus-inducing agents on neural activity in the auditory system. Such agents have been found to cause changes in neural activity that in some ways resemble neuronal responses to sound. This section describes findings bearing on these issues.

NEURAL CORRELATES OF ACOUSTICALLY EVOKED SOUND PERCEPTS THAT RESEMBLE TINNITUS

According to a recent publication, most tinnitus is tonal in character and has a pitch that can be matched to a specific frequency.[1] The frequency of the pitch match is usually quite high, falling in the range of 3 to 8 kHz. As just discussed, this applies also to the form of tinnitus that is induced by noise and salicylate. Thus, we might expect some commonality between the changes in neural activity that are induced experimentally by salicylate and noise and the behaviors that neurons display in response to tones in the 3 to 8 kHz range. Here we describe the neural responses to sounds that may relate to the common forms of tinnitus.

Increases in Neuronal Discharge Rates The most pervasive response to sound is an increase in neural discharge rate. For most auditory nerve fibers, discharge rates increase monotonically as a function of stimulus intensity. The dynamic range over which such monotonicities are observed ranges between 20 and 75 dB.[13,14] However, humans are able to discriminate changes in intensity over a 120 dB range. Thus, the loudness of a tone must be determined by the combined rates across sets of neurons. Alternative codes have been proposed, although the most widely accepted code is the one based on discharge rate. Some classes of neurons, whose discharge rates are more complex, have been identified in the central part of the auditory system. These neurons show nonmonotonic rate-intensity functions. However, these nonmonotonic responses are shaped by inhibition from neighboring neurons, and it is believed that this inhibition may play a role in modulating the dynamic range of a neuron, possibly expanding or narrowing it, depending on the aspects of stimulation that are of interest.

Because most auditory neurons show monotonic increases in discharge rates with acoustic stimulation, it is usually assumed that increases in discharge rate would be an important neural correlate of the loudness of most forms of tinnitus.

Increases in the Number of Active Neurons Increases in stimulus intensity also cause a spread in the wave of excitation along the cochlear partition. This leads to an expansion in the bandwidth over which neurons are activated. In other words, the number of active neurons is increased as the stimulus level increases. A good demonstration of this phenomenon was described by Kim and Molnar.[15] They showed that at low stimulus levels, activation occurred only among neurons with a narrow range of characteristic frequencies (CFs); as the stimulus level was increased, the band of active neurons expanded to include neurons with a wider range of CFs. This recruitment of responding neurons with increases in stimulus level has also been observed in central auditory nuclei using the 2-deoxyglucose (2-DG) metabolic mapping technique.[16] What is unclear is the extent to which information about the number of active neurons is used by the auditory system to encode stimulus intensity. On the one hand, psychophysical studies indicate that even when the spread of excitation across the neural array is removed by masking with bandstop noise (noise with a $\frac{1}{3}$-octave gap), humans can still discriminate changes in intensity over a 120 dB range.[17] On the other hand, the limited dynamic ranges of individual auditory nerve fibers indicate that the encoding of stimulus intensity must involve some process of integration of discharge rates across fibers, which is probably a function of the number of neurons responding. Thus, it seems likely that the number of active neurons represents a potential code of stimulus intensity, which could play a role in the encoding of tinnitus loudness. The pitch of tinnitus could be encoded by the CFs of the dominant neurons whose activity is increased.

Place of Peak Excitation The spatial mapping of frequency that is established along the cochlear partition is preserved in central auditory nuclei and in the auditory cortex in the form of a tonotopic map. Numerous studies at various levels of the auditory system have shown that the place of activation shifts along the tonotopic map with changes in stimulus frequency.[18] The width of the area activated by a tone or narrow band of noise is very restricted for near-threshold stimuli, such that only a few neurons are excited. As the stimulus level increases, the band of excitation expands to activate a larger number of neurons along the tonotopic gradient.[15] Although this spread of excitation is broad for suprathreshold tones, the perception of pitch does not change appreciably with stimulus level. The perceived pitch of the tone is thus most likely determined by the tonotopic locus at which neural activity is greatest. It is unknown why pitches are not heard for all sites that are active within this band of excitation; pitch extraction appears to involve a process of peak selection in which the auditory system rejects all but the locus at which activity is highest. Place theory of pitch encoding is well supported by psychophysical studies demonstrating distinct pitch percepts that shift with the locus of electrical stimulation at the cochlear and brainstem levels.[19,20] Place theory predicts that the pitch of tonal or narrowband noise-like tinnitus is determined by the CFs of the most active neurons, which is determined by the place where activity across the tonotopic gradient reaches a maximum. This seems especially likely for high-pitched tinnitus ($\geq$ 4 kHz), in which coding of sound by the fine temporal structure of the discharges is absent (see the next paragraph).

Induction of Periodicities in Neuronal Discharges In the low-frequency range, the discharges of auditory neurons can be highly regular with distinct periodicities. This is due to the property of phase-locking, whereby impulses are approximately synchronized to the cycles of the stimulus waveform. The periodicity of the response is determined by the frequency of the stimulus. If a neuron were perfectly phase-locked, it would discharge at a rate corresponding exactly to the frequency of the stimulus. In reality, the ability to phase-lock is less than perfect because the firing rate of auditory nerve fibers in response to acoustic stimuli is normally limited to 300 spikes/s. Thus, phase-locking usually falls far short of perfect synchrony, except at the low end of the audible frequency range. For higher-frequency stimuli (above 300 Hz), most auditory nerve fibers fire only once every few cycles on average. Any code for frequency above this limit, therefore, requires that neurons fire in volleys. However, even with volleys, the range over which periodicities could be generated would be limited because phase-locking is very weak above 1 to 2 kHz and is absent above 4 to 5 kHz.[21] It is conceivable that noise exposure could induce periodicities in the spontaneous discharge patterns of auditory neurons. Because of their resemblance to phase-locked responses, such periodicities could generate tonal tinnitus percepts with a perceivable pitch. However, because the discharge rates are limited to only a few hundred spikes/s, it is likely that periodic discharges play a role only in the generation of the less common forms of tinnitus that are matched to low frequencies. Periodic discharges seem unlikely to be correlates of noise- or salicylate-induced tinnitus, which are generally matched to frequencies above 4 kHz.

Increases in Neural Synchrony There is some evidence that acoustic stimulation can cause increases in the degree of synchronization of discharges across the neural population. This has been observed in the auditory nerve[22] and auditory cortex.[23,24] In the auditory cortex, the presence or absence of a steady-state acoustic stimulus was found to be better correlated with the degree of synchrony than with changes in discharge rates; many neurons showed increases in synchrony without any significant changes in firing rate.[23,24] It has been hypothesized that synchrony may underlie the process of "binding," whereby various features of a stimulus are fused into a single percept. One might extend this hypothesis to tinnitus by proposing that pitch and loudness are bound into a single percept by neural synchrony. However, recent work indicates that the degree of synchrony between neurons in the auditory cortex is poorly correlated with stimulus intensity.[23] An alternate hypothesis is that the loudness of tinnitus may be signaled by a joint code combining synchrony and rate information, as has been suggested by Eggermont (see Chapter 13, "The Auditory Cortex and Tinnitus").[23]

Induction of Edge Effects Edge effects are produced by regions of sharply contrasting levels of activity across the neural population. A tonal stimulus elicits a sharp increase in activity at the tonotopic locus representing the frequency of the stimulus. This locus is flanked by neighboring regions in which activity is either not increased or is decreased by lateral inhibition. Edge effects can also be produced by turning sounds off. For example, when a band of noise with a $\frac{1}{3}$-octave gap (bandstop noise) is presented for a few minutes and then turned off, an audible tone (Zwicker tone) with a distinct pitch is heard. The tone lasts for up to 10 seconds, and its pitch corresponds to the center frequency of the $\frac{1}{3}$-octave gap. Such a pitch likely results from adaptation of neurons in response to the noise band and a lack of adaptation at the frequency corresponding to the gap. In this case, the edge effect is created by a post-stimulus decrease in activity (adaptation) in response to the noise, leaving a distinct region, corresponding to the gap, in which activity is normal (no adaptation). Edge effects can also be produced by hair cell injury. In this case, the edge is created by a frequency boundary between tonotopic regions of normal spontaneous activity and decreased activity caused by hair cell damage. Some have hypothesized that the pitch of tinnitus may be produced by such an edge effect. Some evidence for this lies in the fact that tinnitus sometimes has a pitch corresponding to the edge of an accompanying hearing loss. However, as noted above, there is no consistent relationship between the pitch of tinnitus and the spectral distribution of the hearing loss (see Figure 11-1). Thus, edge effects probably have only limited relevance to tinnitus.

In summary, there are numerous potential neural correlates of stimulus-evoked auditory percepts. Almost all appear to play a role in the encoding of the loudness and pitch of tonal stimuli. These provide possible leads into what the neural correlates of tinnitus are likely to resemble. We now turn to studies that actually examined the effects of tinnitus-inducing agents on the auditory system and consider how these compare with the correlates of acoustic stimulation just described. Because tinnitus is the perception of sound without an external acoustic stimulus, the studies to be considered will focus on the effects of these agents on spontaneous activity. These have been carried out primarily with salicylate and intense sound.

NEURAL CORRELATES OF SALICYLATE-INDUCED TINNITUS: INCREASED SPONTANEOUS ACTIVITY

Salicylate has been reported to cause increases in spontaneous discharge rates of auditory nerve fibers.[25,26] This effect is shown in Figure 11-2, taken from Mulheran and Evans.[27] In normal guinea pigs, spontaneous discharge rates show a bimodal distribution, with one population yielding rates below 20 spikes/s and the other yielding rates that range between 40 and 110 spikes/s. Following treatment with 300 to 400 mg/kg of body weight of sodium salicylate, the distribution became trimodal, with a new population yielding rates of 120 spikes/s and higher. This increase seemed to occur at the expense of rates in the middle range because the number of fibers with rates in the range of 40 to 110 spikes/s was reduced by half. Similar results have been reported in two other studies.[26,28] One of these studies suggests that the fibers with in-

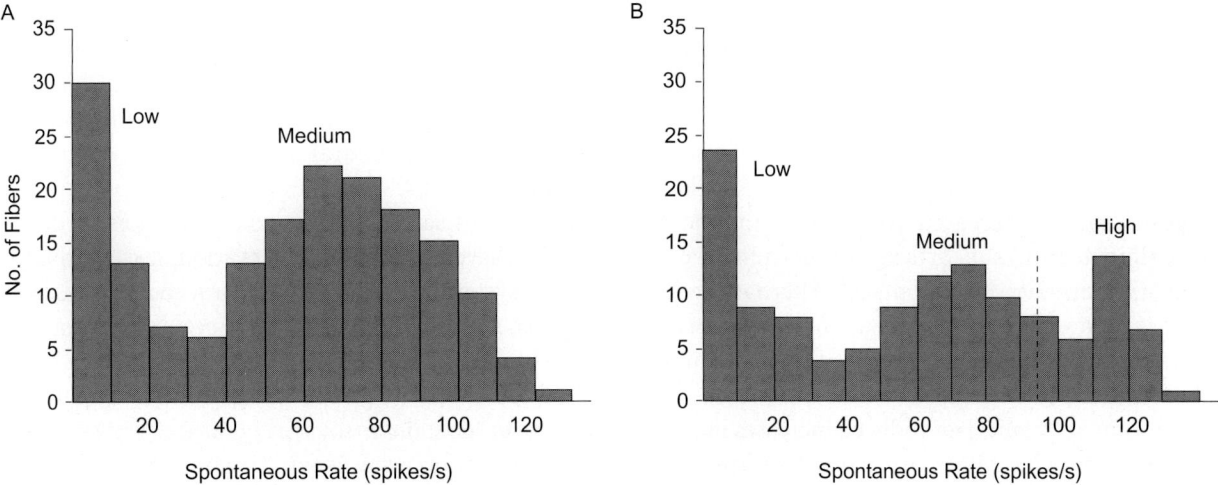

FIGURE 11-2. Histograms showing the incidence of spontaneous discharge rates in control (*A*) and salicylate-treated (*B*) animals. The dose of salicylate administered was between 300 and 400 mg/kg of body weight. Note that salicylate treatment led to an increase in the number of fibers discharging at high rates (≥ 120 spikes/s) and a decrease in the number of fibers discharging at medium rates. Reproduced with permission from Mulheran M and Evans EF.[27]

creased discharge rates were those with high CFs. The authors hypothesized that the high-frequency selectivity of the affected neurons might account for the high pitch of tinnitus induced by salicylate.

Efforts to reproduce these findings in subsequent studies have yielded varying results, although it now appears that some of these variations are attributable to differences in the dose of salicylate used. No significant effects of low to moderate doses (≤ 200 mg/kg) of salicylate were found on mean spontaneous rates in the auditory nerve of guinea pigs[28] or cats,[29] but increasing the dose to 400 mg/kg caused increases in spontaneous rates in the guinea pig.[28] Slight increases in spontaneous rates were also found in the pigeon after intracochlear perfusion of high doses of salicylate.[30]

Salicylate also has potent effects on the central auditory system, even at doses that do not cause a more general toxicity. Kauer and colleagues showed that very high doses of this drug caused an increase in metabolism in the auditory brainstem nuclei of guinea pigs.[31] More recent studies, focusing on the inferior colliculus (IC), have revealed a potent effect of more moderate doses (200–250 mg/kg) of salicylate.[32–35] Within 2 to 3 hours after salicylate injection, mean spontaneous discharge rates for single units increased between two- and threefold above their predrug levels.[32,33] The greatest increases were found among units tuned to high frequencies.[32]

Several aspects of this increased activity suggest that it represents an important neural correlate of tinnitus. The doses of salicylate used to induce the increased discharge rate (200 mg/kg) were within the dose range that has been shown to cause tinnitus in rats (ie, 150–300 mg/kg) without toxic side effects.[36–38] The increased activity was found mainly among units tuned to frequencies between 10 and 16 kHz.[32] This range is consistent with evidence suggesting that salicylate-induced tinnitus in both rats and humans is high in pitch.[3,36,37] The increased activity was reversible using a calcium supplement[32] or lidocaine,[33] factors that are known for their ability to attenuate tinnitus for short periods.

The conscious awareness of annoying sound, which people experience after salicylate ingestion, suggests that the induced tinnitus must involve structures at cortical levels of the auditory system. Indeed, the results of recent studies by Eggermont and his colleagues are consistent with this expectation.[39,40] They compared the influences of salicylate on three auditory cortical areas, including the primary auditory cortex (AI), the secondary auditory cortex (AII), and the anterior auditory field (AAF). The conclusions drawn from these studies were that salicylate causes a decrease in mean spontaneous rates in areas AI and AAF but an increase in rate in area AII (see Chapter 13, "The Auditory Cortex and Tinnitus"). The increased rates in AII occurred among units tuned to high frequencies (between 10 and 16 kHz), in agreement with the results from the IC.[32] This similarity suggests that the increased activity seen in area AII may originate from subcortical auditory centers such as the IC or even lower-level nuclei. Alternatively, the changes seen in AII after salicylate may be a cortical expression of a more general effect of this drug on the extralemniscal (multimodal) pathway.

In summary, salicylate-induced increases in spontaneous activity have been observed at various levels of the auditory system, including the auditory nerve, IC, and AII. This could mean that salicylate has multiple targets along the auditory pathway or that the effects on a single target, possibly the auditory periphery, are relayed to other levels of the auditory system. Future studies are needed to resolve this question.

NEURAL CORRELATES OF NOISE-INDUCED TINNITUS: INCREASED SPONTANEOUS ACTIVITY

The acute and chronic effects of noise exposure on auditory nerve activity have been studied using a wide range of exposure conditions. Young and Sachs reported that spontaneous discharge rates were generally reduced immediately following exposure to sustained tones at moderate levels, but the effects were short-lived, with the activity of most fibers recovering to pre-exposure discharge rates within a few minutes.[41] Salvi and his colleagues observed no acute change in spontaneous rates after a prolonged (5 day) exposure to moderate-level (95 dB) noise.[42] Similar results were obtained when activity was studied 6 months after noise exposure (86 dB), except that mean spontaneous discharge rates of fibers with high CFs (ie, above 2 kHz) were found to be slightly elevated after the longer recovery period.[43] The chronic effects of noise exposure on the auditory nerve of cats have also been studied.[44,45] Between 1 and 2.5 weeks after exposure to narrowband noise at a level of 109 to 121 dB, spontaneous discharge rates were generally decreased. The magnitude of the decrease was found to be proportional to the degree of damage to the tallest stereocilia of inner hair cells (IHCs).[45] Overall, these results indicate that noise exposure generally has both acute and chronic suppressive effects on spontaneous discharge rates of auditory nerve fibers. An exception to this generalization was the slight increase in the upper limit of spontaneous rates observed among high CF fibers by Salvi and Ahroon.[43] The authors suggested that this increase could represent a neural correlate of chronic noise-induced tinnitus.

Studies related to acute and chronic noise-induced tinnitus have been conducted at various levels of the auditory system, including the ventral cochlear nucleus (VCN), IC, and auditory cortex. Several investigations have looked at the effects of intense sound on the VCN. Van Heusden and Smoorenburg found no significant change in the spontaneous firing rates of VCN neurons immediately following exposure to moderate-level noise (half-hour, pink noise [broadband noise with a spectrum that is inversely proportional to frequency], 105 dB).[46] No increase in activation of VCN was apparent a few hours after impulse noise exposure (105 dB) in the 2-DG or c-*fos* experiments of Wallhäuser-Franke and Langner.[47] Salvi and colleagues found that the spontaneous discharge rates of VCN neurons were generally depressed when studied 2 to 12 hours after a prolonged (3.5 to 5 day) exposure to moderate-level (86 dB) noise; however, a small subpopulation of neurons, characterized as "on units," showed either no change in activity or a slight elevation of spontaneous activity after the exposure.[48] These units may correspond to the octopus cells of the posteroventral cochlear nucleus (PVCN). Gerken and colleagues observed decreases in spontaneous activity in chronic recordings from the anteroventral cochlear nucleus (AVCN) and PVCN of cats observed for 15 days following a 48-hour exposure to an intense tone (1 kHz, 110 dB).[49] In the awake rhesus monkey, Lonsbury-Martin and Martin found that most VCN neurons showed either no significant change in or a depression of firing rates immediately following a 3-minute exposure to moderate-level (100 dB) tones, but they found a subpopulation of neurons (those with moderate to high pre-exposure discharge rates) that displayed temporary increases in activity.[50] All changes in spontaneous activity recovered within a few minutes after the offset of the exposure tones. Lonsbury-Martin and Martin suggested that the increased activity displayed by some VCN neurons after exposure tones might represent a neural correlate of the rapidly fading acute form of tinnitus that is commonly observed immediately following similar exposures in humans.[50] However, Gerken's group found that the VCN did not develop acute or chronic increases in activity after intense noise exposure.[49] Thus, if the VCN is a center for the location of correlates of noise-induced tinnitus, the underlying cells would appear to be a relatively small component of the VCN cell population.

In contrast, the DCN generally shows increases in spontaneous activity after intense sound exposure (Figure 11-3). Such increases were initially observed in the DCN of hamsters after they were exposed to an intense 10 kHz tone (125–130 dB) for 4 hours.[51–53] Similar results have been obtained in a number of subsequent studies in other species. Increases in multiunit activity have been observed in the DCN of rats following intense (125–130 dB) tone exposure.[54] Increases in single-unit activity were induced in the chinchilla DCN using a moderate-level (80 dB SPL) 4 kHz tone[55]; the increases were smaller than those observed in the hamster, which were observed after higher levels of acoustic exposure (125–130 dB SPL). This could indicate that there may be a relationship between the level of exposure and the level of hyperactivity in the DCN. Preliminary evidence suggests that the mouse DCN becomes hyperactive following exposure to intense noise (110–115 dB, 6 hours).[56] The effect of noise in causing hyperactivity in the DCN may thus be a general phenomenon across species.

At the midbrain level, two studies examined the effects of noise exposure on spontaneous activity. Salvi reported that the spontaneous discharge rates of single units in the IC were decreased immediately after a brief (8 minute) narrowband noise exposure at a level of 95 dB.[57] Decreased activation in the IC is also suggested by the experiments with 2-DG and c-*fos* a few hours following brief exposure to impulse noise with a peak level of 105 dB.[47] The immediate and chronic effects of free-field noise exposure on ongoing spontaneous multiunit activity in the IC were studied by Gerken and colleagues.[49] The central and pericentral nuclei of the IC showed decreases in activity following a 48-hour intense (110 dB) 1 kHz tone exposure. Most recording sites in the central nucleus of the inferior colliculus (ICc) showed sharp decreases immediately after the exposure; these decreases endured over the entire 15-day observation period. Two examples were presented, however, in which spontaneous activity was increased. These increases were observed in the posterior portion of the IC (ICP). Interestingly, for at least one of these examples, the increase became apparent only after a 5-day period during which activity was depressed. The investigators did not mention these changes in the context of tinnitus. However, it is pos-

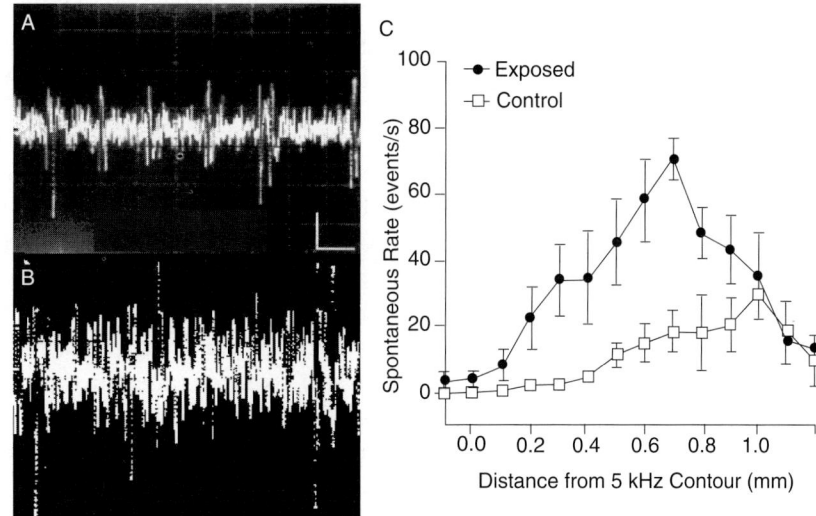

FIGURE 11-3. A comparison of spontaneous activity in control and tone-exposed animals. *A*, Oscillographic trace showing spontaneous activity recorded at the 10 kHz locus of the dorsal cochlear nucleus (DCN) of a control animal. *B*, Spontaneous activity recorded at the corresponding locus of an animal that had been exposed to a 10 kHz tone (125 dB SPL, 4 hours) 1 month previously. *C*, Topographic profiles of mean activity recorded on the DCN surface in control (*lower curve*) and tone-exposed (*upper curve*) animals. Adapted from Kaltenbach JA and McCaslin DL[51] and Kaltenbach JA and Afman CE.[53]

sible that these increases represent a midbrain correlate of tinnitus and could be the IC reflection of hyperactivity that develops in the DCN over several days after intense sound exposure.

Intense noise exposure causes a number of significant changes in the spontaneous activity of auditory cortical neurons. These effects are discussed in detail in Chapter 13, "The Auditory Cortex and Tinnitus," and are summarized only briefly here. Significant increases in spontaneous activity were found in area AI of cats immediately after exposure to tones at levels between 93 and 123 dB SPL; activity in area AII was decreased, whereas that in area AAF did not change significantly.[58] Increases in spontaneous rates were also observed in area AI several months after exposure to an intense (115 dB) tone.[59] It may be significant that these increases were observed in areas of the tonotopic map that showed evidence of reorganization and were associated with increases in the degree of neural synchrony between pairs of neurons within the reorganized areas. This may indicate that there are at least two signals (increased synchrony and increased spontaneous activity) at the cortical level that could give rise to tinnitus.

In summary, exposure to moderate or high levels of sound causes decreases in spontaneous activity in the auditory nerve, VCN, and most parts of the IC. However, increases in spontaneous activity have been found consistently in the DCN and AI, and there is some suggestion that increases may also occur in certain parts of the IC. These findings raise the possibility of a general increase in activity among certain populations of neurons along the entire primary auditory neuroaxis. These results contrast with those observed after salicylate treatment, which generally show increases in activity in the auditory nerve, IC, and AII but not in the VCN and AI.

Other Correlates of Salicylate- and Noise-Induced Tinnitus

Increased Bursting Exposure to some tinnitus-inducing agents alters the temporal properties of auditory neurons. One type of property that has been reported to change after salicylate or noise exposure is bursting activity. This is characterized as sequences of spikes that occur in rapid succession and at regular intervals, sometimes as short as 1 to 2 milliseconds. Bursting behavior after salicylate or noise exposure has been observed in the auditory nerve[25,44,60] and IC.[32] It is possible that the regular discharges that occur in bursts of activity contain periodicities that might be interpreted by the brain as representing certain frequencies. How bursting would lead to the conscious percepts of tinnitus, however, remains unclear because no change in the incidence of bursting activity has been found in area AI or AII of cortex after treatment with salicylate.[40] Patients with tinnitus induced by salicylate generally match the pitch of their tinnitus to frequencies between 7 and 9 kHz.[3] This poses an additional question because this frequency range is well above the presumed 5 kHz limit in which periodicities occur in the discharges of auditory neurons. One possible solution to these obstacles is that the conscious awareness of sound may reside at subcortical levels and that the bursting activity occurs among neurons tuned to high frequencies. Data reported by Chen and Jastreboff are consistent with the latter hypothesis.[32]

Coincident Firing/Neural Synchrony Studies from the laboratory of Eggermont suggest that neurons in area AI become increasingly synchronized in their spontaneous discharges following exposure to tinnitus-inducing agents. Using cross-correlation analysis, they found no increase in the number of neuron pairs showing coincident firing following salicylate treatment; however, a narrowing of the central peak in the cross-correlograms suggested that the degree to which neurons fired synchronously was increased.[40] Similar results have been obtained following exposure to intense sound.[59]

There is also evidence that tinnitus-inducing agents increase the degree of synchronous discharges at subcortical levels of the auditory system. This is suggested by studies based on spectral averaging of electrical activity recorded from the auditory nerve. It is thought that changes in the amplitudes of the spectral peaks from this activity result from changes in the degree of neural synchronization.[22] Martin and colleagues found that increases in the average spectrum of spontaneous auditory nerve activity, recorded with a gross electrode placed either at the round window or on the auditory nerve itself, could be induced acutely in cats and humans by treatment with salicylate.[61] After one high dose of salicylate in cats, an emergence of a 200 Hz peak and a decrease in the 1.7 kHz peak were seen.[61] Similar alterations were also observed in patients suffering from tinnitus.[62]

Spectral averaging of neural activity recorded at the round window was used by Cazals and colleagues to compare the acute and chronic effects of salicylate on spontaneous activity in the auditory nerve.[22] Changes in average spectra were most apparent at 200 Hz and 1 kHz, in agreement with the findings of Martin and colleagues.[61] But the direction and magnitude of the change were strongly dependent on the duration of salicylate exposure. Short-term exposures (a few hours) caused a decrease in spectral amplitude, whereas long-term exposure (a few days to a few weeks) caused an increase. The spectral amplitude at 1 kHz increased to a maximal value after 3 weeks of salicylate exposure. Several considerations support the view that these changes in spectra may be correlates of tinnitus. First, the changes in spectra occurred without an accompanying change in response threshold (measured using the compound action potential), a finding that corresponds to the fact that tinnitus induced by salicylate often precedes a hearing loss. Second, the change in spectrum could be reversed by treatment with the antitinnitus agent lidocaine. Third, similar changes in average spectrum were seen when normal, nonsalicylate-treated animals were stimulated with sound, suggesting that salicylate produces changes in the auditory nerve that mimic the effects of acoustic stimulation. Fourth, the time course of development of the change in spectrum was similar to that of salicylate-induced tinnitus in humans[2,3,63] and rats.[36,37] These considerations suggest that the spectral averaging method may provide a useful and objective measure of a neural correlate of tinnitus.

Changes in Tonotopic Maps It is well known that acoustic injury or other causes of hearing loss result in the reorganization of tonotopic maps of some central auditory regions. In the normal tonotopic map of the auditory cortex, each frequency within the audiometric range is represented by a narrow strip of cells. However, when input to one of these strips is damaged or weakened, adjacent frequency strips can take over the function of the damaged strip. This reorganizes the tonotopic map so that there is an expanded representation of frequencies along the edge of the damaged strip. Map reorganizations have been observed after cochlear trauma in the auditory cortex and IC of cats and guinea pigs.[64–66] Some evidence from magnetic source imaging (magnetoencephalographic) studies suggests that map reorganizations also occur in some patients with tinnitus.[67] Recent studies in the cat indicate that the levels of spontaneous activity recorded in reorganized (ie, expanded) map regions are generally higher than those in normal, unreorganized map regions.[59] One could speculate that the sound percepts associated with tinnitus are due to the increase in activity but that the pitch of those percepts is determined by the CF that dominates the expanded map region.

HYPERACTIVITY OF THE DCN AS A NEURAL CORRELATE OF NOISE-INDUCED TINNITUS

Because noise exposure is the most common cause of the chronic form of tinnitus, it deserves special emphasis. A surprising aspect of the studies reviewed above is that most structures examined following moderate to intense sound exposure showed either no significant change or significant decreases in spontaneous activity. These include the auditory nerve, AVCN, PVCN, ICc, ICP, AII, and AAF. In contrast, increases in activity after exposure were consistently found only in the DCN and AI. This might be interpreted as suggesting that the correlates of noise-induced tinnitus occur among neurons too small or too rare to be found consistently. Alternatively, the percepts of tinnitus might be induced by "edge effects" created by regions of decreased activity. However, this is difficult to reconcile with the fact that the pitch of acute or chronic noise-induced tinnitus does not consistently correspond to the edge of a hearing loss.[9] A third possibility is that noise-induced tinnitus might be represented by the more prominent increases in activity that occur in the DCN and AI. A number of studies have been performed to determine whether DCN hyperactivity is related to tinnitus and to examine what mechanisms might underlie its induction. Studies bearing on these issues are described in this section, whereas those related to the AI are reviewed in Chapter 13, "The Auditory Cortex and Tinnitus."

Relationship of DCN Hyperactivity to Tinnitus

Topographic Pattern of DCN Hyperactivity Resembles That of Stimulus-Driven Activity One of the premises developed in this chapter is that a neural correlate of tinnitus might be expected to show some resemblance to the responses of neurons to a tinnitus-like acoustic stimulus. To investigate whether this is true of DCN hyperactivity, we compared the topographic profiles of activity in exposed animals with activity evoked in the DCN of normal animals responding to a tinnitus-like tone.[53] Activity was recorded in both animal groups, averaged across three rows of recording sites, and the means were plotted as a function of distance across the surface of the DCN. The parameters of the tonal stimulus were selected to approximate a high-pitched, tinnitus-like tone (10 kHz, 20 dB SL). The results of this comparison showed a surprising resemblance between the two topographic profiles (Figure 11-4). Both were characterized by a distinct peak of activity that occurred in the middle region of the DCN. This indicates that the DCN of exposed animals was induced to behave as though it is responding to a tone. An important difference, however, is that the peak of activity that occurred in tone-exposed animals was displaced slightly toward the high-frequency side of the peak representing the 10 kHz stimulus (which was also the frequency of the exposure tone used to induce hyperactivity). Using the tonotopic coordinates obtained in earlier studies of the DCN,[68] we determined that the peak of activity in the tone-exposed animals occurred at a locus corresponding to a frequency of 12 kHz. This is consistent with the observation that the pitch of noise-induced tinnitus is typically higher than that of the exposure.[5,6]

Animals Exposed to Intense Sound Develop Tinnitus
Several studies published in the last few years suggest that animals exposed to intense sound develop tinnitus. A study by Heffner and Harrington examined the auditory percepts of hamsters following intense sound exposure.[69] The procedure used was an adaptation of the paradigm used by Jastreboff to test animals for tinnitus after salicylate treatment.[36,37] Before sound exposure, hamsters were trained for several weeks to discriminate between the presence and absence of a conditioning sound. The ability of the animals to discriminate was signaled by differences in licking behavior. The animals were trained to maintain contact with a waterspout when the conditioning sound was presented and to break contact with the spout when the sound was absent. After several weeks of training, the animals became quite adept at responding correctly to the condition of silence by breaking contact with the spout. This was apparent in the relatively high scores representing the percent correct responses. The animals were then divided into two groups, one of which was exposed to a high-level (125 dB SPL), continuous tone (10 kHz) for 4 hours, whereas the other group was not. Five days after exposures, animals in both groups were again tested. Behavioral data are presented in Figure 11-5. The procedure for this test was similar to that used during training except that no conditioning sound was presented. When this test was performed, unexposed animals tended to break contact with the spout, as they did during training when no sound was presented. This is indicated by their higher behavioral scores (see Figure 11-5B). In contrast, the animals that had been exposed to an intense

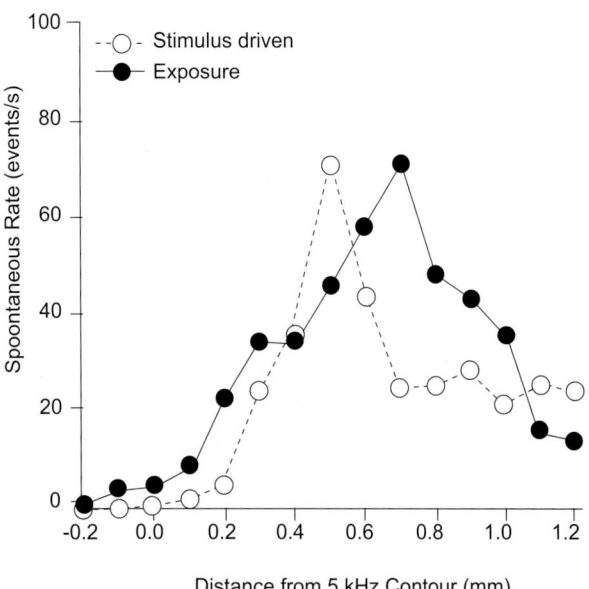

FIGURE 11-4. Comparison of spontaneous activity in tone-exposed animals with activity evoked in the normal dorsal cochlear nucleus during stimulation with a continuous 10 kHz tone at 20 dB SL. The comparison reveals the resemblance between the profile of hyperactivity induced by previous sound exposure and the profile of stimulus-driven activity evoked by a tinnitus-like tone. Note, however, that the peak of hyperactivity is shifted to the right of the locus representing the frequency of the 10 kHz tone, which is also the frequency of the intense exposure tone (125–130 dB SPL, 4 hours) used to induce the hyperactivity. This upward shift is reminiscent of the fact that tinnitus induced by intense sound is usually higher in pitch than the frequency of the exposure tone, as shown in Figure 11-1. Adapted from Kaltenbach JA and Afman CE.[53]

tone 5 days earlier tended to maintain contact with the spout, similar to the way in which they responded to a sound during training. This is indicated by their lower behavioral scores (see Figure 11-5A). Thus, the exposed animals were behaving as though they were hearing a conditioning sound, even though no sound was presented. In other words, they were behaving as though they had tinnitus.

Other studies suggesting that noise exposure causes animals to develop tinnitus include those by Kwon and Brozoski and their colleagues.[55,70] These use various paradigms to assess tinnitus in animals (see Chapter 7, "Animal Models of Tinnitus"). Kwon and colleagues induced tinnitus in animals with a 7.8 kHz tone at a level of 110 dB SPL for a period of 20 minutes.[70] In the study by Brozoski and colleagues, the inducing exposure sound was a 4 kHz tone at 80 dB SPL varied in duration from 30 to 60 minutes.[38] The finding that was common to all of these studies is that animals displayed behavior that was consistent with the interpretation that they had developed tinnitus after the sound exposure.

A more direct look at the relationship between the induced tinnitus and hyperactivity in the DCN was undertaken in a study in which electrophysiologic recordings were conducted in the same animals that had previously been tested for tinnitus.[71] The paradigm for testing animals for tinnitus was the same as that described by Heffner and Harrington.[69] The animals were studied in four rounds of experiments, each consisting of 10 to 15 animals. Half of the animals were exposed to intense sound, whereas the other half were not. The recordings revealed higher levels of activity in exposed animals relative to the unexposed animals (Figure 11-6A). The increased activity was similar to that observed in previous studies (eg, see Figure 11-3), except that the control levels were higher, possibly owing to the frequent exposure of control animals to sound that was required during the behavioral training procedure. The difference between levels of activity was even greater when the comparison was limited to animals falling into the upper and lower quartiles of the score distribution. These correspond to animals with (scores ≤ 60) and without (scores ≥ 70) behavioral evidence of tinnitus (Figure 11-6B). The largest difference in activity levels in the DCN was observed when animals at extreme opposite ends of the score range were compared (Figure 11-6C). These correspond to those with the strongest (scores ≤ 55) and weakest (scores ≥ 80) evidence of tinnitus. Overall, peak activity in the DCN was found to be significantly correlated with the behavioral measures of tinnitus.

Tinnitus and Hearing Loss One of the problems in attempting to find a neural correlate of noise-induced tinnitus is that the procedure of exposing animals to intense sound also causes hearing loss. Indeed, the exposure tone that has been used to induce hyperactivity and tinnitus in the hamster also causes these animals to experience some degree of hearing loss.[69] Thus, it

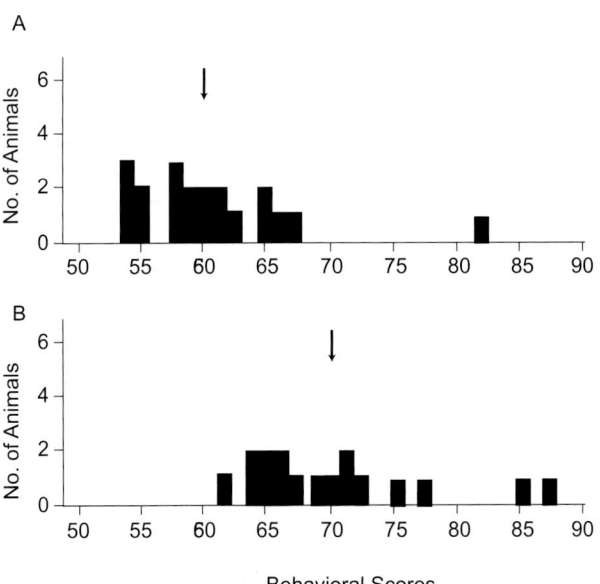

FIGURE 11-5. Behavioral data suggesting that intense sound exposure causes animals to experience tinnitus. Animals were trained for several weeks to break contact with a waterspout in response to silence and to maintain contact with the spout in response to sound. After training, the responses to silence were retested. Control animals that were not tone exposed responded correctly to silence and therefore yielded high scores (B). However, animals that had previously been exposed to an intense tone (125–130 dB SPL, 10 kHz, 4 hours) performed incorrectly in a significant percentage of trials in response to silence and thus yielded lower scores (A). The exposed animals were thus behaving as though they were hearing a sound during the silent test trials, suggesting that they had tinnitus. Reproduced from Kaltenbach JA et al, with permission from Elsevier.[71]

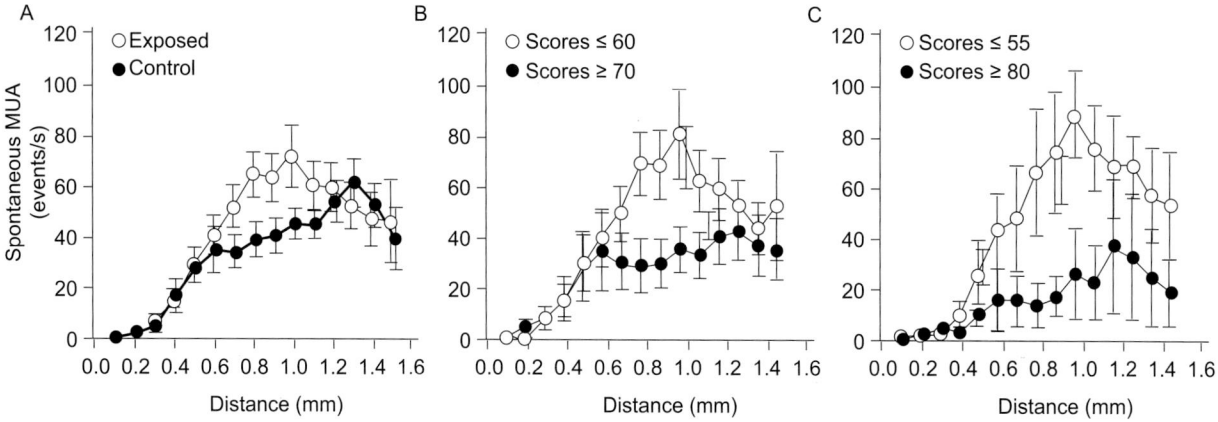

FIGURE 11-6. Relationship between levels of spontaneous activity (MUA = multiunit activity) in the dorsal cochlear nucleus (DCN) and behavioral performance scores. *A*, Comparison of activity levels in tone-exposed (10 kHz, 125–130 dB, 4 hours) and control hamsters. *B*, The upper and lower curves, respectively, were obtained by averaging the levels of activity in the DCN of animals whose behavioral scores fell in the upper and lower quartiles of the behavioral score range shown in the histograms of Figure 11-5. Note the larger difference between activity in the two groups than was seen in the comparison of exposed and control animals. *C*, An even larger difference between activity levels was seen when the comparison was made between animals with the highest and lowest behavioral scores. Reproduced from Kaltenbach JA et al, with permission from Elsevier.[71]

might reasonably be asked whether the psychophysical measures in the behavioral tests or the hyperactivity might be direct correlates of hearing loss rather than tinnitus. The likelihood that hyperactivity in the DCN is a correlate of hearing loss rather than of tinnitus is worth considering because cochlear trauma has been shown to cause decreases in spontaneous activity in the auditory nerve, so it is conceivable that this decrease in peripheral activity could cause a disinhibition of neurons in the DCN, leading to immediate hyperactivity without necessarily causing tinnitus. However, this view now seems unlikely because the development of hyperactivity after exposure follows a different time course from that of the hearing loss. Animals studied 1 month after tone exposure showed evidence of both hearing loss and hyperactivity in the DCN, but when studied 2 days after exposure, increases in neural response thresholds were not associated with hyperactivity in the DCN.[52] Activity observed 2 days after exposure was actually decreased below control levels. This suggests that the inductions of hyperactivity and hearing loss probably involve different mechanisms. This is consistent with the clinical observation that tinnitus and hearing loss are not necessarily associated.

Other Evidence that the DCN Is Involved in Tinnitus

Evidence consistent with the model of the DCN as an important site of tinnitus-related activity has also been obtained from clinical studies of patients with tinnitus caused by acoustic neuromas. Some of the patients received brainstem auditory implants on the surface of the DCN following bilateral resections of the auditory nerves. In most of these patients, the tinnitus was unaffected by the implantation procedure; however, the perceived loudness or severity of their tinnitus was decreased when the implant was used to apply current to the DCN surface.[72,73] This suggests that circuits within the DCN can participate in the modulation of tinnitus.

Changes in the loudness of tinnitus can also be elicited by certain maneuvers of the head and neck musculature,[74–76] a phenomenon that has recently been given the name *somatic tinnitus*.[76] These include clenching of the teeth, moving the jaws, contracting the muscles in the upper neck, or lateral eye gaze. The ability to modulate tinnitus by such maneuvers is also possessed by subjects with profound hearing loss. This implies that the modulation of tinnitus involves structures at central levels of the auditory system. An important aspect of somatic tinnitus is that in subjects with unilateral tinnitus, the modulation of tinnitus loudness can be achieved by contracting muscles on the side ipsilateral to the tinnitus. Levine[76] hypothesized that somatic modulation of tinnitus is mediated by the DCN on the grounds that the DCN is a structure in the lower auditory brainstem that is known to integrate auditory input with ispilateral somatosensory and somatic motor sources[77] (see Chapter 9, "Somatic Tinnitus," and Chapter 10, "Sensory Nuclei in Tinnitus").

Mechanisms Underlying the Induction of Hyperactivity

Role of Hair Cell Injury Hair cell damage appears to be among the factors that trigger hyperactivity in the DCN. The presence of hyperactivity after sound exposure was found to be associated with varying degrees of inner (IHC) and outer hair cell (OHC) loss.[51] No clear relationship was found between the amount of hair cell loss and the level of activity in the DCN. However, this could be related to the limited sample size ($n = 6$) and the fact that all animals studied histologically displayed damage to both IHCs and OHCs. There is evidence that the level of activity in the DCN is determined by the amount of damage to OHCs, but only when damage to IHCs is negligible. This was apparent in studies using the ototoxic agent cisplatin, which is well known for its ability to cause OHC damage.[78,79] Many animals in this study showed varying degrees of OHC loss with little or no injury to IHCs. In these animals, there was a systematic increase in the level of spontaneous activity in the DCN as the percentage of missing OHCs in the basal half of the cochlea increased (Figure 11-7). However, activity was distinctly lower when OHC loss was accompanied by significant injury to IHCs. These findings suggest that OHC loss may trigger the induction of hyperactivity but that this increase can be offset or reversed by IHC damage. Whether a similar mechanism accounts for the emergence of hyperactivity after noise exposure is an issue that is under investigation.

Role of Plasticity There are indications that hyperactivity is a consequence of slowly developing changes in functional connectivity in the DCN. This is suggested by a study showing that the emergence of hyperactivity follows a complex time course.[80] The data from this series of experiments are presented in Figure 11-8A. When activity was recorded 2 days after exposure, no sign of hyperactivity was apparent; spontaneous activity was actually below control levels. At 5 days after exposure, hyperactivity was clearly apparent, covering

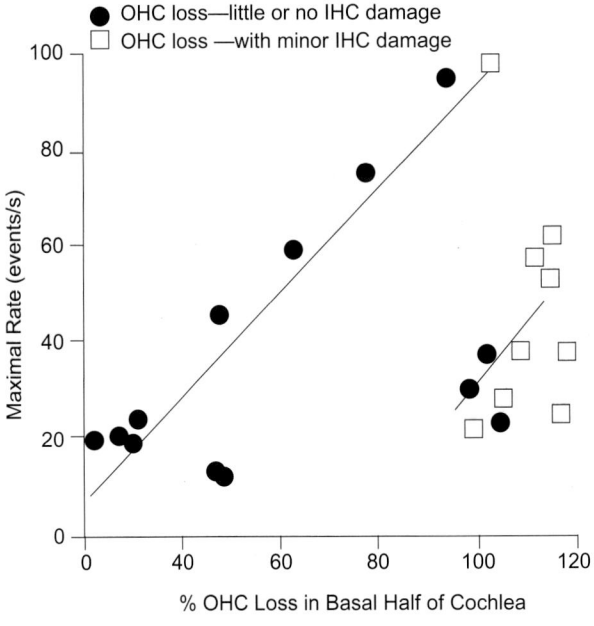

FIGURE 11-7. The relationship between the level of peak activity in the dorsal cochlear nucleus and the amount of outer hair cell (OHC) loss induced in hamsters after receiving five injections, one every other day, of cisplatin (3 mg/kg/d). Note that there was a systematic increase in activity as a function of OHC loss up to approximately 80% OHC loss in the basal half of the cochlea. Above this range, activity showed a sharp reduction. In the range above 80%, OHC loss was associated with significant damage to inner hair cells (IHCs). The curves suggest that OHC loss may be a trigger of hyperactivity, but this hyperactivity may be reversed by damage to IHCs. Adapted from Kaltenbach JA et al.[79]

most of the DCN without any indication of a peak in a particular tonotopic region. When examined at 14 days postexposure, the profile of activity showed a narrowing in the topographic spread, such that a suggestion of a peak was seen at a locus close to that representing the frequency of the exposure tone. This peak was more sharply defined 30 days after exposure, although the level of the peak was not significantly higher than the one at 14 days. The DCN continued to show a profile of hyperactivity after 6 months of postexposure recovery; at this time point, peak activity had shifted to a higher-frequency locus. These findings suggest that the immediate effect of cochlear insult is a reduction of activity in the DCN, but the subsequent emergence of hyperactivity involves plastic readjustments that continue to change over many months following the exposure.

Another indication that plastic readjustments underlie the induction of hyperactivity is its transient relationship to cochlear input. Although the initial insult is mediated by the effects of intense sound on the cochlea, the hyperactivity, once induced, appears to be resistant to the effects of peripheral deafferentation. This was recently demonstrated by comparing activity in the DCNs of exposed and control animals in which peripheral input was removed by cochlear ablation.[81] Approximately 1 month after the exposure, the DCNs were studied electrophysiologically beginning 30 minutes following ablation of the ipsilateral cochlea. The results revealed a persistence of hyperactivity in the DCN of exposed animals. Microdissections performed after the recordings demonstrated that the ablations resulted in complete removal of the soft tissues within the ipsilateral cochlea, including the organ of Corti and spiral ganglion. This result would seem to rule out the possibility that DCN hyperactivity reflects the level of activity in the auditory nerve. It also demonstrates that the induced hyperactivity is independent of peripheral input, suggesting that plastic readjustments in the DCN are probably involved.

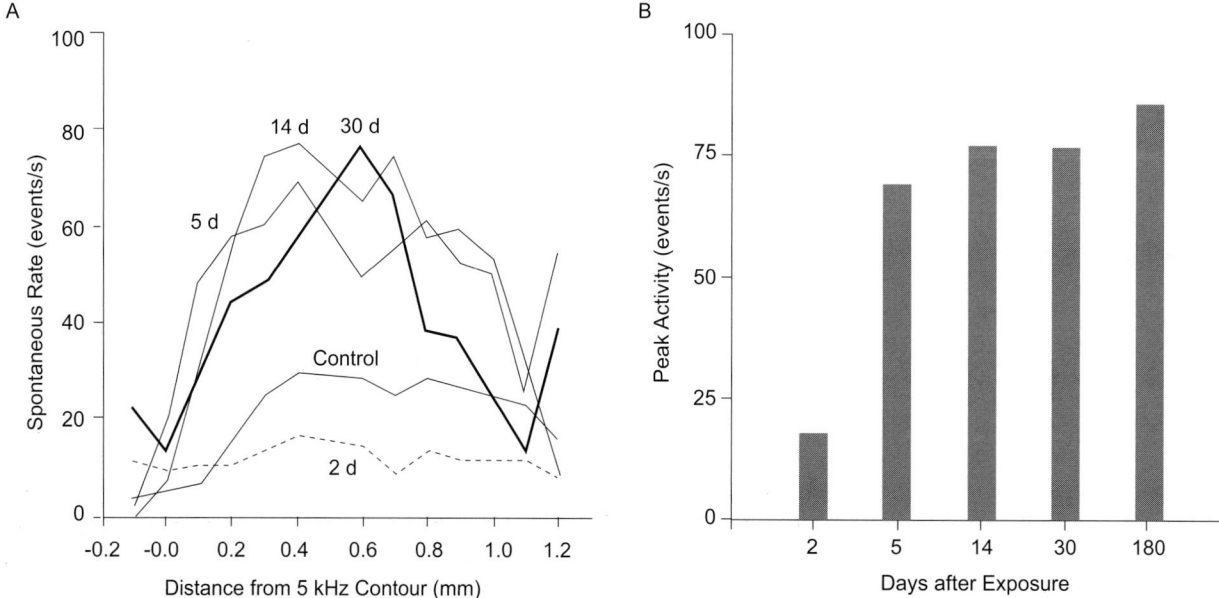

FIGURE 11-8. Evidence that plasticity underlies the induction of hyperactivity in the dorsal cochlear nucleus (DCN) by intense sound exposure. A, For the rather extreme exposure conditions (10 kHz, 125–130 dB SPL, 4 hours), the profile of activity observed across the DCN depends on the postexposure recovery time. Activity recorded 2 days after exposure was depressed below control levels, whereas at all subsequent times, the activity was distinctly higher than control levels. The profile at 5 days shows a broad distribution of hyperactivity across most of the DCN. This profile transformed into one with a more narrowly defined peak at 30 days after exposure. An intermediate profile was observed at 14 days after exposure. B, Peak activity increased most dramatically between 2 and 5 days after exposure. These results demonstrate that the distribution of hyperactivity is shaped by plastic readjustments in the DCN over many weeks after exposure. Adapted from Kaltenbach JA et al.[80]

Role of Excitotoxicity and Related Mechanisms
Excitotoxic effects occur in the cochlear nucleus after noise exposure. For example, noise exposure can cause widespread degeneration throughout the cochlear nucleus and other auditory brainstem structures even when there is relatively little or no auditory nerve fiber degeneration.[82] Excessive levels of the excitotoxic transmitter glutamate and its analogue kainic acid can cause degenerative changes in the cochlear nuclei.[83,84] Preliminary studies in the hamster suggest that some component of hyperactivity induced by intense-tone exposure may develop via an excitotoxic mechanism. We have found that a low level of hyperactivity was induced in the DCN of hamsters after exposure to a moderate-level (80 dB SPL) 10 kHz tone (unpublished results, 2003). Histologic analysis conducted after the recordings revealed no significant loss of hair cells. This is consistent with the results of Brozoski and colleagues, in which hyperactivity was induced in the DCN of chinchillas with an exposure level of 80 dB for only 1 hour.[55] These findings need to be studied in greater detail before a conclusion can be drawn. However, the available data are consistent with the notion that excitotoxicity may be a factor that contributes to some of the hyperactivity that occurs in the DCN after noise exposure.

Cell Types Involved The identification of hyperactive cell group(s) in the DCN of exposed animals is an essential step toward understanding the mechanisms governing the emergence of hyperactivity. Although the relevant work has just begun, a few studies have already shed some light on this issue. One study, recently published by Brozoski and colleagues, focused on the response properties of DCN fusiform cells.[55] Their results showed a small increase in the spontaneous discharge rates of these cells after exposure to a moderate-level (80 dB) tone. This is consistent with our experience that the highest degree of hyperactivity in the DCN of tone-exposed hamsters was found at depths corresponding to the fusiform cell layer.[85] On the other hand, this cell type does not appear to retain any evidence of hyperactivity in DCN slices taken from tone-exposed animals[86]; recordings conducted in each of the DCN layers failed to reveal any differences in the mean discharge rates of DCN neurons. However, two changes were observed in this study. First, there was a new class of spontaneous discharges characterized by low-amplitude spikes occurring at a high frequency that were not observed in slices from control animals. The identity of the cell type from which these small spikes originated has not yet been determined. Second, there was an increase in the number of neurons showing bursting activity. Because bursting activity is thought to arise from DCN cartwheel cells, the higher density of these bursts could signify that the number of active cartwheel cells was increased. Thus, a number of important leads should be studied, but current work suggests that hyperactivity could result from increases in discharge rate, an increase in the number of active neurons, or the activation of a new class of neurons that is normally silent.

INDUCTION OF HYPERACTIVITY AND TINNITUS: SYNTHESIS

Based on the studies just described, we can hypothesize that DCN hyperactivity is a neural correlate of noise-induced tinnitus that is primarily determined by dysfunctions of the OHC system, consisting of the OHCs, the type II spiral ganglion cells, and their target neurons in the cochlear nucleus. Dysfunctions of this system arise through two mechanisms: directly through mechanical trauma to the OHCs themselves or indirectly through excitotoxic injury to central target cells as a consequence of excess stimulation of OHCs and their type II afferents. A common feature of both types of trauma is that they trigger plastic readjustments in the DCN that alter the normal balance of excitation and inhibition. They differ in the speed with which the plastic readjustments occur. When OHCs are severely injured, as would be expected for extremely high-level and/or prolonged sound exposures, the plastic readjustments are slow because the immediate loss of OHCs prevents or reduces hyperstimulation of type II afferents during exposure, thus minimizing excitotoxic injury to DCN neurons. These readjustments may even be preceded by a transient decrease in DCN activity, reflecting damage to IHCs and the attending loss of tonic input from type I afferents. This would lead to tinnitus with a delayed onset, being noticeable only after the DCN begins to readjust to the loss of functional input. In cases of OHC overstimulation without OHC damage, as would be expected for more moderate levels of exposure, injury to DCN neurons would be rapid because the hyperactivation of the OHC–type II afferent projection results in excitotoxic injury to DCN neurons. This would lead to immediate changes in synaptic connectivity. The tinnitus that emerges in this case would have a more immediate onset, one that could be reversible if the induced injury is mild.

One could speculate that the same readjustments triggered by OHC loss could be induced by loss of IHCs. However, as our studies with cisplatin indicate, the hyperactivity induced by OHC loss can be lessened or even reversed by damage to IHCs.[79] Thus, loss of IHCs appears to have some degree of a protective effect against the induction of tinnitus. This may explain why many cases of noise-induced hearing loss are not associated with tinnitus. The model just described is also consistent with the observation that hyperactivity in the DCN does not disappear immediately following cochlear ablation. Apparently, the induction of hyperactivity results from plastic changes in the DCN that lock the hyperactivity into place. What is the nature of the plastic readjustments? They could involve many of the same changes that underlie plasticity in other areas of the brain: synaptic sprouting to fill in vacancies on the cell surface resulting from degeneration of inputting fibers. They could involve denervation supersensitivities resulting from up- or down-regulations of specific neurotransmitter receptors. Or they could involve changes in the properties and/or abundance of certain ion-conductance channels; these would impact on the level of resting activity of DCN neurons. These possibilities are all testable, so it is likely that the answer to the question regarding the nature of the plastic readjustments leading to hyperactivity in the DCN will be answered as research on this subject continues.

SUMMARY AND FUTURE RESEARCH NEEDS

The establishment of well-defined animal models has facilitated rapid progress in understanding the neural basis of tinnitus. Studies in neurophysiology have determined that exposure to tinnitus-inducing agents, such as salicylate and intense sound, causes abnormal activity throughout the auditory system. Evidence has been presented that these agents act peripherally to alter the normal function of the cochlea or auditory nerve, triggering changes at central levels of the auditory system. These changes include increases in spontaneous activity, alterations in temporal firing patterns (increases in bursting activity and synchronous discharges among different neurons), and tonotopic map reorganizations. Evidence has also been presented that at least some of these changes, such as increases in spontaneous activity after intense sound exposure, follow a different time course of development from threshold shift, suggesting that tinnitus-generating mechanisms are not necessarily a direct reflection of hearing loss, although hearing loss may be one of several factors that can trigger tinnitus. The above-cited neurophysiological findings have been complemented by behavioral studies demonstrating that the same agents that cause abnormal activity also cause animals to experience tinnitus-like percepts.

Despite these insights, the understanding of tinnitus mechanisms is still in its early stages of development. A number of fundamental issues need to be addressed to smooth out and complete the picture of how and where tinnitus is generated. First among these is how to reconcile the various theories of tinnitus-generating mechanisms with each other. That is, which of the several types of changes that have been implicated (hyperactivity, changes in temporal properties, and altered tonotopic maps) is (are) most critical in determining the existence of tinnitus? This is the problem of separating the causes from the epiphenomena. A second issue is where the critical changes originate. Are they induced independently at the cortical and subcortical levels of the system, or are they induced at one level and then relayed to other levels? Third, there is a need to investigate the chemical and molecular correlates of hyperactivity in the auditory system. Studies examining changes in gene expression are likely to be helpful in determining whether disturbances in activity are related to changes in the expression of specific receptor and/or ion channel classes. This issue is important because the development of effective drug therapies depends on an understanding of the chemical substrates producing the changes in activity. Fourth, more needs to be learned about which elements within the neuronal circuit are the generators of these disturbances. Although some progress has been made in understanding the cell types underlying noise-induced hyperactivity in the DCN, there is a need to identify hyperactive cell types in other areas of the auditory system and for different types of tinnitus. Finally, do the mechanisms of tinnitus that have been identified with salicylates and noise also underlie other forms of tinnitus, such as those induced by ear infection, head trauma, and other ototoxicities? The progress that has been made in the past decade in understanding the neural basis of tinnitus sets the stage for even more dramatic advances in the next decade.

REFERENCES

1. Vernon JA, Meikle MB. Tinnitus: clinical measurement. Otolaryngol Clin North Am 2003;36:293–305.
2. Day RO, Graham GG, Bieri D, et al. Concentration-response relationships for salicylate-induced ototoxicity in normal volunteers. Br J Clin Pharmacol 1989;28:695–702.
3. McCabe PA, Dey FL. The effect of aspirin upon auditory sensitivity. Ann Otol Rhinol Laryngol 1965;74:312–24.
4. Cazals Y. Auditory sensori-neural alterations induced by salicylate. Prog Neurobiol 2000;62:583–631.
5. Atherley GR, Hempstock TI, Noble WG. Study of tinnitus induced temporarily by noise. J Acoust Soc Am 1968;44:1503–6.
6. Loeb M, Smith RP. Relation of induced tinnitus to physical characteristics of the inducing stimuli. J Acoust Soc Am 1967;42:453–5.
7. Chermak GD, Dengerink JE. Characteristics of temporary noise-induced tinnitus in male and female subjects. Scand Audiol 1987;16:67–73.
8. McFadden D, Plattsmier HS. Suprathreshold aftereffects of exposure to intense sound. In: Hamernik R, Henderson D, Salvi R, editors. New perspectives in noise-induced hearing loss. New York: Raven Press; 1982. p. 347–62.
9. Axelsson A, Barrenas ML. Tinnitus in noise-induced hearing loss. In: Dancer AL, Henderson D, Salvi RJ, Hamernik RP, editors. Noise-induced hearing loss. Boston: Mosby Year Book; 1992. p. 269–76.
10. Axelsson A, Sandh A. Tinnitus in noise-induced hearing loss. Br J Audiol 1985;9:271–6.
11. Man A, Naggan L. Characteristics of tinnitus in acoustic trauma. Audiology 1981;20:70–8.
12. Seligmann H, Podoshin L, Ben-David J, et al. Drug-induced tinnitus and other hearing disorders. Drug Saf 1996;14:198–212.
13. Sachs MB, Abbas PJ. Rate versus level functions for auditory-nerve fibers in cats: tone-burst stimuli. J Acoust Soc Am 1974;56:1835–47.
14. Evans EF, Palmer AR. Relationship between the dynamic range of cochlear nerve fibers and their spontaneous activity. Exp Brain Res 1980;40:115–8.
15. Kim DO, Molnar CE. A population study of cochlear nerve fibers: comparison of spatial distributions of average-rate and phase-locking measures of responses to single tones. J Neurophysiol 1979;42:16–30.
16. Sharp FR, Ryan AF, Goodwin P, Woolf NK. Increasing intensities of wide band noise increase [14C]2-deoxyglucose uptake in gerbil central auditory structures. Brain Res 1981;230:87–96.
17. Viemeister NF. Intensity coding and the dynamic range problem. Hear Res 1988;34:267–74.
18. Irvine DR. The auditory brainstem: a review of the structure and function of auditory brainstem processing mechanisms. Prog Sensory Physiol 1986;7:1–279.
19. Townshend B, Cotter N, Van Compernolle D, White RL. Pitch perception by cochlear implant subjects. J Acoust Soc Am. 1987;82:106–15.
20. Colletti V, Fiorino FG, Carner M, et al. The retrosigmoid approach for auditory brainstem implantation. Am J Otol 2000;21:826–36.
21. Evans EF. Place and time coding of frequency in the peripheral auditory system: some physiological pros and cons. Audiology 1978;17:369–420.
22. Cazals Y, Horner KC, Huang ZW. Alterations in average spectrum of cochleoneural activity by long-term salicylate treatment in the guinea pig: a plausible index of tinnitus. J Neurophysiol 1998;80:2113–20.
23. Eggermont JJ. Sound-induced synchronization of neural activity between and within three auditory cortical areas. J Neurophysiol 2000;83:2708–22.
24. DeCharms RC, Merzenich MM. Primary cortical representation of sounds by the coordination of action-potential timing. Nature 1996;381:610–3.
25. Evans EF, Wilson JP, Borerwe TA. Animal models of tinnitus. In: Evered D, Lawrenson G, editors. Tinnitus. London: Pitman; 1981. p. 108–29.
26. Evans EF, Borerwe TA. Ototoxic effects of salicylates on the responses of single cochlear nerve fibres and on cochlear potentials. Br J Audiol 1982;16:101–8.
27. Mulheran M, Evans EF. A comparison of two experimental tinnitogenic agents: the effect of salicylate and quinine on activity of cochlear nerve fibers in the guinea pig. In: Hazell J, editor. Proceedings of the Sixth International Tinnitus Seminar. London: The Tinnitus and Hyperacusis Centre; 1999. p. 189–92.
28. Kumagai M. [Effect of intravenous injection of aspirin on the cochlea]. Hokkaido J Med Sci 1992;67:216–33.
29. Stypulkowski PH. Mechanisms of salicylate ototoxicity. Hear Res 1990;46:113–46.
30. Shehata-Dieler WE, Richter CP, Dieler R, Klinke R. Effects of endolymphatic and perilymphatic application of salicylate in the pigeon. I: single fiber activity and cochlear potentials. Hear Res 1994;74:77–84.
31. Kauer JS, Nemitz JW, Sasaki CT. Tinnitus aurium: fact or fancy. Laryngoscope 1982;92:1401–7.

32. Chen GD, Jastreboff PJ. Salicylate-induced abnormal activity in the inferior colliculus of rats. Hear Res 1995;82:158–78.
33. Manabe Y, Saito T, Saito H. Effects of lidocaine on salicylate-induced discharges of neurons in the inferior colliculus of the guinea pig. Hear Res 1997;103:192–8.
34. Wallhäuser-Franke E. Salicylate evokes c-*fos* expression in the brain stem: implications for tinnitus. Neuroreport 1997;8:725–8.
35. Wu JL, Chiu TW, Poon PW. Differential changes in Fos-immunoreactivity at the auditory brainstem after chronic injections of salicylate in rats. Hear Res 2003;176:80–93.
36. Jastreboff PJ, Brennan JF, Coleman JK, Sasaki CT. Phantom auditory sensation in rats: an animal model for tinnitus. Behav Neurosci 1988;102:811–22.
37. Jastreboff PJ, Brennan JF, Sasaki CT. An animal model for tinnitus. Laryngoscope 1988;98:280–6.
38. Bauer CA, Brozoski TJ, Rojas R, et al. Behavioral model of chronic tinnitus in rats. Otolaryngol Head Neck Surg 1999;121:457–62.
39. Eggermont JJ, Kenmochi M. Salicylate and quinine selectively increase spontaneous firing rates in secondary auditory cortex. Hear Res 1998;117:149–60.
40. Ochi K, Eggermont JJ. Effects of salicylate on neural activity in cat primary auditory cortex. Hear Res 1996;95:63–76.
41. Young E, Sachs MB. Recovery from sound exposure in auditory-nerve fibers. J Acoust Soc Am 1973;54:1535–43.
42. Salvi RJ, Hamernik RP, Henderson D. Response patterns of auditory nerve fibers during temporary threshold shift. Hear Res 1983;10:37–67.
43. Salvi RJ, Ahroon WA. Tinnitus and neural activity. J Speech Hear Res 1983;26:629–32.
44. Liberman MC, Kiang NY-S. Acoustic trauma in cats. Acta Otolaryngol Suppl (Stockh) 1978;358:1–63.
45. Liberman MC, Dodds LW. Single neuron labeling and chronic cochlear pathology. II. Stereocilia damage and alterations of spontaneous discharge rates. Hear Res 1984;16:43–53.
46. Van Heusden E, Smoorenburg GF. Responses from AVCN units in the cat before and after inducement of an acute noise trauma. Hear Res 1983;11:295–326.
47. Wallhäuser-Franke E, Langner G. Central activation patterns after experimental tinnitus induction in an animal model. In: Hazell J, editor. Proceedings of the Sixth International Tinnitus Seminar. London: The Tinnitus and Hyperacusis Centre; 1999. p. 155–62.
48. Salvi RJ, Hamernik RP, Henderson D. Discharge patterns in the cochlear nucleus of the chinchilla following noise induced asymptotic threshold shift. Exp Brain Res 1978;32:301–20.
49. Gerken GM, Saunders SS, Paul RE. Hypersensitivity to electrical stimulation of auditory nuclei follows hearing loss in cats. Hear Res 1984;13:249–59.
50. Lonsbury-Martin BL, Martin GK. Effects of moderately intense sounds on auditory sensitivity in rhesus monkeys: behavioral and neural observations. J Neurophysiol 1981;46:563–86.
51. Kaltenbach JA, McCaslin DL. Increases in spontaneous activity in the dorsal cochlear nucleus following exposure to high intensity sound: a possible neural correlate of tinnitus. Audit Neurosci 1996;3:57–78.
52. Kaltenbach JA, Godfrey DA, Neumann JB, et al. Changes in spontaneous neural activity in the dorsal cochlear nucleus following exposure to intense sound: relation to threshold shift. Hear Res 1998;124:78–84.
53. Kaltenbach JA, Afman CE. Hyperactivity in the dorsal cochlear nucleus after intense sound exposure and its resemblance to tone-evoked activity: a physiological model for tinnitus. Hear Res 2000;140:165–72.
54. Zhang JS, Kaltenbach JA. Increases in spontaneous activity in the dorsal cochlear nucleus of the rat following exposure to high intensity sound. Neurosci Lett 1998;250:197–200.
55. Brozoski TJ, Bauer CA, Caspary DM. Elevated fusiform cell activity in the dorsal cochlear nucleus of chinchillas with psychophysical evidence of tinnitus. J Neurosci 2002;22:2383–90.
56. Kaltenbach, JA, Heffner, HE, Zhang, J, et al. Neurophysiological mechanisms of noise-induced tinnitus. In: Henderson D, Prasher D, Kopke R, et al, editors. Noise induced hearing loss, basic mechanisms, prevention and control. London: Noise Research Network Publications; 2001. p. 153–68.
57. Salvi RJ. Central components of the temporary threshold shift. In: Henderson D, Hamernik RP, Dosanjh DS, Mills JH, editors. Effects of noise on hearing. New York: Raven; 1976. p. 247–60.
58. Kimura M, Eggermont JJ. Effects of acute pure tone induced hearing loss on response properties in three auditory cortical fields in cat. Hear Res 1999;135:146–62.
59. Seki S, Eggermont JJ. Changes in spontaneous firing rate and neural synchrony in cat primary auditory cortex after localized tone-induced hearing loss. Hear Res 2003;180:28–38.

60. Harrison RV, Prijs VF. Single cochlear fiber responses in guinea pig with long term endolymphatic hydrops. Hear Res 1984;14:79–84.
61. Martin WH, Schwegler JW, Scheibelhoffer J, Ronis ML. Salicylate-induced changes in cat auditory nerve activity. Laryngoscope 1993;103:600–4.
62. Martin W. Spectral analysis of brain activity in the study of tinnitus. In: Vernon JA, Møller AR, editors. Mechanisms of tinnitus. Boston: Allyn and Bacon; 1995. p. 163–80.
63. Mongan E, Kelly P, Nies K, et al. Tinnitus as an indication of therapeutic serum salicylate levels. JAMA 1973;226:142–5.
64. Robertson D, Irvine DR. Plasticity of frequency organization in auditory cortex of guinea pigs with partial unilateral deafness. J Comp Neurol 1989;282:456–71.
65. Harrison RV, Nagasawa A, Smith DV, et al. Reorganization of auditory cortex after neonatal high frequency hearing loss. Hear Res 1991;54:11–9.
66. Rajan R, Irvine DR, Wise LZ, Heil P. Effect of unilateral partial cochlear lesions in adult cats on the representation of lesioned and unlesioned cochleas in primary auditory cortex. J Comp Neurol 1993;338:17–49.
67. Muhlnickel W, Elbert T, Taub E, Flor H. Reorganization of auditory cortex in tinnitus. Proc Natl Acad Sci U S A 1998;95:10340–3.
68. Kaltenbach JA, Lazor J. Tonotopic maps obtained from the surface of the dorsal cochlear nucleus of the hamster and rat. Hear Res 1991;51:149–60.
69. Heffner HE, Harrington IA. Tinnitus in hamsters following exposure to intense sound. Hear Res 2002;170:83–95.
70. Kwon O, Jastreboff MM, Hu S, et al. Modification of single-unit activity related to noise-induced tinnitus in rats. In: Hazell J, editor. Proceedings of the Sixth International Tinnitus Seminar. London: The Tinnitus and Hyperacusis Centre; 1999. p. 459–62.
71. Kaltenbach JA, Zacharek MA, Zhang J-S, Frederick S. Activity in the dorsal cochlear nucleus of hamsters previously tested for tinnitus following intense tone exposure. Neurosci Lett 2004;355:121–5.
72. Soussi T, Otto SR. Effects of electrical brainstem stimulation on tinnitus. Acta Otolaryngol (Stockh) 1994;114:135–40.
73. House WF, Hitselberger WE. Twenty-year report of the first auditory brain stem nucleus implant. Ann Otol Rhinol Laryngol 2001;110:103–4.
74. Møller AR, Møller MB, Yokota M. Some forms of tinnitus may involve the extralemniscal auditory pathway. Laryngoscope 1992;102:1165–71.
75. Rubinstein B. Tinnitus and craniomandibular disorders—is there a link? Swed Dent J Suppl 1993;95:1–46.
76. Levine RA. Somatic (craniocervical) tinnitus and the dorsal cochlear nucleus hypothesis. Am J Otolaryngol 1999;20:351–62
77. Shore SE, Vass Z, Wys NL, Altschuler RA. Trigeminal ganglion innervates the auditory brainstem. J Comp Neurol 2000;419:271–85.
78. Melamed SB, Kaltenbach JA, Church MW, et al. Cisplatin-induced increases in spontaneous neural activity in the dorsal cochlear nucleus and associated outer hair cell loss. Audiology 2000;39:24–9.
79. Kaltenbach JA, Rachel JD, Mathog TA, et al. Cisplatin-induced hyperactivity in the dorsal cochlear nucleus and its relation to outer hair cell loss: relevance to tinnitus. J Neurophysiol 2002; 88:699–714.
80. Kaltenbach JA, Zhang J, Afman CE. Plasticity of spontaneous neural activity in the dorsal cochlear nucleus after intense sound exposure. Hear Res 2000;147:282–92.
81. Zacharek MA, Kaltenbach JA, Mathog TA, Zhang J. Effects of cochlear ablation on noise induced hyperactivity in the hamster dorsal cochlear nucleus: implications for the origin of noise induced tinnitus. Hear Res 2002;172:137–43.
82. Kim J, Morest DK, Bohne BA. Degeneration of axons in the brainstem of the chinchilla after auditory overstimulation. Hear Res 1997; 103:169–91.
83. Schweitzer L, Jensen KF, Janssen R. Glutamate neurotoxicity in rat auditory system: cochlear nuclear complex. Neurotoxicol Teratol 1991;13:189–93.
84. McGinn MD, Faddis BT. Neuronal degeneration in the gerbil brainstem is associated with spongiform lesions. Microsc Res Tech 1998;41:187–204.
85. Kaltenbach JA, Falzarano P. DCN hyperactivity induced by previous intense sound exposure: origin with respect to cell layer. In: Santi PA, editor. Abstracts of the Twenty-third Annual Midwinter Research Meeting of the Association for Research in Otolaryngology. Mt Royal (NJ): Association for Research in Otolaryngology; 2002. p. 208.
86. Chang H, Chen K, Kaltenbach JA, et al. Effects of acoustic trauma on dorsal cochlear nucleus neuron activity in slices. Hear Res 2002;164:59–68.

CHAPTER 12

The Limbic System and Tinnitus

Anthony T. Cacace, PhD

Tinnitus is a ubiquitous phenomenon associated with many different forms of otologic pathology. Recent discoveries showing that tinnitus can involve abnormal interactions among multiple sensory modalities, sensorimotor systems, neurocognitive networks, and brain pathways involved in processing emotional reactions[1] have enhanced our understanding of this phenomenon. Although these contemporary relationships have expanded the biologic basis of tinnitus, many areas require further study. In particular, the neurobiologic underpinnings associated with processing emotional reactions to the tinnitus experience represent a specific domain needing elaboration. The tacit assumption that *the limbic system*, emotion, and tinnitus are closely linked is explored by examining inferences derived from theoretical models, experiments using laboratory animals, functional imaging investigations, and information from other closely aligned disciplines. The assumption of limbic system linkage invariably leads to fundamental questions associated with this term, such as what is the limbic system, and is it a viable concept in contemporary neuroscience? Although many questions emerge in relation to this concept, current debate centers on whether the neural representation of emotion involves individual systems for separate emotions or a more integrated system capable of coding all emotions.[2]

Herein, a profile of ideas is presented linking brain areas with emotions, which have been unfolding from early neuroanatomic studies through to the present day. To put this area into perspective, a brief recapitulation of historical details, based on comprehensive reviews by Mega and colleagues and LeDoux,[3,4] is used to set the stage for current thinking and conceptualizations (see these reviews for relevant citations). The overall intent is to update available information, clarify pertinent issues, encourage debate, and take the optimistic position that this knowledge will lead to a better understanding of the tinnitus experience.

HISTORICAL OVERVIEW

As early as the 1600s, Willis designated the cortical area encircling the brainstem as *cerebri limbus* (Latin, meaning a border); in the late 1800s, the term *grand lobe limbique* was used by Broca to describe the circle of structures forming the medial wall of each hemisphere, including the cingulate gyrus, anterior olfactory region, and hippocampus. Not surprisingly, because these brain structures were common among mammals with well-developed olfactory function, a relationship to the sense of smell was initially emphasized. This led to the concept of the rhinencephalon because corticomedial areas of the amygdala and the entorhinal area of the hippocampus receive inputs from the olfactory bulb. As information accumulated over time, various structural, functional, and behavioral relationships developed that allowed for further refinement in this area. For example, in the late 1800s, Brown and Schäfer found that bilateral temporal lobectomy, which included extirpation of mesial temporal lobe structures, transformed ferocious monkeys into tame and docile animals. The now classic studies by Klüver and Bucy further elaborated on the neural substrates associated with different emotional states. Their investigations showed that bilateral temporal lobe resections in monkeys produced a relatively complex deficit characterized by visual agnosia, hypermetamorphosis, increased orality, hypersexuality, tameness, and placidity (ie, loss of fear). By improving experimental methodology to address criticisms of studies involving temporal lobectomies, it became evident that lesions involving the amygdala played a central role in the expression of emotional reactions related to fear and aggression.[5,6] From neurology clinics came additional information, which began to dissociate theories of hippocampal function from those of other mesial temporal lobe sites. In the early 1900s, Bechterew made the astute observation that bilateral lesions of the hippocampus and other presumed limbic structures (mammillary bodies and anterior thalamus) resulted in alterations in memory. Bechterew noted that long- and short-term memory remained intact, but derangement occurred in the "*process of registering information.*" This study set the stage for distinguishing cognitive from emotional deficits within mesial temporal lobe structures. Within this same time period, Ramón y Cajal systematized the cytoarchitecture of nuclear structures associated with the "*limbic lobe,*" which included the amygdala, septal nuclei, hypothalamus, epithalamus, anterior thalamic nuclei, and parts of the ventral medial portions of the basal ganglia. He also hypothesized a relationship to mnemonic processes and formulated the idea that the hippocampus was involved in forming olfactory memories. Additionally, in the mid-1920s, Cannon proposed that emotions result from the action and reaction of the cerebral cortex and diencephalon. Although reciprocal activation from the diencephalon to basal ganglia was thought to produce motor responses associated with emotional behavior such as crying or laughing, it was also thought to be a way for the cortex to receive conscious appreciation of emotional states.

By combining results from anatomic studies with data derived from patients with emotional disturbances, Papez proposed a mechanism of emotion that was based on a circuit that included the cingulate gyrus, hippocampus, mammillary bodies, and anterior nucleus of the thalamus and allowed for the "*flow of emotion*" leading to internal or external expression. This representation was reported in the mid-1930s and was based on neuropathology involving tumors in the cingulate region (patients showed apathy and decreased motivation) and patients who had contracted rabies. Because the rabies virus was found in the hippocampus, this structure was included as part of the emotional system. However, conspicuously absent from the Papez schema were structures such as the amygdala and septum. In the mid-1940s, Yakovlev proposed that three cortical areas (orbitofrontal cortex, temporal lobe, and insula) and two subcortical structures (amygdala and dorsal medial thalamus) played an important role in motivation and emotional expression. In terms of phylogenetic development, Yakovlev also described three levels or layers of nervous system function: a primitive inner core devoted to arousal and autonomic function, a second surrounding layer that included limbic structures and basal ganglia, and a third layer that included the neocortex and pyramidal system. By the early 1950s, MacLean conjoined the Papez circuit with basal lateral structures described by Yakovlev and collectively coined the term *limbic system*. MacLean's elaboration of Yakovlev's model evolved into the "*triune brain*" and incorporated phylogenetic stages of central nervous system development into this concept. He designated these stages as proreptilian (dealing with basic instincts), paleomammalian (dealing with the limbic system and emotion), and neocortical (dealing with analytic reasoning). In this proposal, the limbic component constituted a phylogenetically ancient ring of medial cortex subserving emotional processing, whereas the more lateral neocortex served primarily a cognitive function.

Thus, the limbic system was an outgrowth of early neuroanatomic investigations, functional correlations, and phylogenetic theory. The frameworks proposed by Papez and MacLean also replaced older concepts, such as the rhinencephalon, by emphasizing that the limbic system was more specifically involved in the elaboration of visceral and emotional expression. In retrospect, however, the main contribution of limbic system theory was in the context of providing an evolutionary explanation of mind and behavior. The construction of this idea was based on the premise that the neocortex is well developed in mammals and that neocortical tissue provided the substrate for highly specialized cognitive faculties such as thinking, reasoning, memory, and problem solving. This is in contrast to the so-called "*old cortex,*" which was thought to mediate more primitive aspects of life, such as emotions.[4]

Whereas the term *limbic system* has been used synonymously as a unifying framework associated with brain areas or circuits subserving emotion, many contemporary investigators have openly expressed dissatisfaction and reservation with this term. As noted above, as early as the 1930s and more recently in the mid-1950s, basic concepts central to limbic system theory began to erode. By extending the findings of Bechterew, Scoville and Milner showed that damage to the hippocampus led to cognitive deficits in long-term memory. Such data were not compatible with those espoused by the triune brain concept, which was based on the premise that the phylogenetically primitive limbic system in general and the hippocampus in particular were not well suited to participate in cognitive functions. Other reasons that the limbic system concept produced discontent among scientists were grounded on the arbitrary nature, confusion, and often questionable justification that resulted by including more and more anatomic areas in this amalgam. Indeed, this discontent culminated with a recommendation by many leading scientists to eliminate or abandon the term entirely. LeDoux has noted several additional problems associated with this concept.[4] These include the lack of objective criteria for deciding what is and what is not a limbic area and the fact that limbic system theory is inadequate for explaining how the brain "*makes*" emotions. Taken together, these criticisms are understandable and noteworthy because the downside of using a vaguely defined neuroanatomic construct is that it imposes undue limitations when it comes to accepting or rejecting domain-specific hypotheses, models, or theories. Indeed, the explosive growth in comparative animal and human studies over the past decade has converged on the importance of the amygdala in the expression and processing of emotions.

RELATIONSHIP BETWEEN TINNITUS AND EMOTION: CENTRAL NERVOUS SYSTEM INTERACTIONS

Within the tinnitus literature per se, limbic system linkage has been inferred from theoretic models,[7] extralemniscal pathway interactions,[8,9] clinical correlations based on functional imaging studies,[10-12] and correlation analysis based on experiments in laboratory animals[13] and indirectly from analogies to the pain literature. However, when potential mechanisms linking tinnitus with emotion are inferred, direct associations to the amygdala have emerged with increased frequency. Linkage that underlies this relationship is based on contemporary neuroanatomic studies documenting the existence of auditory projections from the thalamus and the cortex to the amygdala, which are essential for establishing conditioned reactions to fear (see Sah and colleagues[14] for a review). Additionally, highly processed polysensory inputs also have access to the lateral and basal areas of the amygdala through the prefrontal cortex and perirhinal and entorhinal areas of the hippocampus. Moreover, when complex stimulus representations exist, such as those associated with arousal and attention to biologically relevant stimuli, it has been suggested that there is a greater propensity for these representations to be mediated by corticoamygdalar interactions than by thalamoamygdalar pathways.[15]

Contemporary viewpoints have also emphasized the potential role of the amygdala in processing tinnitus-related neural activity. For example, the observation that the nonclassic or extralemniscal auditory pathway is involved in tinnitus was inferred by studies that showed that electrical stimulation of the somatosensory system could affect the psychophysical dimensions of the tinnitus perception by increasing or decreasing loudness or by altering pitch (reviewed by Møller[16]). These observations are noteworthy because they imply that the generation and/or processing of tinnitus can occur within anatomic pathways that are different from those that normally process sound. Although extralemniscal and classic auditory pathways ascend in parallel from the brainstem to the cortex, Møller emphasizes that divergence occurs in the neuroanatomic and neurophysiological domains. Specifically, it has been reported that the extralemniscal pathway uses relay nuclei in the dorsal and medial thalamus, whereas classic auditory pathways use the ventral thalamic nucleus. Extralemniscal thalamic nuclei project to auditory association cortices and nonsensory structures, whereas thalamic nuclei of the classic pathway project to the primary auditory cortex. Of particular importance to the present discussion is the observation that subcortical thalamic connections from the extralemniscal pathway project directly to the lateral nucleus of the amygdala. Classic pathways also have connections to the amygdala, but they are less direct and involve highly processed neural activity. Moreover, the nuclei of nonclassic pathways perform less specific analysis of sound than those of classic pathways and, as such, may account for differences in the frequency-tuning properties of neurons. Neurons in the classic pathway are sharply tuned, whereas extralemniscal neurons are tuned more broadly. Lastly, in contrast to classic auditory pathways, extralemniscal pathways receive inputs from multiple sensory modalities (somatosensory and visual) and not just from the auditory periphery. Presently, mechanisms underlying how auditory information gets routed to the extralemniscal pathway and redirected to nonauditory areas of the brain, such as the amygdala, remain unknown. However, these relatively new and important relationships open interesting possibilities for understanding abnormal perceptions associated with tinnitus.

Jastreboff provides a generalized framework for conceptualizing tinnitus in the context of known neuroanatomic relationships and psychophysiologic reactions, often referred to as the "*physiological model.*"[17] Key components of this model include links among the sensory, "*limbic*," and autonomic nervous systems. Significantly, the model proposes that fear conditioning plays a major role in sustaining the tinnitus perception. This conceptualization is consistent with prevailing views that fear learning is a product of evolution, which serves as a defense mechanism to promote survival of the organism from impending or future threats,[18] and emphasizes the belief that "*emotions evolved not as conscious feelings, linguistically differentiated or otherwise, but as brain states and bodily responses.*"[19] Current dogma indicates that the amygdala is an essential link in the expression of emotion and motivational responses by processing inputs from multiple sensory modalities (auditory, somatosensory, visual, olfactory, gustatory) and directing output to specific pathways involved in regulating body homeostasis and behavior (eg, hypothalamus, brainstem, striatum, endocrine system, basal forebrain, trigeminal and facial motor nuclei).[19] Therefore, designating the amygdala as the "*sensory gateway to the emotions*" is supported by experimental work in animals and by clinical investigations.[20]

The underlying hypothesis relating tinnitus to emotion is appealing because fear conditioning has strong underpinnings in psychological theory and is linked to a wide range of affective traits and conditions known to have an effect on individuals suffering from this condition, including anxiety disorders and phobias.[21] However, with respect to tinnitus, specifics of the conditioning contingencies have not been well described or established. Nevertheless, it is hypothesized that fear conditioning is initiated when tinnitus is detected and consciously interpreted as a harbinger of a serious medical condition or as a precursor of a potentially distressful event.[7] In relation to mechanisms of action, tinnitus would be considered the stimulus, and the aversive reaction to the stimulus would be considered a negative reinforcer. Pairing the phantom stimulus with negative reactions is thought to engage amygdalar and associated autonomic nervous system components. If left untreated, it is assumed that tinnitus can become pervasive and evolve into a life-altering experience, disturbing sleep, disrupting concentration, and potentially contributing to depression.[22–24] At the extreme, there have been reports linking tinnitus to suicide, although compelling cause-and-effect relationships are difficult to substantiate in the absence of other intervening factors.[25]

Whereas fear conditioning has become a powerful tool for studying processes involved in learning and memory, what makes this approach both appealing and important is that neuroanatomic input and output pathways are relatively well known (Figure 12-1). Additionally, the fear conditioning paradigm allows for questions to be asked about how the brain processes emotional information (ie, detects and responds to danger) without necessarily dealing with or solving the more vexing problem of how or where conscious feelings arise in the central nervous system (ie, issues related to consciousness). In this context, "*…the fear system has been treated as a set of processing circuits that detect and respond to danger, rather than as a mechanism through which subjective states of fear are experienced. With this approach, fear is operationalized, or made experimentally tractable.*"[4] Often applied in research using animals, fear conditioning is based on classical or pavlovian associations, whereby the response to an unconditioned stimulus (US), such as a noxious shock, can activate intrinsic system responses that alter body homeostasis and result in a range of overt behaviors, such as freezing, arousal, and startle.[26] When the US is paired with a neutral stimulus such as a tone, light, or odor and if conditioning is successful, the neutral stimulus acquires the ability to elicit these defensive responses, thereby becoming a conditioned stimulus (CS). Work focusing on the cellular and molecular mechanisms underlying memory consolidation, storage, and plasticity links fear conditioning to the medial and lateral nuclei of the amygdala as a likely site of US-CS convergence.[27,28]

In support of the conditioning paradigm, dissociation designs have been used increasingly in neuropsychological experiments as a way to delineate the functional effects of lesions in different areas of the brain. The double-dissociation design is of particular importance because it has the advantage of demonstrating both the sensitivity of the task and the specificity of the lesion. An example of the double-dissociation principle was demonstrated by Bechara and colleagues in the context of emotional and

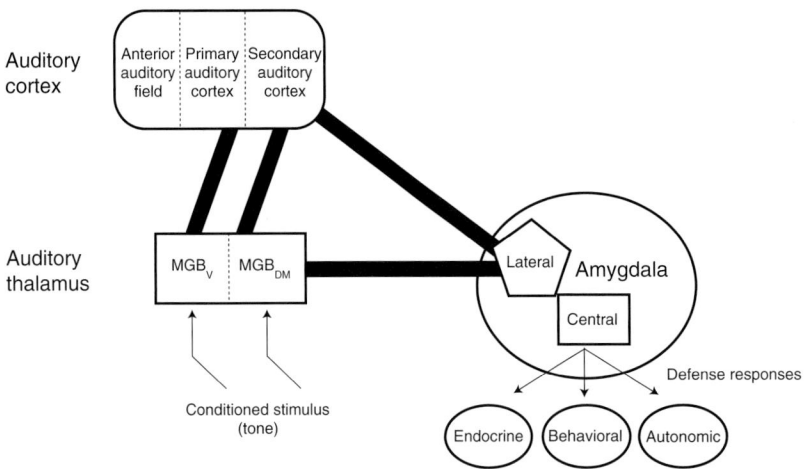

FIGURE 12-1. Schematic block diagram of the neural pathways involved in fear conditioning to acoustic stimuli (see LeDoux[4] for details). In this representation, when the conditioned stimulus is an audible tone, the lateral nucleus of the amygdala is activated by projections from auditory processing areas in the dorsal medial aspect of the medial geniculate body and from the auditory cortex. The lateral nucleus also projects to the central nucleus of the amygdala, which controls the expression of fear through changes in behavior, endocrine function, and/or autonomic responses. Other highly relevant information concerning lemniscal and extralemniscal pathways to the amygdala is described elsewhere (see Møller[16] for details). MGB_{DM} = dorsal medial division of the medial geniculate body; MGB_V = ventral division of the medial geniculate body.

mnemonic processing.[29] In this experiment, three individuals were studied: one individual had bilateral damage to the amygdalae from Urbach-Wiethe disease (lipoid proteinosis), another individual had bilateral damage to the hippocampi, and a third individual had bilateral damage to the amygdalae and hippocampi. Two tasks were used: a conditioning task to a startling sound, in which skin conductance was the dependent variable, and a second task in which declarative knowledge was assessed by probing the individual about aspects of the conditioning task. The result of this investigation showed that the individual with damage to the amygdalae was unable to establish conditioning but was able to acquire declarative facts. In contrast, the individual with bilateral hippocampal damage was able to establish conditioning but was unable to acquire declarative facts. The individual with bilateral lesions to the amygdalae and hippocampi was unable to perform either task. The double dissociation demonstrated by this study provides further support for the view that the amygdala is essential for the association of contextual cues with affect, whereas the hippocampus is critical for learning the relationship among contextual cues.

Although the role of the amygdala in fear conditioning is well established, there are details about specific processes that remain controversial and open to debate. Cahill and colleagues challenged several important issues.[30] The first concern focuses on whether lateral and/or basolateral nuclei of the amygdala are the primary site(s) for encoding and permanently storing learned fear. The issue of contention centers on the inability of prior experiments to distinguish whether lesions primarily affected learning or memory processes or just disrupted the animal's ability to make specific responses. The importance of this concern relates to evidence that the lateral and basolateral nuclei of the amygdala are necessary for expressive behaviors such as unconditioned freezing and fear-potentiated startle. Thus, the inability to distinguish the lesion's effect on memory from other influences on performance (the so-called learning or performance distinction) is a justified criticism.

A second issue concerns interpretation of the effects of intra-amygdala infusion of N-methyl-D-aspartate (NMDA) antagonists on pavlovian fear conditioning. This issue is based on the observation that NMDA antagonists infused into the amygdala prior to conditioning attenuate fear-potentiated startle. Although such findings are consistent with the hypothesis that induction of NMDA-dependent long-term potentiation occurs within the lateral and basolateral nuclei of the amygdala, exclusion of non-memory effects of NMDA antagonists that might disrupt acquisition, such as the effects of attentional or motivational processes, is a necessary consideration.

A final issue concerns whether electrophysiologic data demonstrating the development of long-term potentiation occur in the lateral and basolateral nuclei of the amygdala during fear-potentiated startle or in other areas, such as the medial geniculate nucleus, which sends projections to these regions of the amygdala. Because associative changes in neural responses to the conditioned stimulus and convergence of noxious stimuli are known to occur in the medial geniculate nucleus,[31] delineation between these areas is necessary for proper interpretation. Clearly, the question concerning where in the brain memories are formed and stored continues to be a source of rigorous debate and controversy. Answers to the concerns noted above will help to address some of these important issues. However, this is an area of ongoing research, in which many of the specific details remain unknown, need to be clarified, or are currently under investigation.[32] Progress, however, is being made in these areas.

To summarize, a large body of evidence supports the idea that conditioned fear induced by aversive stimuli is mediated by transmission of information about the CS and US to the amygdala and that fear expression occurs though a cascade of reactions involving the lateral and central nuclei of this structure. As the principal output pathway of the fear system, the central nucleus sends projections to areas of the hypothalamus and brainstem that control specific behavioral, endocrine, and autonomic nervous system responses (eg, arousal, freezing, startle, facial expressions of fear; changes in respiration, blood pressure, electroencephalographic activity).[4,26,28]

Involvement of certain brain areas associated with fear conditioning, fear learning, and plasticity has direct relevance to the nonauditory brain systems involved in tinnitus. Conceptually, unfamiliar sounds and discrepant or novel input tend to produce arousal, increase attention, and potentially initiate fear reactions in those individuals affected. Neurophysiological data suggest that when monkeys are presented with a range of biologically relevant auditory stimuli, neurons in the lateral nucleus of the amygdala respond to unfamiliar sounds but not to familiar sounds associated, for example, with food reward.[33] In the development of specific animal models for studying tinnitus, activation sites in auditory and nonauditory brain areas have been elucidated by metabolic mapping techniques such as 2-deoxyglucose (2-DG), which infers neural activity, or c-*fos* immunocytochemistry studies, which identify gene expression associated with activated neurons.[34–36] Gene expression of nonauditory activation sites following tinnitus induction initially has identified areas of the brain such as the locus ceruleus, midbrain periaqueductal gray area, and lateral parabranchial nucleus. These areas are also known to correlate with behavioral states associated with arousal, anxiety, stress, and pain. Further insight into auditory and nonauditory brain areas involved in tinnitus has used awake gerbils, inducing agents such as salicylate or noise exposure and a combination of 2-DG and c-*fos* labeling as detection methods.[36] Anatomic sites, evaluated by Langner and Wallhäusser-Franke,[13] included the dorsal cochlear nucleus, inferior colliculus, primary auditory cortex, anterior auditory (cortical) field, and lateral, medial, and central nuclei of the amygdala. After tinnitus induction, modest pairwise correlations were found for c-*fos*–labeled cells between the primary auditory cortex and anterior auditory field ($r = .70$); however, much higher correlations were found between the auditory cortex and lateral nucleus of the amygdala ($r = .99$) and the anterior auditory field and central and medial nuclei of the amygdala ($r = .92$ and $.85$, respectively). Also noteworthy were the results of principal component analysis, which showed that ~ 66% of the variance could be explained by interactions between the auditory cortex and amygdala.

Although presently limited in number but not in scope, functional imaging studies are becoming instrumental in gaining insight into the relationship between tinnitus and nonsensory areas such as those involved in emotional and/or cognitive processing. Lockwood and colleagues used positron emission tomography (PET) to study four adults with a constant background tinnitus who had the ability to modulate parameters (such as loudness) of the tinnitus with oral facial maneuvers (OFMs; eg, jaw clenching).[11] In these individuals, tinnitus was unilateral in nature and severe in character, such that it disrupted activities of daily living. Being able to modify differentially a continuous background tinnitus from a resting state provides the conditions necessary to locate brain areas associated with this technique. With this methodology, if the relevant comparisons produce significant differences by statistical analyses, then these sites can be mapped to specific brain areas. In two of the individuals studied, OFMs increased tinnitus loudness (tinnitus localized to the left ear in one participant and the right ear in the other), whereas in the others, OFMs decreased tinnitus loudness (tinnitus localized to right ears in both). Particularly relevant to the current discussion were the two individuals in whom OFMs decreased tinnitus loudness. In these subjects, there was a corresponding reduction in cerebral blood flow (ie, a deactivation), which was localized to the posterior and midportion of the left middle temporal gyrus, determined by subtracting the experimental conditions (rest − OFMs). However, to distinguish differential changes in cerebral blood flow owing to the decrease in tinnitus loudness from changes owing to OFMs, further contrasts (subtractions) were necessary. These contrasts took the following form: [patients (rest − OFMs) − control (rest − OFMs)]. In this analysis, reductions in cerebral blood flow were localized to Brodmann's areas 21 and 41 and the hippocampus on the left side. Although the interpretation of PET-related deactivation effects is not straightforward, these results demonstrate that distinct cortical mechanisms involving auditory and nonauditory mesial temporal lobe structures are engaged when OFMs reduce the loudness perception of tinnitus.

Mirz and colleagues used PET to study brain areas associated with different classes of aversive auditory stimuli to mimic tinnitus.[12] Based on their analysis, they found that aversive acoustic stimuli activated sites in prefrontal and frontal lobe areas, parahippocampal areas, and amygdaloid bodies. These activations were in addition to those expected in the primary auditory cortex in response to acoustic input. Whereas superior and medial frontal gyri and the inferior parietal lobe showed increased activation, no significant activations were found in the cingulate gyrus. These data suggest that brain activation sites associated with aversive auditory stimuli are in partial contrast to those induced by aversive (painful) somatosensory stimuli. Blood and colleagues explored the relationships between musical consonance and dissonance and brain activation associated with these dichotomous inputs.[37] Musical dissonance was correlated with activation in right parahippocampal and precuneus regions. Although it is inferred that music may recruit neural mechanisms associated with pleasant or unpleasant emotional states, it appears that these responses differ from those underlying auditory perceptual representations and those induced by fear.

Neuroanatomic frameworks proposed for understanding certain forms of pain have paralleled models used for gaining insight into tinnitus or vice versa.[38–40] Tinnitus and pain share the common feature that both conditions are often triggered by peripheral injury and result in plastic changes at more central locations in the nervous system.[41,42] In theory, the "*neuromatrix for pain*" was proposed as a way to understand continuously unwanted aversive sensations associated with loss of a body part (ie, "*phantom limb pain*"), a condition thought to arise following deafferentation-induced changes to a central neural representation of an underlying body schema.[40] Briefly, within the pain neuromatrix, three major processing circuits have been implicated: classic somatosensory pathways, neural pathways through brainstem to limbic system areas, and parietal association areas. Partial validation of the pain neuromatrix has also been aided by empiric evidence obtained from functional imaging studies.[42] In a recent review of functional imaging studies associated with pain induced from various forms of aversive or noxious stimuli, Derbyshire showed consistent patterns of activation within a large and broadly distributed network of brain areas.[42] Activated areas include the thalamus, primary and secondary somatosensory cortices, midbrain region of the periaqueductal gray and the lenticular complex, the insula, orbital frontal cortex, prefrontal cortex, and motor and inferior parietal areas. Interestingly, the most consistently activated area across all studies was the anterior cingulate region of the brain. Thus, localization of pain parameters by functional imaging methods allows for commonalities and differences to be compared in a more objective manner.

SUMMARY AND CONCLUSIONS

From its inception to current-day study, the limbic system has evolved into an umbrella term that now encompasses many different brain areas, relationships, and meanings. Although survival of the limbic system concept might be equated with acceptance, the alternative explanation concerning its longevity is more plausible:

This is in part attributable to the fact that both the anatomical concept and the emotional function it was supposed to mediate were defined so vaguely so as to be irrefutable.... On the neural side, the criteria for inclusion of brain areas in the limbic system remain undefined, and evidence that any limbic area, however defined, contributes to any aspect of any emotion has tended to validate the whole concept. Mountains of data on the role of limbic areas in emotion exist, but there is still little understanding of how our emotions might be the product of the limbic system.[4]

Indeed, as research on tinnitus moves forward with the application of powerful and newly developed methods, there is an obvious downside for the continued use of a vaguely defined neuroanatomic construct. Therefore, when pertinent experiments are performed, the appeal is made for researchers to specify neuroanatomic relationships during tinnitus processing rather than to invoke the term *limbic system* and assume that it conveys common knowledge.

REFERENCES

1. Cacace AT. Expanding the biological basis of tinnitus: crossmodal origins and the role of neuroplasticity. Hear Res 2003;175:112–32.
2. Calder AJ, Lawrence AD, Young A. Neuropsychology of fear and loathing. Nat Rev Neurosci 2001;2:352–62.
3. Mega MS, Cummings JL, Salloway S, et al. The limbic system: an anatomic, phylogenetic, and clinical perspective. J Neuropsychiatry Clin Neurosci 1997;9:315–30.
4. LeDoux JE. Emotion circuits in the brain. Annu Rev Neurosci 2000;23:155–84.
5. Weiskrantz L. Behavioral changes associated with ablation of the amygdaloid complex in monkeys. J Comp Physiol Psychol 1956;49:381–91.
6. Meunier M, Bachevalier J, Murray EA, et al. Effects of aspiration versus neurotoxic lesions of the amygdala on emotional responses in monkeys. Eur J Neurosci 1999;11:4403–18.
7. Jastreboff PJ. The neurophysiological model of tinnitus and hyperacusis. In: Hazell J, editor. Proceedings of the Sixth International Tinnitus Seminar. London: The Tinnitus and Hyperacusis Centre; 1999. p. 32–8.
8. Møller AR, Møller MB, Yokota M. Some forms of tinnitus may involve the extralemniscal auditory pathway. Laryngoscope 1992;102:1165–71.
9. Møller, AR, Rollins PR. The non-classical auditory pathways are involved in hearing in children but not adults. Neurosci Lett 2002;319:41–4.
10. Shulman A, Goldstein B. A final common pathway for tinnitus—the medial temporal lobe system. Int Tinnitus J 1995;1:115–26.
11. Lockwood AH, Salvi RJ, Coad, ML, et al. The functional neuroanatomy of tinnitus: evidence for limbic system links and neural plasticity. Neurology 1998;50:114–20.
12. Mirz F, Gjedde A, Sødkilde-Jrgensen H, et al. Functional brain imaging of tinnitus-like perception induced by aversive auditory stimuli. Neuroreport 2000;11:633–7.
13. Langner G, Wallhäusser-Franke E. Computer simulation of a tinnitus model based on labeling of tinnitus activity in the auditory cortex. In: Hazell J, editor. Proceedings of the Sixth International Tinnitus Seminar. London: The Tinnitus and Hyperacusis Centre; 1999. p. 20–5.
14. Sah P, Faber ESL, Lopez de Armentia M, et al. The amygdaloid complex: anatomy and physiology. Physiol Rev 2003;83:803–34.
15. Barbas H. Connections underlying the synthesis of cognition, memory, and emotion in primate prefrontal cortices. Brain Res Bull 2000;52:319–30.
16. Møller AR. Pathophysiology of tinnitus. Otolaryngol Clin North Am 2003;36:249–66.
17. Jastreboff PJ. Tinnitus habituation therapy (THT) and tinnitus retraining therapy (TRT). In: Tyler RS, editor. Tinnitus handbook. San Diego (CA): Singular; 2000. p. 357–76.
18. Fanselow MS. Neural organization of the defensive behavior system responsible for fear. Psychonom Bull Rev 1994;1:429–38.
19. LeDoux JE. The emotional brain. New York: Simon & Schuster; 1996.
20. Aggleton JP, Mishkin M. The amygdala: sensory gateway to the emotions. In: Plutchik R, Kellerman H, editors. Emotion: theory, research, and experience. Vol 3. New York: Academic Press; 1986. p. 281–9.
21. Gray JA, McNaughton N. The neuropsychology of anxiety: an enquiry into the functions of the septohippocampal system. New York: Oxford University Press; 2000.

22. Simpson JJ, Davies WE. Recent advances in the pharmacological treatment of tinnitus. Trends Pharmacol Sci 1999;20:12–8.
23. Erlandsson SI. Psychological profiles of tinnitus patients. In: Tyler RS, editor. Tinnitus handbook. San Diego (CA): Singular; 2000. p. 25–57.
24. McKenna L. Tinnitus and insomnia. In: Tyler RS, editor. Tinnitus handbook. San Diego (CA): Singular; 2000. p. 59–84.
25. Jacobson GP, McCaslin DL. A search for evidence of a direct relationship between tinnitus and suicide. J Am Acad Audiol 2001;12:493–6.
26. Davis M. Neurobiology of fear responses: the role of the amygdala. J Neuropsychiatry Clin Neurosci 1997;9:382–402.
27. Schafe GE, Nader K, Blair HT, Le Doux JE. Memory consolidation of pavlovian fear conditioning: a cellular and molecular perspective. Trends Neurosci 2001;24:540–6.
28. Maren S. Neurobiology of pavlovian fear conditioning. Annu Rev Neurosci 2001;24:897–931.
29. Bechara A, Tranel D, Damasio H, et al. Double dissociation of conditioning and declarative knowledge relative to human amygdala and hippocampus. Science 1995;269:1115–8.
30. Cahill L, Weinberger NM, Roozendaal B, et al. Is the amygdala a locus of "conditioned fear"? Some questions and caveats. Neuron 1999;23:227–8.
31. Weinberger NM. Dynamic regulation of receptive fields and maps in the adult sensory cortex. Annu Rev Neurosci 1995;18:129–58.
32. Medina JF, Repa JC, Mauk MD, et al. Parallels between cerebellum- and amygdala-dependent conditioning. Nat Rev Neurosci 2002;3:122–31.
33. Ono T, Nishijo H. Neurophysiological basis of the Klüver-Bucy syndrome: responses of monkey amygdaloid neurons to biologically significant objects. In: Aggleton AG, editor. The amygdala: neurobiological aspects of emotion, memory and mental dysfunction. New York: Wiley-Liss; 1992. p. 167–90.
34. Sasaki CT, Kauer JS, Babitz L. Differential [14C]2-deoxyglucose uptake after deafferentation of the mammalian auditory pathway—a model for examining tinnitus. Brain Res 1980;194:511–6.
35. Wallhäusser-Franke E, Braun S, Langner G. Salicylate alters 2-DG uptake in the auditory system: a model for tinnitus? Neuroreport 1996;7:1585–8.
36. Wallhäusser-Franke E. Salicylate evokes c-*fos* expression in the brainstem: implications for tinnitus. Neuroreport 1997;8:725–8.
37. Blood AJ, Zatorre RJ, Bermudez P, Evans AC. Emotional responses to pleasant and unpleasant music correlate with activity in paralimbic brain regions. Nat Neurosci 1999;2:382–7.
38. Melzack R. Phantom limbs and the concept of a neuromatrix. Trends Neurosci 1990;13:88–92.
39. Jastreboff PJ. Phantom auditory perception (tinnitus): mechanisms of generation and perception. Neurosci Res 1990;8:221–54.
40. Salvi RJ, Lockwood AH, Burkard R. Neural plasticity and tinnitus. In: Tyler RS, editor. Tinnitus handbook. San Diego (CA): Singular; 2000. p. 123–48.
41. Møller AR. Symptoms and signs caused by neural plasticity. Neurol Res 2001;23:565–72.
42. Derbyshire SW. Exploring the pain "*Neuromatrix.*" Curr Rev Pain 2000;4:467–77.

CHAPTER 13

The Auditory Cortex and Tinnitus

Jos J. Eggermont, PhD

The auditory cortex is necessary for the perception of sounds that require integration of neural events for short periods of time and for temporal pattern discrimination. Bilateral ablation of the auditory cortex still allows discrimination to changes in sound, such as onsets, and changes in intensity and frequency of tones.[1] Part of this latter ability may be the result of reorganization processes in the auditory system that compensate for the loss of cortical processing. This is plausible because after acute blocking of cortical activity with the γ-aminobutyric acid agonist muscimol, rats fail to detect tones or to discriminate frequency.[2] As a consequence, changes in sound stimulation that do not produce measurable changes in the auditory cortex will not lead to a percept. For example, phase-locking of firings in cat auditory nerve fibers to a low-frequency pure tone, without any change in the overall firing rate, starts to occur at sound levels that can be 20 dB below the threshold of hearing.[3] Clearly, these changes in temporal response properties of auditory nerve fibers will not activate the auditory cortex, although they are a perfect correlate of the presence of a stimulus. Only when the firing rate of auditory nerve fibers increases sufficiently above the spontaneous level does the sound become audible. Alternatively, percepts such as tinnitus should be accompanied by measurable changes in auditory cortical activity. Thus, it is important to relate subcortical findings caused by tinnitus-inducing agents to those that are found in the auditory cortex under the same conditions to sort out the sequence of activity that leads to tinnitus.

The auditory cortex is not only a receiving station of subcortical neural activity that reaches it via the lemniscal, tonotopically organized pathway or the nonlemniscal, multimodal pathway,[4] it is also a major control system that affects the processing in subcortical structures.[5] This is reflected in the innervation that the auditory part of the thalamus receives from the auditory cortex (90%) compared with that from the central nucleus of the inferior colliculus (10%). In addition, reflecting on the fact that only 1% of the input to the cortex is extracortical, one could say that "the cortex to a large extent is a thinking machine working on its own output."[6] The thalamic input to the cortex is layer dependent and is highest (about 20% of the total input) in layer IV of the visual cortex.[7] In locally stimulating the primary auditory cortex (AI) electrically with minute currents for short periods of time (less than 15 minutes), lasting changes in the frequency-place maps in the central nucleus of the inferior colliculus (ICc) could be produced,[8] and even the properties of the cochlea could be changed.[9]

This corticofugal action makes it difficult to distinguish feed-forward activity resulting from changes in the functioning of peripheral structures and nuclei from feedback to these structures and nuclei produced by the activity of the auditory cortex. For instance, the dramatically increased spontaneous firing rate in the dorsal cochlear nucleus (DCN) after noise trauma appears 2 to 3 days after the trauma,[10] whereas in the AI, an increase in spontaneous firing rate appears within a few hours after such trauma.[11] This suggests that cortical changes may be instrumental in the increased spontaneous firing rates in the DCN. In return, changes in the DCN might affect the spontaneous activity in the ICc, but the DCN is not the prime mover in the sequence of change. The fact that the DCN is processing both somatosensory and auditory input[12] may also be a factor in the post-trauma plasticity of spontaneous activity in this structure. Another nucleus in the nonlemniscal pathway, the external nucleus of the inferior colliculus (ICx), has shown dramatic changes in spontaneous activity following the application of salicylate, a tinnitus-inducing drug.[13,14] This nucleus, which also receives its major input from the AI and the secondary auditory cortex (AII) and a much reduced input from sub-midbrain structures,[15] does project via the dorsal part of the medial geniculate body to the AII. Thus, also in this case, one could question whether the effect originates in the ICx; I am inclined to put the origin in the auditory cortex.

The number of studies in subcortical parts of the lemniscal pathway related to tinnitus-inducing agents is fairly limited (if we exclude the multimodal DCN). After several hours of noise exposure and long survival times, cat auditory nerve fibers in characteristic frequency (CF) regions with normal thresholds still have normal spontaneous activity and normal interspike interval statistics. Units that no longer respond to sound also have significantly decreased spontaneous firing rates and have a tendency to fire in spike bursts separated by long periods of silence. These abnormally firing fibers might innervate partially damaged inner hair cells,[16] whereas nerve fibers without spontaneous activity likely originate from regions in which all inner hair cells are completely damaged.

Salicylate administration in cats at a dose of 200 mg/kg of body weight produced no significant change in the mean spontaneous rates in the low and high spontaneous firing rate populations of nerve fibers. In some individual cells, however, significant increases in firing rate were seen.[17] Much higher doses of salicylate (400 mg/kg) produced significant increases in spontaneous activity in cat auditory nerve fibers.[18] After injection of 10 to 30 mg/kg of body weight of quinine, guinea pigs showed a significant reduction in the spontaneous firing rate of auditory nerve fibers,[19] as judged from a relative increase in the number of units firing at rates lower than 25 spikes/s compared with controls.

Chinchillas, exposed to an 86 dB SPL, 4 kHz noise band for about 4 days, at 2 to 12 hours postexposure showed markedly decreased spontaneous firing rates for cochlear nucleus neurons with CFs in the region with elevated thresholds.[20] No recordings of spontaneous activity in ICc have been reported following noise trauma or application of tinnitus-inducing drugs. Thus, in the lemniscal pathway, a reduction in spontaneous activity is the rule. As said before, the findings of increased spontaneous firing rates have all been in the DCN and ICx.

Tinnitus in humans is found most often after noise trauma (20%, Oregon Data Archive) either in its transient form or after prolonged stimulation in its permanent form.[21] Tinnitus in humans can also be transiently induced by high doses of salicylate and quinine. Those agents are most often used for application to experimental animals to induce tinnitus. Behavioral tests have been devised to demonstrate that animals can experience tinnitus after being exposed to a tinnitus-inducing agent (mostly salicylate or quinine).[22,23] A common characteristic of salicylate, quinine, and noise trauma is that they all produce a transient hearing loss and sometimes leave a permanent one. In this chapter, studies in the cat auditory cortex are summarized under three different conditions known to induce tinnitus in humans: application of high doses of salicylate or quinine and high levels of sound exposure. The studies involving a single-dose application of the drugs were acute, and the effects were quantified by recording spontaneous activity and frequency tuning curves from the same single units before and after the application. This procedure greatly limits the number of units that can be recorded from the same animal. This limitation was partially offset by recording simultaneously from two or three electrodes in the salicylate and quinine studies and sorting the multiunit (MU) activity at each electrode into single-unit spike trains. The effect of a traumatizing pure-tone exposure was studied in the same way but aided by recording from 16 electrodes, and the remaining effects from 3 weeks to 4 months after the exposure were investigated as well. This allows comparison of the neural correlates of transient and long-standing tinnitus.

Neural correlates of tinnitus should be similar to neural correlates of audible sound, as argued above. Thus, when a sound is made louder, the neurons in the cortex typically increase their firing rates, suggesting that increased spontaneous firing rates should indicate the presence of tinnitus. Raising the sound level from sub- to suprathreshold also increases the neural synchrony,[24] so one could interpret increased neural synchrony also as a correlate of tinnitus. Burst firing is also affected by sound,[25] but, typically, the duration and number of spikes in a burst decrease with increasing sound level. It is, however, not a priori clear if the changes need to happen in primary cortical areas or that the neural correlate of tinnitus could be restricted to the nonlemniscal pathway and thus to the AII.

In this chapter, four aspects of the response of cortical neurons to the tinnitus-inducing agents are highlighted: (1) neural threshold changes as a function of CF, (2) changes in spontaneous firing rates and burst firing, (3) changes in neural synchrony as measured by cross-correlation of the firings in simultaneously recorded neurons, and (4) dose effects.

EFFECTS OF SODIUM SALICYLATE IN THE AI

The following is based on the findings reported previously in part by Eggermont and Ochi and Eggermont.[26,27] We recorded from the same single neurons before and after intraperitoneal injection of sodium salicylate at a dose of 200 mg/kg in seven cats (average weight 1,141 g) using two microelectrodes. This resulted in a CF threshold elevation for neurons recorded in the AI of about 20 to 30 dB after 2 to 3 hours (Figure 13-1A), and it took typically 2 hours before any effect was noted. We were able to record from 21 single neurons before and up to 6 hours after salicylate application. The hearing loss in the frequency range of 7 to 17 kHz appears to be uniform (Figure 13-1B) but with a tendency to be more elevated around 8 kHz. No recordings were made from units with CFs below 6 kHz.

Spontaneous firing rates were little affected by the salicylate. No dependence on time after application was noted (Figure 13-2A), and there was no dependence on CF in the 7 to 17 kHz range (Figure 13-2B), except for a potential increase in the 6 to 9 kHz range. However, there was a significant dependence on CF threshold (Figure 13-2C). Burst firing was quantified by three measures: the percentage of isolated spikes (considered as spikes separated by at least 30 milliseconds from other spikes), the modal interspike interval (ISI), and the mean ISI. The modal ISI (on average 3.2 milliseconds) reflects the most frequent interval during bursts. The percentage of spikes in bursts, which equals (1 − percentage of isolated spikes), was, on average, 34.7%. None of these parameters changed with time after salicylate application.

The degree to which spikes from two different single units are time-locked or, alternatively, fire in synchrony can be quantified by the cross-correlogram (Figure 13-3). The correlogram is a histogram that shows vertically the number of firings of unit B relative to the time of firing of unit A, so that time lag time 0 (horizontal axis) corresponds to perfect time synchrony. To obtain a histogram, a certain bin width has to be chosen. This is usually done on the basis of

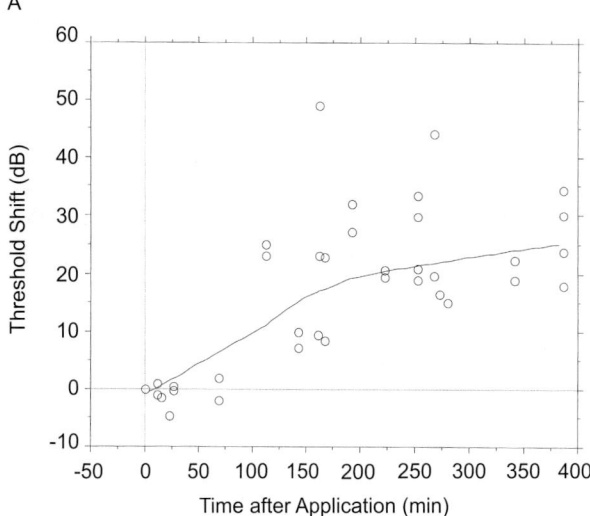

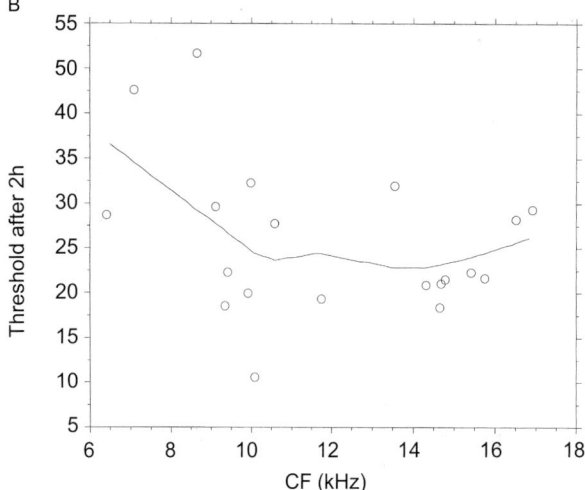

FIGURE 13-1. Characteristic frequency (CF) threshold shifts after application of 200 mg/kg of sodium salicylate shown as a function of time (*A*) and thresholds as a function of CF (*B*). The curves shown are locally weighted scatterplot smoothing curves. Adapted from Ochi K and Eggermont JJ.[27]

the firing rate of the units and the likelihood that a given neuron fires twice in that bin (this should be avoided); the largest possible bin size is selected because this gives the clearest correlograms. The neural synchrony studied in 46 single-neuron pairs for a 10-millisecond bin size was estimated from the peak value of the cross-correlogram, indicated at the top left of each panel (see Figure 13-3), from the width of the central peak at half-amplitude, and from the area under the central peak. For a 10-millisecond bin

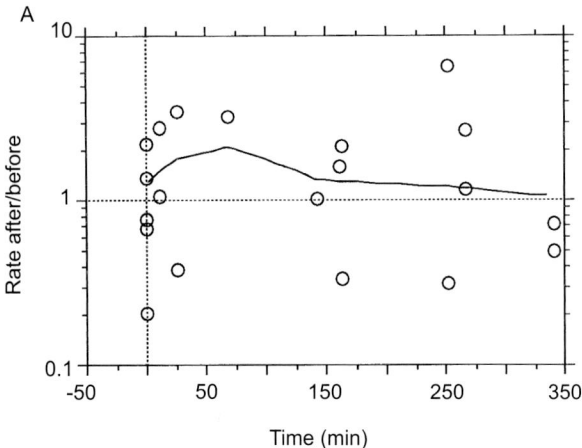
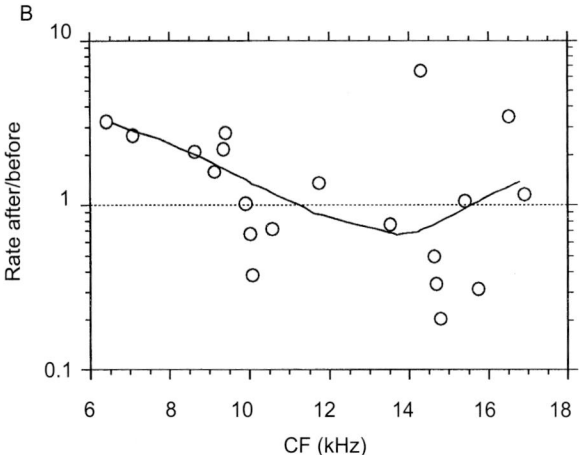
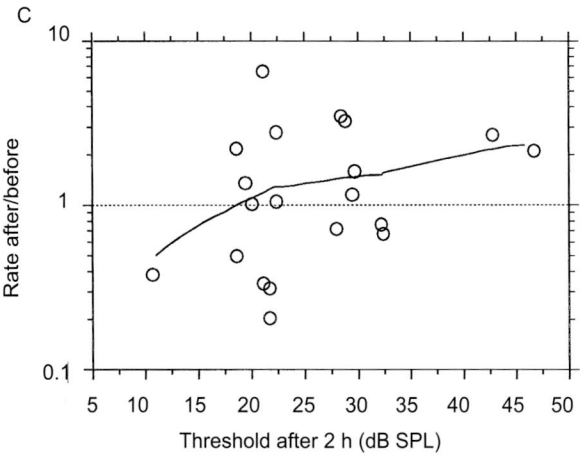

FIGURE 13-2. Spontaneous firing rate ratios as a function of time after application of salicylate (*A*), as a function of characteristic frequency (CF) (*B*), and as a function of CF thresholds 2 hours after application (*C*). Locally weighted scatterplot smoothing curves are drawn in. Adapted from Ochi K and Eggermont JJ.[27]

width, the single-unit pair synchrony is about 0.1, that is, 10% of the time unit B fires within ±5 milliseconds of a spike in unit A. For mixed (single unit on one electrode and MU on the other electrode) pairs, the percentage of synchronized spikes increases, and taking all activity (MU) on each electrode further increases the percentage of synchronized spiking in the correlogram.

In Figure 13-3, one also notices that there are secondary peaks flanking the central peak at lag or lead times of approximately 130 milliseconds. These lag or lead times are equal to the period of the electroencephalographic spindle frequency during light ketamine anesthesia. This period increases after salicylate application,[28] as can be noticed in the MU correlograms. For assessing the effect of salicylate application on the cross-correlogram parameters, single-unit pairs (as in the left-hand column in Figure 13-3) were used, but the single-unit versus MU pairs and MU versus MU pairs showed the same trend. None of these values, peak correlation, peak width, and peak area, changed significantly as a function of time after salicylate administration.

In two cats, we used a dose of 450 mg/kg and, using two microelectrodes, recorded the spontaneous activity of 142 neurons postsalicylate and in 59 neurons presalicylate.[26] In this case, only five of the neurons were recorded pre- and postapplication, and electrodes were used to sample different locations to increase the number of units recorded from, so no pairwise comparisons could be made. The spontaneous firing rate of the population of units in the AI was independent of recording time prior to application but continued to increase up to 5 hours after application ($p < .005$). The number of ISIs less than 100 milliseconds increased two- to threefold, reflecting the increased firing rate. The percentage of pairs that showed significant neural synchrony did not change after the application of salicylate, suggesting that high-dose salicylate does not seem to affect the frequency of shared input between cortical cells, which is the main cause of synchronous firing.[29] A potential problem with these data is that there was a small (1°C) temperature increase following this dose, but the temperature stayed at 38°C, the normal body temperature of the cat. In all of our experiments, we kept the body temperature at 37°C, but these two cats showed a small increase. This "fever" is known as one of the

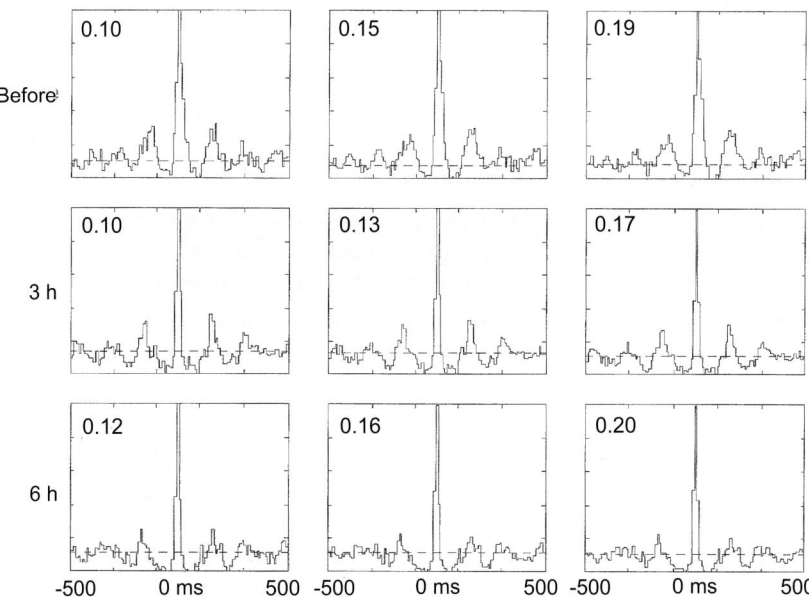

FIGURE 13-3. Examples of cross-correlograms calculated before and 3 and 6 hours after salicylate application. The left-hand column shows correlograms for a single-unit pair, the middle column for a single unit from one electrode with multiunit (MU) activity from the other electrode, and the right-hand column for MU activity on both electrodes. The peak cross-correlation coefficient is indicated in the upper left-hand corner of each panel. Bin size was 10 milliseconds. The dashed line indicates the expected value of the cross-correlation coefficient for independent neurons. Adapted from Ochi K and Eggermont JJ.[27]

toxic effects of salicylate administered in a high dose[30] and produces a confounding factor for the interpretation of the data because elevated temperature could increase spontaneous activity and burst firing. Despite this, the combined data from the two studies suggest a dose-dependent action of sodium salicylate on the spontaneous firing rate of single units in the cat AI,[26,28] similar to that observed in cat auditory nerve fibers.[17,18]

EFFECTS OF QUININE HYDROCHLORIDE IN THE AI

The following is based on the findings reported previously by Ochi and Eggermont.[31] Quinine hydrochloride was injected intramuscularly in seven kittens (average weight 1,015 g) at either 100 mg/kg or 150 mg/kg. Using three microelectrodes, we recorded from 29 single units from before to up to 7 hours after quinine application. Within 1.5 hours, the hearing loss, measured as the shift in single-unit CF threshold, was, on average, 25 dB, regardless of the dose, and the hearing slowly returned to normal in the course of 7 hours after injection (Figure 13-4A). The spontaneous firing rate was independent of the hearing loss (Figure 13-4B), did not show a dose effect (see Figure 13-4B), and did not change as a function of time after application (Figure 13-4C). Burst-firing properties, as reflected in the percentage of spikes in bursts, which equals (1 − the percentage of isolated spikes) and was, on average, 29.9%, the mean ISI (average 12.9 milliseconds), and the modal ISI (average 3.7 milliseconds) were independent of time since application.

In contrast to the effects produced by salicylate, and despite the same average hearing loss produced by quinine and salicylate, the single-unit pair cross-correlation was increased. For 37 single-unit pairs using a bin size of 10 milliseconds, the peak correlation coefficient increased significantly ($p < .01$), as did the area under the central correlation peak, A ($p < .01$), for the high dose but not for the low dose (Figure 13-5). The width of the central peak at half-amplitude in the correlogram did not change significantly.

DIFFERENTIAL EFFECTS OF SALICYLATE AND QUININE IN THE AI, ANTERIOR AUDITORY FIELD, AND AII

Here the results are compared from 36 recording sites in 12 cats from which stable MU data were obtained over a period of at least 12 hours so that a large number of pre- and postapplication recordings could be obtained. In most of these experiments, simultaneous recordings were made from the AI, anterior auditory field (AAF), and AII; in some cats, we inserted two electrodes in the AI and one in the AAF. In contrast to the previous studies on the effects of salicylate and quinine in AI, these data were based on multiple single-unit spike trains. In these experiments, MU spike trains were sorted for single units, and the well-sorted units were then combined to form a multiple single-unit spike train. The following is based on the findings reported previously in part by Eggermont and Kenmochi.[32] Because the results are based on two drugs, different doses, and three cortical areas, we have a multitude of potential comparisons.

First, combining cortical areas and plotting CF threshold shifts relative to the average preapplication values per electrode (Figure 13-6, A and B), one observes that low doses of quinine (100 mg/kg) do not produce threshold increases, that the sodium salicylate (200 mg/kg) produces a moderate threshold increase up to, on average, 30 dB, and that the high quinine dose (150 mg/kg) produced threshold shifts of up to 80 dB after 1 hour, which decrease with time. In contrast, it is noted that these high threshold conditions do not produce, on average, an increase in

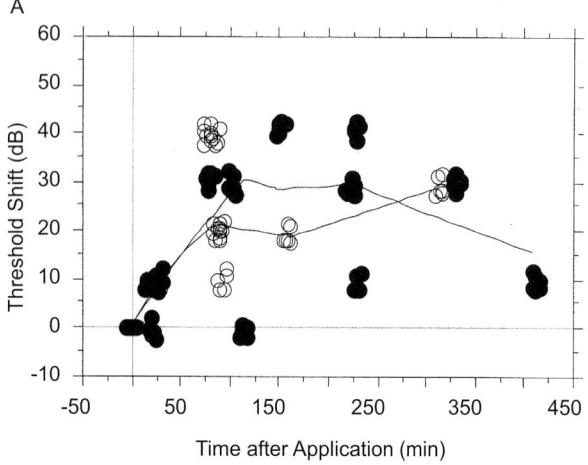
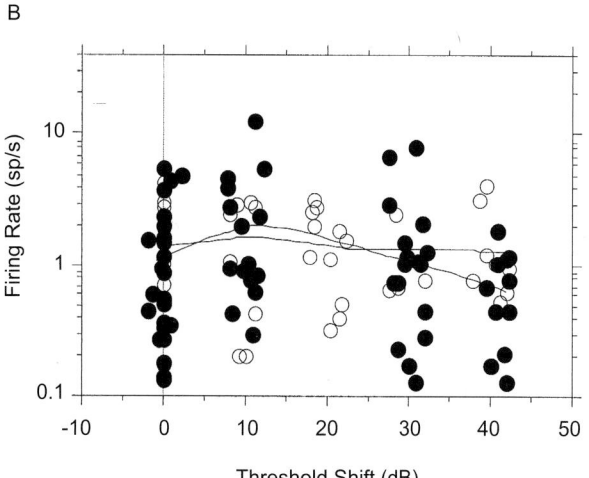
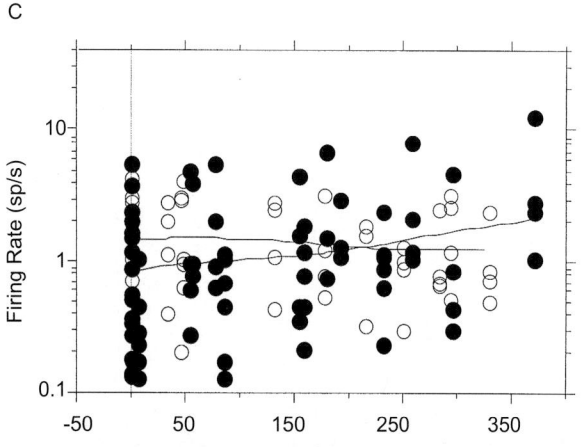

FIGURE 13-4. Threshold shift and changes in spontaneous firing rate after application of quinine show no dose effect. Adapted from Ochi K and Eggermont JJ.[31] Open circles = 100 mg/kg; filled circles = 150 mg/kg.

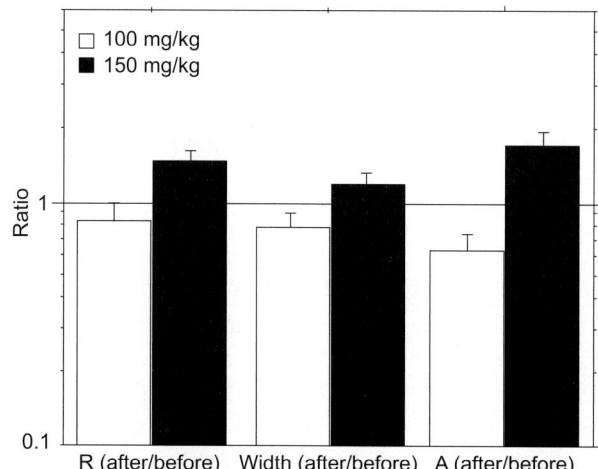

FIGURE 13-5. Changes in peak cross-correlation coefficient (shown here as a ratio) after quinine application are dose dependent. Error bars indicate standard error of the mean. A = area under the central correlation peak; R = peak cross-correlation coefficient. Adapted from Ochi K and Eggermont JJ.[31]

spontaneous activity (see Figure 13-6B), as shown in the ratio of firing rates, where 1 indicates no change. Most firing rate increases are found for the low-dose quinine application, and there is quite a range of change in spontaneous firing rates.

Plotted as a function of CF (across areas), one observes that the CF thresholds after application tend to be lowest around 6 kHz (Figure 13-7A), where normal thresholds are also lowest in cats. Threshold shifts (Figure 13-7B) of more than 20 dB are occurring in the frequency range of 4 to 15 kHz, and the ones produced by salicylate tend to be less than 30 dB, whereas for the high quinine dose, they are much higher. Figure 13-8, A and B, shows that spontaneous firing rates after application are highest in the frequency range of 6 to 15 kHz and that units with significant

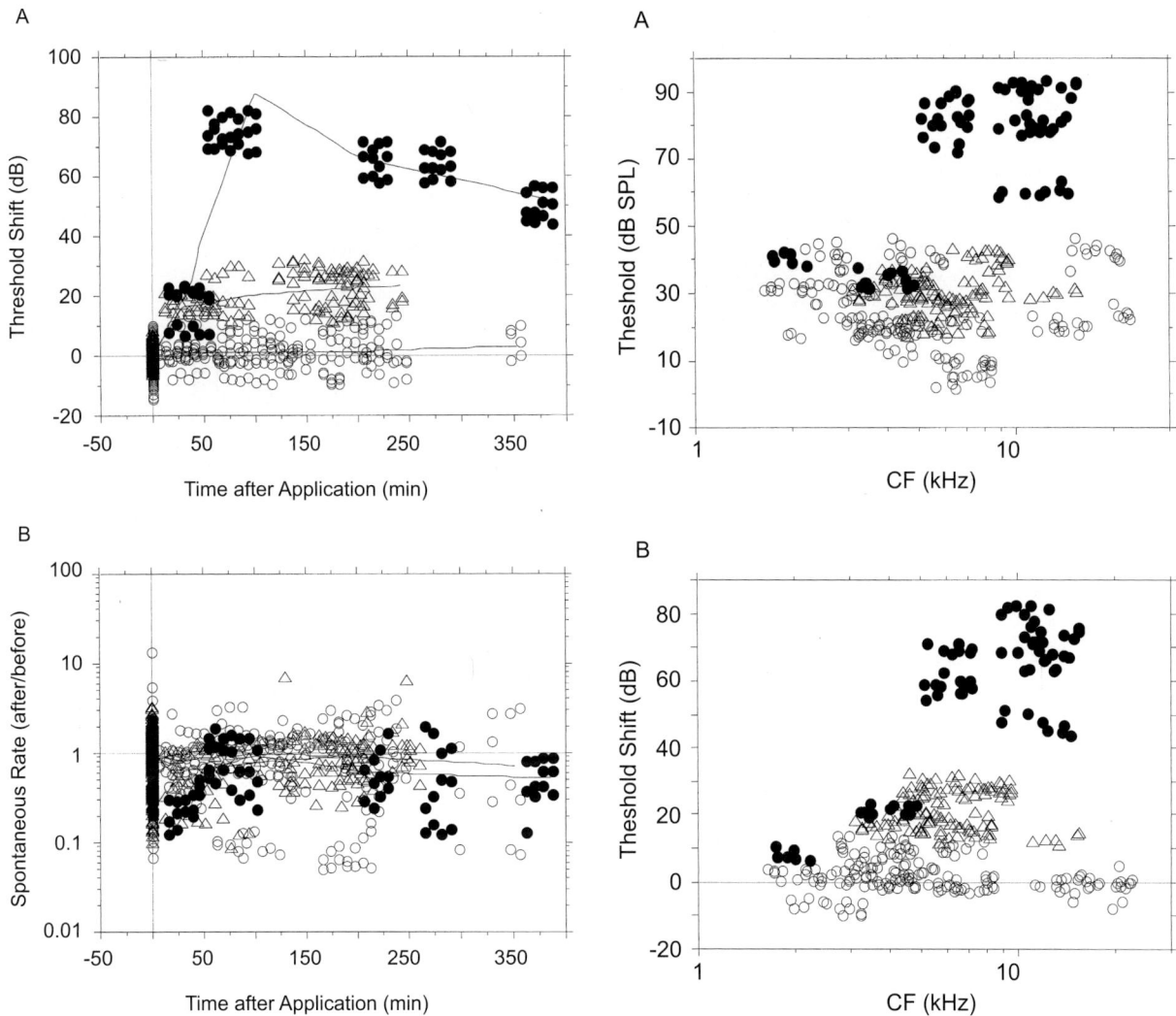

FIGURE 13-6. Changes in characteristic frequency threshold (A) and spontaneous firing rate (B) after quinine and salicylate application. Data are pooled across three cortical areas. Low dose stands for 100 mg/kg for quinine (*open circles*); high dose applies to 150 mg/kg quinine (*filled circles*). Salicylate was applied at a dose of 200 mg/kg (*triangles*). Adapted from Eggermont JJ and Kenmochi M.[32]

FIGURE 13-7. Characteristic frequency (CF) thresholds (A) and CF threshold shifts (B) as a function of CF after salicylate or quinine application. Data are pooled across three cortical areas. Adapted from Eggermont JJ and Kenmochi M.[32] Open circles = low-dose quinine; filled circles = high-dose quinine; triangles = salicylate.

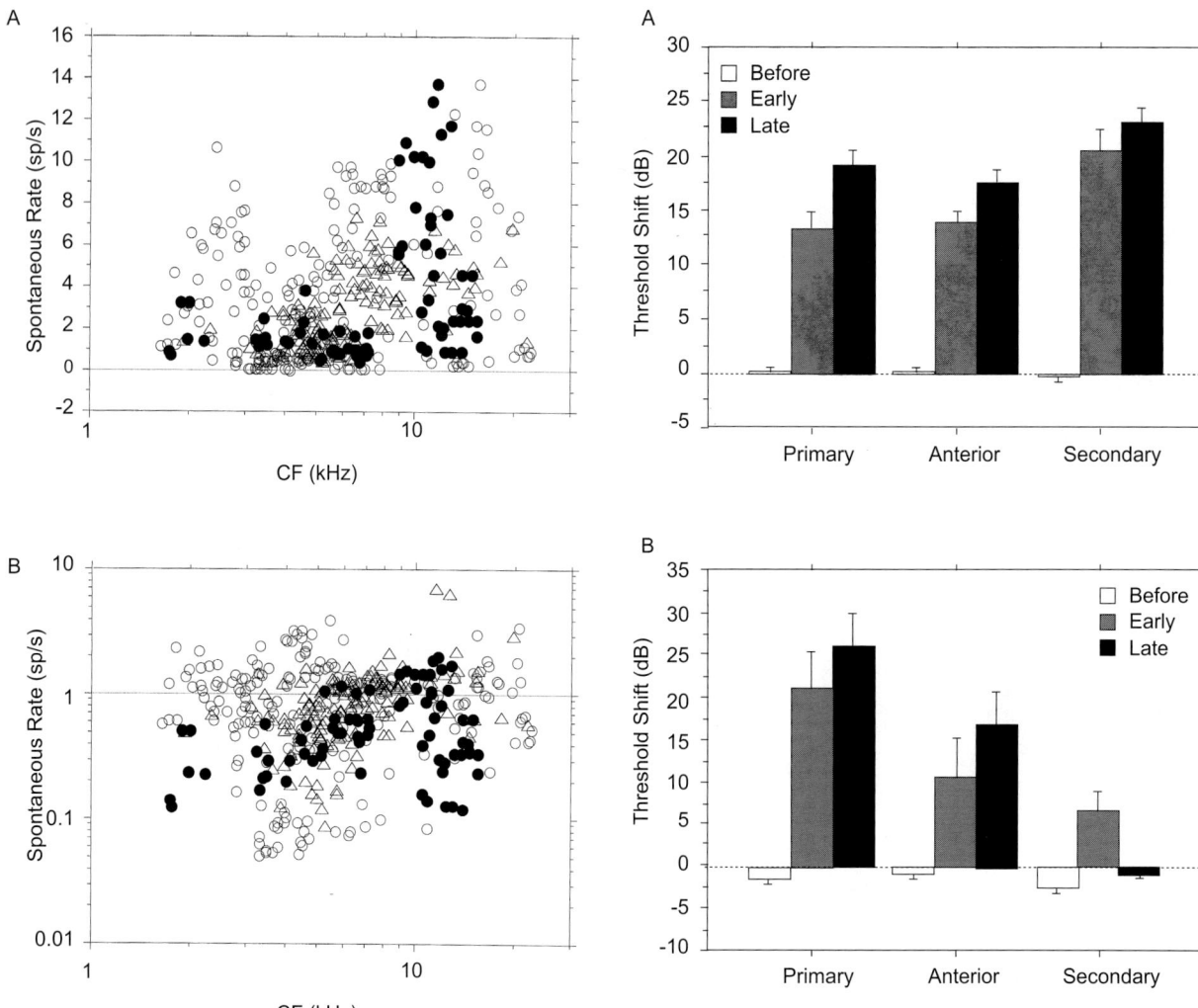

FIGURE 13-8. Spontaneous firing rate (*A*) and change in spontaneous firing rate (expressed as a ratio) (*B*) as a function of characteristic frequency (CF) after salicylate or quinine application. Data are pooled across three cortical areas. Adapted from Eggermont JJ and Kenmochi M.[32] Open circles = low-dose quinine; filled circles = high-dose quinine; triangles = salicylate.

FIGURE 13-9. Average threshold shifts in three different cortical areas at two instances after application of salicylate (*A*) and quinine (*B*). Error bars indicate standard error of the mean. Adapted from Eggermont JJ and Kenmochi M.[32]

increases in spontaneous firing rate are found in the 3 to 6 and 15 to 25 kHz range and dominantly after quinine application.

Threshold shifts for salicylate (Figure 13-9A) were significant ($p < .0001$) for times up to 90 minutes (early) and between 90 and 360 minutes after application (late), and there were significant threshold increases from the early to the late period in the AI and AAF ($p < .05$) but not in the AII. For quinine (Figure 13-9B), threshold shifts were significant for the early and late periods ($p < .0001$) in the AI and AAF but only for the early period in the AII ($p < .005$). There were no significant increases from the early to the late period in the AI and AAF but a significant decrease in the AII ($p < .05$).

Spontaneous activity following salicylate application, illustrated by the ratio of the post- and preapplication firing rates (Figure 13-10A), was not significantly changed in the AI, was significantly reduced ($p < .0001$) in the early and late periods in the AAF, and was significantly ($p < .005$) increased in the late period in the AII. Following quinine application

(Figure 13-10B), there was a significant reduction in firing rate in the late period in the AI ($p < .005$), no change in the AAF, and a significant ($p < .0001$) increase in firing rate in the late period in the AII. Thus, for the two drugs combined, our data suggest that a significant increase in spontaneous firing rate following application is limited to the AII.

In reanalyzing the data, I found an unexpected relationship between threshold changes and changes in spontaneous firing rates. Intuitively, one would expect that the changes in spontaneous firing rates would be found for those units with CFs in the range of frequencies showing a hearing loss. However, I found a significant ($p < .05$) negative correlation between the CF threshold shift and spontaneous firing rate change for the AAF and AII, as could already be surmised from Figure 13-6. This is further illustrated in Figure 13-11, which shows a scattergram of the square root of the ratio of spontaneous firing rates after and before the application of salicylate or quinine as a function of the corresponding threshold shift. Thus, increases in spontaneous firing rates (ratios > 1) in the AAF and AII tend to be largest for units with threshold shifts < 30 dB. The regression lines suggest a significant decrease in the ratio for increasing threshold in the AII and AAF, but only the post-pre ratio of spontaneous firing rate in the AII is, on average, > 1 for threshold shifts between −10 and 30 dB.

Neural synchrony, based on MU activity, was calculated between electrodes in different areas. Overall, there was no significant effect of salicylate or quinine on the peak cross-correlation coefficient; none of the pairwise correlations between neural activity recorded in the AI, AAF, and AII were significantly changed.

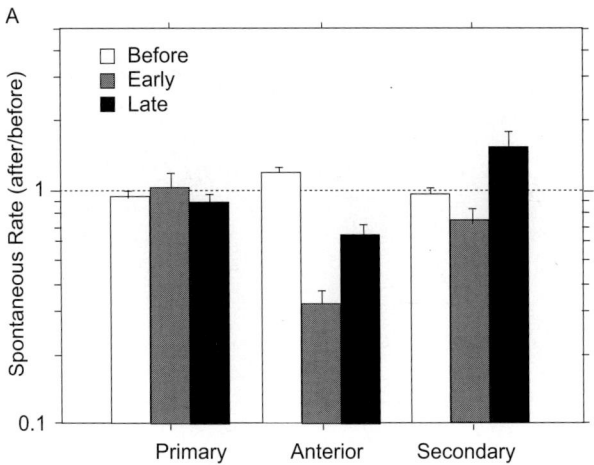

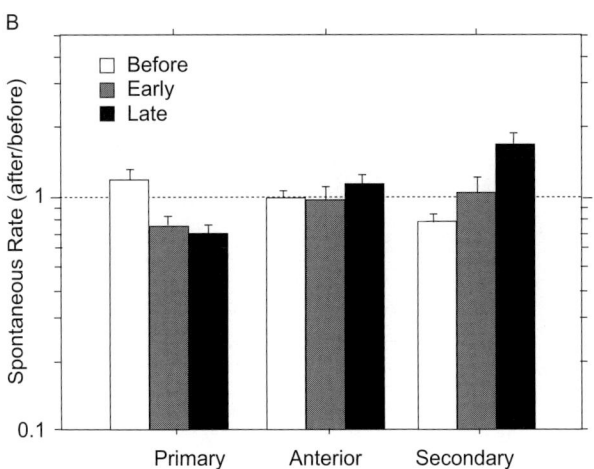

FIGURE 13-10. Changes in spontaneous firing rate (expressed as a ratio) in three different cortical areas at two instances after application of salicylate (*A*) and quinine (*B*). Error bars indicate standard error of the mean. Adapted from Eggermont JJ and Kenmochi M.[32]

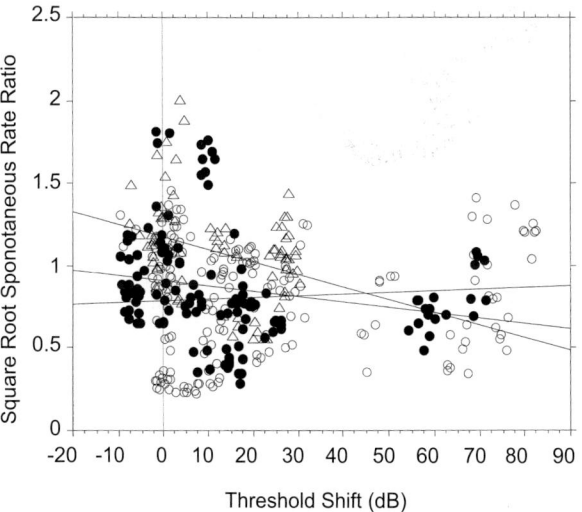

FIGURE 13-11. Square root of the spontaneous firing rate plotted as a function of characteristic frequency threshold shift in three cortical areas. Linear regression lines are drawn in. Adapted from Eggermont JJ and Kenmochi M.[32] Open circles = primary auditory cortex; filled circles = anterior auditory field; triangles = secondary auditory cortex.

ACUTE TRAUMA TONE EXPOSURE–INDUCED EFFECTS

This section is based on a study by Noreña and Eggermont.[11] After a 1-hour exposure to a 5 or 6 kHz tone presented at a level of 115 to 120 dB SPL, the hearing loss was measured using the shift in auditory brainstem response (ABR) thresholds at 6 hours after the exposure compared with prior to the exposure. The average hearing loss in five cats was about 40 dB in the range of 6 to 32 kHz (Figure 13-12). Recordings in these and nine other cats were done from the AI using two multielectrode arrays of eight electrodes each to increase the yield of units that can be sampled in each cat before and up to 6 hours after exposure to the trauma tone. We recorded from 124 MU clusters. Basing the hearing loss on shifts in CF thresholds of cortical neurons is complicated after the localized hearing loss owing to the pure-tone trauma because the CFs of the neurons shift to lower values after the exposure without much threshold shift (on average only 12 dB) as a result of the unmasking of new excitatory inputs.[11] CF threshold shifts as a function of the difference between the pretrauma CF and the trauma tone frequency are illustrated in Figure 13-13A. The

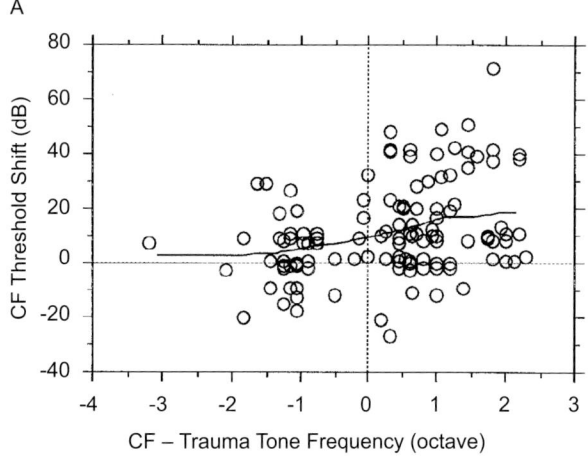

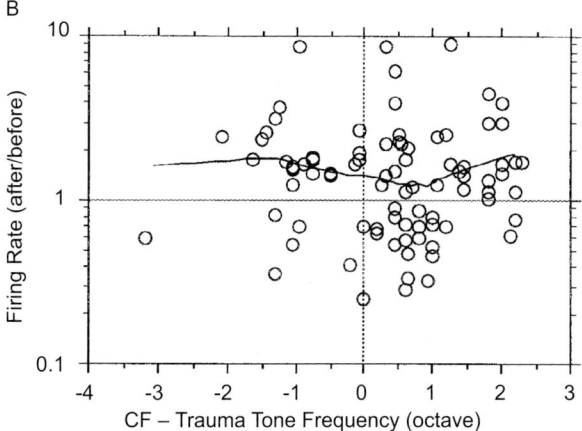

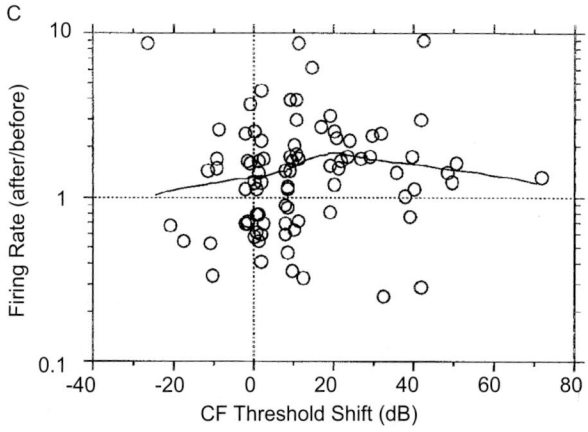

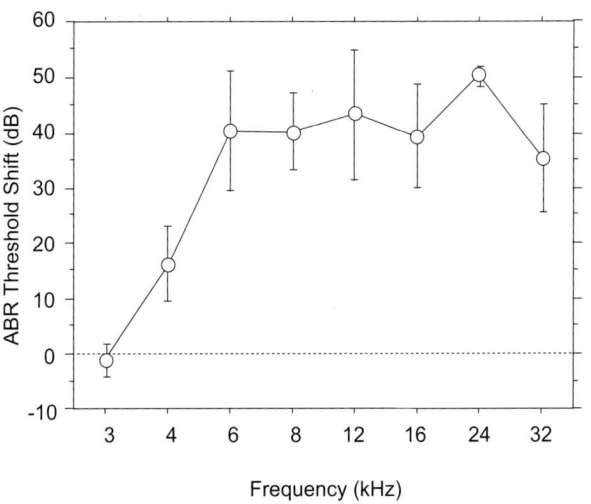

FIGURE 13-12. Peripheral threshold shifts 6 hours after a 1-hour exposure to a 5 kHz tone presented at 115 to 120 dB SPL (compared with pre-exposure conditions) as measured with the auditory brainstem response (ABR). Error bars indicate standard error of the mean. Adapted from Noreña AJ and Eggermont JJ.[11]

FIGURE 13-13. Characteristic frequency (CF) threshold shift (*A*) and changes in spontaneous firing rate (*B*) as a function of the difference between pre-exposure CF and the trauma tone frequency. *C* shows the dependence of changes in spontaneous firing rate on CF threshold shift. Adapted from Noreña AJ and Eggermont JJ.[11]

average CF threshold shift a few hours after the trauma was 5.6 dB for CFs below and 15.6 dB for CFs above the trauma tone frequency. Both changes were significantly different from 0 ($p < .01$), and the difference between the shifts of units with CFs above and below the trauma tone frequency was also significant ($p < .005$). The change in spontaneous firing rate, quantified as a post-pre ratio (Figure 13-13B), was also significantly different below (mean 2.045; $p < .01$) and above (mean 2.01; $p < 0.005$) the trauma tone frequency. The changes in spontaneous firing rate were largest for moderate CF threshold increases, that is, around 20 dB (Figure 13-13C). Thus, pure tone–induced trauma produced a twofold increase in spontaneous firing rate that was clearly present a few hours after the end of the exposure.

Peak cross-correlation coefficients (R) were calculated for 771 electrode pairs, using a bin width of 2 milliseconds, and were based on MU activity on each electrode. Figure 13-14A shows the change in R, as a post-pre ratio, as a function of the difference between the geometric mean of the pre-exposure CFs at the two electrodes and the trauma tone frequency. No trend was observed in these changes that showed, on average, a 54% increase over the pre-exposure values. This increase was not significantly different below and above the trauma tone frequency or, when the correlation pairs were split according to both CFs below, both CFs above, or one CF below and one CF above the trauma tone frequency. The changes in the geometric mean firing rate of the two MU recordings explained about 25% of the changes in the peak cross-correlation coefficient (Figure 13-14B).

LONG-STANDING EFFECTS OF TRAUMA TONE EXPOSURE

The data presented here are based on Eggermont and Komiya and Seki and Eggermont.[33-35] In the first study, five juvenile cats (5 weeks old) were exposed to a 6 kHz pure tone at 126 dB SPL for 1 hour, which was repeated the following week. Two to 5 months later, that is, when the cats were adult-like in all cortical response properties,[36] the AI was mapped, and spontaneous neural activity was recorded. In the exposed cats, in one litter, the highest CF found was 10 kHz, and in the other litter, it was 8 kHz. Figure 13-15A shows the hearing loss as measured using ABRs in comparison with controls, and one observes, on av-

erage, a threshold increase of 30 dB for frequencies above 10 kHz. Figure 13-15B shows the spontaneous firing rates in the exposed cats, and one observes the increased rates for CFs above 7 kHz. This increase was significant ($p < .05$) compared with the nonreorganized parts (CF < 7 kHz) and also compared with a set of normal controls ($p < .05$). The range of CFs (see Figure 13-15B) is clearly much smaller than the range

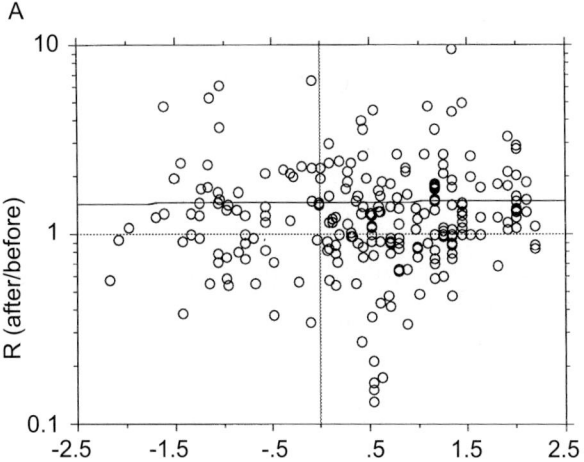

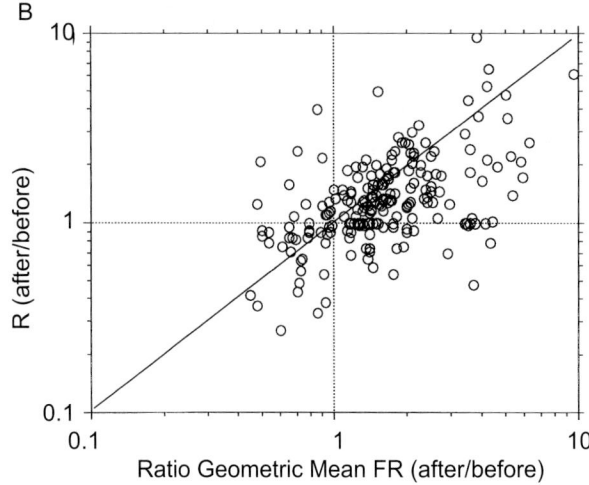

FIGURE 13-14. A, Peak cross-correlation coefficient, R, as a function of the difference between pre-exposure characteristic frequency (CF) and the trauma tone frequency. A linear regression line is drawn in. B, Changes in R as a function of changes in the geometric mean firing rate (FR) of the units used in the calculation. There is a tendency for a reduction in R despite increased firing rates. Adapted from Noreña AJ and Eggermont JJ.[11]

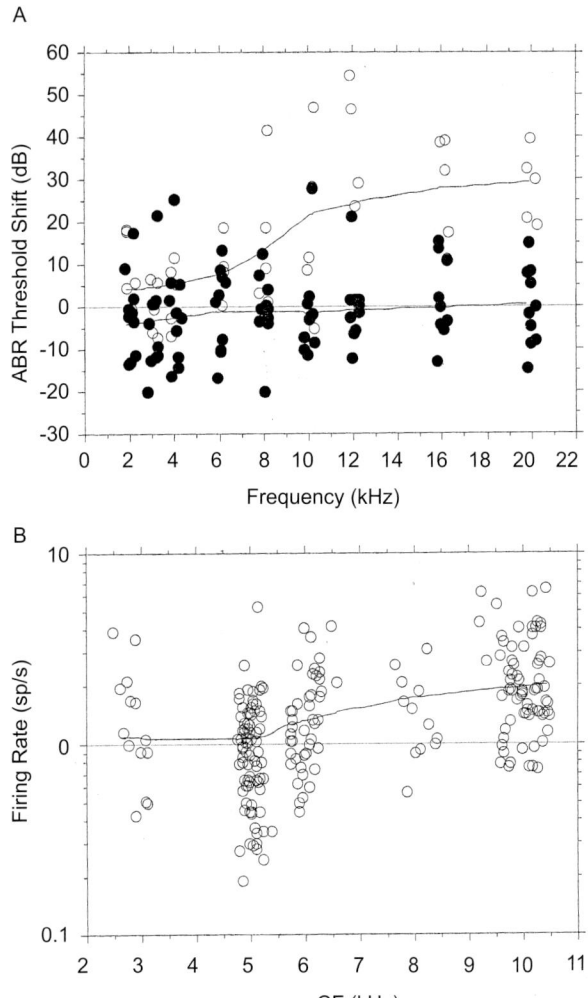

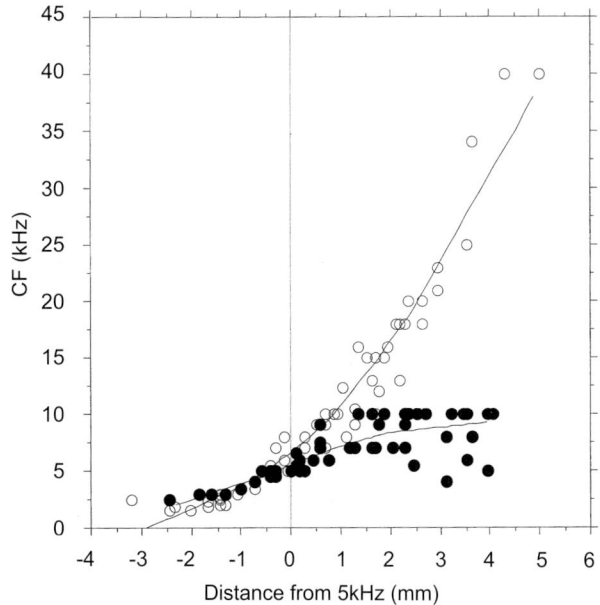

FIGURE 13-16. Characteristic frequency (CF) gradients parallel to the midline (ie, perpendicular to the isofrequency sheets) for control cats (*open circles*) and exposed juvenile cats (*filled circles*). A large region (up to 3 mm in length) appears to have CFs much lower than in the controls. Adapted from Eggermont JJ and Komiya H.[33]

FIGURE 13-15. *A*, Auditory brainstem response (ABR) threshold shift measured at least 2 months after a trauma induced by exposure at an age of 5 weeks to a 6 kHz pure tone at 126 dB SPL for 1 hour and repeated the following week. *B*, Changes in spontaneous firing rate as a function of characteristic frequency (CF). Note the absence of CFs higher than 10.5 kHz. Adapted from Eggermont JJ and Komiya H.[33] Open circles = trauma group; filled circles = control group.

of ABR frequencies (see Figure 13-15A); the reason for this is the reorganization of the tonotopic map. As a result of that, there were no CFs with frequencies above 10 kHz (Figure 13-16) over a 4 mm distance from the 5 kHz point (taken along a direction perpendicular to the isofrequency sheets). Normally, this range would include CFs up to 30 kHz. No changes in burst-firing properties were found. R values, based on single-unit pairs, were not significantly increased in reorganized parts compared with nonreorganized parts. However, the percentage of significant correlations increased in the reorganized part to 100%.

This initial study was followed with one in which 11 cats were exposed to a 6 kHz tone at 115 dB SPL for 2 hours, which produced, on average, smaller and more variable amounts of hearing loss (Figure 13-17A). The average hearing loss from 8 to 32 kHz was 20 dB, but the range at 8 kHz (0.5 octave above the trauma tone frequency) was from 0 to 57 dB.

In animals with variable hearing loss, recorded from at least 3 weeks after the exposure, one can distinguish between its effects based on the changes in the cortical tonotopic map. This map can be reorganized after sufficiently large high-frequency hearing loss (as illustrated in Figure 13-16), which is typically more than 20 dB.[34,37,38] The definition for reorganization that we used in case of hearing losses just exceeding 20 dB is a functional one. Because the studies by Seki and Eggermont used arrays of eight microelectrodes with an interelectrode distance of 0.5 mm,[34,35] a CF shift of more than one octave between neighboring electrodes or a significant reduction in the frequency gradient was used as an indicator for reorganization. Because the trauma tone frequency was 6 kHz, typically, the reorganized region is expected above 8 kHz, but not infrequently, tuning curves with two low-intensity tips were found. The two CFs were invariantly between 4 and 6 kHz and between 8 and 14 kHz, with only slight differences in thresholds. So, depending on which tip threshold was lowest, that value was assigned to the unit. Spontaneous firing rates obtained in the exposed cats were thus distinguished on the basis of originating from a reorganized part or from a nonreorganized part of the AI and compared with values obtained in a large number of control cats. Only in five cats was a reorganization in the tonotopic map found, and these had average hearing losses in the 8 to 32 kHz range of more than 20 dB.

Figure 13-17B shows the square root of the spontaneous firing rate plotted as a function of CF for all exposed cats in this second study. For the entire frequency range, the firing rate of neurons in reorganized areas (1.44 ± 0.92 sp/s) was significantly ($p < .005$) higher compared with controls (1.20 ± 0.71 sp/s), and so was the firing rate of units in nonreorganized areas (1.55 ± 0.71 sp/s; $p < .0001$). Limiting ourselves to the CF range above the trauma tone frequency, significant differences were again found for the same conditions. This suggests that exposure without reorganization can increase the spontaneous firing rate for CFs above and below the trauma tone frequency. Overall, there was no significant difference between the firing rates in reorganized and nonreorganized areas. However, for the five cats showing reorganization of the cortical tonotopic map, the mean firing rates (2.87 ± 3.59 sp/s, $n = 191$) of the units in reorganized parts of the cortex were significantly ($p < .005$) higher than those in the nonreorganized parts (1.80 ± 1.93 sp/s, $n = 82$).

The spontaneous firing rates were significantly correlated with the threshold at CF (Figure 13-18) but in a different way for units in reorganized parts (positive correlation $r^2 = .17$), compared with those in nonreorganized parts ($r^2 = .21$) and controls ($r^2 = .08$). In reorganized cortex, the CF thresholds ranged from 10 to 50 dB SPL, extending about 10 dB above the normal range in controls. Typically, spontaneous firing rates in this group were significantly increased only when the CF threshold was above 30 dB SPL. In nonreorganized cortex, thresholds at CF could be found between −10 and 55 dB SPL. Thus, when CF thresholds exceed 30 dB SPL, neurons in reorganized areas show higher spontaneous activity than do neurons in nonreorganized areas.

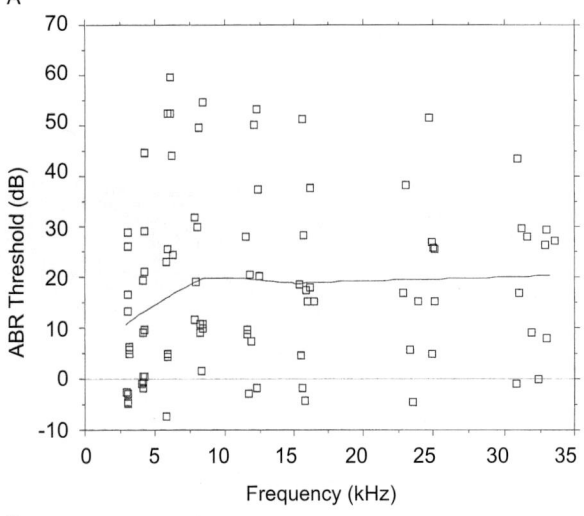

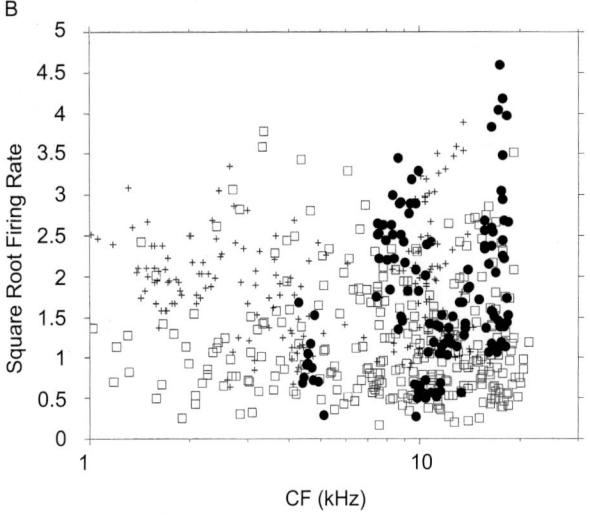

FIGURE 13-17. *A*, Auditory brainstem response (ABR) thresholds measured in 11 cats at least 3 weeks after exposure to a 6 kHz tone at 115 dB SPL for 2 hours. *B*, Square root of the spontaneous firing rate as a function of characteristic frequency (CF) for reorganized (*filled circles*) and nonreorganized (*plus signs*) parts of exposed cats and control cats (*squares*). Adapted from Seki S and Eggermont JJ.[35]

Neural synchrony was calculated between electrode pairs, that is, based on MU activity using a 2-millisecond bin width. It appeared that peak cross-correlation coefficients (R) for both electrodes in the reorganized part or for one electrode in the reorganized part and the other electrode in the nonreorganized cortex were not significantly different. So, for the purpose of this chapter, they were combined.

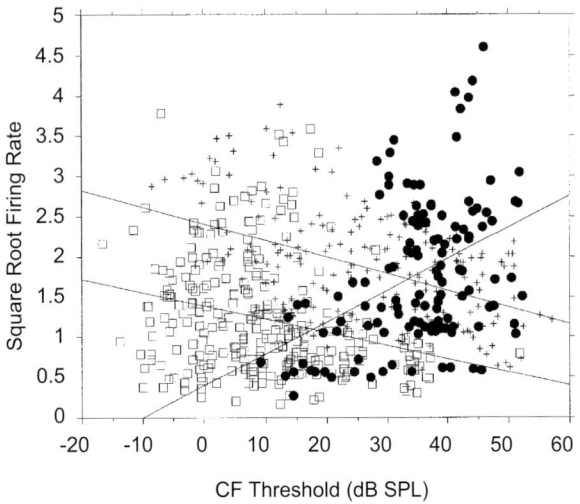

FIGURE 13-18. Square root of the spontaneous firing rate measured in 11 cats at least 3 weeks after exposure to a 6 kHz tone at 115 dB SPL for 2 hours as a function of characteristic frequency (CF) threshold for reorganized (*filled circles*) and nonreorganized (*plus signs*) parts of exposed cats and control cats (*squares*). Adapted from Seki S and Eggermont JJ.[35]

Figure 13-19A shows the findings split according to whether the pairs included reorganized cortex (at least one electrode) or nonreorganized cortex (both electrodes) or were from control cats. R values were not significantly dependent on CF for control cats ($r^2 = .00004$; $p = .9$). Across the entire CF range, the R values for pairs involving reorganized areas (0.15 ± 0.07) were significantly ($p < .0001$) higher than for pairs in nonreorganized areas (0.13 ± 0.05) and also significantly ($p < .0005$) higher than for controls (0.13 ± 0.06). There was no significant difference ($p = .5$) between R values for pairs in nonreorganized cortex and controls.

Neural synchrony in this study was again positively correlated with spontaneous firing rate; on average, 20% of the variance in R was explained by the spontaneous firing rate (Figure 13-19B).

COMMONALITIES AMONG DRUG- AND TRAUMA TONE–INDUCED EFFECTS

The findings that I obtained in my studies conducted in the last decade and that are reviewed in this chapter are briefly summarized in Tables 13-1 to 13-3. Most of the data were collected in the AI,

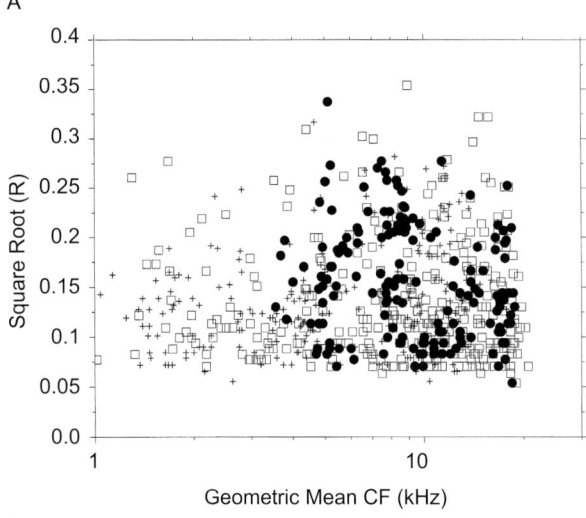
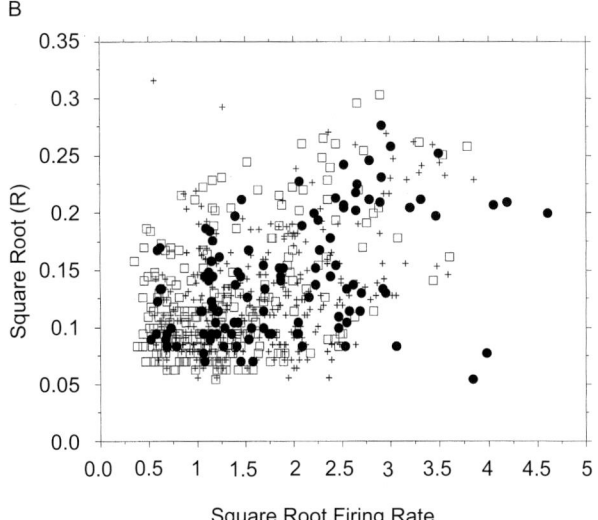

FIGURE 13-19. Square root of the peak cross-correlation coefficient R, measured in 11 cats at least 3 weeks after exposure to a 6 kHz tone at 115 dB SPL for 2 hours as a function of the geometric mean of the characteristic frequencies (CFs) of the participating units (*A*) and the square root of their spontaneous firing rates (*B*). Adapted from Seki S and Eggermont JJ.[35] Filled circles = reorganized parts of exposed cats; plus signs = nonreorganized parts of exposed cats; squares = control cats.

and I focused on three basic parameters of spontaneous activity. The first was spontaneous firing rate, the second was spontaneous burst firing, and the third was neural synchrony. Table 13-1 shows the average changes found for the various treat-

TABLE 13-1. Changes in the Primary Auditory Cortex by Tinnitus-Inducing Agents

	Salicylate		Quinine		Acute Effects of Trauma Tone		Long-standing Effects of Trauma Tone	
	200 mg/kg	450 mg/kg	100 mg/kg	150 mg/kg	Early	Late	Nonreorg	Reorganized
Spontaneous firing rates	≈	↑	≈	≈	≈	↑	↑	↑
Burst firing	≈	≈	≈	≈	≈	≈	≈	≈
Neural synchrony	≈	≈	≈	↑	↑	↑	≈	↑

≈ = no significant change with respect to pretreatment values or to normal controls; ↓ and ↑, respectively, indicate a significant decrease or increase in the spontaneous activity property.

ments in the AI. None of the treatments resulted in any significant change in spontaneous burst-firing properties. One observes that application of salicylates produced a measurable effect only for a dose of 450 mg/kg, namely an increase in spontaneous firing rate. This dose was, in effect, too high for the cat because it induced a small fever; therefore, the number of cats that received this dose was only two. For quinine, a dose of 200 mg/kg proved to be lethal for most cats; therefore, the highest dose used was 150 mg/kg. This dose produced a significant increase in neural synchrony. Thus, the effects of salicylate and quinine on the AI are modest indeed. The acute effects of noise trauma in the AI manifest themselves within minutes after the exposure in a significant increase of neural synchrony. A few hours after the exposure, neural synchrony is further increased, and spontaneous activity also increased significantly. The long-standing effects of pure-tone trauma include a significant increase in spontaneous firing rates regardless of the presence of cortical tonotopic map reorganization, whereas changes in neural synchrony were restricted to reorganized parts of the cortex.

Table 13-2 shows findings involving, in addition to the AI, the AAF and AII. The findings show that after salicylate (200 mg/kg) or quinine (150 mg/kg) application, the spontaneous firing increased significantly in the AII. The immediate effects after pure-tone exposure included a significant increase in the firing rate in the AI but not in the other cortical areas. Pairwise correlations between activity recorded on electrodes in different cortical areas showed no significant change. This suggests that tinnitus-inducing agents do not affect interarea neural synchrony, at least not in the early phase (within 6 hours) after the application. So transient tinnitus may be a percept that occurs without "synchrony binding," that is, potentially limited to changes in only one of the cortical areas studied.

In addition, I presented the amount of hearing loss introduced by the tinnitus-inducing agent either as a shift in ABR thresholds compared with control or pretreatment values or as a shift in the CF thresholds of cortical neurons. All of my treatments produced at least 20 dB hearing loss, on average, in the high frequencies. I found that changes in spontaneous activity were negatively correlated with the increases in CF thresholds, except when the cortical tonotopic map was reorganized (see Table 13-3).

TABLE 13-2. Cortical Area Differences

	Salicylate			Quinine			Acute Effects of Trauma Tone		
	AI	AAF	AII	AI	AAF	AII	AI	AAF	AII
Spontaneous firing rates	≈	↓	↑	↓	≈	↑	↑	≈	↓
	AIxAAF	AAFxAII	AIxAII	AIxAAF	AAFxAII	AIxAII	AIxAAF	AAFxAII	AIxAII
Neural synchrony (interarea)	≈	≈	≈	≈	≈	≈	≈	≈	≈

AAF = anterior auditory field; AI = primary auditory cortex; AII = secondary auditory cortex; ≈ = no significant change with respect to pretreatment values or to normal controls; ↓ and ↑, respectively, indicate a significant decrease or increase in the spontaneous activity property.

There were clear dose effects: a high drug dose leads to either increased spontaneous rate or increased synchrony. High sound levels lead to reorganization of the cortical tonotopic map, but effects on spontaneous firing rate do not seem to depend on reorganization alone. Spontaneous firing rate is highest for low CF thresholds following drug- or noise-induced hearing loss without reorganization. This suggests that units that acquire new CFs (unmasked excitations) are less inhibited or neurons of which CF and threshold were less affected also acquired less inhibition from areas in which high threshold changes occurred.

Neural synchrony is not independent of spontaneous firing rate; changes in the latter account for about 25% of the variance of changes in R.

ROLE OF NEURAL SYNCHRONY IN PERCEPTION

Ever since we included changes in neural synchrony in our description of changes produced by tinnitus-inducing agents, there have been questions as to why neural synchrony would play a role in the perception of tinnitus. This is not an issue restricted to the study of tinnitus. There is a large body of literature, mainly originating from studies of the visual cortex, that suggests a role of neural synchrony in perceptual binding.[39] Typically, neurons, even those that are separated by a large cortical distance, which respond to a particular stimulus feature, show synchrony in their firings. This synchrony in the visual system is often accompanied by oscillations in the local field potentials in the frequency range around 40 Hz. Although, in the auditory cortex, neural cross-correlation studies are not performed routinely, except in my laboratory, one can summarize the findings as showing a significant increase in neural synchrony between neural spiking in separate cortical areas during stimulation compared with spontaneous firing. The amount of cortical neural synchrony in the cat auditory cortex[24] or, for that matter, in the frog auditory midbrain[40] did not depend on the stimulus level. Thus, the stepwise change in neural synchrony between sub- and suprathreshold conditions may help, together with the increase in firing rate, in signaling the presence of sound. Neural synchrony has also been implicated in signaling the presence of a continuous tone[41–43] in the absence of any difference in firing rate from the spontaneous condition. Thus, neural synchrony may signal both a change from silence to sound and the presence of an ongoing stimulus. The latter may be important in the perception of tinnitus.

Recently, simultaneous recording from cell pairs in the thalamus and a cortical target cell has made an interesting addition by studying the effect of synchronous inputs of thalamic neurons on the ability to fire a cortical cell.[44,45] It was found that thalamocortical efficacy after synchronous thalamic activity (both reference neurons firing) was nearly twice as large as the efficacy obtained when pairs of thalamic neurons discharged asynchronously. This suggests that neural synchronization may play a critical role in the transmission of sensory information from the somatosensory thalamus to the cortex. It is likely that increased synchronization of auditory cortical neurons similarly will enhance the transmission of information to subsequent stages in auditory processing.

In my studies, neural synchrony was correlated with the spontaneous firing rate, such that the squared correlation coefficient was around 20 to 25%. This can be interpreted in two ways; the first is that changes in neural synchrony are determined largely by changes in spontaneous firing rate. However, our previous studies into the immediate effects of an acoustic trauma indicate that initial increases in neural synchrony and spontaneous firing rate are uncorrelated, whereas, after a few hours, they became

TABLE 13-3. Relationship to Hearing Loss

	Salicylate (AII)	Quinine (AII)	Pure-Tone Trauma (AI)	
			Nonreorganized	Reorganized
Spontaneous firing rates	↓	↓	↓	↑
Neural synchrony	≈	≈	≈	≈

≈ = no significant change with respect to pretreatment values or to normal controls; ↓ and ↑, respectively, indicate a significant decrease or increase in the spontaneous activity property.

correlated.[11] I interpret this to indicate that neural synchrony changes are priming subsequent changes in firing rate, likely by the mechanisms suggested above. I have suggested previously that binding in auditory perception occurs through synchronous firing of different neurons to auditory stimulus contours.[46] Auditory stimulus contours mark changes and transitions in sound, and the auditory cortex appears to be particularly sensitive to these dynamic aspects of sound, such as onsets, offsets, voice-onset time, and low-rate amplitude modulation. Because contours are temporally represented, this binding would assemble neurons that share common changes and thus provide a binding mechanism for auditory stimuli.

We have seen that after application of tinnitus-inducing agents, there is no evidence for increased neural synchrony between different cortical areas, in contrast to the effect of sound stimulation, which did show preferential increases in synchronization between cortical areas.[24]

Obviously, our knowledge of the effects of tinnitus-inducing agents on cortical neural activity is incomplete. Despite this present level of ignorance, it seems that the cortical representation of phantom sounds is different from that of external sounds; this applies particularly to the joint representation of external and phantom sounds across cortical areas.

ACKNOWLEDGMENTS

This work was supported by the Alberta Heritage Foundation for Medical Research, a Canadian Institutes of Health Research-New Emerging Teams (CIHR-NET) grant, the American Tinnitus Association, and the Campbell McLaurin Chair for Hearing Deficiencies. Arnaud Noreña commented on an earlier version of the chapter.

REFERENCES

1. Neff WD, Diamond IT, Casseday JH. Behavioral studies of auditory discrimination: central nervous system. In: Keidel WD, Neff WD, editors. Handbook of sensory physiology. Vol V/2. Auditory system. Berlin: Springer-Verlag; 1975. p. 307–400.
2. Talwar SK, Musial PG, Gerstein GL. Role of mammalian auditory cortex in the perception of elementary sound properties. J Neurophysiol 2001;85:2350–8.
3. Javel E, McGee JA, Horst JW, Farley GR. Temporal mechanisms in auditory stimulus coding. In: Edelman GM, Gall WE, Cowan WM, editors. Auditory function. Neurobiological bases of hearing. New York: J. Wiley & Sons; 1988. p. 515–58.
4. Graybiel AM. The thalamo-cortical projection of the so-called posterior nuclear group: a study with degeneration methods in the cat. Brain Res 1973;49:229–44.
5. Suga N, Gao E, Zhang Y, et al. The corticofugal system for hearing: recent progress. Proc Natl Acad Sci U S A 2000;97:11807–14.
6. Braitenberg V. Thoughts on the cerebral cortex. J Theor Biol 1974;46:421–47.
7. Douglas RJ, Martin KA. The neocortex. In: Shepherd GM, editor. The synaptic organization of the brain. New York: Oxford University Press; 1998. p. 389–438.
8. Yan W, Suga N. Corticofugal modulation of the midbrain frequency map in the bat auditory system. Nat Neurosci 1998;1:54–8.
9. Xiao Z, Suga N. Modulation of cochlear hair cells by the auditory cortex in the mustached bat. Nat Neurosci 2002;5:57–63.
10. Kaltenbach JA, Zhang J, Afman CE. Plasticity of spontaneous neural activity in the dorsal cochlear nucleus after intense sound exposure. Hear Res 2000;147:282–92.
11. Noreña AJ, Eggermont JJ. Changes in spontaneous neural activity immediately after an acoustic trauma: implications for neural correlates of tinnitus. Hear Res 2003;183:137–53.
12. Young ED. Cochlear nucleus. In: Shepherd GM, editor. The synaptic organization of the brain. New York: Oxford University Press; 1998. p. 121–57.
13. Jastreboff PJ, Sasaki CT. Salicylate-induced changes in spontaneous activity of single units in the inferior colliculus of the guinea pig. J Acoust Soc Am 1986;80:1384–91.
14. Manabe Y, Yoshida S, Saito H, Oka H. Effects of lidocaine on salicylate-induced discharge of neurons in the inferior colliculus of the guinea pig. Hear Res 1997;103:192–8.
15. Oliver DL, Huerta MF. Inferior and superior colliculi. In: Webster DB, Popper AN, Fay RR, editors. The mammalian auditory pathway: neuroanatomy. New York: Springer Verlag; 1992. p. 168–221.
16. Liberman MC, Kiang NY-S. Acoustic trauma in cats. Cochlear pathology and auditory-nerve activity. Acta Otolaryngol Suppl (Stockh) 1978;358:1–63.
17. Stypulkowski PH. Mechanisms of salicylate ototoxicity. Hear Res 1980;46:113–46.
18. Evans EF, Wilson JP, Borerwe TA. Animal models of tinnitus. Ciba Found Symp 1981;85:108–38.

19. Mulheran M. The effect of quinine on cochlear nerve fibre activity in the guinea pig. Hear Res 1999;134:145–52.
20. Salvi RJ, Hamernik RP, Henderson D. Discharge patterns in the cochlear nucleus of the chinchilla following noise induced asymptotic threshold shift. Exp Brain Res 1978;32:301–20.
21. Tinnitus archive. Available at http://www.ohsu.edu/ohrc-otda (accessed April 8, 2004).
22. Jastreboff PJ, Brennan JF, Sasaki CT. Phantom auditory sensation in rats: an animal model for tinnitus. Behav Neurosci 1988;102:811–22.
23. Bauer CA, Brozoski TJ, Rojas R, et al. Behavioral model of chronic tinnitus in rats. Otolaryngol Head Neck Surg 1999;121:457–62.
24. Eggermont JJ. Sound induced correlation of neural activity between and within three auditory cortical areas. J Neurophysiol 2000;83:2708–22.
25. Bowman DM, Eggermont JJ, Smith GM. Effect of stimulation on burst firing in cat primary auditory cortex. J Neurophysiol 1995;74:1841–55.
26. Eggermont JJ. Salicyl-induced changes in the spontaneous activity in cat auditory cortex. In: Aran JM, Dauman R, editors. Tinnitus 91. Amsterdam: Kugler Publications; 1992. p. 293–8.
27. Ochi K, Eggermont JJ. Effects of salicylate on neural activity in cat primary auditory cortex. Hear Res 1996;95:63–76.
28. Kenmochi M, Eggermont JJ. Salicylate and quinine affect the central nervous system. Hear Res 1997;113:110–6.
29. Eggermont JJ, Sininger Y. Correlated neural activity and tinnitus. In: Vernon JA, Møller AR, editors. Mechanisms of tinnitus. Boston: Allyn and Bacon; 1995. p. 21–34.
30. Jung TKT, Rhee CK, Lee CSL, et al. Ototoxicity of salicylate, nonsteroidal anti-inflammatory drugs and quinine. Otolaryngol Clin North Am 1993;26:791–810.
31. Ochi K, Eggermont JJ. Effects of quinine on neural activity in cat primary auditory cortex. Hear Res 1997;105:105–18.
32. Eggermont JJ, Kenmochi M. Salicylate and quinine selectively increase spontaneous firing rates in secondary auditory cortex. Hear Res 1998;117:149–60.
33. Eggermont JJ, Komiya H. Moderate noise trauma in juvenile cats results in profound cortical topographic map changes in adulthood. Hear Res 2000;142:89–101.
34. Seki S, Eggermont JJ. Changes in cat primary auditory cortex after minor-to-moderate pure-tone induced hearing loss. Hear Res 2002;173:172–86.
35. Seki S, Eggermont JJ. Changes in spontaneous firing rate and neural synchrony in cat primary auditory cortex after localized tone-induced hearing loss. Hear Res 2003;180:28–38.
36. Eggermont JJ. Differential maturation rates for response parameters in cat primary auditory cortex. Audit Neurosci 1996;2:309–27.
37. Rajan R. Receptor organ damage causes loss of cortical surround inhibition without topographic map plasticity. Nat Neurosci 1998;1:138–43.
38. Rajan R. Plasticity of excitation and inhibition in the receptive field of primary auditory cortical neurons after limited receptor organ damage. Cereb Cortex 2001;11:171–82.
39. Singer W, Gray CM. Visual feature integration and the temporal correlation hypothesis. Annu Rev Neurosci 1995;18:555–86.
40. Eggermont JJ. Coding of free field intensity in the auditory midbrain of the leopard frog. I. Results for tonal stimuli. Hear Res 1989;40:147–66.
41. DeCharms RC, Merzenich MM. Primary cortical representation of sounds by the coordination of action-potential timing. Nature 1996;381:610–3.
42. Eggermont JJ. Firing rate and firing synchrony distinguish dynamic from steady state sound. Neuroreport 1997;8:2709–13.
43. Noreña A, Eggermont JJ. Neural correlates of an auditory after image in primary auditory cortex. J Assoc Res Otolaryngol 2003;4:312–28.
44. Alonso JM, Martinez LM. Functional connectivity between simple cells and complex cells in cat striate cortex. Nat Neurosci 1989;1:395–403.
45. Roy SA, Alloway KD. Coincidence detection or temporal integration? What the neurons in somatosensory cortex are doing. J Neurosci 2001;21:2462–73.
46. Eggermont JJ. Between sound and perception: reviewing the search for a neural code. Hear Res 2001;157:1–42.

CHAPTER 14

Cortical Plasticity and Tinnitus

Christoph E. Schreiner, PhD, MD, Steven W. Cheung, MD

Cortical plasticity refers to the brain's ability to re-organize its functional capacity by reconfiguring its information processing machinery and the programs for learning.[1,2] This enables the organism to meet new environmental challenges with novel skills and strategies and allows the brain to compensate for the effects of injury and insult to its own integrity or that of its end-organs. However, under certain circumstances, some forms of plasticity may create undesirable sensory and motor effects. Examples are the sensation of phantom limbs, the pain following amputation, and the development of focal dystonia, a degradation in the ability to perform specific coordinated movements.[3,4] Tinnitus in its many forms may also be an auditory reflection of pathologic plasticity processes in the brain in response to anomalous conditions in the auditory system or in neural systems that affect auditory processing.[5–12] The symptom of tinnitus, by definition, represents an abnormal and undesirable state of the auditory system and, thus, is related to negative expressions of plasticity. There is indirect evidence of brain plasticity in tinnitus, but that role may not be the same for each type of tinnitus. Transient, rapid-onset tinnitus, for example, following a brief episode of low blood pressure or exposure to very loud sounds, may not involve the same central auditory mechanisms that may be active in slow-onset chronic tinnitus, which is often encountered after permanent hearing loss. Other forms of tinnitus may not involve plastic changes in the auditory system but could be a reflection of influence from an adjacent neural system, for example, through abnormal crossmodal connections in transient, gaze- or movement-evoked tinnitus. Furthermore, the plasticity of brain structures may also contribute to the emotional impact that the sensation of tinnitus may evoke in some patients.

In this chapter, we review some of the evidence that neural plasticity is involved in chronic tinnitus, discuss some of the forms of expression of plasticity in the function of the central part of the auditory system, survey some components that may modulate the plasticity of neural circuitry and their potential role in the generation of tinnitus, and, finally, speculate on how plasticity might be used to alleviate tinnitus symptoms.

TINNITUS

PHYSIOLOGIC CORRELATES

The physiologic substrate for tinnitus and its locus of expression in the nervous system are not known. Several patterns of neural activity and various locations have been suggested.[7–9,13–18] Because the perception of chronic tinnitus considered here is not caused by identifiable acoustic events, it has been assumed that an altered form of spontaneous activity must be present.[8,9,13,14,16,19–24] Different forms of tinnitus are likely to have different pathophysiologic triggers, including changes in firing pattern and focal, global, or diffuse deafferentiation of the peripheral part of the auditory system.[7–9,13,25] They may also have different neural substrates and sites of manifestations. Cellular studies in animal models and recent evidence from human field potential and imaging studies have bolstered that assumption and suggested several potential neuronal substrates of tinnitus. Among the main candidate attributes of neural activity considered (and discussed in other chapters of this book) are increased (or decreased) local spontaneous activity, an expanded network of neurons showing synchronized activity, increased numbers of neurons representing the perceived tinnitus frequency, and changes in the temporal pattern of spontaneous activity in frequency representation associated with the tinnitus pitch, for example, bursting spike activity.[7–9,13,16,21,23,26–28] Into the last group also falls the idea that thalamocortical dysrhythmia may be a key element not only in the induction of tinnitus but also in other disorders, such as epilepsy and neurogenic pain.[18] Dysrhythmia has been characterized as an increased theta rhythmicity and coherence between low- and high-frequency thalamocortical oscillations.[18] If this disturbance of the normal activity pattern is limited to a narrow frequency range in the thalamocortical tonotopic system, this might evoke a phantom sensation of a specific pitch. Other locations that have been suggested as primary sites of tinnitus generation include nuclei of the brainstem (eg, the dorsal cochlear nucleus), nuclei of the lemniscal or tonotopic pathway from the inferior colliculus to the primary auditory cortex, and nuclei of the nonlemniscal or nonclassic pathway.[21–23,26,29,30]

EVIDENCE OF INVOLVEMENT OF CENTRAL SITES

It is now widely believed that tinnitus arises in the central part of the auditory system, although its primary trigger may lie at more peripheral (cochlear and hair cell) levels.[7–10,13,26] Evidence of crossmodal interactions with tinnitus has prompted the idea that tinnitus is generated at central nervous system loci different from those normally processing sound.[7,8,31] This view is supported by the observation that median nerve stimulation can modify tinnitus.[8] However, in the context of this discussion, we distinguish between chronic tinnitus, with triggers residing within the auditory pathway, on the one hand, and modulation of tinnitus by nonauditory means and transient induction of an auditory sensation through crossmodal mechanisms on the other hand.[7,8] Although the latter does have a place in the discussion of tinnitus, crossmodal initiation of an auditory sensation does not necessarily require altered mechanisms within the auditory system but may reflect normal auditory processing of advertent or inadvertent nonauditory input.

Evidence of cerebral auditory involvement in tinnitus expression comes from several objective methods in humans. The main advantage of these methods is that they can be correlated with the introspective report of patients regarding the presence and nature of the tinnitus percept. Electroencephalographic assessment before and after the sudden disappearance of tinnitus perception revealed quantitative differences in the power spectrum, especially in the 16 Hz band, at specific scalp electrode locations.[32] In a potentially related finding, tinnitus-associated activity interfered with the intensity dependence of the N100 magnitude in a frequency-specific manner.[33,34] Similarly, magnetoencephalographic studies indicated a covariance between the presence of tinnitus and an abnormal amplitude ratio of the M200 and M100 waves.[35,36] These studies support the notion of the involvement of auditory cortex in tinnitus expression, although they cannot identify the generation site and pathophysiologic substrate.

Suppression of tinnitus with lidocaine provided further correlative evidence for the engagement of cortical stations. In functional magnetic resonance imaging and positron emission tomographic studies, lidocaine application in patients with tinnitus diminished the tinnitus percept and also reduced global regional cortical blood flow.[5,37–40] Conversely, increases in tinnitus loudness were associated with a small increase in regional cerebral blood flow. The global cortical sites activated by tinnitus when compared to reduced tinnitus under lidocaine and masking conditions were in the right hemisphere association cortex.[5,37,38] Evidence of unilateral activation further suggests central generator(s) for tinnitus.[38] It can also be interpreted as evidence of activation of nonprimary auditory pathways associated with attention, emotion, and memory.[21,26,29,37] The effectiveness of lidocaine in altering tinnitus signals points to effects on neurotransmission that can modify synchrony, spontaneous activity, and bursting discharge patterns, that is, several of the candidate physiologic substrates of tinnitus.[9,10,37]

An origin of tinnitus central to the inferior colliculus is also suggested by metabolic 2-deoxyglucose mapping and immediate early-gene expression experiments. The auditory cortex was activated without concomitant activity in the cochlear nuclei and inferior colliculus after sound trauma or salicylate exposure.[21,26,30]

Of course, these signs of the engagement of cortical stations in tinnitus do not allow the conclusion that the observed effects demark the site of origin of this percept. Rather, they suggest that those structures are affected in the context of their normal functional capacity of sensory processing.

TINNITUS AND PLASTICITY

Neural plasticity may play a significant role in the development of chronic tinnitus and associated symptoms such as hyperacusis, affective disorders, phonophobia, and depression.[8,15] Evidence of plasticity in human or nonhuman subjects with hearing loss is abundant.[11,20,23,24,41–51] In contrast, direct evidence of the involvement of plasticity in the genesis and maintenance of tinnitus is still sparse. A fundamental problem is distinguishing reorganization following hearing loss from that necessary for tinnitus generation because much hearing loss is not accompanied by tinnitus. In humans, measures of cortical reorganization are still indirect and constrained by spatial and temporal resolution limits in noninvasive imaging. Studies that control for the severity of human hearing loss are difficult to design because of individual variation. In animals, reliable and reproducible induction of hearing loss is more feasible; however, the diagnosis of tinnitus is challenging because it requires extensive psychophysical evaluations.[52–54] Accordingly, few studies have established a link between the attributes of reorganization and the verified presence of tinnitus. In a magnetoencephalographic study, the frequency representation associated with the pitch of the subject's tinnitus was displaced from the tonotopically organized primary auditory cortex (AI) to an adjacent area.[6] It was concluded that tinnitus might relate to plastic changes in the auditory cortex, perhaps beyond the AI, much as phantom limb sensation is correlated with concomitant somatosensory cortical reorganization.[3] Of special interest is that the observed reorganization was limited to the frequency range that corresponded to the tinnitus pitch and that the degree of departure from normal tonotopic organization correlated with subjective tinnitus strength.[6] However, the observed plastic changes may be more appropriately related to the hearing deficit and, therefore, only indirectly to tinnitus.

Plasticity within auditory areas, then, may be related to tinnitus. However, plasticity in activating the connections between areas conveying or enabling emotional influences (eg, via the limbic system) and memory (eg, via the prefrontal system) may also shape the affective impact of the percept. For example, c-*fos* activity after sound trauma or salicylate, common triggers for tinnitus, was highly correlated between the AI and the lateral amygdala, a key auditory-limbic interface.[26,30,55–57] The mechanisms and conditions that trigger the expression of plasticity at the many different levels and stages of neural processing are unclear. However, the effects of plasticity are not limited to one site but have local and remote consequences owing to the rich, reciprocal connectivities that characterize the organization of the central nervous system.[58] This implies multiple types of plasticity and several loci for modulation of its expression.

Several questions, then, need to be addressed: (1) What sites and mechanisms lead to the enduring perception of a phantom sound? (2) How does plasticity shape the processes that result in tinnitus? and (3) Can plasticity mechanisms abolish or modify the phantom perception? The answers to these questions are still elusive, although progress has brought us closer to resolving them.

CORTICAL PLASTICITY

Before considering the potential roles of synaptic plasticity in tinnitus generation, we must discuss briefly the stages and conditions that can affect neural responses and their relationship to different mechanisms, usually subsumed under the rubric of plasticity. The discussion is limited to sensory brain processes, although other modalities and the motor system show similar principles of plasticity.[1,2]

At least two temporal domains of plasticity are defined. Short-term plasticity reflects rapidly induced processes and may last from fractions of seconds to several minutes. In contrast, long-term plasticity may require a longer induction time, but the changes may endure for hours, days, or months.[1,59,60]

Short-term plasticity regulates the properties of practically all types of synapses. Forms of short-term plasticity that affect synaptic transmission include facilitation, augmentation, post-tetanic potentiation, and synaptic depression.[61,62] Combinations of these processes, dependent on details of the timing of activation, determine the reliability and flexibility of network operations.

Long-term plasticity occurs in the brain under several main conditions. Developmental plasticity is associated with the immature brain as it begins to process sensory information. We omit this form of plasticity because tinnitus has been studied primarily in the mature brain. However, some properties of developmental plasticity may differ sufficiently from mature plasticity processes to warrant special consideration in the search for causes and remedies in childhood tinnitus. Activity-dependent plasticity refers to brain reorganization owing to changes in the body that, in turn, change input information to the brain.[1,2] Examples include sensory changes after reduction in eyesight or hearing or limb amputations that alter the balance of afferent input to the brain.[63–66] Such input changes are likely helpful for understanding tinnitus caused by peripheral hearing loss. Plasticity of learning and memory occurs when behaviorally significant changes in the environment alter sensory input statistics to the brain or behavioral conditions that affect sensory information processing. Examples are improvements in hearing while learning to play a musical instrument and in somatic sensation during learning of braille.[67–69] Such plasticity may be relevant for the understanding of tinnitus in two ways. It could affect the nature and intensity of emotive or autonomic affect affixed to the tinnitus percept. Further, learned plasticity, if understood more completely, may be exploited to reduce such negative associations. Finally, injury-induced plasticity refers to reorganizational processes (eg, sprouting, transneuronal de- and regeneration) after damage to the brain.[70–73]

Mechanisms of Plasticity

Understanding the mechanisms of plasticity, that is, how brain circuits organize and adjust to experience or sensory stimulation, is crucial for developing clinical strategies to ameliorate tinnitus. Understanding plasticity requires analysis of the synaptic mechanisms and neural pathways. Several cellular and molecular mechanisms potentially contribute to the different types of plasticity mentioned above. For example, synaptic short-term plasticity is regulated by many molecular mechanisms, including the activation of Ca^{2+} channels, which affect the neurotransmitter vesicle availability and control presynaptic contributions from metabotropic and ionotropic receptors.[1,2,61,74–78]

Network effects that may not be expressions of synaptic plasticity also come into play.[79–82] Periods of rapid, transient change in receptive fields occur in the auditory cortex after behavioral training to an adapting tone or to a different stimulus context.[80–82] A related phenomenon may be the Zwicker tone, an auditory illusion induced with notched noise that has been suggested as a model for transient tinnitus.[27] Although short-term synaptic plasticity may influence these effects, other influences include changes of central network balance owing to alterations in the peripheral input pattern. Different input conditions may have immediate effects owing to masking or unmasking and change the pattern of excitatory and inhibitory balance.[79] Lateral inhibitory network models show that if the spontaneous input to a region of the network is reduced, the edges between the normal and the reduced spontaneous regions are enhanced and transformed into focal activity by nonlinear corticothalamic effects.[42,83–86] In relation to this, positive feedback from within the auditory cortex and from emotion- and attention-modulating systems has been postulated in the generation of tinnitus as a consequence of an effort to enhance sensitivity in frequency regions with reduced input.[26,29,30] Otherwise hidden projections can be revealed by stimulus-induced reduction of inhibition (as with notched noise), thus unmasking latent but silent thalamocortical and horizontal, corticocortical connections that are otherwise blocked by inhibition.[87] This effect parallels that seen in focal peripheral lesions, in vascular compression of the auditory nerve, and in percepts associated with notched noise, all of which alter spontaneous activity and might thus contribute to the induction of tinnitus.[8,14,15,27]

Persistent plastic changes in synaptic efficacy are accomplished by adjustments in the strength of connections between ensembles of neurons. The main candidates for cortical plasticity are thalamocortical and horizontal connections, with most synapses originating from intra- and interlaminar neurons. A promising candidate for learning and memory is changes in synaptic efficacy. Maintaining the efficacy of new thalamocortical and horizontal, corticocortical connections requires a form of synaptic stabilization. Changes in neuronal connectivity through synapse unmasking and addition could create a permissive state for new connections by disinhibition of latent excitatory inputs.[70] Changes in synaptic efficacy can be rapid or protracted in activity-dependent modification of synaptic transmission, as reflected in long-term potentiation and long-term depression.[1,2,74–76] Structural changes in the reorganization of the cortical network, for example, an increase in the number of synapses via synaptogenesis, will require more time.[1,2,70,88,89] Plastic changes often distort cortical sensory or motor maps.[1,46,60,66] For example, limb denervation shifts the map border in the somatosensory cortex between limb and face representation.[89,90] This change can be associated with altered synaptic efficacy, sprouting of new connections, and altered neuronal intrinsic properties (eg, reduction in input resistance).[70,89,90] This demonstrates the coordinated involvement of many different factors that lead to macroscopic changes in cortical organization.[58] How such changes may be associated with tinnitus remains to be established. In cellular studies, plasticity mechanisms are dependent on correlation-based rules that strengthen or weaken synaptic efficacy. In particular, correlated pre- and postsynaptic activity produces long-term changes in synaptic strength.[1,2,75,76,91,92] Glutamatergic receptors play a crucial role in synaptic plasticity. Activation of N-methyl-D-aspartate (NMDA) receptors is required for the manifestation of perceptual learning through synaptic modification.[88] The NMDA receptor is available to glutamate only when the postsynaptic membrane is depolarized in a temporally coordinated manner. The ensuing calcium influx elicits several processes that ultimately modify synaptic strength. Activation of NMDA receptors is a necessary but not sufficient condition to induce activity-dependent plasticity. Regulation of other glutamate receptors, such as trafficking of alpha-amino-3-hydroxy-5-methyl-4-isoxazole propionic acid (AMPA) receptors, also contributes to persistent changes in synaptic transmission.[93]

Intracortical microstimulation increases the local correlation between the activity of many neurons and thus enhances the ability of synapses to change a cell's response properties.[94–96] Receptive fields of cells near the electrically stimulated site emerge with properties similar to those at the stimulation site. Farther from the stimulation site (up to several hundred microns), the emergent receptive field properties dominate, whereas the original inputs to those zones are suppressed.[94–96] Perhaps chronic cortical activity associated with tinnitus may likewise affect local reorganization as a consequence of tinnitus.

ACTIVITY-DEPENDENT PLASTICITY

As defined above, activity-dependent long-term neuroplasticity usually refers to brain reorganization owing to peripheral changes, in turn changing inputs to the brain. Such plasticity is essential for understanding the origins of tinnitus because it may create the conditions in central auditory structures, especially the cortex, that underlie and sustain the activity profile that is perceptually manifested as tinnitus.

The potential reorganization of receptive fields and sensory maps in activity-dependent plasticity is a consequence of deprivation of inputs. Deafferented areas become responsive to sensory inputs formerly represented only within cortical sectors near those representing the lesioned input source. For example, peripheral nerve transection or digit amputation reorganizes the initially unresponsive area in the somatosensory cortex by enabling previously ineffective input from neighboring skin to emerge.[1,79,89,90] Similarly, acoustic trauma specific to certain frequency regions increases the driven firing rate at the edges of spectral receptive fields.[9,97–99] Decreased excitatory drive, owing to peripheral damage, can decrease inhibition, which, in turn, broadens frequency-receptive fields, increases firing rate, and elicits tonotopic map reorganization.[28,43,48,50,51,98,99] Hearing loss produces perceptual changes such as hypersensitivity, hyperactivity, and enhanced difference limens near the cutoff frequency of the loss.[42,100] This may reflect denervation supersensitivity, a reduction of inhibition, and an increase in activity.[101,102] Alternatively, an increased number of neurons tuned to the lesion's edge frequency may have developed.[10,28] Increased activity is also seen outside the lemniscal pathway, including the dorsal cochlear nucleus, the external nucleus of the inferior colliculus, and the second auditory cortical field, and is a likely contributor to the various perceptual effects associated with tinnitus.[8,9,24,29]

Expanded frequency representation at lesion borders appears to be a common change in focal hearing loss.[16,28,50,51] The area of cortical overrepresentation is not the region with profound damage (scotoma) but a region with only slightly elevated threshold near the denervated frequencies.[28,44,103] Several models suggest that cortical GABAergic circuits are down-regulated by removal of sensory input.[44,104,105] As a consequence, otherwise weak cortico-cortical excitatory input may emerge and contribute to the long-term reorganization and expansion of frequencies that often abut the perceived (chronic) tinnitus frequency.

Some of these effects are already present soon after trauma. Acute pure-tone trauma can elicit release from inhibition and an expansion of receptive fields, likely through unmasking of previously inhibitory responses.[23,44] However, acute trauma effects and chronic effects are not identical, suggesting that long-term plasticity is involved in cortical reorganization.[9,10,23,44]

LEARNING-INDUCED PLASTICITY

Many studies show that spatiotemporal cortical representations are remodeled by experience.[1,106–110] This "representational" plasticity could manifest the basic adaptive processes underlying central nervous system contributions to learning. Such plasticity may be a key in the development of treatment strategies for tinnitus.

Improvement or, more generally, alterations of perceptual abilities with training likely embody cortical (and thalamic) representational remodeling.[1,77,106–112] Learning-induced changes in a cortical network are seen when inputs reach this system during an attended behavior. Many studies demonstrate receptive field plasticity in auditory cortical neurons during classic conditioning.[77,113,114] Significant changes in discharge activity in these cells follow the associative pairing of an acoustic conditioned stimulus with an unconditioned stimulus. Because the extent of these physiologic changes is absent in the sensitization and extinguishing phases of training, the associative process may be salient in discharge plasticity.[77,113,114]

Auditory cortical neural plasticity and the spatial distribution of receptive field properties are demonstrated in learning conditions, for example, operant detection, discrimination training, and exposure to altered sensory inputs. Thus, the location and extent of the spatial distribution of characteristic frequencies in AI neurons are altered by frequency-discriminative training.[106] Other features, such as temporal and spectral integration properties, are also flexible.

Cortical neurons function adaptively, changing their representation dynamically as learning recruits and allocates neurons to represent salient features.[111,115] This process requires intense training that engages reward systems through several of the neuromodulatory networks. Accordingly, a motivational drive combined with a behaviorally important context is necessary for the robust expression of use-dependent reorganization.[1,2]

Behavioral context modulates the type of plasticity expressed. The responses of AI neurons to a standard, nonrewarded tone habituate, whereas responses to rewarded target tones increase during acquisition in frequency or temporal discrimination tasks in monkeys.[109,110] Changes in spectral and temporal receptive fields correlate with the probability that a particular signal predicted a reward. Nonreinforced or rarely reinforced signals were represented weakly, with reduced response strength and area of representation, whereas consistently reinforced signals were represented more robustly, with higher firing rates and receptive fields expanded to encompass the rewarded stimulus properties. This outcome is similar to phenomena in learning studies using classic (pavlovian) conditioning procedures: the sensory contexts that trigger rewarded motor responses are enhanced.[109,110] The different behavioral context (rewarded or nonrewarded) suggests that neuromodulators increase the representation or salience of the cue in the cortex (see below). In this context, if tinnitus is construed as a stimulus, aversive reaction acts as a negative reinforcer. It might be possible to reverse functional changes in the auditory system that are linked to tinnitus by invoking the basic principles of plasticity. One such attempt is tinnitus retraining therapy, which teaches patients to habituate their reaction to tinnitus and, eventually, its percept.[116,117] Because nonauditory limbic pathways and the autonomic nervous system contribute to the emotive aspects of tinnitus, they must also be modified by learning-induced plasticity.

Injury-Induced Plasticity

Damage to the cortex alone can also lead to extensive plasticity and, occasionally, to a tinnitus percept. Compensatory sensory and motor plasticity after stroke and gradual functional impairment in regions that have developed epileptic foci are often seen after trauma.[72,118–120] Although the development of tinnitus in those circumstances is not common, such cases exist, for example, a hemorrhage adjacent to the AI, resulting in tinnitus.[71] This has been interpreted as a pathologic activation of nonspecific neural networks for auditory perception. In another instance, a unilateral, high-pitched tinnitus was the manifestation of a seizure emanating from a lesion in the superior temporal gyrus and inferior part of the supramarginal gyrus.[121] Both cases suggest that cortical changes alone may suffice for tinnitus, without contribution from peripheral influences such as input deprivation or ascending altered spontanenous activity. However, such reports do not exclude subcortical changes that may contribute to the generation of a tinnitus perception. Damage to the corticofugal system could alter ascending spontaneous activity, perhaps eliciting tinnitus.

MODULATION OF PLASTICITY

Neuromodulation is a key factor in neural coding and storage of environmental information, with a critical role in cortical plasticity.[122] Adaptive changes depend on sensory input and on the functional state of the cortex, which are controlled by nonsensory inputs, such as the neuromodulatory inputs that influence arousal, attention, and motivation. Neuromodulatory transmitters act pre- and postsynaptically, control excitability, gate information processes, enhance signal-to-noise ratios, and modulate activity-dependent synaptic modifications, for example, through facilitation of NMDA receptor–gated processes that underlie receptive field and map reorganization.[66,123]

Several neuromodulatory systems exist.[123] Nonauditory sites with neuromodulatory roles include the nucleus basalis (NB) (acetylcholine [ACh] system), the locus ceruleus (noradrenergic system), the ventral tegmentum (dopaminergic system), and raphe nuclei (serotonin system). The functions of these areas are associated with arousal, emotion, and nociception. Several lines of evidence indicate that these systems participate in the expression and/or emotional association of the tinnitus percept or in fear, depression, and phonophobia.[7,8,29,124] Studies of metabolic activity and early-gene expression in animals with tinnitus show involvement of the amygdala and of the locus ceruleus, that is, stations subserving regulation of attention and emotion.[21,26,30]

Analysis of these widespread modulatory systems for treatment for tinnitus or its emotional manifestation could advance therapeutic outcomes. Direct and indirect manipulations of the neuromodulatory system have been attempted, especially in the context of activity-induced representational plasticity. These affect plasticity processes in perceptual learning. Augmentation of NMDA receptor effects on perceptual learning by systemic amphetamine application increased dopamine, serotonin, and noradrenaline (NA) levels and reflected up-regulation of several neuromodulatory systems.[125]

CHOLINERGIC SYSTEM

The cholinergic (ACh) system is involved in many aspects of behavioral and physiologic regulation, such as sensory processing, learning, memory, mood, attention, sleep, and arousal.[126] Application of ACh to the cortex modifies frequency and intensity tuning in a stimulus-specific modulation of auditory information processing.[127–129] The cholinergic system may be involved in stimulus feature–directed perceptual learning by allowing an extensive and rapid physiologic modification in the sensory cortex. Cholinergic basal forebrain input promotes activity-dependent synaptic modifications in the auditory cortex.[130,131] NB neurons receive amygdaloid and other limbic projections.[132] NB lesions reduce cortical plasticity, whereas electrical NB stimulation enhances receptive field and map reorganization.[130–133] Spectrotemporal simple stimuli paired with NB stimulation alter cortical topography; more complex stimuli enhance context-dependent (sequence sensitive) facilitation and increase synchrony without affecting AI coarse frequency mapping.[134] Other changes include a reduction in spontaneous activity and latency. NB-induced cortical changes are mediated by widespread cholinergic projections to the cortex and the amygdala. Therefore, cortical plasticity induced by paired NB stimulation may entail parallel changes in subcortical systems.[58,135] The ACh system has potential significance for tinnitus therapies because its action is stimulus feature directed and because the amygdala is critical for emotional processing.[21,26,30,55]

SEROTONIN SYSTEM

The serotoninergic system may also be implicated in auditory learning, as well as in memory and emotion.[123] Serotonin- (5-hydroxytryptamine) positive axons in the cortex arise from two raphe nuclei. Their immunopositive axon terminals reach pyramidal cells and inhibitory interneurons in all cortical layers. Like other such neuromodulators, direct application of serotonin to cortical neurons can enhance or depress activity. Much like the ACh mechanism, serotonin is associated with NMDA receptor–gated synaptic modifications. Decreased serotonin reduced plasticity, for example, in expression of ocular dominance columns, and enhanced allodynia and hypersensitivity in denervation-associated models of central chronic pain.[102,136–139]

Tinnitus could involve a serotonin pathway dysfunction: local deprivation may trigger a change in synaptic organization and neurotransmission and alter receptor configuration to the neural patterns supporting tinnitus.[138] Further, serotonin receptor decrease enhances audiogenic seizure susceptibility through decreased inhibitory activity.[140] A reduced anticonvulsant effect of serotoninergic stimulation might weakly enhance local epileptogenic activity in areas with reduced serotonin receptor density, leading to increased synchrony and a characteristic temporal profile. Treatment with local application of serotonin agonists or reuptake inhibitors could reduce these signs. Systemic application of such drugs, which are used in the treatment of depression and schizophrenia, may reduce the level of aversive impact of the tinnitus percept. However, a controlled study with selective serotonin reuptake inhibitors has provided only weak support for such a hypothesis.[141]

Dopaminergic System

Dopamine constitutes another substrate for cortical neuromodulation.[123,142] Dopaminergic projections arise from the ventral tegmental area (VTA) and terminate in the cortex differentially in areas and layers. This system plays a role in cognition; affective, motor, and endocrine function; and long-term memory consolidation. Dopamine potentiates NMDA responses, as seen in larger membrane potential amplitudes and shorter latencies. Its application depresses activity, enhances synaptic modification, and may strongly facilitate long-term depression. Thus, dopamine release may contribute to active "unlearning," as demonstrated in the formation of behaviorally relevant associations during auditory conditioning.[137,142] It may be essential for contingency-based associative learning.

VTA stimulation following exposure to a tone results in overrepresentation of the tone frequency in the AI (forward pairing).[143] In contrast, VTA stimulation preceding a narrowband noise reduces the frequency band in the AI (backward pairing).[144] This has been interpreted as a contingency-based mechanism, that is, enhanced cortical representation with positive contingencies and a decrease with negative contingencies.

Activation of the cholinergic and dopaminergic systems alters auditory cortical plasticity with regard to stimulus-specific receptive plasticity that resembles that seen in behavioral conditioning.[139] However, the systems do not have comparable motivational effects.

Noradrenergic System

Much like the ACh system, the NA system can play a permissive role in developmental plasticity and learning.[123,139] The locus ceruleus is the sole origin of NA afferents to the cortex.[145–147] Axons that contain dopamine β-hydroxylase, the NA-synthesizing enzyme, are in all neocortical regions and layers. NA affects attention, arousal, and vigilance. Direct application reduces spontaneous activity and enhances signal-to-noise ratio and plasticity in the visual and piriform cortex.[148,149] NA depletion may abolish plasticity.[148] The ceruleocortical NA system is implicated in selective attention. A modulatory NA influence on sensory responses might underlie its role in learning and memory by improving stimulus selection and processing.[150]

The differential functions and interactions of these four neuromodulatory systems for tinnitus induction, expression, and, potentially, manipulation remain to be explored in depth. They might open a window on our understanding and control of a pathology with strong affective elements.

CONCLUSIONS

We have considered some of the mechanisms and expressions of cortical plasticity, with special attention to the central auditory consequences of peripheral hearing loss. The evidence suggests that plasticity is associated with tinnitus. It is unknown if an altered cortical substrate is necessary or sufficient for a tinnitus percept. In the section on tinnitus and plasticity, three questions were posed. Although answers to these questions remain open, a picture is developing that suggests that solutions may soon emerge.

The first question was "What sites and mechanisms lead to tinnitus?" As discussed here and elsewhere in this volume, the likelihood is high that central auditory structures, foremost the auditory cortex, in conjunction with influences from nonauditory, limbic structures, sustain the percept of canonic chronic tinnitus. The processes expressing the percept could be those in normal hearing but amplified by elevated or characteristically patterned activity from subcortical stations. Alternatively, chronic, central tinnitus could be the expression of modified cortical perceptual machinery with self-sustaining attributes. In either case, electrophysiologic inquiries will provide vital answers about its nature and neural substrate.

The second question was "What is the role of plasticity in shaping the processes that result in tinnitus?" Altering the central auditory processing networks is an unavoidable consequence of hearing loss. Nevertheless, it is unresolved whether tinnitus is a consequence of plasticity or if local plasticity is induced by tinnitus. To resolve this question, it is critical to distinguish between plasticity associated with hearing loss and changes associated with tinnitus. Experimental designs that include behavioral verification of tinnitus and of the extent and nature of the hearing loss are indispensable.

The third question was "Can plasticity mechanisms be invoked to modify the phantom perception?" We surveyed four neuromodulatory systems that can profoundly influence the induction and expression of cortical plasticity. Each system affects plasticity in somewhat different ways, including aspects of stimulus features, the affective valence of the stimulus, motivation, and contingency-based conditions.[151] Neuromodulation of the central auditory substrates of tinnitus perception may require the activation of all or a subset of several neuromodulatory systems.[152] Concurrent activation of the modulatory systems, and likely their coordinated action, requires an awake and attending subject. Therefore, behavioral training, perhaps augmented by pharmacologic intervention, may be the most promising regimen to modify the central nervous substrate of tinnitus and, consequently, its percept.

ACKNOWLEDGMENT

We thank Drs. Jeffery A. Winer and Gerald Langner for their insightful comments on the manuscript.

REFERENCES

1. Buonomano DV, Merzenich MM. Cortical plasticity: from synapses to maps. Annu Rev Neurosci 1998;21:149–86.
2. Calford MB. Dynamic representational plasticity in sensory cortex. Neuroscience 2002;111:709–38.
3. Flor H, Elbert T, Knecht S, et al. Phantom-limb pain as a perceptual correlate of cortical reorganization following arm amputation. Nature 1995;375:482–4.
4. Byl NN. Focal hand dystonia may result from aberrant neuroplasticity. Adv Neurol 2004;94:19–28.
5. Lockwood AH, Salvi RJ, Coad ML, et al. The functional neuroanatomy of tinnitus: evidence for limbic system links and neural plasticity. Neurology 1998;50:114–20.
6. Muehlnickel W, Elbert T, Taub E, Flor H. Reorganization of auditory cortex in tinnitus. Proc Natl Acad Sci U S A 1998;95:10340–3.
7. Cacace AT. Expanding the biological basis of tinnitus: crossmodal origins and the role of neuroplasticity. Hear Res 2003;175:112–32.
8. Møller AR. Pathophysiology of tinnitus. Otolaryngol Clin North Am 2003;36:249–66.
9. Eggermont JJ. Central tinnitus. Auris Nasus Larynx 2003;30 Suppl:S7–12.
10. Eggermont JJ. The auditory cortex and tinnitus. In: Snow JB, editor. Tinnitus: theory and management. Hamilton (ON): BC Decker; 2004. p. 172–89.
11. Syka J. Plastic changes in the central auditory system after hearing loss, restoration of function, and during learning. Physiol Rev 2002;82:601–36.
12. Salvi RJ, Lockwood AH, Burkhard R. Neural plasticity and tinnitus. In: Tyler RS, editor. Tinnitus handbook. San Diego (CA): Singular, Thompson Learning; 2000. p. 123–48.
13. Jastreboff PJ. Phantom auditory perception (tinnitus): mechanisms of generation and perception. Neurosci Res 1990;8:221–54.
14. Møller AR. Similarities between severe tinnitus and chronic pain. J Am Acad Audiol 2000;11:115–24.
15. Møller AR. Symptoms and signs caused by neural plasticity. Neurol Res 2001;23:562–72.
16. Seki S, Eggermont JJ. Changes in spontaneous firing rate and neural synchrony in cat primary auditory cortex after localized tone-induced hearing loss. Hear Res 2003;180:28–38.
17. Shulman A. A final common pathway for tinnitus—the medial temporal lobe system. Int Tinnitus J 1995;1:115–26.
18. Llinas RR, Ribary U, Jeanmonod D, et al. Thalamocortical dysrhythmia: a neurological and neuropsychiatric syndrome characterized by magnetoencephalography. Proc Natl Acad Sci U S A 1999;96:15222–7.
19. Kaltenbach JA, McCaslin DL. Increase in spontaneous activity in the dorsal cochlear nucleus following exposure to high intensity sound: a possible neural correlate of tinnitus. Audit Neurosci 1996;3:57–78.
20. Komiya H, Eggermont JJ. Spontaneous firing activity of cortical neurons in adult cats following pure tone trauma induced at 5 weeks of age. Acta Otolaryngol (Stockh) 2000;120:750–6.
21. Wallhaeusser-Franke E, Braun S, Langner G. Salicylate alters 2-DG uptake in the auditory system: a model for tinnitus? Neuroreport 1996;7:1585–8.
22. Jastreboff PJ, Sasaki CT. Salicylate-induced changes in spontaneous activity of single units in the inferior colliculus of the guinea pig. J Acoust Soc Am 1986;80:1384–91.
23. Noreña AJ, Eggermont JJ. Changes in spontaneous neural activity immediately after an acoustic trauma: implications for neural correlates of tinnitus. Hear Res 2003;183:137–53.

24. Kaltenbach JA. Hyperactivity in the dorsal cochlear nucleus after intense sound exposure and its resemblance to tone-evoked activity: a physiological model for tinnitus. Hear Res 2000;48:111–24.
25. Zenner HP, Ernst A. Cochlear-motor, transduction and signal-transfer tinnitus: models for three types of cochlear tinnitus. Eur Arch Otorhinolaryngol 1993;249:447–54.
26. Wallhaeusser-Franke E, Mahlke C, Oliva R, et al. Expression of c-fos in auditory and non-auditory brain regions of the gerbil after manipulations that induce tinnitus. Exp Brain Res 2003;153:649–54.
27. Noreña AJ, Eggermont JJ. Neural correlates of an auditory afterimage in primary auditory cortex. J Assoc Res Otolaryngol 2003;4:312–28.
28. Rajan R, Irvine DRF. Features of, and boundary conditions for, lesion-induced reorganization of adult auditory cortical maps. In: Salvi RJ, Henderson D, Fiorin F, et al, editors. Auditory system plasticity and regeneration. New York: Thieme Medical Publishers; 1996. p. 224–37.
29. Møller AR, Møller MB, Yokata M. Some forms of tinnitus may involve the extralemniscal pathway. Laryngoscope 1992;102:1165–71.
30. Zhang JS, Kaltenbach JA, Wang J, Kim SA. Fos-like immunoreactivity in auditory and nonauditory brain structures of hamsters previously exposed to intense sound. Exp Brain Res 2003;153:655–60.
31. Pinchoff RJ, Burkhard RF, Salvi RJ, et al. Modulation of tinnitus by voluntary jaw movements. Am J Otol 1998;19:785–9.
32. Weiler EWJ, Brill K, Tachiki KH, Wiegand R. Electroencephalography correlates in tinnitus. Int Tinnitus J 2000;6:21–4.
33. Kadner A, Viirre E, Wester DC, et al. Lateral inhibition in the auditory cortex: an EEG index of tinnitus? Neuroreport 2002;13:443–6.
34. Jacobson GP, McCaslin DL. A re-examination of the long latency N1 response in patients with tinnitus. J Am Acad Audiol 2003;14:393–400.
35. Hoke M, Pantev C, Luetkenhoner B, Lehnertz K. Auditory cortical basis of tinnitus. Acta Otolaryngol Suppl (Stockh) 1991;491:176–81.
36. Hoke M, Feldmann H, Pantev C, et al. Objective evidence of tinnitus in auditory evoked magnetic fields. Hear Res 1989;37:281–6.
37. Mirz F, Gjedde A, Skodkilde-Jorgensen H, Pedersen CB. Functional brain imaging of tinnitus-like perception induced by aversive auditory stimuli. Neuroreport 2000;11:633–7.
38. Reyes SA, Salvi RJ, Burkhard RF, et al. Brain imaging of the effects of lidocaine on tinnitus. Hear Res 2002;171:43–50.
39. Weissman JL Hirsch BE. Imaging tinnitus: a review. Radiology 2000;216:342–9.
40. Andersson G, Lyttens L, Hirvela C, et al. Regional cerebral blood flow during tinnitus: a PET case study with lidocaine and auditory stimulation. Acta Otolaryngol (Stockh) 2000;120:967–72.
41. Kral A, Hartmann R, Tillein J, et al. Hearing after congenital deafness: central auditory plasticity and sensory deprivation. Cereb Cortex 2002;12:797–807.
42. Thai-Van H, Micheyl C, Moore BC, Collet L. Enhanced frequency discrimination near the hearing loss cut-off: a consequence of central auditory plasticity induced by cochlear damage? Brain 2003;126:2235–45.
43. Robertson D, Irvine DR. Plasticity of frequency organization in auditory cortex of guinea pigs with partial unilateral deafness. J Comp Neurol 1989;282:456–71.
44. Rajan R. Plasticity of excitation and inhibition in the receptive field of primary auditory cortical neurons after limited receptor organ damage. Cereb Cortex 2001;11:171–82.
45. Kaltenbach JA, Zhang J, Afman CE. Plasticity of spontaneous neural activity in the dorsal cochlear nucleus after intense sound exposure. Hear Res 2000;147:282–92.
46. Rauschecker JP. Mechanisms of compensatory plasticity in the cerebral cortex. Adv Neurol 1997;73:137–46.
47. Willott JF, Lu SM. Noise induced hearing loss can alter neural coding and increase excitability in the central nervous system. Science 1982;216:1331–2.
48. Kamke MR, Brown M, Irvine DRF. Plasticity in the tonotopic organization of the medial geniculate body in adult cats following restricted unilateral cochlear lesions. J Comp Neurol 2003;459:355–67.
49. Schwaber MK, Garraghty PE, Kaas JH. Neuroplasticity of the adult primate auditory cortex following cochlear hearing loss. Am J Otol. 1993;14:252–8.
50. Rajan R, Irvine DR, Wise LZ, Heil P. Effect of unilateral partial cochlear lesions in adult cats on the representation of lesioned and unlesioned cochleas in primary auditory cortex. J Comp Neurol 1993;338:17–49.

51. Harrison RV, Nagasawa A, Smith DW, et al. Reorganization of auditory cortex after neonatal high frequency cochlear hearing loss. Hear Res 1991;54:11–9.
52. Heffner HE, Harrington IA. Tinnitus in hamsters following exposure to intense sound. Hear Res 2002;170:83–95.
53. Bauer CA, Brozoski TJ, Rojas R, et al. Behavioral model of chronic tinnitus in rats. Otolaryngol Head Neck Surg 1999;121:457–62.
54. Jastreboff PJ, Brennan JF, Sasaki CT. Phantom auditory sensation in rats: an animal model for tinnitus. Behav Neurosci 1988;102:811–22.
55. LeDoux JE. Emotion circuits in the brain. Annu Rev Neurosci 2000;23:155–84.
56. Campeau S, Davis M. Involvement of subcortical and cortical afferents to the lateral nucleus of the amygdala in fear conditioning measured with fear-potentiated startle in rats trained concurrently with auditory and visual conditioned stimuli. J Neurosci 1995;15:2312–27.
57. Gallagher M, Chiba AA. The amygdala and emotion. Curr Opin Neurobiol 1996;6:221–7.
58. Winer JA, Lee CC, Imaizumi K, Schreiner CE. Challenges to a neuroanatomical theory of plasticity. In: Syka J, Merzenich MM, editors. Functional organization and plasticity of auditory cortex. New York: Klüver Academic/Plenum Publishers; 2004. [In press]
59. Atienza M, Cantero JL, Dominguez-Marin E. The time course of neural changes underlying auditory perceptual learning. Learn Mem 2002;9:138–50.
60. Ahissar E, Ahissar M. Plasticity in auditory cortical circuitry. Curr Opin Neurobiol 1994;4:580–7.
61. Zucker RS, Regehr WG. Short-term synaptic plasticity. Annu Rev Physiol 2002;64:355–405.
62. Finnerty GT, Roberts LSE, Connors BW. Sensory experience modifies the short-term dynamics of neocortical synapses. Nature 1999;400:367–71.
63. Nishimura H, Hashikawa K, Doi K, et al. Sign language 'heard' in the auditory cortex. Nature 1999;397:116.
64. Calford MB, Tweedale R. Immediate and chronic changes in response of somatosensory cortex in adult flying-fox after digit amputation. Nature 1988;332:446–8.
65. Dietrich V, Nieschalk M, Stoll W, et al. Cortical reorganization in patients with high frequency cochlear hearing loss. Hear Res 2001;158:95–101.
66. Rauschecker JP. Cortical map plasticity in animals and humans. Prog Brain Res 2002;138:73–88.
67. Pantev C, Engelien A, Candia V, Elbert T. Representational cortex in musicians. Plastic alterations in response to musical practice. Ann N Y Acad Sci 2001;930:300–14.
68. Gizewski ER, Gasser T, de Greiff A, et al. Cross-modal plasticity for sensory and motor activation patterns in blind subjects. Neuroimage 2003;19:968–75.
69. Goldreich D, Kanics IM. Tactile acuity is enhanced in blindness. J Neurosci 2003;23:3439–45.
70. Kleim JA, Barbay S, Cooper NR, et al. Motor learning-dependent synaptogenesis is localized to functionally reorganized motor cortex. Neurobiol Learn Mem 2002;77:63–77.
71. Yoneoka Y, Fujii Y, Nakada T. Central tinnitus: a case report. Ear Nose Throat J 2001;80:864–6.
72. Calabresi P, Centonze D, Pisani A, et al. Synaptic plasticity in the ischaemic brain. Lancet Neurol 2003;2:622–9.
73. Jenkins WM, Merzenich MM. Reorganization of neocortical representations after brain injury: a neurophysiological model of the bases of recovery from stroke. Prog Brain Res 1987;71:249–66.
74. Sippy T, Cruz-Martin A, Jeromin A, Schweizer FE. Acute changes in short-term plasticity at synapses with elevated levels of neuronal calcium sensor-1. Nat Neurosci 2003;6:1031–8.
75. Markram H, Lübke J, Frotscher M, Sakmann B. Regulation of synaptic efficacy by coincidence of postsynaptic APs and EPSPs. Science 1997;275:213–5.
76. Egger V, Feldmeyer D, Sakmann B. Coincidence detection and changes of synaptic efficacy in spiny stellate neurons in rat barrel cortex. Nat Neurosci 1999;2:1098–105.
77. Edeline J. Learning-induced physiological plasticity in the thalamocortical sensory systems: a critical evaluation of receptive field plasticity, map changes and their potential mechanisms. Prog Neurobiol 1999;57:165–224.
78. Shen M, Kim MJ. Postsynaptic signaling and plasticity mechanisms. Science 2002;298:776–80.
79. Wall PD. The presence of ineffective synapses and circumstances which unmask them. Philos Trans R Soc Lond B Biol Sci 1977;278:361–72.
80. Fritz J, Shamma S, Elhilali M, Klein D. Rapid task-related plasticity of spectrotemporal receptive fields in primary auditory cortex. Nat Neurosci 2003;6:1216–23.
81. Phillips DP, Hall SE. Multiplicity of inputs in the afferent path to cat auditory cortex neurons revealed by tone-on-tone masking. Cereb Cortex 1992;2:425–33.

82. Blake DT, Merzenich MM. Changes of AI receptive fields with sound density. J Neurophysiol 2002; 88:3409–20.
83. Kral A, Majernik V. On lateral inhibition in the auditory system. Gen Physiol Biophys 1996;15:109–27.
84. Gerken GM. Central tinnitus and lateral inhibition: an auditory brainstem model. Hear Res 1996;97:75–83.
85. Bruce IC, Sachs MB, Young ED. An auditory-periphery model of the effects of acoustic trauma on auditory nerve responses. J Acoust Soc Am 2003; 113:369–88.
86. Langner G, Wallhaeusser-Franke E. Computer simulation of a tinnitus model based on labeling of tinnitus activity in the auditory cortex. In: Hazell J, editor. Proceedings of the Sixth International Tinnitus Seminar. London: The Tinnitus and Hyperacusis Centre; 1999. p. 20–5.
87. Jacobs KM, Donoghue JP. Reshaping the cortical motor map by unmasking latent intracortical connections. Science 1991;251:944–7.
88. Fox K. Anatomical pathways and molecular mechanisms for plasticity in the barrel cortex. Neuroscience 2002;111:799–814.
89. Florence SL, Taub HB, Kaas JH. Large-scale sprouting of cortical connections after peripheral injury in adult macaque monkeys. Science 1998;282:1117–21.
90. Hickmott PW, Merzenich MM. Local circuit properties underlying cortical reorganization. J Neurophysiol 2002;88:1288–301.
91. Hebb DO. The organization of behaviour. New York: Wiley; 1949.
92. Cruikshank SJ, Weinberger NM. Receptive-field plasticity in the adult auditory cortex induced by hebbian covariance. J Neurosci 1996;16:861–75.
93. Malinow R, Malenka RC. AMPA receptor trafficking and synaptic plasticity. Annu Rev Neurosci 2002; 25:103–26.
94. Recanzone GH, Merzenich MM, Dinse HR. Expansion of the cortical representation of a specific skin field in primary somatosensory cortex by intracortical microstimulation. Cereb Cortex 1992;2:181–96.
95. Spengler F, Dinse HR. Reversible relocation of representational boundaries of adult rats by intracortical microstimulation. Neuroreport 1994;5:949–53.
96. Valentine PA, Eggermont JJ. Intracortical microstimulation induced changes in spectral and temporal response properties in cat auditory cortex. Hear Res 2003;183:109–25.
97. Wang J, Salvi RJ, Powers N. Plasticity of response properties of inferior colliculus neurons following acute cochlear damage. J Neurophysiol 1996; 75:171–83.
98. Salvi RJ, Wang J, Ding D. Auditory plasticity and hyperactivity following cochlear damage. Hear Res 2000;147:261–74.
99. Wang J, Ding D, Salvi RJ. Functional reorganization in chinchilla inferior colliculus associated with chronic and acute cochlear damage. Hear Res 2002;168:238–49.
100. Gerken GM, Saunders SS, Paul RE. Hypersensitivity to electrical stimulation of auditory nuclei follows hearing loss in cats. Hear Res 1984;13:249–60.
101. Cannon WB, Rosenbleuth A. The supersensitivity of denervated structures. New York: Macmillan; 1949.
102. Hains BC, Willis WD, Hulsebosch CE. Serotonin receptors 5-HT1A and 5-HT3 reduce hyperexcitability of dorsal horn neurons after chronic spinal cord hemisection injury in rat. Exp Brain Res 203; 149:174–86.
103. Rajan R. Receptor organ damage causes loss of cortical surround inhibition without topographic map plasticity. Nat Neurosci 1998;1:138–43.
104. Jones EG. Cortical and subcortical contributions to activity-dependent plasticity in primate somatosensory cortex. Annu Rev Neurosci 2000;23:1–37.
105. Krnjevic K. Role of GABA in cerebral cortex. Can J Physiol Pharmacol 1997;75:439–51.
106. Recanzone G, Schreiner CE, Merzenich MM. Plasticity in the frequency representation of primary auditory cortex following discrimination training in adult owl monkeys. J Neurosci 1993;13:87–103.
107. Recanzone GH, Merzenich MM, Schreiner CE. Changes in the distributed temporal response properties of SI cortical neurons reflect improvements in performance on a temporally based tactile discrimination task. J Neurophysiol 1992;67:1071–91.
108. Diamond DM, Weinberger NM. Role of context in the expression of learning-induced plasticity of single neurons in auditory cortex. Behav Neurosci 1989;103:471–94.
109. Beitel RE, Schreiner CE, Cheung SW, et al. Reward-dependent plasticity in the primary auditory cortex of adult monkeys trained to discriminate temporally modulated signals. Proc Nat Acad Sci U S A 2003;10:1083–9.
110. Blake DT, Strata F, Churchland AK, Merzenich MM. Neural correlates of instrumental learning in primary auditory cortex. Proc Nat Acad Sci U S A 2002; 99:10114–9.

111. Diamond DM, Weinberger NM. Role of context in the expression of learning-induced plasticity of single neurons in auditory cortex. Behav Neurosci 1989;103:471–94.
112. Clark SA, Allard T, Jenkins WM, Merzenich MM. Syndactyly results in the emergence of double digit receptive fields in somatosensory cortex in adult owl monkeys. Nature 1988;332:444–5.
113. Disterhoft JF, Stuart DK. Trial sequence of changed unit activity in auditory system of alert rat during conditioned response acquisition and extinction. J Neurophysiol 1976;39:266–81.
114. Bakin JS, Weinberger NM. Classical conditioning induces CS-specific receptive field plasticity in the auditory cortex of the guinea pig. Brain Res 1990;536:271–86.
115. Ahissar E, Vaadia E, Ahissar M, et al. Dependence of cortical plasticity on correlated activity of single neurons and on behavioral context. Science 1992;257:1412–5.
116. Jastreboff PJ, Jastreboff MM. Tinnitus retraining therapy (TRT) as a method for treatment of tinnitus and hyperacusis patients. J Am Acad Audiol 2000;11:162–77.
117. Jastreboff PJ, Hazell JW. A neurophysiological approach to tinnitus: clinical implications. Br J Audiol 1993;27:7–17.
118. Byl N, Roderick J, Mohamed O, et al. Effectiveness of sensory and motor rehabilitation of the upper limb following the principles of neuroplasticity: patients stable poststroke. Neurorehabil Neural Repair 2003;17:176–91.
119. Richardson MP, Strange BA, Duncan JS, Dolan RJ. Preserved verbal memory function in left medial temporal pathology involves reorganisation of function to right medial temporal lobe. Neuroimage 2003;20 Suppl 1:S112–9.
120. Scharfman HE. Epilepsy as an example of neural plasticity. Neuroscientist 2002;8:154–73.
121. Hurst RW, Lee SI. Ictal tinnitus. Epilepsia 1986;27:769–72.
122. Hasselmo ME. Neuromodulation and cortical function: modeling the physiological basis of behavior. Behav Brain Res 1995;67:1–27.
123. Gu Q. Neuromodulatory transmitter systems in the cortex and their role in cortical plasticity. Neuroscience 2002;111:815–35.
124. Møller AR, Rollins PR. The non-classical auditory pathways are involved in hearing in children but not in adults. Neurosci Lett 2002;319:41–4.
125. Dinse HR, Ragert P, Pleger B, et al. Pharmacological modulation of perceptual learning and associated cortical reorganization. Science 2003;301:91–4.
126. Shute CC, Lewis PR. Cholinergic pathways. Pharmacol Ther 1975;1:79–87.
127. Ashe JH, McKenna TM, Weinberger NM. Cholinergic modulation of frequency receptive fields in auditory cortex: II. Frequency-specific effects of anticholinesterases provide evidence for a modulatory action of endogenous ACh. Synapse 1989;4:44–54.
128. McKenna TM, Ashe JH, Weinberger NM. Cholinergic modulation of frequency receptive fields in auditory cortex: I. Frequency-specific effects of muscarinic agonists. Synapse 1989;4:30–43.
129. Metherate R, Weinberger NM. Cholinergic modulation of responses to single tones produces tone-specific receptive field alterations in cat auditory cortex. Synapse 1990;6:133–45.
130. Bakin JS, Weinberger NM. Induction of a physiological memory in the cerebral cortex by stimulation of the nucleus basalis. Proc Natl Acad Sci U S A 1996;93:11219–24.
131. Kilgard MP, Merzenich MM. Cortical map reorganization enabled by nucleus basalis activity. Science 1998;279:1714–8.
132. Mesulam MM, Mufson EJ, Wainer BH, Levey AI. Central cholinergic pathways in the rat: an overview based on an alternative nomenclature (Ch1-Ch6). Neuroscience 1983;10:1185–201.
133. Hars B, Maho C, Edeline JM, Hennevin E. Basal forebrain stimulation facilitates tone-evoked responses in the auditory cortex of awake rat. Neuroscience 1993;56:61–74.
134. Kilgard MP, Pandya PK, Vazquez J, et al. Sensory input directs spatial and temporal plasticity in primary auditory cortex. J Neurophysiol 2001;86:326–38.
135. Bear MF, Singer W. Modulation of visual cortex plasticity by acetylcholine and noradrenaline. Nature 1986;320:172–6.
136. Rogawski MA, Aghajanian GK. Norepinephrine and serotonin: opposite effects on the activity of lateral geniculate neurons evoked by optic pathway stimulation. Exp Neurol 1980;69:678–94.
137. Stark H, Scheich H. Dopaminergic and serotonergic neurotransmission systems are differentially involved in auditory cortex learning: a long-term microdialysis study of metabolites. J Neurochem 1997;68:691–7.
138. Simpson JJ, Davies WE. A review of evidence in support of a role for 5-HT in the perception of tinnitus. Hear Res 2000;145:1–7.

139. Kasamatsu T. Studies on regulation of ocular dominance plasticity: strategies and findings. In: Albowitz B, Albus K, Kuhnt U, et al, editors. Structural and functional organization of the neocortex. Berlin: Springer-Verlag; 1994. p. 68–80.
140. Brennan TJ, Seeley WW, Kilgard M, et al. Sound-induced seizures in serotonin 5-HT2C receptor mutant mice. Nat Genet 1997;16:387–90.
141. Robinson SK, Viirre ES, Bailey KA, et al. Randomized placebo controlled trial of selective serotonin reuptake inhibitors in the treatment of tinnitus. [In preparation]
142. Jay TM. Dopamine: a potential substrate for synaptic plasticity and memory mechanisms. Prog Neurobiol 2003;69:375–90.
143. Bao S, Chan VT, Merzenich MM. Cortical remodeling induced by activity of ventral tegmental dopamine neurons. Nature 2001;412:79–83.
144. Bao S, Chan VT, Zhang L, Merzenich MM. Suppression of cortical representation through backward conditioning. Proc Nat Acad Sci U S A 2003;100:1405–8.
145. Devilbiss DM, Waterhouse BD. Norepinephrine exhibits two distinct profiles of action on sensory cortical neuron responses to excitatory synaptic stimuli. Synapse 2000;37:273–82.
146. Rogawski MA, Aghajanian GK. Modulation of lateral geniculate neurone excitability by noradrenaline microiontophoresis or locus coeruleus stimulation. Nature 1980;287:731–4.
147. Lecas JC. Noradrenergic modulation of tactile responses in rat cortex. Current source-density and unit analyses. C R Acad Sci III 2001;324:33–44.
148. Kasamatsu T. Adrenergic regulation of visuocortical plasticity: a role of the locus coeruleus system. Prog Brain Res 1991;88:599–616.
149. Bouret S, Sara SJ. Locus coeruleus activation modulates firing rate and temporal organization of odour-induced single-cell responses in rat piriform cortex. Eur J Neurosci 2002;16:2371–82.
150. Sara SJ. Noradrenergic modulation of selective attention: its role in memory retrieval. Ann N Y Acad Sci 1985;444:178–93.
151. Yukie M. Connections between the amygdala and auditory cortical areas in the macaque monkey. Neurosci Res 2002;42:219–29.
152. Imamura K, Kasamatsu T. Interaction of noradrenergic and cholinergic systems in regulation of ocular dominance plasticity. Neurosci Res 1989;6:519–36.

EDITORIAL COMMENTARY

Kaltenbach and colleagues cite evidence of increased spontaneous activity in the dorsal cochlear nucleus and primary auditory cortex, alteration in temporal firing patterns (increases in burst firing and synchronous discharging of different neurons), and tonotopic reorganization as neural correlates of tinnitus owing to intense sound or salicylate. They make the case for hearing loss and tinnitus involving different mechanisms even though the mechanism for the generation of tinnitus may be initiated by hearing loss. The time courses of the development of hyperactivity in the dorsal cochlear nucleus and hearing loss after exposure to intense sound are different and suggest that they evolve from different mechanisms. Kaltenbach and colleagues point out that emergence of hyperactivity in the dorsal cochlear nucleus after intense sound exposure involves plastic changes that continue to evolve for many months.

They note that there is no consistent relationship between the pitch of tinnitus and the spectral distribution of the hearing loss and relate the pitch of tinnitus to the activation of neurons with high characteristic frequencies. Kaltenbach and colleagues speculate that the sound percepts of tinnitus are due to increased spontaneous activity and perhaps increased synchrony in the auditory cortex and that the pitches of those percepts are determined by the characteristic frequencies that dominate in the expanded (reorganized) region.

Cacace emphasizes the central role of the amygdala in the processing and expression of emotion and cites the increasing frequency with which emotion owing to tinnitus is linked to the amygdala.

Auditory projections from the thalamus and cortex to the amygdala are thought to be important for developing conditioned reactions, with the latter being more prominent. Cacace notes that fear-conditioned reactions may primarily affect learning and memory processes or may disrupt the ability to perform effectively. In tinnitus, conditioning through fear enables the amygdala to regulate homeostasis and behavior, potentially resulting in anxiety and phobias.

Cacace points out that fear conditioning, fear learning, and plasticity affect nonauditory brain sites, such as the locus ceruleus, periaqueductal gray area, and lateral parabranchial nucleus, areas known to be associated with arousal, anxiety, stress, and pain.

Eggermont delineates spontaneous neural hyperactivity and hypoactivity in the lemniscal (tonotopically organized) and nonlemniscal (multimodal) parts of the brain in response to tinnitus-inducing agents (salicylates, quinine, and intense sound) and concludes that in the lemniscal pathway, a reduction in spontaneous activity is the rule. The findings of increased spontaneous activity have all been in the dorsal cochlear nucleus that receives multimodal (auditory and somatosensory) input and the nonlemniscal external nucleus of the inferior colliculus.

He emphasizes the small percentage of cortical innervation from subcortical centers and the huge intracortical innervation. Also, the cortical input to the auditory part of the thalamus is much larger than its input from the central nucleus of the inferior colliculus. It is generally inferred that the sites responsible for the initiation, generation, and maintenance of tinnitus are activated in an ascending or afferent progression toward the auditory cortex. Eggermont points out the temporal relationship of the increased spontaneous activity in the auditory cortex appearing in hours and in the dorsal cochlear nucleus in days after exposure to intense sound, as well as the corticofugal pathways to the lemniscal and nonlemniscal nuclear centers. He suggests the possibility that the initiation of increased spontaneous activity after exposure to intense sound comes from the auditory cortex rather than the other way around.

For salicylate and quinine administrations, his and his colleagues' data demonstrate that a significant increase in spontaneous firing is limited to the secondary auditory cortex. After intense sound, clear increases in spontaneous activity have been found in the primary auditory cortex, and these increases are accompanied by increases in neural synchrony. Because these changes occur within minutes of acoustic trauma, it is unlikely that they are all induced through the nonlemniscal pathway. Drug-induced tinnitus and sound-induced tinnitus may have different neural substrates, at least as to cortical areas involved. Tinnitus, in contrast to activity evoked by external sounds, does not show synchrony between cortical areas.

Eggermont raises the questions in the generation of tinnitus of whether the initiation occurs in the primary auditory cortex or whether the neural correlates of tinnitus could be restricted to the secondary auditory cortex and the nonlemniscal pathway.

Schreiner and Cheung emphasize that it is difficult to differentiate between the plastic changes owing to hearing loss and those associated with tinnitus. They point out that plasticity in activating connections between auditory areas and the limbic system may shape the affective impact of tinnitus.

Schreiner and Cheung indicate that although activity-dependent plasticity is most likely involved in the development of tinnitus, learning-induced plasticity, particularly involving the limbic and autonomic nervous systems, may be critical in the development of therapeutic strategies for tinnitus. They have documented that stroke and trauma to the auditory cortex initiate injury-induced plasticity, which may account for rare forms of tinnitus without peripheral influences of input deprivation or altered spontaneous activity.

Schreiner and Cheung point out that neuromodulatory systems probably participate in the emotional associations of tinnitus and in the fear, depression, and phonophobia often found in individuals with tinnitus. They indicate that direct and indirect manipulation of these systems could be used in the treatment of tinnitus, particularly in the context of activity-dependent plasticity. The cholinergic system has potential importance in therapy for tinnitus because its action is stimulus feature directed and because the amygdala is critical for emotional processing. The systemic application of drugs influencing the serotoninergic system, such as the selective serotonin reuptake inhibitors, may reduce the aversive impact of tinnitus.

It remains uncertain whether tinnitus is a consequence of plasticity or if local plasticity is induced by tinnitus. To distinguish between plasticity associated with hearing loss and plasticity associated with tinnitus, Schreiner and Cheung advocate that experimental designs should include behavioral verification of tinnitus and of the hearing loss.

They conclude that behavioral training, augmented with pharmacotherapy, may be the most promising treatment strategy for tinnitus.

James B. Snow Jr

CHAPTER 15

Otologic Evaluation

P. Ashley Wackym, MD, David R. Friedland, MD, PhD

The complete evaluation of the patient with a complaint of tinnitus is important for identifying causes that may be amenable to medical or surgical intervention. This is particularly relevant in cases of pulsatile tinnitus, which often have an underlying organic pathology.[1] The otologic physical examination, therefore, is directed at identifying abnormalities of the cochleovestibular system and the head and neck, which can present with tinnitus as the primary complaint.[2,3] In addition, the office examination can suggest ancillary tests, such as the audiologic assessment, electrophysiologic tests, and radiography, that may aid in the evaluation. This chapter reviews an otologic examination that can be performed in the office or bedside setting with little or no specialized equipment. The components of this examination may not be as sensitive as some of the computerized or electrophysiologic tests, but they can identify important abnormalities of the peripheral cochleovestibular apparatus and aid in the evaluation of tinnitus. This chapter also reviews some of the neuroradiographic findings underlying some of the commonly seen causes of pulsatile tinnitus.

HISTORY TAKING

The evaluation of the tinnitus sufferer always begins with a thorough history because many causes of tinnitus have distinct presentations.[4] A standardized form helps in the evaluation process by directing the questions and ensuring completeness (Figure 15-1). Important factors to determine are associated otologic problems such as otalgia, hearing loss, otorrhea, hearing fluctuation, hyperacusis, recruitment, aural fullness, and vestibular symptoms. These often indicate that the tinnitus is a secondary phenomenon of a primary otologic disorder. Further investigation when presented with positive findings on this review of otologic symptoms would include evaluations for infection, presbycusis and other hearing losses, inner ear trauma, and retrocochlear pathology.

A thorough description of the tinnitus experienced by the patient is essential to establishing a differential diagnosis because patients use the term "ringing" to describe a myriad of nonpulsatile sounds, ranging from a high-pitched tone to the sound of crickets to sizzling sounds to a buzzing or humming like the 60 cycle/s hum from electrical wires. There can also be a wide range of pulsatile sounds associated with a variety of lesions. The nature of the tinnitus can often provide the initial indication of whether there is a primary cochlear lesion or a problem referable to a neighboring structure. Some additional qualities that should be determined include the following: Is the tinnitus always present, or does it occasionally go away? Is it continuous or pulsatile? Does it fluctuate in pitch and intensity? Is it low or high pitched? What type of sound is it? What makes it better or worse? Among some patterns of tinnitus are the frequent association of low-toned, nonpulsatile, seashell-like fluctuating tinnitus with Meniere's disease; intermittent, nonpulsatile, high-pitched tinnitus with seasonal allergies, eustachian tube dysfunction or some medications; pulsatile tinnitus with extracochlear lesions; and continuous, "electric-buzzing" tinnitus with industrial noise exposure. Often, however, additional history is necessary to formulate a differential diagnosis.

It is important in evaluating the patient with tinnitus to identify cochleotoxic exposures to noise and chemicals. A thorough noise exposure history includes military, occupational, and recreational exposures. A military history should identify the duration and level of noise experienced, such as serving in the artillery, using small weapons or large guns, or serving on an aircraft carrier. Audiograms from the service are useful in assessing new changes in the older

| CC: _____ | Referring Physician: _____ |

HPI:	
	Age: _____

Allergies: _____	PMH:	Surgery:
Medications:		
ROS:		

Otologic Symptoms	**Associated History**	
☐ Otalgia (R) (L)	Noise Exposure:	
☐ Otorrhea: (R) (L)	Chemo Tx:	IV Abx:
☐ Hearing Loss: (R) (L)	Family Hx:	Cane/Walker:
☐ Hearing Fluctuation: (R) (L)	Stressors:	Hearing Aids:
☐ Tinnitus: (R) (L)	Caffeine:	Sodium:
☐ Aural Pressure: (R) (L)	Tobacco:	ETOH:
☐ Recruitment/Hyperacusis: (R) (L)		
☐ Lightheadedness:	**Diagnostics**	
☐ Vertigo/Disequilibrium:	Audio:	
☐ Sinonasal Problems:	ENG/Rotary:	
☐ Migraines/Scotomas:	Radiology:	
☐ Ear Surgery:		
☐ Ear Infections:	Other:	

FIGURE 15-1. Sample template for acquiring a complete history from the patient with a complaint of tinnitus. It is important to correlate otologic signs and symptoms with changes in tinnitus. Inquiring as to potential ototoxic exposures is likewise important. Reproduced with permission, copyright © 2003 P. Ashley Wackym, MD. CC = chief complaint; ChemoTx = history of chemotherapy; ENG = electronystagmography; ETOH = alcohol use; HPI = history of present illness; Hx = history; IV Abx = history of potentially ototoxic intravenous antibiotics; L = left ear; PMH = past medical history; R = right ear; ROS = review of systems.

patient. Occupational histories should include the type of noise, daily duration of exposure, duration of use of ear protection, and type of protection (eg, foam plugs, headphone style, or noise cancellation devices). Attention should be paid to the nature of the occupation and the potential for unilateral or differential cochlear damage. For example, truckers in the United States commonly have greater noise-induced hearing loss and, subsequently, tinnitus in the left ear because it is closer to the window and traffic noise. Similarly, a right-handed carpenter may have worse hearing and tinnitus in the right ear because the head shadows the left ear from the acoustic energy of the hammering. Recreational exposures are most often overlooked but likely account for a significant portion of an individual's noise experience. Questions regarding hunting, target shooting, woodworking, motorcycle riding, lawn mowing, farming, loud music, and night clubs should be routinely asked. Degrees of exposure are important, and even the difference between deer hunting (few shots) and duck hunting (many shots) can account for additional hearing losses.

Potentially cochleotoxic chemical exposures should also be investigated because they can cause inner ear damage and lead to tinnitus.[5–8] Occupational exposure to styrenes, insecticides, and heavy metals is cochleotoxic and can cause damage synergistically with noise in the workplace. Similarly, some medications, such as aminoglycosides, loop diuretics, aspirin, and quinines, can affect the inner ear and produce tinnitus.

The association of tinnitus with disturbances of balance can indicate inner ear, retrocochlear, or central pathology. True vertigo is commonly caused by primary vestibular abnormalities but can also be due to brainstem or cerebellar infarction or dysfunction. Disequilibrium may be related to an uncompensated vestibular insult but is also found in central sensory integration problems, extremity neuropathies, drug toxicities, endocrine and metabolic disorders, and infections. Lightheadedness is a common complaint and is usually posturally related, thus indicating an orthostatic or autonomic component. Its association with tinnitus, however, may also indicate low blood sugar, anemia, or medication side effects.

Additional information to obtain includes current and past medications, medical problems (eg, diabetes, hypertension, arrhythmias), and prior surgeries (particularly otologic surgery or high blood loss procedures). Head trauma, alcohol and illegal drug use, occupational exposure to neurotoxic chemicals, chemotherapy, and radiation may also contribute to produce tinnitus.

GENERAL EXAMINATION

The physical examination, like the history, can be guided by a standardized template to aid in organizing the evaluation (Figure 15-2). The initial examination of the patient should focus on appearance and basic function. For example, how a patient walks into the examination room can suggest associated vestibular pathology.[9] Factors such as the use of assistive devices (eg, canes, walkers, wheelchairs), pace of walking, normal or wide-based gait, large or narrow radius turns, and whether the head is held stiff and in line with the body are clues to overall function. Patients with unilateral labyrinthine lesions may turn normally to the good side but take a wide-radius turn toward the affected side. The patient's head position, whether in an examination chair, stretcher, or hospital bed, can be very helpful. For example, an acute unilateral vestibular lesion affecting the otolith organs can induce a head-tilt to the side of the lesion.[10] This is associated with ocular roll and vertical deviation owing to the asymmetric otolith activation.[11] Affect and mood are also important in the evaluation because depression and somatization disorders are intimately associated with many complaints of disabling tinnitus.[12,13]

OTOLOGIC EXAMINATION

The otologic examination is important to rule out acute and chronic disease processes that can affect inner ear function. In the poor historian, look for postauricular and craniotomy incisions. Examine the tympanic membrane for signs of chronic eustachian tube dysfunction, perforation, acute infection, chronic suppurative otitis media, and cholesteatoma. The nose, oral cavity, and pharynx should also be examined to identify processes that can affect the eustachian tube, such as acute or chronic rhinosinusitis, hypertrophic lymphoid tissue, and nasopharyngeal masses. Oral examination should include assessment of the temporomandibular joints because there is an increased incidence of tinnitus in temporomandibular joint disorders.[14–16] A summary of the basic office or bedside physical examination methods that can be employed in the evaluation of the patient with tinnitus is presented in Table 15-1.

Cranial Nerves

A cranial nerve examination is important in evaluating the patient for associated lesions. Such findings may suggest a stroke or intracranial or skull base neoplasm. Generally, the olfactory nerve is not tested, but cranial nerves (CNs) II to XII are examined. The optic nerve is readily tested by having the patient read an eye chart or even newsprint with each eye. The oculomotor (CN III), trochlear (CN IV), and abducens (CN VI) nerves are tested by having the patient track the examiner's finger in left-right, up-down, and diagonal directions. The trigeminal nerve (CN V) can be tested for sensation with pinprick of the face or gentle touching of the cornea with a cotton fiber to elicit a blink reflex. Care must be taken to distinguish the afferent (CN V) from efferent (CN VII) limbs of this protective mechanism. The facial nerve (CN VII) is tested by having the patient show his or her teeth, pucker as though kissing, move the midface or nose (as though smelling something foul), close the eyes tightly, and raise the eyebrows. Facial nerve weakness is recorded using the House-Brackmann scale.[17] Isolated weakness is suggestive of a peripheral lesion distal to the stylomastoid foramen. The cochleovestibular nerve (CN VIII) can be assessed with bedside vestibular tests and the use of tuning forks, which are discussed in the following section. The glossopharyngeal nerve (CN IX) is difficult to test in isolation and is often evaluated

General				Appearance:	☐ WNWD	☐ other _____
T _____		P _____		Alertness:	☐ awake/alert	☐ somnolent
BP _____		Wt _____		Speech/Voice:	☐ normal	☐ other _____

Otologic
Pinna: ☐ wnl ☐ lesion ☐ erythema ☐ edema ☐ tender
EACs: ☐ wnl ☐ cerumen ☐ other: _____
TMs: ☐ wnl ☐ retracted ☐ bulging ☐ perforated ☐ fluid ☐ opaque/erythema
☐ Fistula/Hennebert: (R) (L) (+) (-)   ☐ Whisper(R) (L) (+) (-)

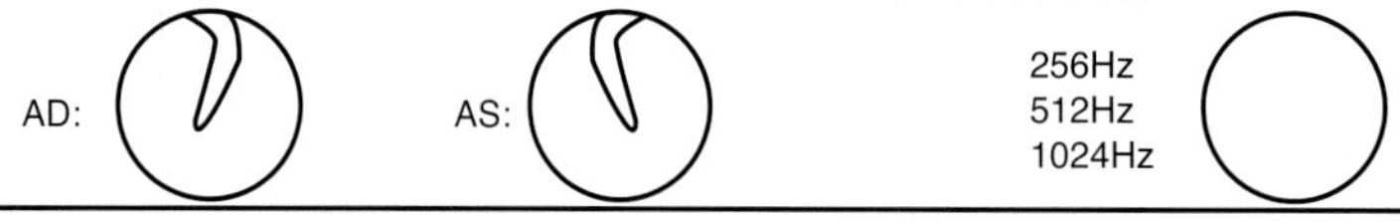

AD: AS: 256Hz / 512Hz / 1024Hz

Neuro/Vestibular
CN II – XII: ☐ intact ☐ other: _____   Frenzel Lenses:
Facial Nerve: ☐ intact ☐ H-B Grade _____   ☐ Spontaneous Nystagmus   none (R) (L)
Oculomotor: ☐ EOMI ☐ other: _____   ☐ Gaze Evoked Nystagmus   none (R) (L)
Head Thrust: (R) (L) (+) (-)   ☐ Positional Nystagmus   none (R) (L)
Other Vestibular Tests: ☐ Dix-Hallpike   (+) (-) (R) (L)
☐ DVA ☐ Romberg   ☐ Head Shake   none (R) (L)
☐ Fukada Step ☐ Finger-Nose   ☐ Valsalva   none (R) (L)
☐ Sharpened Romberg Gait: _____   ☐ Hyperventilation   none (R) (L)

Head and Neck
Oral Cavity   Nose
Mandible/maxilla: ☐ wnl ☐ other: _____   Nares: ☐ wnl ☐ other: _____
Dentition: ☐ wnl ☐ other: _____   Septum: ☐ wnl ☐ other: _____
Palate: ☐ wnl ☐ other: _____   Turbs: ☐ wnl ☐ other: _____
Tonsils: ☐ wnl ☐ grade: _____   Mucosa: ☐ wnl ☐ other: _____
Mucosa: ☐ wnl ☐ lesion: _____
TMJ: ☐ wnl ☐ other: _____   Neck: ☐ wnl ☐ adenopathy ☐ thyroid

Medical Decision Making:

Follow-up:

Send Copies to: _____   Provider: _____ MD/NP

FIGURE 15-2. Sample template for the performance of a complete otologic physical examination. The otologic section includes a diagram of each tympanic membrane (TM) to document perforations or other abnormalities. The tuning fork diagram is explained in Figure 15-3. The neurovestibular section enables the documentation of Frenzel tests with the direction of any nystagmus. The head thrust template allows the examiner to note positive refixation saccades (+) and the side of their occurrence. If more than just the horizontal semicircular canal (HSCC) was tested, this can also be documented. Reproduced with permission, copyright © 2003 P. Ashley Wackym, MD. AD = auris dexter (right ear); AS = auris sinister (left ear); BP = blood pressure; CN = cranial nerve; DVA = dynamic visual acuity; EAC = external auditory canal; EOMI = extraocular motion intact; H-B Grade = House-Brackmann facial nerve paralysis scale (I–VI); L = left; NP = nurse practitioner; P = pulse rate; R = right; T = temperature; TMJ = temporomandibular joint; turbs = turbinates; wnl = within normal limits; WNWD = well-nourished, well-developed; wt = weight.

with vagal nerve (CN X) motor and sensory function in palatal elevation and gag reflex on both sides. Spinal accessory nerve (CN XI) function can be tested with a shoulder shrug maneuver against resistance. Hypoglossal nerve (CN XII) function is tested by tongue protrusion and movement to the left and right. Abnormalities in the cranial nerve examination should be further evaluated with respect to the potential site

TABLE 15-1. Précis of Several Components of the Otologic Examination

Clinical Examination	Significance of Test
Tuning fork examinations	
Rinne	Distinguishes conductive from sensorineural hearing loss in association with an abnormal Weber examination
Weber	Lateralization can suggest a contralateral labyrinthine insult and hence a vestibular imbalance
Head thrust	Elicitation of a refixation saccade suggests ipsilateral vestibular hypofunction in the canal oriented in the plane of thrust
Frenzel tests	
Spontaneous nystagmus	Fast phase of nystagmus will beat away from the hypofunctional, usually the pathologic, ear
Gaze-evoked nystagmus	Nystagmus will increase in amplitude and frequency when gaze is shifted toward the normal active side (away from the lesioned side)
Head shake	Inducible nystagmus is abnormal, and the fast phase will be away from the lesioned side
Valsalva's maneuvers	
Glottic	Increases intracranial pressure and can suggest central abnormalities or superior canal dehiscence
Nose-pinch	Increases middle ear pressure and suggests perilymphatic fistula or superior canal dehiscence
Hyperventilation nystagmus	Can unmask a vestibular schwannoma or accentuate cerebellar disease
Vibration-induced nystagmus	Induction of nystagmus suggests hypofunction in the ear opposite to the fast phase

of the lesion and may entail consultation (ophthalmology, neurology) or radiographic studies (magnetic resonance imaging [MRI], computed tomography [CT] of the brain, skull base, or neck).

TUNING FORK TESTING

In the simplest of the bedside tests of auditory nerve function, a tuning fork is used. Numerous variations (eg, Bing, Rinne, Weber, Schwabach) have been described to help determine the threshold of hearing and frequency of loss and distinguish conductive from sensorineural hearing losses.[18–22] Several studies have demonstrated the Rinne test to be the most sensitive and reliable for clinical screening.[23–25] The most reliable frequency appears to be around 512 Hz, but multiple frequencies can be used.[23] The lower frequencies are advantageous in the evaluation of the dizzy patient because Meniere's disease often causes low-frequency hearing fluctuation. Two methods of performing the Rinne test have been described. The simpler involves placing the stem of the vibrating fork on the mastoid (bone conduction) and then placing the tines near the ear (air conduction) and asking the patient which is louder. An oblique orientation of the tuning fork tines to the external ear canal can reduce the intensity, so care should be taken to align the outer surface of the tips of the tines perpendicular to the axis of the ear canal. If there is doubt as to the result or equivocation on the patient's part, an alternative method can be used. This entails placing the tuning fork stem against the mastoid until the patient can no longer hear the tone. The fork is then moved into the air-conduction position, and perception is tested. If the tone is heard, this indicates a normal examination or a possible sensorineural hearing loss. If stimulation by bone conduction is perceived louder than by air conduction, a conductive hearing loss is suggested. Errors can be avoided by the appropriate use of masking. The reverse order of presentation of the tone, air to bone, can also be performed.

An adjunct to the Rinne test is the Weber test. The Weber test consists of placing the tuning fork stem on the patient's forehead or, for greater transmission, on an upper incisor tooth. The patient is then asked if he or she hears the tone in one ear or in the middle of the head. Perception of the tone in both ears constitutes a normal examination. Lateralization of the tone implies a conductive hearing loss on the side with tone perception or a sensorineural hearing loss in the contralateral ear. Performing this test in conjunction with the Rinne test can help distinguish between these types of losses. Often patients will comment that they hear the tone bilaterally but more in one ear than in the other. This should not be considered a sign of asymmetric hearing loss and is likely representative of the patient's ear preference and subjective perception. Patients with mixed hearing losses are difficult to evaluate accurately with Weber testing. An easy means of documenting the tuning fork examination is presented in Figure 15-3.

Auscultation

Auscultation is an important part of any physical examination and can be useful in evaluating the patient with tinnitus. The patient with pulsing or "clicking" complaints may have an objective tinnitus that is audible to the examiner. The use of a stethoscope for auscultation of the neck and periauricular region can detect the bruit of carotid stenosis, vascular compression, and arteriovenous malformations (AVMs). Such bruits are often the source of pulsatile tinnitus but may also be signs of vascular compromise, leading to inner ear and brainstem pathology manifesting as subjective "ringing" tinnitus.

Listening directly to the offending ear with a Toynbee tube may also aid in diagnosing tinnitus of eustachian tube and myoclonic origin, as well as paragangliomas. Patients complaining of an intermittent, rhythmic tinnitus may suffer from palatal myoclonus, stapedial muscle spasms, tensor tympani muscle spasm, or a patulous eustachian tube. During such episodes, contractions and associated opening of the eustachian tube can be heard by the examiner. Subsequent direct observation of the tympanic membrane, eustachian tube orifice, or palate may identify the source. Flexible and rigid nasopharyngoscopy can provide high-resolution views of the eustachian tube orifice to aid in diagnosing the patulous tube and visualizing myoclonic activity.

Vestibular Tests

Simple bedside testing in the tinnitus sufferer can often identify associated vestibular abnormalities that indicate further evaluation. For example, tinnitus in one ear with an ipsilateral reduced vestibular response may suggest retrocochlear pathology and prompt MRI for a cerebellopontine angle lesion. This section presents several tests that can be quickly performed in the clinic to help assess vestibular function.

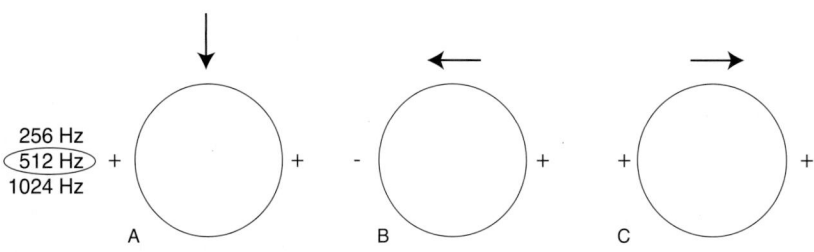

FIGURE 15-3. Easy diagram for documenting the tuning fork examination. The circle represents the patient's head (facing toward the examiner). The plus sign is used to denote a normal Rinne test (air > bone) and the minus sign to denote an abnormal test (bone > air). An arrow is placed to indicate any lateralization on Weber testing. The frequency of tuning fork used is circled. Examples given include a normal examination (A), a conductive hearing loss on the right (B), and a sensorineural hearing loss on the right (C). Reproduced with permission, copyright © 2003 P. Ashley Wackym, MD.

Head Thrust The vestibulo-ocular reflex is extremely rapid and reliable and serves to maintain gaze during head movement. The "head thrust" test exploits this reflex to identify a peripheral vestibular weakness.[26,27] The examiner holds the patient's head with both hands and asks the patient to fix his or her gaze on a stationary object (usually the tip of the examiner's nose). While maintaining gaze, the examiner rapidly turns the patient's head approximately 15 to 20° to the side.[10] Each side is tested while the examiner observes the patient's eyes. A competent vestibular system will allow the patient to maintain fixed gaze without eye deviation. A rapid thrust to a lesioned or hypofunctional side will result in inappropriate eye movements. Specifically, the patient will be unable to maintain fixed gaze and demonstrate a "catch-up" or "refixation" saccade at the end of the movement as his or her eye reacquires the target. With repeated thrusts to a hypofunctional side, patients will improve their performance, so the initial thrusts are the most informative. Typically, the thrusts are performed in the horizontal or yaw plane and thus test the lateral semicircular canals. Head thrusts performed obliquely can be used to test the anterior semicircular canal (downward thrust) and the contralateral posterior canal (backward thrust). Generating high-frequency thrusts in these planes is difficult for most examiners and is not as reliable. The overall reliability of the head thrust examination is less than that of caloric testing and is most useful for acute or profound hypofunction.[28] Care should be taken in performing this procedure on any patient with a history of cervical disease.

Cerebellar Tests Simple cerebellar tests can help distinguish between peripheral and central vestibular abnormalities. Basic tasks include asking the patient to touch alternately his or her nose and the examiner's finger. The examiner places his or her finger both ipsilateral and contralateral to the test hand. Both hands should be tested to identify a unilateral cerebellar abnormality. Other cerebellar tests include rapid alternating movements such as tapping the palmar and dorsal surfaces of one hand on the other in rapid succession. Again, both hands should be tested to identify unilateral lesions.

Spontaneous and Gaze-Evoked Nystagmus Frenzel lenses are essential and easily portable adjuncts to the otologic examination. These glasses typically have 10+ diopter lenses that prevent visual fixation and suppression of nystagmus. They also serve as magnifiers and are usually illuminated to allow better visualization of the patient's iris, which facilitates detecting linear and, particularly, torsional nystagmus. Several tests and observations are made while the patient is wearing these lenses.

Initial observations should be made with the patient seated and looking forward. The patient should be examined for spontaneous nystagmus, and the fast phase component should be noted. The direction of the nystagmus is determined by the direction of the fast phase, and the nystagmus should be described as left or right beating or up- or downbeating and as horizontal, vertical, or torsional with its associated directions (eg, clockwise, counterclockwise). The presence of spontaneous nystagmus is most suggestive of an acute peripheral vestibular process but can be seen with congenital nystagmus or central abnormalities. The fast phase of nystagmus is toward the more active side and thus away from the lesioned side. The presence of vertical nystagmus is strongly suggestive of a cerebellar lesion and should prompt further evaluation for posterior fossa abnormalities.

After assessing for spontaneous nystagmus, the patient is instructed to gaze to the left, right, and upward. Each gaze direction is held for about 5 seconds, and the patient is instructed to return his or her gaze to midline. This process makes use of Alexander's law, which states that gaze in the direction of the fast phase of nystagmus will increase the amplitude and frequency of the nystagmus. A low-grade spontaneous nystagmus can be unmasked by gaze away from an acute peripheral lesion (toward the normal, active side). Inducible nystagmus with upward gaze is typically vertical and, as noted, suggests cerebellar disease. Abnormal eye movements on return to midline gaze (ie, rebound nystagmus) are also indicative of a cerebellar lesion.[29]

Head Shake Examination Ewald's second law states that excitatory responses of the vestibulo-ocular reflex are more pronounced than the inhibitory responses. That is, when the head is turned to one side, the excitatory response elicited in the ipsilateral horizontal canal is farther above baseline than the inhibitory response in the contralateral canal, which is below baseline. Thus, if an individual's head is shaken back and forth rapidly, each side will sum the excitatory responses, and the inhibitory responses will essentially be masked. If there is an asymmetry in vestibular function, the sum of the excitatory responses will reflect this, resulting from relative hypofunction of the weaker side. To exploit this phenomenon clinically, the head shake test is performed.[30,31] As with all head maneuvers, the patient should first be questioned about cervical disease. The patient is seated opposite the examiner with Frenzel lenses in place, and his or her head is rapidly shaken side to side for 10 to 15 seconds. If there is a unilateral weakness, the patient will manifest horizontal nystagmus beating away from the hypofunctional side. In this examination, the result in the individual with bilateral vestibular hypofunction may appear to be normal. Similar to the head thrust examination, this test is not as sensitive as caloric testing for determining asymmetric vestibular function.

Vibration-Induced Nystagmus Warm caloric stimulation is the classic means of causing excitation in the semicircular canals. An alternative means of producing low-frequency stimulation of the vestibular end-organs is with vibration.[32] The placement of a vibratory stimulus, typically a handheld massage device, on the mastoid can cause vestibular activation. Similar to bone-conduction audiometry, the stimulus affects both labyrinths, and an asymmetry will be manifest as fast beating nystagmus away from the side of the lesion. Alternatively, the vibratory stimulus can be placed on the forehead or occiput. Significant asymmetry has to be present to generate nystagmus, and not all individuals are susceptible to vibratory vestibular stimulation. The use of Frenzel lenses will make any inducible nystagmus easier to identify.

Valsalva's Maneuver–Induced Nystagmus The results of Valsalva's maneuvers can be suggestive of perilymphatic fistulae or of superior canal dehiscence. Two forms of Valsalva's maneuvers may be performed: the nose-pinch or glottic closure. The nose-pinch forces air into the eustachian tube and increases pressure within the middle ear. The patient should be instructed to pinch his or her nose and to try to "pop" the ears gently. A young child can be encouraged to perform this maneuver by attempting to inflate a balloon held to one naris. This may elicit momentary nystagmus or oscillopsia in cases of labyrinthine fistula. Alternatively, pneumatic otoscopy can be performed to elicit Hennebert's sign for fistula evaluation. The glottic closure can be elicited by asking the patient to bear down as though lifting something heavy or giving birth. This does not transmit pressure to the middle ear but rather increases intracranial pressure by reducing venous return. In cases of superior canal dehiscence, this has been shown to be associated with the induction of oscillopsia.[33,34]

Hyperventilation-Induced Nystagmus In contrast to Valsalva's maneuver, hyperventilation serves to reduce CO_2 levels and reduces intracranial pressure. Typically, the patient wears Frenzel lenses and is asked to breathe deeply and rapidly for 30 seconds while seated comfortably to prevent falling and injury. Hyperventilation-induced nystagmus has been reported in some cases of vestibular schwannoma (acoustic neuroma). The mechanism is thought to reflect a temporary reduction of pressure on the vestibular nerve and improved axonal conduction.[35] Hyperventilation-induced nystagmus is also useful in accentuating the downbeating nystagmus seen with cerebellar lesions.[28] Asking the patient to compare the induced "lightheadedness" with his or her experience of dizziness during attacks is another means of assessing the nature of the complaints and whether they represent true vertigo.

DIAGNOSTIC STUDIES

Additional diagnostic studies are routinely employed to narrow the differential diagnosis of tinnitus. The audiologic strategies used to evaluate patients with tinnitus are presented in Chapter 16, "Audiologic Assessment"; however, limited discussion, particularly of vestibular testing, is appropriate in the context of the otologic evaluation. Likewise, imaging of tinnitus is presented in Chapter 18, "Imaging Tinnitus"; therefore, the focus will be on MRI, CT, and angiographic tools used to diagnose specific diseases, with a structural basis, that can produce tinnitus.

AUDIOLOGIC ASSESSMENT

The hallmark of the evaluation of the patient with a complaint of tinnitus is the audiogram, and the practitioner should become familiar with hearing loss patterns and their association with tinnitus. Additional tests should be performed based on the findings on the physical examination and review of systems. Electro- or videonystagmography is useful in the patient with tinnitus who has vertigo or if a unilateral vestibular weakness is suspected. Auditory brainstem responses can help in evaluation of a retrocochlear lesion in the patient with an asymmetric sensorineural hearing loss or reduced vestibular response. Evoked electromyography for facial nerve weakness is important for determining severity and planning potential surgical intervention. Vestibular evoked myogenic potentials are increasingly used in the evaluation of otologic disorders such as Meniere's disease and superior canal dehiscence syndrome and may be beneficial if these conditions are suspected.

RADIOGRAPHIC IMAGING

Patients with pulsatile tinnitus or findings on examination and testing that suggest otologic or neurotologic pathology should have radiographic imaging to evaluate them for temporal bone and intracranial lesions.[36,37] The principal imaging modalities include MRI and high-resolution CT. In addition, angiography is often used as a diagnostic, therapeutic, or surgical adjunct for vascular tumors and abnormalities. As a general rule, assessment of processes suspected of affecting the brain, brainstem, cerebellum, or cranial nerves is best accomplished with MRI. For example, the gold standard for diagnosis of vestibular schwannoma is a gadolinium-enhanced MRI of the internal auditory canals. In contrast to MRI use, processes that are felt to be within the temporal bone are best assessed with CT, which better delineates the relationship between structures of the middle and inner ears and the carotid and jugular systems. The use of intravenous contrast is reserved for suspicion of neoplasm but is not necessary for assessment of vascular structures and their abnormalities. For example, the diagnosis of a glomus jugulare is best made by identifying irregular bone erosion around the jugular fossa rather than by contrast-enhanced features. In some instances, CT and MRI are used together for diagnosis and surgical planning. This section reviews many of the causes of pulsatile tinnitus and their radiographic evaluation and appearance (Table 15-2).

As noted above, otologic symptoms, in addition to the nature of the presenting tinnitus, are important in diagnosing and evaluating the patient. The presence of pulsatile tinnitus with a conductive hearing loss is highly suggestive of a reversible and treatable process involving the middle ear. Most commonly, this pattern represents eustachian tube dysfunction and consequent problems ranging from tympanic membrane retraction to serous otitis media to cholesteatoma. The otoscopic examination is thus important in the evaluation to rule out an infectious or pressure-related cause of the tinnitus and conductive hearing loss. If the otoscopic examination is normal or suggests a middle ear abnormality other than fluid or tympanic membrane retraction, further evaluation with CT is recommended.

Conductive hearing loss and pulsatile tinnitus from middle ear dysfunction occur with encroachment on the ossicular chain by vascular and cerebral structures (Figures 15-4 to 15-10). A mass in the middle ear may arise locally but more commonly reflects herniation of a surrounding neurovascular structure. CT evaluation may identify a mass protruding through the middle fossa floor and impacting the ossicular chain (see Figure 15-4). To establish the relationship of the mass to the brain, MRI should be performed (see Figure 15-5). In the illustrated case, the mass represented an encephalocele that was reduced through a middle fossa craniotomy. Vascular abnormalities tend to protrude

TABLE 15-2. Differential Diagnosis of Pulsatile Tinnitus

Idiopathic stapedial muscle spasm

Palatal myoclonus

Patulous eustachian tube

Temporal lobe encephalocele

Vascular abnormalities
    Arteriovenous shunts
        Congenital arteriovenous malformations
        Post-traumatic dural arteriovenous malformations
        Acquired arteriovenous shunt
        Glomus jugulare
        Glomus tympanicum
    Arterial bruits
        High-riding carotid artery
        Carotid stenosis
        Persistant stapedial artery
    Microvascular compression syndrome
    Venous hums
        Dehiscent jugular bulb
        Hypertension
        Transverse sinus obstruction

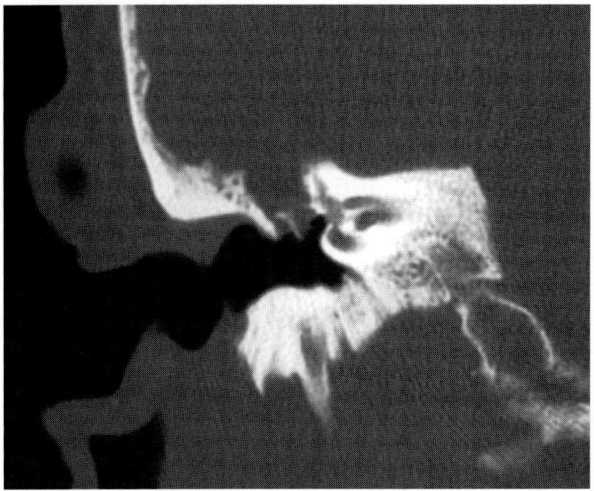

FIGURE 15-4. Unilateral encephalocele. Evaluation of a patient with a 15 to 20 dB conductive hearing loss and pulsatile tinnitus led to the diagnosis of right temporal lobe encephalocele. Coronal computed tomography using bone windows shows a defect in the middle cranial fossa floor and herniation of soft tissue through it. The soft tissue surrounds the ossicular chain (*center*). Normal oval window, vestibule, and basal turn of the cochlea can be seen (*center, right*). Reproduced with permission, copyright © 2003 P. Ashley Wackym, MD.

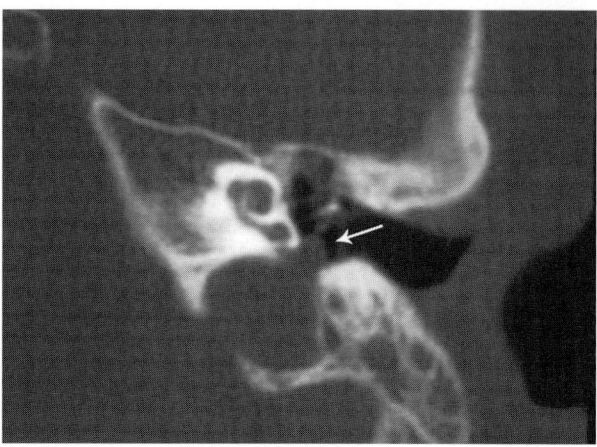

FIGURE 15-6. Dehiscent jugular bulb and pulsatile tinnitus. Axial computed tomographic scan with bone window technique shows a dehiscence within the anterolateral bony margin of the jugular foramen with protrusion of a soft tissue density mass from the foramen into the mesotympanum (*arrow*). Reproduced with permission, copyright © 2003 P. Ashley Wackym, MD.

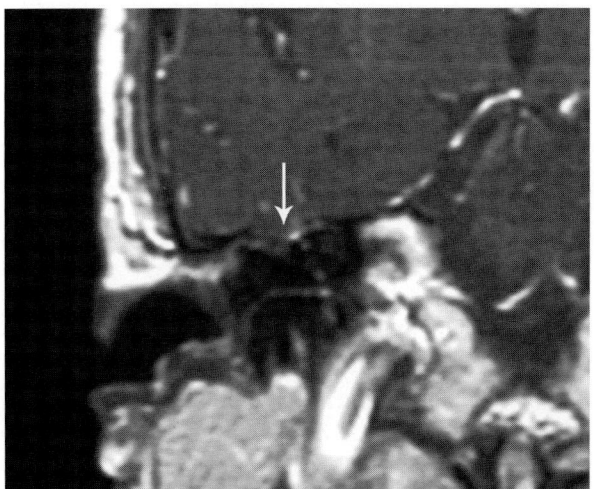

FIGURE 15-5. Unilateral encephalocele. T_1-weighted gadolinium-enhanced coronal magnetic resonance image shows temporal lobe parenchyma herniated through the dura into the epitympanum (*arrow*). Enhanced dura can be seen to the left and right of the encephalocele. Reproduced with permission, copyright © 2003 P. Ashley Wackym, MD.

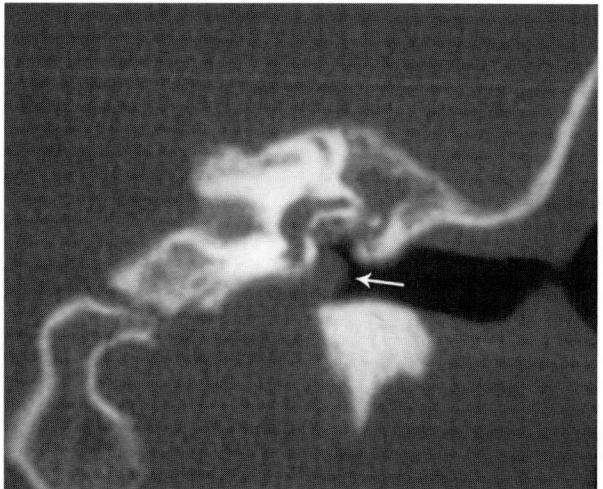

FIGURE 15-7. Dehiscent jugular bulb and pulsatile tinnitus. Coronal bone window computed tomographic scan at the level of the oval window shows protrusion of soft tissue from the jugular foramen into the middle ear cavity. The protruding jugular bulb (*arrow*) extends superiorly over the cochlear promontory toward the stapes footplate. Note opacification of the epitympanum with chronic inflammatory debris. Reproduced with permission, copyright © 2003 P. Ashley Wackym, MD.

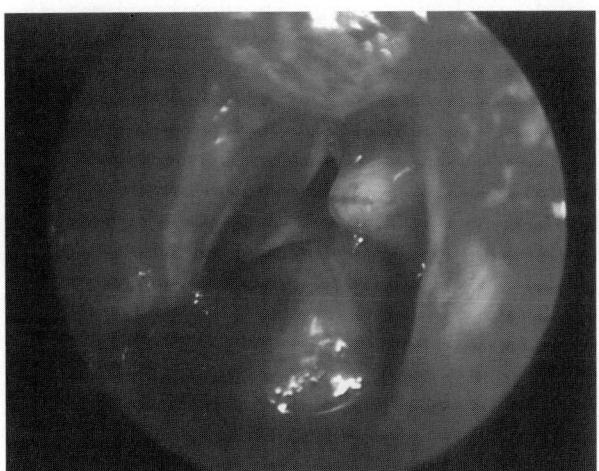

FIGURE 15-8. Dehiscent jugular bulb and pulsatile tinnitus. Intraoperative endoscopic photograph shows the relationship of the dehiscent jugular bulb, the stapes superstructure, and the lenticular process of the incus. Vascular pulsations related to the cardiac cycle were directly transmitted to the ossicular chain. Reproduced with permission, copyright © 2003 P. Ashley Wackym, MD.

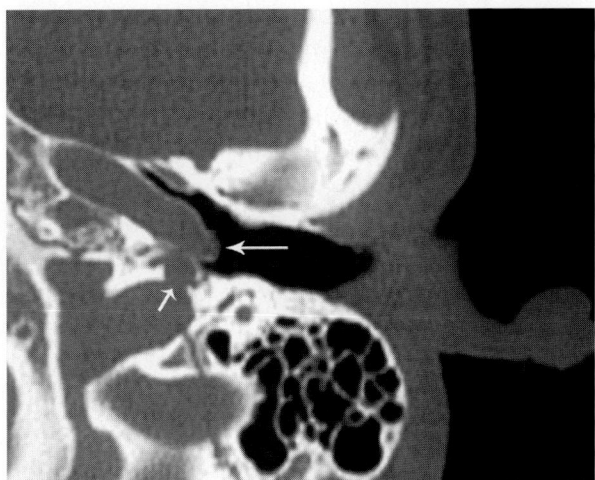

FIGURE 15-10. Dehiscent carotid artery and pulsatile tinnitus (arterial bruit). A 15-year-old child was referred for evaluation of unilateral (left) pulsatile tinnitus. Axial computed tomographic scan with bone window technique shows a dehiscence within the posterolateral bony margin of the carotid canal with protrusion of a portion of the carotid artery into the mesotympanum (*long arrow*). Also note a dehiscence within the anterolateral bony margin of the jugular foramen with protrusion of a portion of the jugular bulb into the mesotympanum (*short arrow*). Reproduced with permission, copyright © 2003 P. Ashley Wackym, MD.

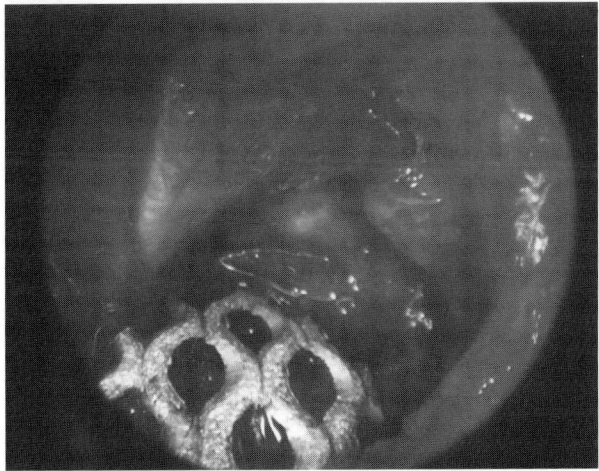

FIGURE 15-9. Dehiscent jugular bulb and pulsatile tinnitus. Endoscopic photograph after decompression of the dehiscent jugular bulb shows reduction of the dehiscence away from the ossicular chain and fixation with titanium mesh. Reproduced with permission, copyright © 2003 P. Ashley Wackym, MD.

from the hypotympanic region, and, occasionally, a blue-hued mass can be seen through the tympanic membrane. A CT scan may demonstrate a dehiscent jugular bulb with extension of a mass over the promontory, even to the ossicular chain (see Figures 15-6 to 15-9). This can be managed surgically with improvement in both the conductive hearing loss and the severity of the tinnitus. The carotid artery may also be dehiscent into the middle ear and may present as a vascular mass (see Figure 15-10). Pulsations and protrusion from the anterior hypotympanum should alert the clinician to this vascular abnormality and prevent the potentially devastating bleeding complications associated with myringotomy.

Arteriovenous malformations (AVMs), particularly dural AVMs, can produce pulsatile tinnitus. In many cases, objective pulsatile tinnitus can be identified in these patients. When a history of intermittent pulsatile tinnitus is relayed, having the patient increase cardiac output by vigorously walking and then performing auscultation with a stethoscope and Toynbee tube may allow subjective pulsatile tinnitus to become objective for the examiner owing to a higher rate of blood flow. Figure 15-11 shows an example of a dural AVM involving the jugular foramen that is being fed principally by the ascending pharyngeal artery and is draining into the jugular bulb. The patient was successfully treated for this lesion with superselective embolization. Other dura-based AVMs along the temporal bone may develop sufficiently turbid blood flow to be perceived by the patient. Such lesions often require a combination of transarterial embolization, stereotactic radiation, and/or surgery for effective control.[38]

In addition to vascular malformations, vascular neoplasms of the temporal bone can produce pulsatile tinnitus. Glomus tympanicum and glomus jugulare tumors often have as their initial presentation complaints of pulsatile tinnitus. The glomus tympanicum tumor typically arises from chemoreceptors over the promontory or along Jacobson's nerve (Figures 15-12 to 15-14). This tumor is commonly seen as a vascular blush behind the tympanic membrane, and if it contacts the membrane, it can be made to blanch with pneumatic otoscopy. The glomus jugulare tumor erodes bone at the jugular foramen, which is a diagnostic feature on CT (Figure 15-15). Associated deficits of the lower cranial nerves can commonly be identified on physical examination. Angiography is frequently used in the evaluation and management of glomus jugulare tumors and can identify principal arterial feeders, which usually arise from the ascending pharyngeal artery (Figure 15-16).

When CT and physical examination fail to demonstrate an intratemporal lesion to explain pulsatile tinnitus, MRI of the posterior fossa can be useful. Other causes for pulsatile tinnitus include vascular compression of the cochleovestibular nerve (Figures 15-17 and 15-18).[39] This can also be accompanied by intermittent attacks of vertigo (eg, disabling positional vertigo).[40] Transtemporal approaches to the cerebellopontine

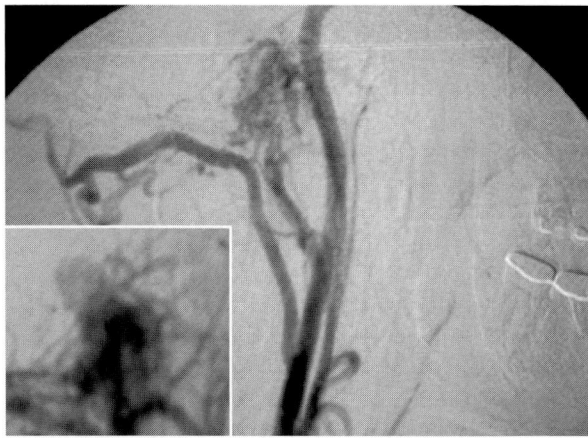

FIGURE 15-11. Dural arteriovenous malformation (AVM) and pulsatile tinnitus. Angiogram of an AVM within the dura near the jugular bulb. The primary arterial supply is from the ascending pharyngeal artery in this patient. *Inset*, left, shows that the venous drainage is via the jugular bulb. Vascular lesions in this region should be distinguished from glomus jugulare and glomus vagal tumors by magnetic resonance imaging and computed tomography, as shown in Figure 15-15. Reproduced with permission, copyright © 2003 P. Ashley Wackym, MD.

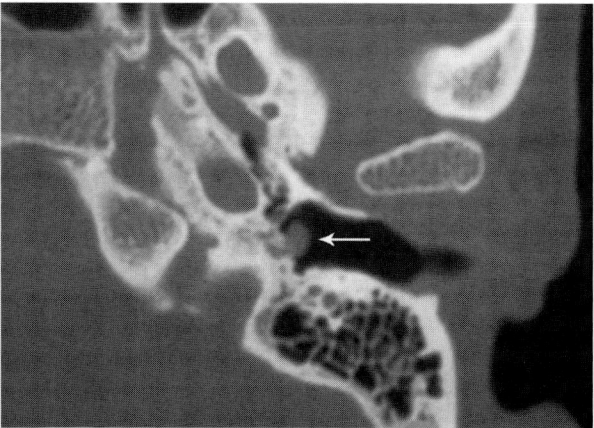

FIGURE 15-12. Glomus tympanicum tumor and pulsatile tinnitus. Evaluation of left-sided pulsatile tinnitus demonstrated a vascular mass touching the tympanic membrane, within the left middle ear. Axial computed tomographic scan with bone window technique shows a soft tissue mass within the mesotympanum (*arrow*). Reproduced with permission, copyright © 2003 P. Ashley Wackym, MD.

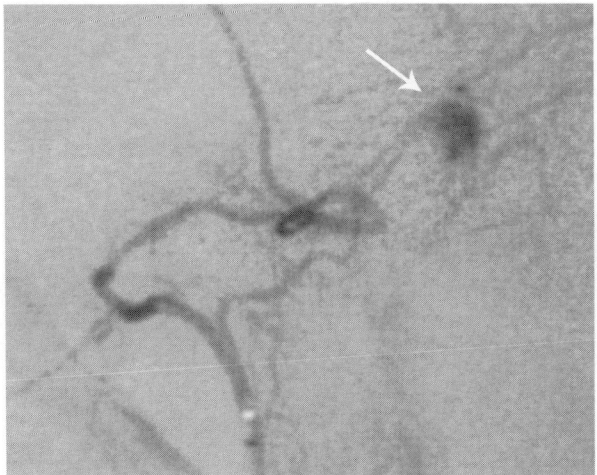

FIGURE 15-13. Glomus tympanicum tumor and pulsatile tinnitus. Pre-embolization angiogram shows a significant tumor blush (*arrow*), suggesting abundant vascular supply from the ascending pharyngeal artery arising from the external carotid artery. Subsequent embolization prepared the patient for surgical resection. Interestingly, the patient experienced marked reduction in her pulsatile tinnitus after embolization. Reproduced with permission, copyright © 2003 P. Ashley Wackym, MD.

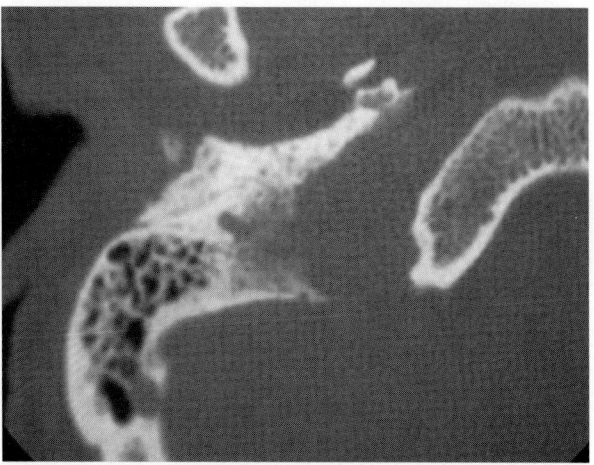

FIGURE 15-15. Glomus jugulare tumor and pulsatile tinnitus. High-resolution computed tomography through the jugular foramen reveals characteristic erosion of the surrounding bone and loss of a sharp cortical bone margin. Intravenous contrast is not critical to establishing this diagnosis. Reproduced with permission, copyright © 2003 P. Ashley Wackym, MD.

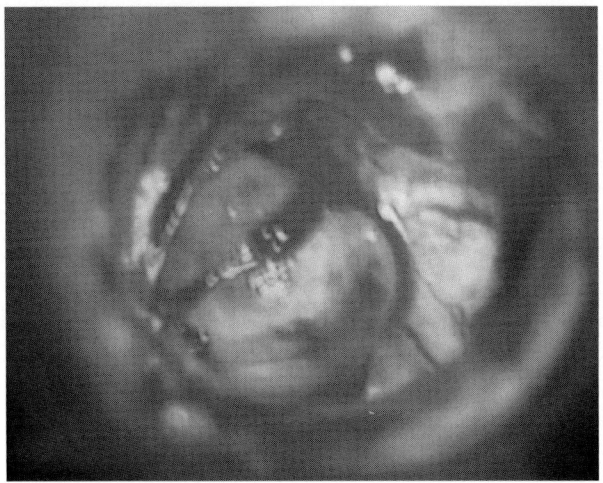

FIGURE 15-14. Glomus tympanicum tumor and pulsatile tinnitus. Intraoperative photograph shows that the embolized tumor has a smooth capsule and is adjacent to the stapes and long process of the incus. Reproduced with permission, copyright © 2003 P. Ashley, MD.

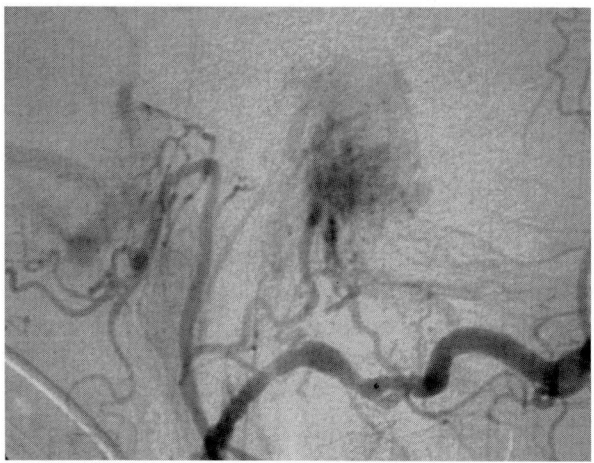

FIGURE 15-16. Glomus jugulare tumor and pulsatile tinnitus. Angiogram of a jugular foramen lesion showing the rich vascularity of glomus tumors. Preoperative angiography with embolization helps control the arterial feeders aiding in the surgical resection. Reproduced with permission, copyright © 2003 P. Ashley Wackym, MD.

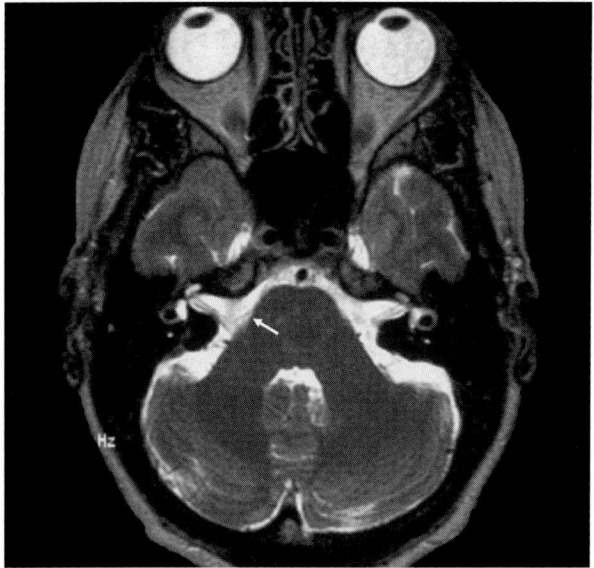

FIGURE 15-17. Microvascular compression syndrome. A woman presented with intractable right unilateral tinnitus. She had been managed medically for several years and did not have a vestibular schwannoma based on previous magnetic resonance imaging (MRI) studies. T_2-weighted MRI shows a vessel crossing the right root entry zone of the eighth nerve complex (*arrow*). Normal cochlea, vestibular apparatus, and cochlear and inferior vestibular nerves are shown. Reproduced with permission from Wackym PA et al.[39]

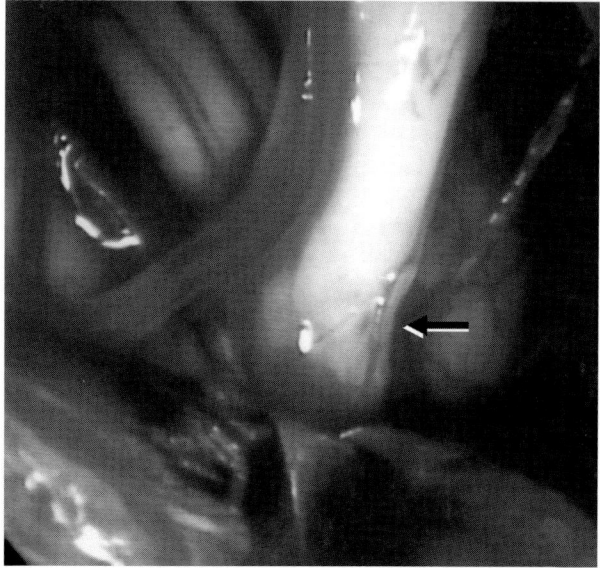

FIGURE 15-18. Microvascular compression syndrome. The patient whose magnetic resonance image is shown in Figure 15-17 underwent microvascular decompression using endoscopic techniques. After mobilization of the vein crossing the root entry zone, indentation and demyelination of the cochlear nerve can be seen (*arrow*). Reproduced with permission from Wackym PA et al.[39]

angle may enable removal of the offending vessel from the cochlear nerve while preserving hearing.

CONCLUSION

The complete examination of the patient with tinnitus is important for identifying aural lesions that may be treatable and curable. This is particularly important in the patient with pulsatile forms of tinnitus. In nonpulsatile tinnitus, identifying associated cochleovestibular abnormalities may prompt further electrophysiologic or radiographic testing. For the patient with, currently, incurable tinnitus, the performance of a complete and thorough otologic evaluation reassures the patient that all issues have been addressed and imparts trust in the physician-patient relationship.

REFERENCES

1. Sismanis A. Pulsatile tinnitus. Otolaryngol Clin North Am 2003;36:389–402.
2. Schwaber MK. Medical evaluation of tinnitus. Otolaryngol Clin North Am 2003;36:287–92.
3. Seabra JC. The medical audiological evaluation of tinnitus patients. Int Tinnitus J 1999;5:53–6.
4. Noell CA, Meyerhoff WL. Tinnitus. Diagnosis and treatment of this elusive symptom. Geriatrics 2003;58:28–34.
5. Makitie AA, Pirvola U, Pyykko I, et al. The ototoxic interaction of styrene and noise. Hear Res 2003;179:9–20.
6. Morata TC, Campo P. Ototoxic effects of styrene alone or in concert with other agents: a review. Noise Health 2002;4:15–24.

7. Seligmann H, Podoshin L, Ben-David J, et al. Drug-induced tinnitus and other hearing disorders. Drug Saf 1996;14:198–212.
8. Rybak LP. Hearing: the effects of chemicals. Otolaryngol Head Neck Surg 1992;106:677–86.
9. Stolze H, Klebe S, Petersen G, et al. Typical features of cerebellar ataxic gait. J Neurol Neurosurg Psychiatry 2002;73:310–2.
10. Eggers SD, Zee DS. Evaluating the dizzy patient: bedside examination and laboratory assessment of the vestibular system. Semin Neurol 2003;23:47–58.
11. Wolfe GI, Taylor CL, Flamm ES, et al. Ocular tilt reaction resulting from vestibuloacoustic nerve surgery. Neurosurgery 1993;32:417–20; discussion 420–1.
12. Dobie RA. Depression and tinnitus. Otolaryngol Clin North Am 2003;36:383–8.
13. Marciano E, Carrabba L, Giannini P, et al. Psychiatric comorbidity in a population of outpatients affected by tinnitus. Int J Audiol 2003;42:4–9.
14. Tuz HH, Onder EM, Kisnisci RS. Prevalence of otologic complaints in patients with temporomandibular disorder. Am J Orthod Dentofacial Orthop 2003;123:620–3.
15. Ren YF, Isberg A. Tinnitus in patients with temporomandibular joint internal derangement. Cranio 1995;13:75–80.
16. Morgan DH. Tinnitus of TMJ origin: a preliminary report. Cranio 1992;10:124–9.
17. Smith IM, Murray JA, Cull RE, Slattery J. A comparison of facial grading systems. Clin Otolaryngol 1992;17:303–7.
18. Pearce JM. Early days of the tuning fork. J Neurol Neurosurg Psychiatry 1998;65:728–33.
19. Ng M, Jackler RK. Early history of tuning-fork tests. Am J Otol 1993;14:100–5.
20. Hinchcliffe R. Tuning fork tests. Br J Audiol 1988;22:153–6.
21. Huizing EH. The early descriptions of the so-called tuning-fork tests of Weber, Rinne, Schwabach, and Bing. III. The development of the Schwabach and Bing tests. ORL J Otorhinolaryngol Relat Spec 1975;37:92–6.
22. Huizing EH. The early descriptions of the so-called tuning-fork tests of Weber, Rinne, Schwabach, and Bing. II. The "Rhine test" and its first description by Polansky. ORL J Otorhinolaryngol Relat Spec 1975;37:88–91.
23. Burkey JM, Lippy WH, Schuring AG, Rizer FM. Clinical utility of the 512-Hz Rinne tuning fork test. Am J Otol 1998;19:59–62.
24. Miltenburg DM. The validity of tuning fork tests in diagnosing hearing loss. J Otolaryngol 1994;23:254–9.
25. Thijs C, Leffers P. Sensitivity and specificity of Rinne tuning fork test. BMJ 1989;298:255.
26. Della Santina CC, Cremer PD, Carey JP, Minor LB. Comparison of head thrust test with head autorotation test reveals that the vestibulo-ocular reflex is enhanced during voluntary head movements. Arch Otolaryngol Head Neck Surg 2002;128:1044–54.
27. Goebel JA. The ten-minute examination of the dizzy patient. Semin Neurol 2001;21:391–8.
28. Fife TD, Tusa RJ, Furman JM, et al. Assessment: vestibular testing techniques in adults and children: report of the Therapeutics and Technology Assessment Subcommittee of the American Academy of Neurology. Neurology 2000;55:1431–41.
29. Hood JD. Further observations on the phenomenon of rebound nystagmus. Ann N Y Acad Sci 1981;374:532–9.
30. Wei D, Hain TC, Proctor LR. Head-shaking nystagmus: associations with canal paresis and hearing loss. Acta Otolaryngol (Stockh) 1989;108:362–7.
31. Hain TC, Fetter M, Zee DS. Head-shaking nystagmus in patients with unilateral peripheral vestibular lesions. Am J Otolaryngol 1987;8:36–47.
32. Hamann KF, Schuster EM. Vibration-induced nystagmus—a sign of unilateral vestibular deficit. ORL J Otorhinolaryngol Relat Spec 1999;61:74–9.
33. Minor LB. Superior canal dehiscence syndrome. Am J Otol 2000;21:9–19.
34. Minor LB, Solomon D, Zinreich JS, Zee DS. Sound- and/or pressure-induced vertigo due to bone dehiscence of the superior semicircular canal. Arch Otolaryngol Head Neck Surg 1998;124:249–58.
35. Minor LB, Haslwanter T, Straumann D, Zee DS. Hyperventilation-induced nystagmus in patients with vestibular schwannoma. Neurology 1999;53:2158–68.
36. Corr P, Tsheole-Marishane L. Pulsatile tinnitus. Br J Radiol 2001;74:669–70.
37. Marsot-Dupuch K. Pulsatile and nonpulsatile tinnitus: a systemic approach. Semin Ultrasound CT MR 2001;22:250–70.
38. Lewis AI, Rosenblatt SS, Tew JM Jr. Surgical management of deep-seated dural arteriovenous malformations. J Neurosurg 1997;87:198–206.
39. Wackym PA, King WA, Meyer GA, et al. Endoscope-assisted surgery of the trigeminal, facial, cochlear or vestibular nerve. In: Wackym PA, Rice DH, Schaefer SD, editors. Minimally invasive surgery of the head, neck and cranial base. Philadelphia: Lippincott Williams and Wilkins; 2002. p. 101–16.
40. Brackmann DE, Kesser BW, Day JD. Microvascular decompression of the vestibulocochlear nerve for disabling positional vertigo: the House Ear Clinic experience. Otol Neurotol 2001;22:882–7.

CHAPTER 16

Audiologic Assessment

James A. Henry, PhD

Patients with hearing difficulties have a clear course of action if and when they decide to pursue a clinical evaluation of their condition. Ear and hearing specialists practice in every major city in this country, and their services are comparable. These patients can receive a medical evaluation from an otolaryngologist (or otologist) and an audiologic assessment from an audiologist. The type of training these professionals receive is consistent, and assessment procedures are fairly standardized. Patients thus know what to expect and will generally receive a high level of services that are fairly uniform across clinics.

The professional consistency that exists for managing hearing difficulties does not exist for managing "the other" auditory disorder, tinnitus. Patients with tinnitus do not have a clear course of action and often resort to Internet searches and long-distance telephone calls in the attempt to find help. The information they receive will be vastly different depending on their source of information and advice. The lack of professional standards for clinical tinnitus management is explainable because tinnitus management is not a major focus of most professional training programs. Until training standards are developed and implemented, this scenario is not likely to change.

Tinnitus management includes two broad components: assessment of the disorder and therapeutic intervention. The present chapter focuses on providing guidelines to perform a psychoacoustic test battery for the patient with tinnitus, which is an important aspect of the assessment component. Most of the methods that are described are not new; they have the benefit of many years of development and application. The primary purpose is to provide clinical professionals with the tools to perform a tinnitus psychoacoustic assessment using standard audiologic testing instrumentation.

ROLE OF THE AUDIOLOGIST

A strong case can be made that audiologists are in the best position of all health care professionals to serve as the primary treatment provider for patients with tinnitus: (1) audiologists are trained in all types of auditory disorders (tinnitus being the conspicuous exception), giving them an understanding of the functional aspects of the auditory system; (2) audiologists are skilled in the fitting of hearing aids, which are often used effectively in the treatment of tinnitus (see Chapter 22, "Role of Hearing Aids in Management for Tinnitus"); (3) the use of sound to treat tinnitus is common (especially with tinnitus masking and tinnitus retraining therapy [TRT]), and audiologists have the background in acoustics and psychoacoustics to understand the concepts relevant to acoustic forms of tinnitus therapy; (4) audiologists work closely with otolaryngologists, comprising a pairing of professional auditory disciplines that would be important for addressing a phantom auditory symptom; (5) audiologists usually receive training in counseling techniques to provide aural rehabilitation, and counseling is an essential aspect of virtually all tinnitus management programs[1–3]; and (6) audiologists routinely assess hearing function; thus, they possess the expertise and auditory testing equipment to perform psychoacoustic evaluations of tinnitus.

Although audiologists have the benefit of training and skills that position them well to provide tinnitus treatment, their typical lack of graduate-level training in this area leaves them unprepared to assume such a role. Audiologists must therefore be self-motivated to acquire specialized expertise to provide direct tinnitus services in their scope of practice. The "training" that is available to audiologists in this regard is limited to occasional workshops and the extant tinnitus literature. The present chapter can help fill this void with respect to psychoacoustic assessment of tinnitus.

RATIONALE FOR PERFORMING TINNITUS ASSESSMENT

A number of tinnitus measures can be obtained, but the results of these tests are not generally considered useful for diagnostic or therapeutic purposes. The value of obtaining tinnitus psychoacoustic measures is thus commonly questioned. In spite of the perceived lack of justification, however, tinnitus clinicians routinely perform at least rudimentary tests in the attempt to quantify their patients' tinnitus perceptions. From the perspective of maintaining high medical standards, a comprehensive tinnitus assessment would be insufficient without obtaining measures that quantify the symptom.

There is inherent clinical value in quantifying a patient's symptoms that are associated with any type of health-related complaint. All medical disciplines attempt to quantify their patients' disorders through diagnostic procedures. Whenever intervention is required, the symptoms must be thoroughly described to implement appropriately therapeutic strategies. Tinnitus is no different. During the 1980s, tinnitus professionals made great strides in their attempts to establish standardized methods of diagnosis and treatment. Treatment using tinnitus masking was at the forefront of therapeutic techniques, and a battery of tinnitus measures was considered important to establish an individualized masking program.[4–6] Tinnitus masking is an approach that focuses on the use of sound to achieve tinnitus relief, and it was clinically relevant to define the interactions between tinnitus and external sounds to develop the most effective masking protocol for a given patient.[7,8]

Other methods of tinnitus treatment became popular in the late 1980s and early 1990s that did not rely on the use of customized sound as the primary basis of treatment. In particular, the cognitive-behavioral approach to tinnitus management[9] and TRT[10] came into use. For these methods, psychoacoustic measures of tinnitus are inconsequential diagnostically, and test results are useful primarily for counseling purposes. Cognitive-behavioral therapy emphasizes a description of the psychological impact of tinnitus as the critical diagnostic factor.[11] With TRT, tinnitus measurements are of no consequence to the design of appropriate intervention.[12]

With prevailing therapies defaming the need for tinnitus psychoacoustic assessment, it is important to justify why these measures should be performed routinely and in a standardized fashion. Most generally, standardization of a psychoacoustic tinnitus test battery would establish uniformity in the quantification of tinnitus symptoms across all clinical and research groups. Standardization would further promote (1) the development of meaningful diagnoses of the underlying causes of tinnitus; (2) better design of treatments to address tinnitus symptoms and psychological effects; (3) better understanding of the effects of treatment on the perceptual characteristics of tinnitus; (4) a uniform method to quantify subjective symptoms as a tool to counsel patient and family; (5) development of methods to identify accurately the presence of tinnitus to assess for tinnitus "malingering"; (6) elucidation of potential psychoacoustic "rules" that would define the systematic effects of acoustic stimuli on the tinnitus percept; (7) better understanding of tinnitus mechanisms; and (8) consistent methodology for obtaining tinnitus measures that would be essential for litigation purposes.

HISTORICAL DEVELOPMENT OF TINNITUS ASSESSMENT PROCEDURES

This section provides a brief overview of historical studies with respect to the development of techniques that have been used to assess psychoacoustically and to treat acoustically patients with tinnitus. Later sections provide greater detail as necessary.

EARLY ATTEMPTS TO MEASURE TINNITUS AND TREAT PATIENTS USING SOUND

The spectral characteristics of tinnitus have been recognized as fundamentally important for many years. Reportedly, as early as 1821, different types of masking sounds were used to treat tinnitus according to whether it was high or low pitched.[13] Vernon and Meikle[5] and Feldmann[14] reviewed various additional attempts to mask tinnitus prior to the availability of electronic devices. The advent of electroacoustic equipment enabled the use of calibrated acoustic stimuli to measure tinnitus pitch and loudness and to mask tinnitus.[15] Psychoacoustic methods for describing tinnitus were first reported by Wegel and by Josephson, who both performed tinnitus loudness and pitch matching with pure tones.[16,17] In addition, Wegel showed "masking curves" that were obtained by determining the levels of pure tones necessary to mask tinnitus.[16]

Development of Tinnitus Loudness and Pitch Matching Techniques

In the 1930s and 1940s, Edmund Fowler made a number of important contributions to tinnitus measurement. He was the first to describe a method for measuring loudness recruitment by balancing the loudness of tones between ears, which he termed the *alternating binaural loudness balance* (ABLB).[18,19] He applied the ABLB technique to test for tinnitus loudness by balancing the loudness of a tone presented to one ear with the loudness of the tinnitus perceived in the contralateral ear.[20] The level of the comparison tone, expressed in decibels above hearing threshold (HL) that is the sensation level (SL), represented the tinnitus loudness as experienced by the patient. Fowler argued that it was important to match the loudness and pitch of tinnitus using contralateral tones.[21] For pitch matching, he stressed the importance of presenting matching tones at levels equal to the perceived tinnitus loudness. Fowler commented that patients described their tinnitus as very loud, yet the tinnitus could usually be matched at only 5 to 10 dB SL.[22,23] These basic techniques of Fowler's were adapted and used in many subsequent studies.[24–35]

Tinnitus Masking Studies

Numerous studies have evaluated the effects of various sounds on tinnitus to understand systematic tinnitus masking effects.[35–43] The results of these studies have shown consistently that the predictable frequency dependence seen in conventional tone-on-tone masking is usually not applicable to tinnitus masking. Tinnitus masking is thus categorically different from conventional masking.

Phenomenon of Residual Inhibition

Residual inhibition is defined as the temporary suppression or elimination of tinnitus that is often observed following auditory stimulation.[7,44] This so-called "after-effect of masking" was first reported by Spaulding and later by Josephson.[17,45] The phenomenon was formally studied by Feldmann[36] and was referred to as residual inhibition by Vernon and Schleuning.[46] Residual inhibition has been developed as a routine clinical procedure, and the effect occurs with 80 to 90% of patients who receive the appropriate type of auditory stimulation.[8,47–49]

Attempts to Standardize Tinnitus Psychoacoustic Assessment

Formal efforts to promote the establishment of standardized tinnitus evaluation were expended over 20 years ago by the Ciba Foundation in London and the National Academy of Sciences.[50,51] These efforts recommended a clinical tinnitus assessment battery that would include pitch matching, loudness matching, tinnitus maskability, and residual inhibition. In association with the Ciba Symposium, Vernon and Meikle provided procedural details for these four tests.[52] The tinnitus assessment procedures advocated by Vernon and Meikle have remained "more or less" the standard, although special equipment is required to perform their techniques. Currently, there is no specialized tinnitus testing equipment that is commonly used or advocated for routine clinical tinnitus evaluations. Most audiologists who do tinnitus evaluations use their audiometers in some manner to obtain some or all of these measures. The recommended tests are thus not performed uniformly.

One way to achieve standardization in this haphazard arena of tinnitus assessment is to computer-automate the tinnitus testing procedures, which has been a main objective of clinical research in our laboratory. An automated clinical procedure for tinnitus evaluation should be capable of evaluating all parameters of tinnitus that are relevant to rehabilitation, and significant progress has been made toward this end. This project has been ongoing since 1995, when a pilot-testing system was developed.[53] Since then, the system has undergone numerous upgrades, resulting in a series of studies that have documented the system's performance.[54–58] Our current efforts are to develop a clinically practical, uniform method for obtaining a battery of tinnitus measures in the clinical environment.

TEST–RETEST RELIABILITY OF TINNITUS MEASURES

Matching tinnitus to a pure tone would appear to be a straightforward task. If this were the case, good test–retest reliability of test results would be expected. A number of factors, however, complicate such testing. As described above, there is the consistent observation that tinnitus does not share the same psychophysical characteristics as external acoustic stimuli.[27,34,36,39,59] Although studied by many investigators, none have discovered any rules to define the effects of external sounds on the perception of tinnitus, unlike the field of psychoacoustics, which has defined many rules for the perception of sound.

TINNITUS LOUDNESS MATCHING

The reliability of tinnitus loudness matches has been reviewed elsewhere.[54,60] In general, tinnitus loudness matches have been shown to be produced reliably by most individuals with chronic tinnitus, and repeated measures are usually obtained within a few decibels of each other both within and between sessions.[54] Equivalent reliability also seems to be the case when loudness matches are obtained at test frequencies that are in a different region than the perceived tinnitus frequency.

TINNITUS PITCH MATCHING

Obtaining consistent tinnitus pitch matches has posed a significantly greater challenge than for loudness matching.[60] Historically, every clinical study that has reported repeated pitch matches has shown high variability of the repeated responses.[34,58–61] Penner and Bilger argued that this high variability suggests that tinnitus is either a fluctuating signal, a broadband signal, or both, and there is evidence to support their premise.[62] Almost half of a large clinical population of patients with tinnitus reported fluctuating tinnitus.[47] Fluctuating tinnitus would involve changes in pitch, loudness, and/or timbre. About half of a large group of patients from the same clinic reported tinnitus consisting of multiple sounds,[63] which would certainly be expected to reduce pitch match reliability. Also, the majority of patients with tinnitus have hearing loss, which is well known to reduce frequency resolving ability.[64]

Penner and Bilger note that the variability of tinnitus pitch matches often spans several octaves, as demonstrated by a number of studies.[62] Our studies have focused on this issue by obtaining multiple pitch matches both within and between sessions, and our findings have been consistent with their observations.[61] Clinicians should thus be aware that a single pitch match might not accurately represent the range of responses that would likely be obtained if testing were repeated. For this reason, clinical pitch match procedures should incorporate repeated tests.

RELIABILITY OF TINNITUS MASKABILITY AND RESIDUAL INHIBITION

No known studies have performed repeated measures of tinnitus maskability or residual inhibition to determine the reliability of the responses. This is surprising because these tests were advocated in the early 1980s for routine tinnitus assessment. It will be essential to determine the reliability of these measurements for these tests to be used routinely in the clinic.

PROCEDURES FOR CONDUCTING A TINNITUS TEST BATTERY

AUDIOMETRIC ASSESSMENT

Most patients with tinnitus also have hearing loss; thus, standard audiologic testing would be routine for these patients. The combined testing should enable an adequate assessment of the auditory system with respect to hearing sensitivity, loudness tolerance, and tinnitus.

Audiometric evaluation should include the following tests (in approximately this order):
1. Pure-tone thresholds
2. Speech recognition thresholds
3. Tinnitus loudness and pitch matching
4. Minimum masking levels (MMLs)
5. Residual inhibition
6. Loudness discomfort levels (LDLs) to speech and pure tones
7. Word recognition scores
8. Distortion-product otoacoustic emissions (DPOAEs)
9. Immittance (reflex and reflex decay only if tolerated comfortably by patient)

The rationale for this order of testing involves two primary concerns. First, a patient's tinnitus perception can be altered by acoustic stimulation. The likelihood of such alteration increases with increasing stimulus intensity. The above testing order, therefore, includes only threshold testing prior to the tinnitus tests. Second, many patients with tinnitus are hypersensitive to sound. This condition, loosely referred to as "hyperacusis," has been reported to occur in about 40% of patients with tinnitus.[12,65] Although there are no consensual criteria for identifying hyperacusis, many patients with tinnitus have loudness hypersensitivity to some degree, and patients should be tested for their LDLs prior to the presentation of louder sounds during testing. One exception to this rule is that testing for MMLs and residual inhibition can potentially involve uncomfortable levels of broadband noise. Patients should, therefore, be instructed to report if the broadband noise becomes uncomfortably loud, and these two tests should be terminated if that occurs.

TINNITUS LOUDNESS AND PITCH MATCHING

The assumption underlying tinnitus loudness and pitch matching is that the patient is capable of selecting a tone that is considered a "good match" with the tinnitus in terms of both pitch and loudness. From the examiner's standpoint, the patient's selection identifies the frequency and decibels (hearing level or sound pressure level) of the matching tone. As discussed above, patients with tinnitus can generally provide repeated loudness matches within a few decibels, but repeated pitch matching tends to produce results spanning multiple octaves.

Considerations Regarding Presentation of Matching Tones Matching tinnitus to a pure tone is generally an easier task when the tone is presented to the ear contralateral to the tinnitus than to the ipsilateral ear. Contralateral presentation of tones facilitates a perceptual separation between the tinnitus and the matching tone that is optimal for distinguishing each sound separately while both are present. Tinnitus loudness and pitch matching procedures thus typically involve unilateral presentation of tones to the "stimulus ear," which is the ear contralateral to the "tinnitus ear." To identify the tinnitus ear, the patient is asked to report the ear that contains the "louder" or "more predominant" tinnitus. If the patient reports that the tinnitus is symmetrically lateralized (heard as an equivalent sound in each ear) or centrally located (heard as a single sound approximately in the middle of the head), selection of the stimulus ear can be an arbitrary decision. In all cases, however, the examiner must attempt to achieve as much perceptual separation as possible between the tonal stimulus and the tinnitus sound to be matched.

In some cases, the tinnitus may be described as consisting of two or more distinct sounds. If multiple sounds are heard in one ear, the procedure of contralateral tone presentation can be done first to match one of the sounds, followed by the same procedure repeated for any additional sounds. If there are different sounds to be matched in each of the two ears, contralateral stimulus presentation will switch from one ear to the other accordingly.

Although contralateral presentation of matching tones is recommended as the standard procedure, ipsilateral presentation may be more appropriate in some situations. The most basic concern is that a patient's perception of pitch in the stimulus ear might be distorted in some way. For example, greater hearing loss increases the probability of reduced frequency discrimination. The extreme of such a condition would be the inability to distinguish differences between any tones, meaning that all tones would sound the same. The auditory condition of "diplacusis" (double hearing) describes a distorted sense of pitch such that a pure tone is heard as two tones or as noise or buzzing.[66] The patient may perceive the same auditory stimulus differently between ears (diplacusis binauralis), which could result in different matching results depending on which ear is used. Between-ear differences in auditory perception can include pitch differences (diplacusis dysharmonica) and differences in growth of loudness (recruitment). Substantial hearing loss in the contralateral ear or asymmetric hearing should lead the examiner to consider any of these concerns.

If a patient is suspected for any reason of having a distorted perception of pure tones, the patient can be pretested for his or her ability to differentiate between "louder" and "softer" tones and between "higher-" and "lower-pitched" tones using a pretesting procedure that has been previously described.[58] This pretesting protocol can also be used for any patient who might have difficulty understanding the difference between "pitch" and "loudness."

A great deal of time can be spent performing these matching procedures, and the extent to which an examiner matches each tinnitus sound reported by a patient will depend on the need to provide such detailed results. Such precise identification of each tinnitus sound would not normally be considered a necessity for a clinical intake assessment owing to time constraints. For legal cases, however, a complete description of the patient's tinnitus will require identification of each tinnitus sound as much as possible.

Overview of Vernon and Meikle's "Standard" Procedures The loudness and pitch matching protocol described in detail in the next section is based on Vernon and Meikle's procedures (1981),[52] which followed the basic recommendations of the Ciba Foundation in London[50] and the National Academy of Sciences.[51] Vernon and Meikle's protocol has received extensive clinical use and is often considered the standard for loudness and pitch matching. Performing these procedures, however, requires specialized instrumentation that is not available to most audiologists. In addition, testing time can be fairly lengthy for routine clinical application. For these reasons, the description of the full protocol that is described below will be followed by a modified protocol that could be performed more rapidly using a clinical audiometer.

Vernon and Meikle's loudness and pitch matching protocol involves three separate procedures.[52] Testing alternates systematically among threshold testing, loudness matching, and pitch matching to achieve (1) a pitch match and (2) a loudness match at the pitch match frequency. The general strategy of testing is to gradually approach the tinnitus frequency by presenting successive pairs of tones and, from each tone pair, having the patient select the tone that is "closest in pitch" to the perceived tinnitus frequency. Because patients are often thought to confuse the concepts of pitch and loudness during testing, all tones used for pitch matching should be presented only at their loudness-matched levels. Thus, loudness matches must be obtained prior to pitch matching, and loudness matches are always preceded by threshold testing at the same frequency.

Loudness matches and hearing thresholds are obtained with 1 dB resolution. This level of precision is necessary because a loudness match will usually be obtained within 10 dB of the hearing threshold and will often be within a few decibels of threshold. As an aside, an important concept to understand is that loudness matching across a range of test frequencies yields loudness match functions. The shapes of such functions vary among individuals and are seen most clearly when loudness matches are plotted in decibel sensation level (dB SL).[67] It has been observed that most patients reveal "merging" functions, that is, loudness matches that are large at low frequencies and decrease to small values at high frequencies (Figure 16-1). For some patients, a "parallel" function is obtained, meaning that all of the loudness matches are at about the same sensation level. Although these loudness match functions are not diagnostic, it is apparent that the clinical tinnitus population can be separated into several major categories according to the shapes of their functions. Etiologic factors may someday be revealed that account for these differences.

Testing starts at 1,000 Hz, which is a frequency generally well below the typical pitch match frequency. In a large sample of tinnitus clinic patients who were tested with Vernon and Meikle's procedures, 75% of the patients provided pitch matches above 4,000 Hz, and 55% had pitch matches above 6,000 Hz.[68,69] The progression of test frequencies thus typically moves upward to approach gradually the perceived tinnitus pitch. Test frequencies are divisible by 1,000 Hz, which provides for greater frequency resolution in the higher frequencies (corresponding with progressively decreasing distances between points on the basilar membrane). When the tinnitus has been identified to the closest 1,000 Hz, finer frequency adjustments can be made if the patient is able to identify the tinnitus pitch with greater resolution.

Specifics of Vernon and Meikle's Procedures As explained above, testing normally occurs in the "stimulus ear," that is, the ear contralateral to the ear with the predominant tinnitus. The patient's tasks include threshold testing, loudness matching, and pitch matching. Testing starts by obtaining a hearing threshold at 1,000 Hz in the stimulus ear. Hearing threshold procedures are adapted from the modified Hughson-Westlake ascending-descending audiometric test technique.[70] The threshold is first bracketed to

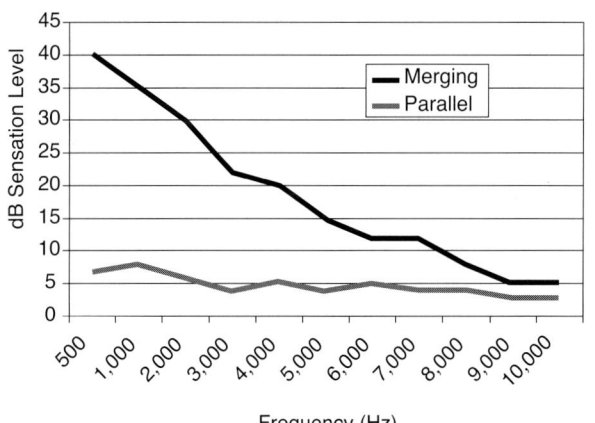

FIGURE 16-1. Loudness match functions representing two primary categories of patients with tinnitus. Some patients show "merging" functions for which their loudness matches (in dB SL) are relatively high at lower frequencies and gradually become smaller at higher frequencies. "Parallel" functions reveal loudness matches that are approximately the same across the range of test frequencies.

within 5 dB using increasing steps of 5 dB and decreasing steps of 10 dB. The threshold with 1 dB resolution is determined using increasing steps of 1 dB and decreasing steps of 2 dB. Although responses will tend to be more variable with such small steps, two responses should be obtained at the lowest level for that level to be recorded as the auditory sensitivity threshold.

A tinnitus loudness match is next obtained at 1,000 Hz. Each tone is presented for 2 to 3 seconds, and the first tone is presented at 10 dB above threshold. After each presentation, the patient is asked, "Should the tone be louder or softer to be the same loudness as your tinnitus?" If the tone is reported to be louder than the tinnitus, the level is decreased by 5 dB. Otherwise, the level is increased in 5 dB increments until the tone is louder than the tinnitus. The level is then reduced by 5 dB and adjusted up or down in 1 dB increments until the patient reports a loudness match.

Considering the average patient with tinnitus with mild-to-moderate hearing loss, starting levels for loudness matching should be (1) 10 to 20 dB SL for frequencies through 2,000 Hz, (2) 5 to 15 dB SL for 3,000 to 8,000 Hz, and (3) 0 to 5 dB for 9,000 to 16,000 Hz. Two concerns, however, are instructive for selecting the initial levels of tones for loudness matching. First, loudness matches can vary systematically for a given patient depending on the test frequency. Recall that most patients exhibit a "merging" function for their loudness matches across frequencies. Typically, lower-frequency loudness matches are made at higher levels above threshold, and higher-frequency matches are made at lower levels. Second, repeated presentation of tones at levels louder than the tinnitus can increase the potential for changing the perceived tinnitus loudness. For these reasons, the levels of tones that are presented for loudness matching do not always follow a prescribed pattern but should be made in accordance with a patient's responses. The loudness match obtained at 1,000 Hz serves as a guide for the starting level used at 2,000 Hz. The starting tone at 2,000 Hz should be 5 to 10 dB below the loudness match level obtained at 1,000 Hz. For example, if the loudness match at 1,000 Hz is 25 dB SL, testing at 2,000 Hz should start at 15 to 20 dB SL. For subsequent test frequencies, each starting level should continue to be 5 to 10 dB below the previous frequency's loudness match level. Increases in level at each frequency should then be made to stay below the tinnitus loudness or to exceed it by no more than a few decibels. If hearing sensitivity is greatly reduced at higher frequencies, even greater caution should be exercised owing to the increased potential for loudness recruitment.

The first steps of testing are to determine the threshold and loudness matches at 1,000 Hz, followed by the same at 2,000 Hz. Testing then transitions to the first stage of pitch matching, which uses 1,000 and 2,000 Hz tones at the loudness-matched levels. These two tones are presented alternately in the same ear, using the two-alternative forced choice (2AFC) method. Each tone is presented for 3 to 4 seconds with an intertone interval of 0.5 to 1 second. Before the tones are presented, patients are given the following instructions: "You will listen to two tones, one following the other. Tell me whether the first or the second tone sounds closest in pitch to your tinnitus." Because the preponderance of patients have a perceived tinnitus pitch above 4,000 Hz, they will usually choose the higher-frequency tone (2,000 Hz).

Next, a threshold and loudness match are obtained at 3,000 Hz. Pitch matching is then done as before using the pair of loudness-matched tones at 2,000 and 3,000 Hz. Testing continues in this manner until the patient chooses the lower-frequency tone from a tone pair. Choosing the lower-frequency tone signals that the tinnitus pitch has been bracketed to within the frequency range encompassed by the last two frequencies used for pitch matching. This also signals the next step to evaluate for "octave confusion."

Octave confusion refers to a common mistake made by patients when matching the pitch of their tinnitus to external tones.[24,71] When the patient confirms that a tone is at least "very close" to the pitch of the tinnitus, the 2AFC procedure is used to compare the pitch-matched tone to tones one octave higher and one octave lower. It is suggested to start with the lower-frequency octave pair, followed by the higher-frequency pair. When this is done, patients may report that one of the octave tones is the closest match. Prior to performing the 2AFC procedure between octave frequencies, a threshold and a loudness match are obtained at the octave frequency to be tested. This testing is, of course, contingent on the equipment's capability to produce the octave tones. The higher-frequency octave is often not an option.

In some cases, a patient's tinnitus will be matched to a tone below 1,000 Hz. When the first pair of tones (1,000 and 2,000 Hz) is presented for pitch matching, patients with such low-frequency tinnitus would choose 1,000 Hz as closest to the tinnitus pitch. Test frequencies below 1,000 Hz would include progressively lower octave frequencies (500, 250, and 125 Hz). The first test frequency below 1,000 Hz would thus be 500 Hz. A threshold and loudness match would be obtained at 500 Hz, and the 2AFC procedure would be used for pitch matching between the 500 and 1,000 Hz tones. Testing can be done further at 250 and 125 Hz if the testing equipment has such capability. Pitch matching at these lower frequencies would also culminate in octave confusion testing.

Following octave confusion testing, test frequencies can be varied around the final octave-confirmed frequency to determine if more precise pitch match resolution is possible. For this final stage of pitch matching, the frequency is simply varied according to examiner judgment (at the same output level), and the patient is asked if any of the new frequencies improve on the previous pitch match. Patients have been known to select a pitch match with 1 Hz precision, although it would have to be questioned if such a response would be reliable on repeated testing. Again, such testing is entirely dependent on equipment capabilities.

As mentioned above, the loudness and pitch matching procedures recommended by Vernon and Meikle[52] require specialized testing instrumentation. Such equipment has been available commercially (eg, Danavox, Starkey, and Norwest companies), but these devices have been out of production for years. Also, audio bench equipment (eg, tone generators, attenuators, amplifiers, filters) can be adapted to perform tinnitus matching with these procedures. At present, however, there is no such instrumentation available commercially, and bench equipment is not realistic for the typical clinic. Using the principles that have been described for loudness matching and pitch matching, a reasonably close approximation of testing can be performed using a clinical audiometer.

Loudness and Pitch Matching Protocol Using a Clinical Audiometer Most audiologists do not have access to the kind of equipment that would be required to conduct loudness and pitch matching, as described above. Yet audiologists who encounter patients with tinnitus must obtain these measures as part of the intake assessment. Clinical audiometers are not designed for tinnitus testing, but they are adaptable for this purpose.

Most generally, audiometers present calibrated pure tones at octave and half-octave frequencies between 125 and 8,000 Hz. Some audiometers will test at frequencies up to 12,000 Hz or even 16,000 Hz. Output levels can be varied in increments of 5 dB, and some audiometers enable test increments of 1 or 2 dB. Audiometers are not designed to facilitate the type of 2AFC testing that is used for pitch matching, which requires alternating presentation of tones that differ in frequency and output level. Two-channel audiometers can, however, be set up to perform 2AFC testing in this manner. Considering these technical limitations and the need for clinical expediency, procedures are described below for conducting tinnitus loudness and pitch matching with an audiometer.

The objective of tinnitus loudness and pitch matching with an audiometer is to determine (1) the frequency of a tone that the patient reports to be a good match with the perceived tinnitus pitch and (2) the decibel level (dB SL) of the tone at the pitch match frequency that the patient reports to be a good match with the perceived tinnitus loudness. The overall strategy is to present tones that increase in frequency to approach gradually the tinnitus frequency. Each tone should be presented at a level that approximates the tinnitus loudness. Patients should also clearly understand the difference between the terms "pitch" and "loudness." If there is confusion, an understanding of these concepts can be evaluated using any variation of the pretesting procedure that was referred to above.[58]

Patients undergoing a tinnitus assessment will have already been tested for their pure-tone hearing thresholds at audiometric test frequencies. Loudness matching is not done at every frequency, but the examiner must use his or her best judgment to present tones for pitch matching at levels that would be equivalent to or slightly below the perceived tinnitus loudness. Recalling that most patients will exhibit a "merging" loudness match function (see Figure 16-1), a basic rule of thumb is to present initial loudness matching tones at (1) 10 to 20 dB SL at frequencies at which hearing sensitivity is essentially normal and (2) 5 to 10 dB SL at frequencies at which there is hearing loss. These suggested levels will vary according to the degree of hearing loss and according to the individual patient's perception of the loudness of the tones in relation to the tinnitus loudness.

The tinnitus pitch is first bracketed to within an octave, and testing starts at 1,000 Hz. For most patients, a 1,000 Hz tone can be perceived as definitively lower in pitch than the tinnitus frequency. This easily perceived difference assists the patient in understanding the pitch matching task. When the 1,000 Hz tone is first presented, the examiner should adjust the tone to a level that approximates the loudness of the patient's tinnitus by asking the patient, "Is the loudness of the tone about the same loudness as your tinnitus?" When an approximate loudness match has been obtained, the patient is asked, "Is the pitch of your tinnitus higher or lower than the pitch of the tone?" If the patient responds "higher," the next tone is presented at 2,000 Hz. The examiner attempts again to approximate the loudness of the tinnitus with the tone and again asks if the tinnitus is higher or lower in pitch than the tone. Testing progresses in this manner until the tinnitus pitch has been bracketed to within an octave, at which point, interoctave frequencies are tested in the same way. A pitch match is thus obtained to the closest half-octave.

Because of the potential for octave confusion, the examiner presents the pitch-matched tone in alternation with tones an octave higher and an octave lower and asks the patient to identify the tone that best matches the tinnitus pitch. When an octave-confirmed pitch match has been identified, a loudness match is obtained to the smallest decibel resolution that is possible with the audiometer.

Loudness matching at the pitch match frequency should be done in accordance with the loudness match parameters outlined above, which are based on Vernon and Meikle's procedures.[52] The pitch-matched tone will have already been presented at a level that is close to the perceived tinnitus loudness. The level of the tone should be varied in small steps while asking the patient to report the level that provides the closest match to the tinnitus loudness.

Tinnitus Matching to Bands of Noise Following the identification of a pitch match, the next phase of testing is to determine if the patient's tinnitus sounds more like a pure tone or more like a band of noise. Limited "noise matching" can be done with an audiometer, and more detailed noise-band matching can be done with special equipment.

When a tinnitus pitch match has been obtained with an audiometer and confirmed by octave confusion testing, narrowband noise is presented that is centered at the pitch match frequency. The patient is asked if the noise sounds more like the tinnitus than the previous tone that was identified as a pitch match. If the noise does not sound more like the tinnitus, then the tone is considered the final match. If the noise is reported to be a closer match, then broadband noise (speech noise or white noise) is presented. Thus, to achieve the best match, the patient can choose between three stimulus options: the pure-tone pitch match, the narrow band of noise centered at the pitch match frequency, or the broadband noise. If the patient chooses either of the noise stimuli, the level of the selected noise is then matched to the loudness of the tinnitus.

If the testing equipment enables the presentation of variable bands of noise, a more precise noise-band match can be provided for patients who select narrowband noise as a better match than a pure tone. With special equipment, the narrowest band of noise, centered at the pitch match frequency, is selected first. If the noise is a closer match than the tone, the band is then widened in sequential steps to determine the width of the band that provides the best match.

Minimum Masking Level

The MML refers to the minimum level of broadband noise that completely masks an individual's tinnitus. MML testing is commonly done with tinnitus clinic patients and is considered especially important for clinics that use the treatment approach of tinnitus masking.[4,72] Treatment success with masking is thought to be a predictable function based on the findings of MML testing—the lower the MML, the more likely it is that the masking will be successful. Although MML results are not a factor in prescribing treatment with TRT, MML data have been reported to correlate with treatment efficacy using this approach.[73] For patients treated with TRT, MMLs were observed generally to decrease in conjunction with an improved condition.

Use of the term "masking" with respect to tinnitus has been challenged owing to the findings of many studies that have shown that masking of tinnitus does not follow the psychoacoustic rules that were established for the masking of one sound by another. These studies, cited above, have shown that the usual frequency dependence seen in conventional tone-on-tone masking is not characteristic of most attempts to mask tinnitus. Masking of tinnitus thus appears to be categorically different from conventional masking.

Jastreboff and Jastreboff have suggested that the reduction of tinnitus perception may be more appropriately termed "suppression."[74]

MMLs can be obtained both monaurally and binaurally. Monaural MML testing can be an especially challenging task for patients, who are expected to ignore the tinnitus on the opposite side of the head and to report when the tinnitus on the stimulus side becomes inaudible. Patients often experience difficulties in differentially tracking the tinnitus perception in one ear only during presentation of a masking stimulus to that ear. Therefore, unless there are special treatment considerations requiring MML information from individual ears, obtaining monaural MMLs is not normally recommended.

Broadband noise is used as the masking stimulus for obtaining binaural MMLs. Vernon and colleagues recommended the use of a 2 to 12 kHz band of noise for performing this test.[75] Without special equipment, however, the broadest band available from an audiometer should be used for MML testing.

Testing for MML starts with the establishment of monaural hearing thresholds for the noise stimulus. Noise threshold testing is done as for pure tones, and each threshold is obtained to the closest 1 dB increment. The noise is then set for binaural presentation, and the levels of noise presented to each ear will be relative to the noise threshold obtained in each ear, respectively. For example, if the noise threshold is 5 dB greater in the left ear than in the right ear, each binaural presentation of noise will reflect this difference.

After noise thresholds have been obtained, the binaural noise for establishing MML is presented to each ear at levels 1 dB above the respective thresholds (ie, at 1 dB SL). The noise presentation should last long enough for the patient to determine whether the tinnitus can still be heard in the presence of the noise. If the tinnitus is inaudible, the binaural MML is recorded as 1 dB SL. If the tinnitus can still be heard at that level, the noise is raised in 1 dB steps, and at each level, the patient reports whether the tinnitus is still audible.

TESTING FOR RESIDUAL INHIBITION

Residual inhibition testing is done immediately following the establishment of the binaural MML. As for MML testing, a 2 to 12 kHz noise band is recommended by Vernon and colleagues.[75] With an audiometer, however, the same broadband noise used for MML testing is used to test for residual inhibition.

To start the test, the noise levels established for MML are raised 10 dB. The patient is told, "There will be noise presented for exactly one minute. The noise will then be shut off, and you will be asked if there is any kind of change in your tinnitus." To obtain an unbiased response, it is important that patients are not given the expectation that their tinnitus loudness will be reduced following the stimulus.

After 60 seconds of the noise presented at MML + 10 dB, the examiner waits a few seconds and then asks, "Does your tinnitus sound the same as before, or is there any difference?" If the patient reports that it sounds the same, the test is over, and the patient has not experienced residual inhibition. If the patient reports that the tinnitus is softer, the examiner asks the patient to report the loudness of the tinnitus in relation to the "usual loudness" of the tinnitus. The percentage levels that should be used to obtain this information from the patient include 10, 25, 50, 75, and 90% of the usual loudness. If the tinnitus is "completely gone," the percentage is zero, which would indicate "complete" residual inhibition. Any level of tinnitus loudness between 10 and 90% is considered "partial" residual inhibition. During the period in which residual inhibition is experienced, the patient is asked at brief intervals to note the percentage level of the tinnitus until the tinnitus has recovered to its usual loudness. The total duration of residual inhibition is recorded, as well as the duration during each percentage category.

REPORTING RESULTS OF A TINNITUS ASSESSMENT

When reporting the results of loudness and pitch matching, the report should always include the tonal pitch match and the loudness match at the tonal pitch match frequency. If one of the noise stimuli provides a better match than does the tone, this should be noted, along with the level of the noise that matches the patient's tinnitus loudness. Additional information that is helpful for the report is to indicate the patient's judgment as to the quality of the tonal pitch match and/or the noise match. Descriptive terms can include "exact match," "very close," "somewhat close," and "not a match."

To report MML results, the type of noise stimulus used is specified. Test results indicate whether the patient's tinnitus could be masked. If so, the noise thresholds are reported in dB HL, and the binaural MML is reported in dB SL. For residual inhibition, the type of noise used is reported as the same used for MML testing, and the presentation level is reported. The patient's responsiveness to testing is noted as either responding or not responding to the test protocol. If the patient experienced residual inhibition, it is specified as "partial" or "complete." If the patient experienced a period of complete residual inhibition, the duration of the complete residual inhibition should be reported, along with the duration of the combined period of complete and partial residual inhibition.

ADDITIONAL AUDIOLOGIC TESTS FOR PATIENTS WITH TINNITUS

Evaluation for Hyperacusis

An additional problem that is encountered with many patients with tinnitus is hypersensitivity to sound. Unfortunately, this condition, commonly referred to as hyperacusis, has multiple definitions. There is, therefore, no standard diagnostic procedure to identify the condition. Until such a standard emerges, there are tools that the examiner can use to test for reduced loudness tolerance in patients with tinnitus. At the least, it is necessary to perform a loudness sensitivity assessment to ensure that suprathreshold audiologic testing does not cause auditory discomfort. When tested, some patients will reveal a significant clinical condition of hyperacusis that requires specific intervention.

If the patient does not have a loudness tolerance problem, the assessment will be very brief. If testing reveals such a problem, more complete questioning should ensue to specify the nature and extent of the problem. Questions have been developed for this purpose as part of the initial assessment for TRT. These questions, which are available on-line (<http://www.vard.org/jour/03/40/2/pdf/henry.pdf>), are appropriate for all patients with tinnitus, regardless of the type of treatment that they will receive.[76] If the patient is not aware of a loudness sensitivity problem, answering only the first question (Are sounds bothersome or unpleasant to you when they seem normal to other people around you?) will make this evident. In addition to the questions, the patient should be tested for LDLs at audiometric frequencies. The results of LDL testing should corroborate the patient's responses to the questions about loudness sensitivity.

Loudness Discomfort Levels

An LDL is the threshold level of discomfort for a sound. LDL testing can be done for any type of sound, including pure tones, speech stimuli, and broadband noise. For clinical expediency, LDLs are minimally measured at octave frequencies between 1,000 and 8,000 Hz. If a loudness sensitivity problem is noted, testing can be done at additional audiometric frequencies and with other types of auditory stimuli.

There can be considerable variation in how patients respond to LDL testing; thus, it is important to ensure that patients understand the testing instructions. Patients are instructed to report when they would "not want to listen to the tone for more than a few seconds." The intent of testing is to find the level at which any further increase in loudness would result in discomfort. Some patients will erroneously identify LDLs far below levels that are actually uncomfortable owing to fear of hearing sounds that would be painful. Other patients will endure uncomfortably loud sounds because they misinterpret the instructions. For these reasons, and because patients' within-session LDLs are often inconsistent,[77,78] LDL testing should be repeated. Prior to performing the repeat testing, the examiner should reinstruct as to the objective of testing, and the patient should repeat the instructions to the examiner.

Each ear should be tested separately. Test frequencies are ordered from lowest to highest, and tones are presented for 1 to 2 seconds each. The initial tone at 1,000 Hz is presented at the estimated most comfortable level, and 50 dB HL is generally appropriate. The level is raised in 5 dB increments until the patient signals that the LDL has been reached. Starting levels at remaining frequencies should be about 20 dB below the previous frequency's LDL. For example, if the first LDL at 1,000 Hz is 90 dB HL, testing at 2,000 Hz should start at about 70 dB HL. Good judgment is required to perform testing rapidly while avoiding patient discomfort. The final results of testing should be reported as the second set of measures, and the test–retest reliability should be noted.

Otoacoustic Emissions

The results of otoacoustic emission (OAE) tests are accepted as evidence of the functioning of outer hair cells.[79,80] The hypothesis that outer hair cell dysfunction can be the cause of tinnitus has led to many attempts to link tinnitus with OAE results.[81] Although some interesting relationships between the two have been observed, there are no definitive studies showing that OAE measures are diagnostic for patients with tinnitus (see Chapter 6, "Otoacoustic Emissions and Tinnitus"). These measures are also not obtainable at all frequencies in a high percentage of patients with tinnitus because any hearing loss exceeding approximately 40 dB HL precludes OAE responses.

Although not diagnostic or predictive of treatment efficacy, patients with tinnitus should nonetheless receive OAE testing as part of a comprehensive audiologic evaluation. The results of OAE testing can further be useful as a counseling tool. Indeed, DPOAE testing is recommended for patients evaluated for TRT as part of the TRT directive counseling protocol.[82] An explanation of DPOAE results would be educational for any patient with tinnitus to assist in understanding outer hair cells as a potential site of tinnitus generation.

ASSESSMENT OF TINNITUS FOR LEGAL CLAIMS

For many patients, the primary purpose of the tinnitus assessment is not to receive clinical management but to provide documentation to support a claim for financial compensation. The tinnitus specialist must therefore possess the skills to conduct such an assessment and to make qualified judgments as to the legitimacy of such claims. The examiner's task is to verify if the patient's claim is accurate and honest. Performing a tinnitus assessment for litigation purposes is a complex matter. There are several components to the assessment, and each component requires an informed decision based entirely on subjective information furnished by the individual making the claim.

COMPONENTS OF THE ASSESSMENT

Presence of Tinnitus The primary component in assessing an individual's claimed tinnitus for legal documentation purposes is to establish the very presence of tinnitus. For patients who have loud, unremitting tinnitus, this is a straightforward issue. Their tinnitus is clearly audible in almost any acoustic environment. Other patients, however, have less prominent tinnitus that might be undetectable in most everyday situations, or the tinnitus might be of an intermittent or "recurring" nature. The basic question that must be answered is whether the individual's tinnitus condition would be considered pathologic. Making such a judgment is particularly difficult in light of the classic study of Heller and Bergman, who demonstrated that tinnitus perception was induced in 94% of non-tinnitus individuals when placed in a sound-insulated environment.[83] It would thus seem that practically anyone could claim to have at least recurrent tinnitus, depending on the level of ambient noise. There is, unfortunately, no clearly defined boundary between "normal" phantom auditory sensations and pathologic tinnitus.

Severity of Tinnitus Meikle has defined tinnitus severity as the "nature and extent of patients' tinnitus-related problems."[84] In spite of many published outcome instruments that are used to obtain tinnitus severity ratings, consensual methodology for assessing tinnitus severity has not been established.[85–87] The fact that tinnitus prevalence is about five times higher than the number of patients who seek treatment[88–92] suggests that the majority of individuals who experience tinnitus do not consider their tinnitus to be a significant or debilitating problem.

Etiology of Tinnitus Based on data from a population of over 2,000 patients who attended the Oregon Tinnitus Clinic, about 40% of these patients could not identify any known events associated with their tinnitus onset. For patients who could identify such an association, there were four broad categories of tinnitus etiology: (1) noise related, (2) head and neck trauma, (3) head and neck illness, and (4) other medical conditions. More specific causes that would fit under these four categories have been described elsewhere.[93,94] It is generally accepted that the most common cause of tinnitus is noise exposure.[62,95]

Permanency of Tinnitus Vernon has noted the necessity of establishing the permanency of tinnitus.[96] The pertinent question would be how long the patient must experience pathologic tinnitus before the tinnitus can be considered a permanent condition. If the tinnitus has been present constantly for less than about 6 months, the tinnitus could be more labile, with the possibility of resolution. If it has been present for 6 to 12 months or longer, it is more likely to be a permanent irreversible condition. Vernon proposes that a minimum of 2 years duration is necessary before considering tinnitus to be permanent.

MAKING THE CLINICAL JUDGMENT

At the present time, there is no objective measure to prove the existence of tinnitus or to verify its reported severity. Making an assessment of tinnitus is akin to pain assessment, which depends on subjective scaling, self-report, and medical history. Assessing a patient's tinnitus for litigation purposes relies on an overall assessment that establishes the reliability of tinnitus psychoacoustic measures, consistency of verbal responses and medical records, and sufficient duration of tinnitus to determine permanency. There is the further question of severity, which may or may not be a factor in assessing a claim. For example, the US Veterans Affairs health care system, in assessing veterans' claims for tinnitus, does not consider the severity of the tinnitus in making the decision. The only two factors for awarding a "service-connected" tinnitus disability for veterans are that the tinnitus must be at least recurrent (intermittent) and the tinnitus must be related to military service.

Each component of the assessment relies solely on the patient's responses to either verbal or written questions or to psychoacoustic tests. Throughout the assessment, the examiner must be vigilant to the possibility that any of the self-reported measures are susceptible to exaggeration. The objective is to establish whether the patient's responses are consistent, plausible, and credible.[97]

The results of audiologic testing are often thought to provide the most valid evidence to support tinnitus claims. Although there are documented tests for detecting exaggerated hearing loss,[98] no such tests exist to assess patients suspected of feigning tinnitus. Vernon has often been cited for his "two dB rule" as providing acceptable court evidence to address whether an individual has tinnitus as claimed.[96] Vernon suggests that loudness matching should be performed five or six times within a test session, with other testing interspersed between the repeated tests. Each loudness match is obtained to the nearest 1 dB, and if the repeated results agree to within 2 dB, that degree of reliability is considered evidence for the presence of tinnitus. Recent studies, however, have challenged the validity of Vernon's approach. Jacobson and Henderson evaluated differences in tinnitus loudness matches between individuals with tinnitus and individuals without tinnitus.[99] The results of that study showed that individuals without tinnitus provided loudness matches at a higher level than did patients with tinnitus, but the reliability of the loudness matches was not significantly different. We conducted a study of 45 individuals with tinnitus and 45 individuals without tinnitus that included repeated loudness matches. Preliminary results have shown that the nontinnitus subjects were able to provide repeated loudness matches that were at least as reliable as those of the tinnitus group.[100]

Preliminary analyses of data from our own study seem to suggest that the results from a number of tinnitus psychoacoustic tests should be evaluated in aggregate to optimize the accuracy of determining whether a patient has tinnitus as claimed. The rationale is that an individual without tinnitus would have particular difficulty responding appropriately and reliably to all tests in a tinnitus test battery that includes loudness matching, pitch matching, and testing for MML and residual inhibition. Combined results from these four tests could provide an individual response "profile" that would be evaluated in combination with other factors that would be relevant to supporting a tinnitus claim. Dobie has proposed additional factors that should be considered: plausible and consistent history, credibility of the patient, early documentation of tinnitus, a tinnitus complaint that is "unsolicited," and hearing loss that is not exaggerated.[101]

REFERRAL OF THE PATIENT WITH TINNITUS

The testing procedures in this chapter do not negate the necessity of referring patients with tinnitus appropriately to an otolaryngologist or otologist to receive a complete ear examination. This would normally be a recommendation for any patient with tinnitus as part of the initial evaluation.[94] There are, however, certain issues that would suggest that physician referral may not be an absolute necessity for every patient with tinnitus. First, otologic surgery is an option only for a very small proportion of patients with tinnitus whose tinnitus has a surgically correctable cause. Second, a physician may not be available who has specialized expertise in evaluating and treating tinnitus. Third, the patient may choose not to see a physician even when a referral is made. It is therefore incumbent on the examining audiologist to be familiar with the symptoms that knowledgeable physicians look for in the initial tinnitus evaluation. A thorough review of these symptoms has been provided by Perry and Gantz.[94]

A tinnitus examination by a physician will result in radiologic and laboratory testing only if the physician determines that there is a reasonable chance that there is a correctable cause of the tinnitus.[94] Perry and Gantz suggest that further examination by a physician is obviated when there is (1) a history of noise exposure, (2) evidence of bilateral, nonpulsatile tinnitus (ie, sensorineural tinnitus), and (3) an audiogram that is consistent with sensorineural tinnitus. These suggestions can serve as general referral guidelines for the examining audiologist whenever a physician referral is not automatic.

There is further the matter that some patients might benefit from pharmaceutical intervention, which would also require referral to a physician. It should be noted, however, that Dobie has reviewed the randomized clinical trials that have been conducted to evaluate drugs that have been used for tinnitus treatment and has determined that none of them offered any definitive advantage over placebo.[102] Patients should, therefore, be referred for potential drug treatment only if nondrug forms of treatment are unsuccessful or if the condition is of such severity that medication might be warranted. Further, patients should be referred if there is reason to believe that the cause of tinnitus distress might be mainly attributable to an underlying emotional condition that could benefit from psychiatric management. In addition, patients with tinnitus with sleep problems should be considered for antidepressant therapy.

CONCLUSION

There are many reasons why uniform tinnitus assessment techniques are needed, as reviewed above in the introductory section. This need has been recognized for many years, but efforts thus far have not resulted in a standardized testing protocol. There is at present no formalized effort to establish standardized testing, and an appeal is made once again for leaders in the field to coordinate the development of consensual testing methodology for the clinical quantification of the perceptual characteristics of tinnitus.

The tinnitus assessment procedures advocated by Vernon and Meikle[52] function well in a clinic that has specialized testing equipment and the availability of clinician time to perform the procedures. Both of these criteria are not realized in most tinnitus clinics. This chapter attempts, therefore, to outline details of a battery of tinnitus test procedures that would be appropriate for general clinical application by audiologists or by other professionals who might have audiologic testing skills and access to testing equipment. The recommended procedures can serve to guide a tinnitus assessment that would suffice for most clinical or legal purposes.

REFERENCES

1. Hall JW, Ruth RA. Outcome for tinnitus patients after consultation with an audiologist. In: Hazell J, editor. Proceedings of the Sixth International Tinnitus Seminar; London: The Tinnitus and Hyperacusis Centre; 1999. p. 378–80.
2. Sweetow R. Cognitive aspects of tinnitus patient management. Ear Hear 1986;7:390–6.
3. Sweetow RW. Cognitive-behavior modification. In: Tyler RS, editor. Tinnitus handbook. San Diego (CA): Singular Publishing Group; 2000. p. 297–311.
4. Henry JA, Schechter MA, Nagler SM, Fausti SA. Comparison of tinnitus masking and tinnitus retraining therapy. J Am Acad Audiol 2002;13:559–81.
5. Vernon JA, Meikle MB. Tinnitus masking. In: Tyler RS, editor. Tinnitus handbook. San Diego (CA): Singular Publishing Group; 2000. p. 313–56.
6. Vernon JAE. Tinnitus treatment and relief. Needham Heights (MA): Allyn & Bacon; 1998.
7. Vernon J. Relief of tinnitus by masking treatment. In: English GM, editor. Otolaryngology. Philadelphia: Harper & Row; 1982. p. 1–21.
8. Vernon JA. Current use of masking for the relief of tinnitus. In: Kitahara M, editor. Tinnitus. Pathophysiology and management. Tokyo: Igaku-Shoin; 1988. p. 96–106.
9. Jakes SC, Hallam RS, Rachman S, Hinchcliffe R. The effects of reassurance, relaxation training and distraction on chronic tinnitus sufferers. Behav Res Ther 1986;24:497–507.
10. Jastreboff PJ. Phantom auditory perception (tinnitus): mechanisms of generation and perception. Neurosci Res 1990;8:221–54.

11. Henry JL, Wilson PH. The psychological management of chronic tinnitus. Needham Heights (MA): Allyn & Bacon; 2001.
12. Jastreboff PJ. Tinnitus habituation therapy (THT) and tinnitus retraining therapy (TRT). In: Tyler RS, editor. Tinnitus handbook. San Diego (CA): Singular Publishing Group; 2000. p. 357–76.
13. Stephens SDG. Historical aspects of tinnitus. In: Hazell JWP, editor. Tinnitus. London: Churchill Livingstone; 1987. p. 1–19.
14. Feldmann H. Masking of tinnitus—historical remarks. In: Feldmann H, editor. Proceedings of the Third International Tinnitus Seminar Munster. Karlsruhe (Germany): Harsch Verlag; 1987. p. 224–8.
15. Jones IH, Knudsen VO. Certain aspects of tinnitus, particularly treatment. Laryngoscope 1928;38:597–611.
16. Wegel RL. A study of tinnitus. Arch Otolaryngol 1931;14:158–65.
17. Josephson EM. A method of measurement of tinnitus aurium. Arch Otolaryngol 1931;14:282–3.
18. Fowler EP. A method for the early detection of otosclerosis. Arch Otolaryngol 1936;24:731–41.
19. Fowler EP. The diagnosis of diseases of the neural mechanism of hearing by the aid of sounds well above threshold. Laryngoscope 1937;47:289–300.
20. Fowler EP. The use of threshold and louder sounds in clinical diagnosis and the prescribing of hearing aids. New methods for accurately determining the threshold for bone conduction and for measuring tinnitus and its effects on obstructive and neural deafness. Trans Am Otol Soc 1938;28:154–71.
21. Fowler EP. Head noises—significance, measurement and importance in diagnosis and treatment. Arch Otolaryngol 1940;32:903–14.
22. Fowler EP. The "illusion of loudness" of tinnitus—its etiology and treatment. Laryngoscope 1942;52:275–85.
23. Fowler EP. Control of head noises. Their illusions of loudness and of timbre. Arch Otolaryngol 1943;37:391–8.
24. Graham JT, Newby HA. Acoustical characteristics of tinnitus: an analysis. Arch Otolaryngol 1962;75:82–7.
25. Hazell JW, Wood SM, Cooper HR, et al. A clinical study of tinnitus maskers. Br J Audiol 1985;19:65–146.
26. Kodama A, Kitahara M. Clinical and audiological characteristics of tonal and noise tinnitus. ORL J Otorhinolaryngol Relat Spec 1990;52:156–63.
27. Penner MJ. Variability in matches to subjective tinnitus. J Speech Hear Res 1983;26:263–7.
28. Penner MJ. Magnitude estimation and the "paradoxical" loudness of tinnitus. J Speech Hear Res 1986;29:407–12.
29. Penner MJ. Judgments and measurements of the loudness of tinnitus before and after masking. J Speech Hear Res 1988;31:582–7.
30. Reed GF. An audiometric study of two hundred cases of subjective tinnitus. Arch Otolaryngol 1960;71:94–104.
31. Roeser RJ, Price DR. Clinical experience with tinnitus maskers. Ear Hear 1980;1:63–8.
32. Tyler RS. The psychophysical measurement of tinnitus. In: Aran JM, Dauman R, editors. Tinnitus 91: proceedings of the Fourth International Tinnitus Seminar. Amsterdam: Kugler Publications; 1992. p. 17–26.
33. Tyler RS, Conrad-Armes D. The determination of tinnitus loudness considering the effects of recruitment. J Speech Hear Res 1983;26:59–72.
34. Tyler RS, Conrad-Armes D. Tinnitus pitch: a comparison of three measurement methods. Br J Audiol 1983;17:101–7.
35. Tyler RS, Conrad-Armes D. Masking of tinnitus compared to masking of pure tones. J Speech Hear Res 1984;27:106–11.
36. Feldmann H. Homolateral and contralateral masking of tinnitus by noise-bands and by pure tones. Audiology 1971;10:138–44.
37. Formby C, Gjerdingen DB. Pure-tone masking of tinnitus. Audiology 1980;19:519–35.
38. Mitchell C. The masking of tinnitus with pure tones. Audiology 1983;22:73–87.
39. Hazell JWP. Measurement of tinnitus in humans. Ciba Found Symp 1981;85:35–48.
40. Shailer MJ, Tyler RS, Coles RRA. Critical masking bands for sensorineural tinnitus. Scand Audiol 1981;10:157–62.
41. Penner MJ. Masking of tinnitus and central masking. J Speech Hear Res 1987;30:147–52.
42. Penner MJ, Klafter EJ. Measures of tinnitus: step size, matches to imagined tones, and masking patterns. Ear Hear 1992;13:410–6.
43. Mitchell CR, Vernon JA, Creedon TA. Measuring tinnitus parameters: loudness, pitch, and maskability. J Am Acad Audiol 1993;4:139–51.
44. Vernon JA, Meikle MB. Measurement of tinnitus: an update. In: Kitahara M, editor. Tinnitus. Pathophysiology and management. Tokyo: Igaku-Shoin; 1988. p. 36–52.
45. Spaulding JA. Tinnitus: with a plea for its more accurate musical notation. Arch Otolaryngol 1903;32:263–72.
46. Vernon J, Schleuning A. Tinnitus: a new management. Laryngoscope 1978;88:413–9.
47. Meikle M, Walsh ET. Characteristics of tinnitus and related observations in over 1800 tinnitus patients. In:

Shulman A, Ballantyne J, editors. Proceedings of the Second International Tinnitus Seminar. Ashford (KY): Invicta Press; 1984. p. 17–21.
48. Tyler RS, Babin RW, Neibuhr DP. Some observations on the masking and post-masking effects of tinnitus. In: Shulman A, Ballantyne J, editors. Proceedings of the Second International Tinnitus Seminar. Ashford (KY): Invicta Press; 1984. p. 150–6.
49. Vernon JA. Some observations on residual inhibition. In: Paparella MM, Meyerhoff WL, editors. Sensorineural hearing loss, vertigo and tinnitus. Ear Clinics International. Vol 1. Baltimore: Williams & Wilkins; 1981. p. 138–44.
50. Evered D, Lawrenson G, editors. Tinnitus. Ciba Found Symp 1981;85.
51. McFadden D. Tinnitus facts, theories and treatments. Washington (DC): National Academy Press; 1982.
52. Vernon JA, Meikle MB. Tinnitus masking: unresolved problems. Ciba Found Symp 1981;85:239–56.
53. Henry JA, Fausti SA, Mitchell CR, et al. An automated technique for tinnitus evaluation. In: Reich GE, Vernon JA, editors. Proceedings of the Fifth International Tinnitus Seminar 1995. Portland (OR): American Tinnitus Association; 1996. p. 325–6.
54. Henry JA, Flick CL, Gilbert AM, et al. Reliability of tinnitus loudness matches under procedural variation. J Am Acad Audiol 1999;10:502–20.
55. Henry JA, Flick CL, Gilbert AM, et al. Fully-automated system for tinnitus loudness and pitch matching. In: Hazell J, editor. Proceedings of the Sixth International Tinnitus Seminar; London: The Tinnitus and Hyperacusis Center; 1999. p. 520–1.
56. Henry JA, Fausti SA, Mitchell CR, et al. Computer-automated clinical technique for tinnitus quantification. Am J Audiol 2000;9:36–49.
57. Henry JA, Flick CL, Gilbert A, et al. Reliability of hearing thresholds: computer-automated testing with ER-4B canal phone earphones. J Rehabil Res Dev 2001;38:567–81.
58. Henry JA, Flick CL, Gilbert AM, et al. Comparison of two computer-automated procedures for tinnitus pitch-matching. J Rehabil Res Dev 2001;38:557–66.
59. Burns EM. A comparison of variability among measurements of subjective tinnitus and objective stimuli. Audiology 1984;23:426–40.
60. Henry JA, Meikle MB. Psychoacoustic measures of tinnitus. J Am Acad Audiol 2000;11:138–55.
61. Henry JA, Flick CL, Gilbert A, et al. Comparison of manual and computer-automated procedures for tinnitus pitch-matching. J Rehabil Res Dev 2004;41:121–38.
62. Penner MJ, Bilger RC. Psychophysical observations and the origin of tinnitus. In: Vernon JA, Moller AR, editors. Mechanisms of tinnitus. Needham Heights (MA): Allyn & Bacon; 1995. p. 219–30.
63. Meikle MB, Vernon J, Johnson RM. The perceived severity of tinnitus. Otolaryngol Head Neck Surg 1984;92:689–96.
64. McFadden D, Wightman FL. Audition: some relations between normal and pathological hearing. Annu Rev Psychol 1983;34:95–128.
65. Coles RRA. Tinnitus: epidemiology, aetiology and classification. In: Reich GE, Vernon JA, editors. Proceedings of the Fifth International Tinnitus Seminar 1995. Portland (OR): American Tinnitus Association; 1996. p. 25–9.
66. Stach BA. Comprehensive dictionary of audiology. Baltimore: Williams & Wilkins; 1997.
67. Meikle MB, Henry JA, Mitchell CM. Methods for matching the loudness of tinnitus using external tones. In: Reich GE, Vernon JA, Proceedings of the Fifth International Tinnitus Seminar 1995. Portland (OR): American Tinnitus Association; 1996. p. 178–9.
68. Meikle M, Griest S. Computer data analysis: Tinnitus Data Registry. In: Shulman A, editor. Tinnitus: diagnosis/treatment. Philadelphia: Lea & Febiger; 1991. p. 416–30.
69. Meikle MB, Creedon TA, Griest SE. Tinnitus Archive. 2nd ed. Available at: http//www.tinnitusarchive.org (accessed March 13, 2004).
70. Carhart R, Jerger JF. Preferred method for clinical determination of pure-tone thresholds. J Speech Hear Disord 1959;24:330–45.
71. Vernon JA, Johnson RM, Schleuning AJ, Mitchell CR. Masking and tinnitus. Audiol Hear Ed 1980;6:5–9.
72. Vernon JA. Tinnitus: causes, evaluation, and treatment. In: English GM, editor. Otolaryngology. Philadelphia: JB Lippincott; 1992. p. 1–25.
73. Jastreboff PJ, Hazell JWP, Graham RL. Neurophysiological model of tinnitus: dependence of the minimal masking level on treatment outcome. Hear Res 1994;80:216–32.
74. Jastreboff PJ, Jastreboff MM. Tinnitus retraining therapy. Semin Hear 2001;22:51–63.
75. Vernon J, Griest S, Press L. Attributes of tinnitus and the acceptance of masking. Am J Otolaryngol 1990;11:44–50.

76. Henry JA, Jastreboff MM, Jastreboff PJ, et al. Guide to conducting tinnitus retraining therapy initial and follow-up interviews. J Rehabil Res Dev 2003;40:157–78.
77. Byrne D, Dirks D. Effects of acclimatization and deprivation on non-speech auditory abilities. Ear Hear 1996;17(3 Suppl):29S–37S.
78. Hawkins DB, Walden B, Montgomery A. Description and validation of an LDL procedure designed to select SSPL90. Ear Hear 1987;8:162–9.
79. Burch-Sims PG, Ochs MT. The anatomic and physiologic bases of otoacoustic emissions. Hear J 1992;45:9–10.
80. Brownell WE. Outer hair cell electromotility and otoacoustic emissions. Ear Hear 1990;11:82–92.
81. Henry JA, Flick CL, Gilbert AM, et al. Masking curves and otoacoustic emissions in subjects with and without tinnitus. In: Hazell J, editor. Proceedings of the Sixth International Tinnitus Seminar. London: The Tinnitus and Hyperacusis Center; 1999. p. 345–9.
82. Jastreboff PJ, Jastreboff MM. Tinnitus retraining therapy (TRT) as a method for treatment of tinnitus and hyperacusis patients. J Am Acad Audiol 2000;11:162–77.
83. Heller MF, Bergman M. Tinnitus aurium in normally hearing persons. Ann Otol Rhinol Laryngol 1953;62:73–83.
84. Meikle MB. A conceptual framework to aid the diagnosis and treatment of severe tinnitus. Aust N Z J Audiol 2003;24:59–67.
85. Dobie RA. Randomized clinical trials for tinnitus: not the last word? In: Patuzzi R, editor. Proceedings of the Seventh International Tinnitus Seminar. Perth: Physiology Department, University of Western Australia; 2002. p. 3–6.
86. Meikle MB, Griest SE. Tinnitus severity and disability: prospective efforts to develop a core set of measures. In: Patuzzi R, editor. Proceedings of the Seventh International Tinnitus Seminar. Perth: Physiology Department, University of Western Australia; 2002. p. 157–61.
87. Tyler RS. Tinnitus disability and handicap questionnaires. Semin Hear 1993;14:377–83.
88. Brown SC. Older Americans and tinnitus: a demographic study and chartbook. GRI monograph series A, No. 2. Washington (DC): Gallaudet Research Institute, Gallaudet University; 1990.
89. Hinchcliffe R. Prevalence of the commoner ear, nose and throat conditions in the adult rural population of Great Britain. Br J Prev Soc Med 1961;15:128–40.
90. Leske MC. Prevalence estimates of communicative disorders in the U.S.: language, hearing and vestibular disorders. ASHA 1981;23:229–37.
91. Office of Population Census and Surveys. General household survey: the prevalence of tinnitus 1981. In: OPCS Monitor, Reference GHS83/1. London: Office for National Statistics; 1983.
92. Davis AC. Hearing in adults. London: Whurr Publishers, Ltd.; 1995.
93. Vernon JA, Møller AR. Mechanisms of tinnitus. Needham Heights (MA): Allyn & Bacon; 1995.
94. Perry BP, Gantz BJ. Medical and surgical evaluation and management of tinnitus. In: Tyler RS, editor. Tinnitus handbook. San Diego (CA): Singular Publishing Group; 2000. p. 221–41.
95. Axelsson A, Barrenas M-L. Tinnitus in noise-induced hearing loss. In: Dancer AL, Henderson D, Salvi RJ, Hamnernik RP, editors. Noise-induced hearing loss. St. Louis: Mosby-Year Book, Inc.; 1992. p. 269–76.
96. Vernon JA. Is the claimed tinnitus real and is the claimed cause correct? In: Reich GE, Vernon JA, editors. Proceedings of the Fifth International Tinnitus Seminar 1995. Portland (OR): American Tinnitus Association; 1996. p. 395–6.
97. Dobie RA. Medical-legal evaluation of hearing loss. 2nd ed. San Diego (CA): Singular Publishing Group; 2001.
98. Martin FN. Pseudohypacusis. In: Katz J, editor. Handbook of clinical audiology. Baltimore: Williams & Wilkins; 1994. p. 553–67.
99. Jacobson GP, Henderson JA. Toward the development of a subjective measure of the presence of tinnitus: preliminary observations [abstract]. In: Abstracts of the 22nd MidWinter Research Meeting of the Association for Research in Otolaryngology. Mount Royal (NJ): Association for Research in Otolaryngology; 1999. p. 172.
100. Rheinsburg BE, Henry JA, Ellingson RM, Schechter MA. Automated tinnitus measurement to assess tinnitus malingering. Presented at the 15th Annual Convention & Expo—American Academy of Audiology, San Antonio, TX, April 3, 2003.
101. Dobie RA. Medico-legal aspects of tinnitus. In: Patuzzi R, editor. Proceedings of the Seventh International Tinnitus Seminar. Perth: Physiology Department, University of Western Australia; 2002. p. 25–8.
102. Dobie RA. A review of randomized clinical trials in tinnitus. Laryngoscope 1999;109:1202–11.

CHAPTER 17

Tinnitus Questionnaires

Craig W. Newman, PhD, Sharon A. Sandridge, PhD

The use of self-report measures within the context of a comprehensive tinnitus evaluation has gained popularity among clinicians for several reasons. First, a weak relationship exists between tinnitus sensation and its impact on the individual. In this connection, several investigators have reported low correlations among psychoacoustic measures of tinnitus loudness and pitch and perceived tinnitus severity and annoyance.[1,2] Accordingly, psychoacoustic measures are inadequate for describing individuals' reactions to the perceived tinnitus sensation(s). Second, tinnitus is fundamentally a self-report phenomenon.[3] Similar to chronic pain, tinnitus is not readily apparent to others except through the complaints of the sufferer. This is in direct contrast to hearing loss, which is often first experienced by others, such as friends, family, and/or coworkers, who are directly affected by communication breakdowns. Third, tinnitus questionnaires help identify those individuals who are particularly bothered by their tinnitus and who may benefit from intervention.[4] That is, these tools may serve as a means to triage patients, indicating which individuals may require intensive rehabilitative management versus those who simply need minimal counseling. Fourth, by conducting an item analysis of the questionnaires, specific problems may be identified that are encountered by the patient. In this way, the clinician can address directly specific areas of concern or discover maladaptive thoughts and behaviors. This might be helpful in recommending, for example, cognitive-behavioral therapy as part of the total management process.[5] Finally, tinnitus questionnaires can be used in a pre- and post-treatment paradigm to evaluate treatment efficacy. The latter is especially important in light of today's need in the health care environment to demonstrate to third-party payers the clinical effectiveness of treatment protocols.

In addition to clinical applications, tinnitus questionnaires have been useful for a variety of research purposes.[4] For example, tinnitus questionnaires may provide a basis for understanding the relationship between personality and psychopathology and their impact on the day-to-day living of individuals, including distress, handicap, and perceived social support.[6] Further, tinnitus questionnaires provide a method for researchers to standardize or quantify tinnitus as a criterion for subject selection. That is, self-report measures allow investigators to select only those patients indicating a certain degree of tinnitus severity (as defined in the research protocol) to be included in the study. Furthermore, self-report measures allow investigators to evaluate the effectiveness, over the short or the long term, of a particular experimental treatment. In fact, Dobie highlighted the need to include measures of tinnitus consequence as primary outcome variables in randomized clinical trials for tinnitus treatment.[7]

Whether it is for research or clinical purposes, quantifying the impact of tinnitus on everyday life is critical. Perhaps it is just as critical, if not more so, as measuring the psychoacoustic dimensions of tinnitus sensation. Given that, the World Health Organization (WHO) classification scheme for describing the consequences of health conditions[8,9] has been recommended as an appropriate conceptual framework for developing a tinnitus evaluation model.[10–12] Table 17-1 summarizes the individual components of the WHO model as it corresponds to tinnitus. As shown, *impairment* relates to the actual perception of the tinnitus sensation. In this regard, a variety of psychoacoustic methods have been developed to quantify tinnitus pitch, loudness, maskability, and other dimensions of the tinnitus experience.[11] In contrast, *disability/activity limitation* and *handicap/participation restriction* focus on the consequences of the impairment. That is, disability/activity limitations and handicap/participation

TABLE 17-1. Domains of Function and Measurement Tools Based on the World Health Organization Model for Describing Consequences of Health Conditions

Category	Impairment	Disability/Activity Limitation	Handicap/Participation Restriction
Definition	Dysfunction of the auditory system resulting in the perception of tinnitus (ie, sensation of sounds)	Effect of impairment on reducing an individual's ability to function in a normal manner	Psychosocial manifestations of impairment and disability resulting in the need for extra effort and reduced independence
Representative dimensions	Pitch, loudness, maskability, residual inhibition	Loss of concentration; sleep disturbance; reduced speech perception; reduced sound localization ability; associated health issues such as vertigo/unsteadiness, headache, hyperacusis; associated psychological problems such as distress, annoyance, intrusiveness, loss of control	Relationships with family, friends, and/or coworkers; avoidance of situations, including quiet or noisy places or environments
Measurement tools	Psychoacoustic measures including pitch and loudness matching, minimum masking levels, and tests of residual inhibition Magnitude estimations (eg, 1–10 scales for pitch or loudness) and visual analog measures	Open-ended and fixed-item tinnitus questionnaires, psychological tests, and diaries	Open-ended and fixed-item tinnitus questionnaires, diaries

Adapted from the World Health Organization[8,9] and Tyler R.[10,11]

restriction reflect to what degree the tinnitus affects the individual's routine abilities and lifestyle.[10] Thus, tinnitus questionnaires are the primary tools for evaluating the disabling and handicapping effects of tinnitus, providing insight into how the tinnitus sensation (impairment) generates a disability at the personal level that ultimately produces a handicap at the societal level.

This chapter presents a review of the more commonly used self-report tinnitus questionnaires. The chapter, however, begins with a brief review of some of the important psychometric properties that must be considered when evaluating the usefulness of a particular tinnitus questionnaire for a specific purpose. It is our intent to provide a useful and practical reference guide for clinicians and researchers seeking information about the availability of tinnitus questionnaires measuring one or more of the following constructs: distress, disability, handicap, negative and positive thought processes, and coping styles and strategies. Finally, the application of tinnitus questionnaires is discussed, including their usefulness in determining treatment candidacy, in subject selection for research purposes, and as outcome variables in clinical trials.

PSYCHOMETRIC ADEQUACY

The purpose of this section is to assist the reader in becoming an informed consumer of the literature. In doing so, readers will be able to select the most appropriate questionnaire for their specific clinical or research application.

First and foremost, the selection of any tinnitus questionnaire should be guided by the appropriateness of the items comprising the inventory. The purpose and context of the tool should be evaluated related to its intended application. For example, if the principal application of the tinnitus questionnaire is to monitor the outcome of a specific treatment protocol, a number of questions should be addressed: Which consequences of tinnitus are important to explore? Are the scale items sensitive to the effects of intervention? How much change is considered clinically significantly different following intervention? Can the individual's score be compared with a normative database? Does the tinnitus questionnaire have high test–retest reliability and stability? Does the administration mode (eg, paper/pencil, interview format, computer assisted) affect the precision and accuracy of the results?

Thus, the decision to use a particular questionnaire needs to be made after a critical review of the evidence in support of that instrument. Unfortunately, it is beyond the scope of this chapter to present an in-depth discussion of all of the psychometric characteristics that should be assessed prior to the selection of a particular scale. Readers are referred to Hyde for such an in-depth discussion.[13] A few key areas of psychometric standards that are helpful when evaluating a "candidate" tool, however, are reviewed briefly below:

- *Overall methodology of development, validation, and norming.* The theoretic constructs underlying the development of the questionnaire and how each of the constructs is conceptualized must be analyzed. That is, what is the questionnaire assessing? Is it assessing the disability (or activity limitation) or handicap (or participation restriction) that the WHO model[8,9] describes? Or is it assessing other constructs, such as coping style or maladaptive thoughts and behaviors? In addition, is the scale standardized? If so, scores can be compared across individuals, time, and clinical settings. Moreover, normative data in the form of estimated population means, standard deviations, and percentiles provide the user with information about what is considered typical or atypical for the target population or for a given individual.[14]
- *Reliability.* The concept of reliability relates to the precision of measurement and is assessed by examining the consistency or stability of the measure. There are several aspects to reliability. Internal consistency reliability deals with the interitem consistency of responses or relationships among scale items. For example, if a tinnitus questionnaire has a relatively large number of items addressing the emotional consequences of tinnitus (eg, Does your tinnitus make you angry? Does your tinnitus make you upset? Does your tinnitus make you feel frustrated?), it is reasonable to expect that the scores on each item would be correlated with scores on all of the other items within the emotional domain. Cronbach's α is the statistical method for calculating internal consistency.

  Another aspect of reliability, reproducibility, can be evaluated in two dimensions. Test–retest reliability assesses short-term, day-to-day fluctuations in test scores. In contrast, retest stability measures changes that occur in scores over longer periods of time.[14] Reproducibility is critical when using the tool to document changes over time. For example, if a patient is enrolled in a sound therapy program (eg, habituation or masking), changes in tinnitus over time may need to be documented. If reproducibility has not been evaluated for each time interval, documented changes in perceived tinnitus problems may not be due to the treatment per se but rather to measurement error of the questionnaire being used for monitoring purposes. Pearson product-moment correlations are often used to estimate reliability.
- *Validity.* The ability of the instrument to yield relevant and useful inferences and decisions in specific contexts that are "truthful," "correct," or "real" reflects the validity of the instrument.[13,15] A variety of validation strategies are used by scale developers, including content validity, criterion-related validity, and construct validity. Content validity demonstrates the extent to which the items comprising the scale sample the important or relevant behaviors or characteristics to be measured, known as the target domains. Criterion-related validity measures how well the inventory correlates with some outside validating criterion or gold standard. Construct validity evaluates the degree to which an instrument either empirically or rationally purports to measure some theoretic construct (ie, a model that proposes observable variables and predicts relationships) or explanation of the behavior or characteristic to be assessed.[15]
- *Responsiveness.* This characteristic reflects the ability of the instrument to yield changes in observed values following an individual's response to some

external factor, such as clinical or experimental intervention. For example, responsiveness relates directly to changes in perceived tinnitus severity, distress, or annoyance that could be measured by a tinnitus questionnaire using a pre- and postadministration format.

- *Feasibility.* Feasibility concerns the practical application of the instrument in the real-world context. The instrument must be acceptable to the respondents and its target situation of use whether for research, clinical, or administrative purposes.[13] For example, tinnitus questionnaires used in a busy clinical practice must be brief and easy to administer, score, and interpret.

SPECIFIC TINNITUS QUESTIONNAIRES

Many questionnaires assessing some aspect of tinnitus consequences are available. This section presents a review of the more commonly used questionnaires. Qualitative and quantitative approaches are examined.

QUALITATIVE APPROACHES

Qualitative tinnitus questionnaires are not score driven. That is, the responses are descriptive in nature and are not assigned a predetermined response value per item. Thus, there are no "total scores" obtained from these questionnaires. Examples of qualitative questionnaires include the initial intake interview, open-ended methods for obtaining information regarding patient's complaints, and daily monitoring diaries.

Intake Interview Questionnaires A detailed history and primary source of data about the nature of the patient's complaints can be obtained through the initial intake. In addition, the case history format helps establish rapport between the clinician and patient and the tone for subsequent intervention. The goal of the intake interview is to arrive at a thorough understanding of the nature of the tinnitus by exploring a broad range of inquiry, including causal, descriptive, and diagnostic variables. Further, a detailed history is especially important in medicolegal cases in that it contributes to the consistency and plausibility of the individual's report.[16]

Many practitioners use published case history questionnaires[4,16–18] or develop their own for clinical use. Table 17-2 summarizes the major components of a tinnitus case history. Note that Table 17-2 is not a

TABLE 17-2. Major Categories Comprising a Tinnitus Case History Questionnaire

Perceptual features
  Location
  Tinnitus descriptor (eg, hissing, ringing, pulsing, etc)
  Magnitude estimation of pitch and loudness (eg, 1–10 scale)
  Changes in pitch, loudness, and/or quality
Duration
  Initial onset
  Length of time when tinnitus became noticeable/bothersome
  Tinnitus awareness (eg, constant, intermittent)
  Recent experiences
Exacerbating factors
  Sound environment (eg, quiet vs noise)
  Diet
  Stress
  Time of day
  Medication
  Activity (eg, change in body position, physical exertion)
  Alcohol
  Smoking
  Sleep disturbance
Reducing factors
  Sound environment (eg, quiet versus noise)
  Diet
  Medications
  Alcohol
  Smoking
  Sleep
Psychosocial and functional consequences
  Annoyance
  Sleep disturbance
  Depression
  Concentration difficulty
  Interference with speech understanding
  Suicidal ideation
  Increased mental/emotional stress
  Effects on family/friends/coworkers
  Interference/avoidance of social situations
  Positive/negative thoughts about tinnitus
  Acceptance
Hearing
  Assessment of impairment, disability, and handicap
  Hearing aid use
  Sound intolerance (eg, hyperacusis, phonophobia)
Treatment history
  Medical
  Surgical
  Rehabilitative
  Benefits from treatment
  Current expectations

Item categories adapted from Henry JL and Wilson PH,[4] Schechter MA and Henry JA,[16] Henry JA et al,[17] and Stouffer JL and Tyler RS.[18]

case history form but rather a listing of the important elements discerned from a number of published intake questionnaires. Generally speaking, the intake questionnaire should include such information as (1) the history and descriptive characteristics of the tinnitus; (2) specific behavioral, social, interpersonal, and emotional consequences of tinnitus; (3) factors that may either exacerbate or reduce tinnitus severity; and (4) previous tinnitus treatments.

Tinnitus Problems Questionnaire The Tinnitus Problems Questionnaire (TPQ) developed by Tyler and Baker employs a completely open-ended format.[19] The patient is simply asked to respond to the following statement: "Please make a list of the difficulties that you have as a result of your tinnitus. List them in order of importance, starting with the biggest difficulties. Write down as many of them as you can."

The primary advantage of any open-ended questionnaire is that it allows the patient to list specific problems that are encountered without the constraints imposed by a fixed-item scale. For example, the use of questionnaires that have a fixed list of tinnitus-related problems, such as the Tinnitus Handicap Inventory (THI)[20] and the Tinnitus Reaction Questionnaire (TRQ),[21] may contain items that are either irrelevant to or infrequently experienced by the tinnitus sufferer. Potentially, the validity of the fixed-item scale could be questioned given the fact that irrelevant items carry the same weight as those that are relevant to the individual patient. The primary disadvantage of an open-ended questionnaire is that the responses cannot be quantified across time or patients.[10] Therefore, it is recommended that the combined use of the open-ended questionnaire, along with a structured inventory, may provide the most useful clinical information for a given individual.

Using data obtained from 72 members of a tinnitus self-help group completing the TPQ, Tyler and Baker determined that tinnitus problems relate primarily to one of four general categories: effects on hearing, effects on lifestyle, effects on general health, and emotional problems.[19] Table 17-3 displays the 15 most common difficulties attributed to tinnitus, along with their assignment to one of the four major categories. Sanchez and Stephens applied the TPQ to a sample of patients being seen for tinnitus in a clinical setting.[22] Responses from a total of 436 patients confirmed the findings reported earlier by Tyler and Baker.[19] That is, 9 of the 15 most frequent complaints

TABLE 17-3. Top 15 Difficulties Attributed to Tinnitus and Associated General Consequence Categories for 72 Respondents from a Tinnitus Self-Help Group

Difficulty	Percentage of Total Respondents	General Category
Getting to sleep	56.9	Effects on lifestyle
Persistence of tinnitus	48.6	Effects on lifestyle
Understanding speech	37.5	Effects on hearing
Despair, frustration, depression	36.1	Emotional problem
Annoyance, irritation, inability to relax	34.7	Emotional problem
Concentration, confusion	33.3	Emotional problem
Dependence on drugs	23.6	Effects on general health
Pain/headache	18.0	Effects on general health
Worse on awakening in morning	16.6	Effects on lifestyle
Insecurity, fear, worry	16.6	Emotional problem
Avoid noisy situations	15.3	Effects on lifestyle
Withdraw, avoid friends	13.8	Effects on lifestyle
Giddiness, balance, fuzzy head	13.8	Effects on general health
Understanding television	11.1	Effects on hearing
Avoid quiet situations	11.1	Effects on lifestyle

Adapted from Tyler RS and Baker LJ.[19]

were comparable between the two samples. It is noteworthy that complaints relating to hearing and sleep disturbance were the most prominent for both groups.

The TPQ has been instrumental in the development of fixed-list quantitative measures. That is, tinnitus complaints obtained from open-ended questionnaires have formed the corpus of the items used in the developmental stages of quantitative questionnaires.

Daily Diaries Daily monitoring of tinnitus may be used as a technique for assessing the occurrence or patterns of tinnitus complaints over time. For example, daily monitoring diaries can track a variety of tinnitus attributes, including self-rated changes in pitch, loudness, annoyance, and sleep disturbance. Other factors, such as noise exposure, medication use, and diet, can be recorded to determine relationships between changes in tinnitus perception and everyday life events. Although helpful in designing cognitive-behavioral therapy sessions, the use of daily monitoring also poses several limitations.[4] These include response bias, exaggeration, and increasing attention to the tinnitus. The latter is especially problematic when patients are obsessive about monitoring their tinnitus at regular intervals throughout the day. In fact, continued shifts in attention to the tinnitus may be counterproductive when using sound therapy in a habituation rehabilitative model (eg, tinnitus retraining therapy [TRT]). When used appropriately, however, daily monitoring diaries may be useful by enlightening the clinician to the difficulties experienced by the patient, the coping strategies used by the patient, and the consequences of tinnitus on the individual's psychosocial functioning.

Quantitative Approaches

Quantitative tinnitus questionnaires are score driven. That is, the responses can be summed and/or averaged, resulting in a total score or subscale scores. They fall into two broad categories: those that quantify tinnitus distress, disability, and handicap and those that tap into coping styles and strategies. Table 17-4 summarizes the categories, functions, responses, and complaints assessed

TABLE 17-4. Dimensions of Function Assessed by Tinnitus Questionnaires

Dimension	STSS	TQ	THI	THQ	TH/SS	TRQ	TSS	TCQ	TCSQ
Catastrophic response			X			X			
Effective coping style									X
Effects on hearing		X		X			X		
Emotional distress		X	X	X	X				
Engagement in negative cognitions and thoughts								X	
Engagement in positive cognitions and thoughts								X	
General distress						X	X		
General severity	X								
Intrusiveness		X					X		
Maladaptive coping style									X
Mental functioning			X						
Patient outlook/perceived attitudes				X	X				
Physical consequences of tinnitus			X	X					
Sleep disturbance		X					X		
Social support					X				
Social/occupational interference			X	X	X	X			
Somatic complaints		X							

STSS = Subjective Tinnitus Severity Scale[23]; TCQ = Tinnitus Cognitions Questionnaire[43]; TCSQ = Tinnitus Coping Style Questionnaire[44,45]; THI = Tinnitus Handicap Inventory[20]; THQ = Tinnitus Handicap Questionnaire[29]; TH/SS = Tinnitus Handicap/Support Scale[41]; TQ = Tinnitus Questionnaire[24]; TRQ = Tinnitus Reaction Questionnaire[21]; TSS = Tinnitus Severity Scale.[42]

by the various quantitative tinnitus questionnaires. Each questionnaire is presented using the same format: a description of the questionnaire, how the questionnaire is scored and interpreted, the psychometric adequacy of the questionnaire, and, finally, the strengths and weaknesses of the instrument.

Many of the scales in this category contain items that overlap. That is, many scales do not solely assess distress, disability, or handicap but rather assess a combination of the aforementioned domains. Therefore, the questionnaires have not been divided separately by scales of distress, disability, or handicap but grouped under this section.

Subjective Tinnitus Severity Scale Description The 16-item Subjective Tinnitus Severity Scale (STSS) was devised by Halford and Anderson to provide a simple questionnaire to assess tinnitus "severity."[23] Severity is defined in terms of intrusiveness, prominence, and distress, although there is no subset of items identified for each of these domains. Each question is answered with either a "yes" or "no" response.

Scoring and Interpretation. Each item is worth 1 point. Ten of the 16 items earn a point if the response is "yes" (eg, "Are you almost always aware of your tinnitus?"), whereas the other six items earn a point if the response is "no" (eg, "When you are busy, do you quite often forget about your tinnitus?"). Accordingly, scores range from 0 to 16, with higher scores reflecting greater overall severity.

Psychometric Adequacy. The STSS yielded high internal consistency reliability, as indicated by a Cronbach's α of .84. Criterion validity was assessed by demonstrating significant correlations with two independent clinician ratings of severity. Weak yet statistically significant correlations were observed between severity scores and several audiometric variables (loudness match at 1,000 Hz, sensation level at 1,000 Hz, threshold at tinnitus frequency, and loudness match at tinnitus frequency).

Strengths and Weaknesses. The STSS is a brief questionnaire that is simple to administer and score. Two major limitations, however, are noteworthy. First, no classification scheme was developed, making it difficult to categorize the tinnitus severity for a given individual with any precision. Second, test–retest reliability was not assessed, limiting its applicability for measuring treatment outcome.

Tinnitus Questionnaire Description The 52-item Tinnitus Questionnaire (TQ) developed by Hallam and colleagues is also known as the Tinnitus Effects Questionnaire.[24] This instrument was designed to measure the dimensions of patients' complaints about their tinnitus, namely sleep disturbance (eg, "It takes me longer to get to sleep because of the noises."), emotional distress (eg, "The way the noises sound is really unpleasant."), and auditory perceptual difficulties (eg, "Because of the noises, it is more difficult to listen to several people at once."). Each question relates directly to the "noises" in the ear as the major cause or source of distress. Further, the authors included items that reflect inappropriate or a lack of coping skills, which they refer to as "absolutist" beliefs (eg, "It is unfair that I have to suffer with my noises.").

Scoring and Interpretation. Individuals indicate their level of agreement to each statement using one of three response alternatives: true (2 points), partly true (1 point), or not true (0 points). Affirmative responses to an item (indicated by true) are identified as complaints about tinnitus, with the exception of the following items: 1, 7, 32, 40, 44, and 49. These six statements are reverse-scored because they are considered "positive" statements (eg, "I can sometimes ignore the noises even when they are there."). Possible scores range from 0 to 104 points, with higher scores reflecting greater tinnitus complaints.

Psychometric Adequacy. Studies by Hallam, Henry and Wilson, Hiller and Goebel, and Hiller and colleagues provide the psychometric characteristics of the TQ.[25–28] This instrument has been found to have high internal consistency reliability (Cronbach's α = .91–.95) and high test–retest reliability (r = .91–.94).[26] The high test–retest reliability suggests good stability over time. High correlations were also found between the TQ and measures of tinnitus handicap (Tinnitus Handicap Questionnaire [THQ])[29] and tinnitus distress (TRQ).[21] Interestingly, factor analyses conducted in Germany[27] and Australia[26] were consistent with the factors originally identified by Hallam and colleagues in the United Kingdom supporting the instrument's validity.[24]

Strengths and Weaknesses. The TQ has been found to measure a number of different dimensions of tinnitus complaints and is a stable measure over time. In this connection, the TQ would be useful as an outcome measure in determining the effectiveness of treatment. Hiller and Goebel,[27] as well as Henry and Wilson,[4] suggest that subscale scores may be of more use to clinicians in identifying the severity of major complaints of tinnitus rather than using the total score. No data, however, are available to assist the clinician in determining what is considered a clinically and statistically significant change in scores following intervention for a given patient, therefore limiting its use as a pre- or post-test measure.

Tinnitus Handicap Inventory Description Newman and colleagues devised the 25-item THI.[20] The items were grouped a priori into three subscales. The functional subscale (11 items) evaluates role limitations in the areas of mental (eg, "Because of your tinnitus, is it difficult for you to concentrate?"), social/occupational (eg, "Because of your tinnitus, do you not enjoy social activities such as going out to dinner or to the movies?"), and physical functioning (eg, "Because of your tinnitus, do you have trouble falling to sleep at night?"). The emotional subscale (nine items) includes items representing a broad range of affective responses to tinnitus, including anger, frustration, irritability, and depression. The catastrophic subscale (five items) probes the most severe reactions to tinnitus, such as desperation, loss of control, inability to cope, inability to escape from tinnitus, and fear of having a grave disease.

SCORING AND INTERPRETATION. For each item on the inventory, the patient responds with "yes" (4 points), "sometimes" (2 points), or "no" (0 points). The responses are summed, with a total score ranging from 0 to 100 points. Higher scores represent greater perceived handicap. In a subsequent study, Newman and colleagues developed handicap severity categories based on quartiles calculated for the total THI score.[30] These categories are no handicap (0–16 points), mild handicap (18–36 points), moderate handicap (38–56 points), and severe handicap (58–100 points).

PSYCHOMETRIC ADEQUACY. The THI has excellent internal consistency reliability (Cronbach's α = .93) and high test–retest reliability for the total score (r = .92), as well as the subscales (ranging from .84–.94). Similarly, the coefficient of repeatability was determined to be high for the total score and the three subscales. The 95% confidence interval was 20 points for the total scale, suggesting that a 20-point or greater difference needs to be observed between test and retest for a change (eg, pre- and post-treatment administration) to be considered statistically and clinically significant. Convergent validity was assessed using the THQ,[29] whereas construct validity was assessed using the Beck Depression Inventory,[31] Modified Somatic Perception Questionnaire,[32] symptom rating scales (eg, sleep disturbance, annoyance), and perceived tinnitus pitch and loudness. More recently, Baguley and colleagues indicated that the THI demonstrated high convergent validity with the TQ.[24,33]

STRENGTHS AND WEAKNESSES. The THI is useful in a busy clinical practice because it is brief and easily administered and assesses the domains of function that can be remedied by available medical, surgical, and rehabilitative interventions. In light of the response format and scoring, the THI can be used as a companion scale to the Hearing Handicap Inventory for the Elderly (HHIE), the Hearing Handicap Inventory for Adults (HHIA),[34,35] and the Dizziness Handicap Inventory (DHI).[36] Using these three inventories in concert might be useful for quantifying handicap for a variety of patient groups, especially those with Meniere's disease. The test–retest data are important for attempting to quantify changes in perceived handicap following treatment; however, the retest was conducted, on average, 20 days after the initial administration, suggesting that further study should include retest stability over longer time intervals. In this way, it would be possible to evaluate statistically significant changes in perceived handicap over the medium and long term. A Danish translation of the THI (THI-DK) was developed by Zachariae and colleagues using a sample of 50 patients presenting with tinnitus as the primary complaint.[37] Similar to the THI, the THI-DK appears to be a reliable and valid measure of tinnitus handicap. The distinctness of the subscales (ie, functional, emotional, and catastrophic), however, has been questioned.[37,38] In fact, Baguley and Andersson recommend that the THI be considered a unifactorial scale, that is, only the total score should be used for clinical purposes.[38] In addition, a Spanish version of the THI is now available.[39]

Tinnitus Handicap Questionnaire Description Kuk and colleagues developed the 27-item THQ.[29] It was developed to be broad in scope but sensitive to patients' perceived degree of tinnitus handicap. Based on a factor analysis using principal components extraction, three factors or subscales emerged. Factor 1, consisting of 15 items, reflects the physical (eg, "I am unable to relax because of my tinnitus."), emotional (eg, "Tinnitus makes me feel insecure."), and social (eg, "I find it difficult to explain what tinnitus is to others.") consequences of tinnitus. Factor 2, composed of eight items, probes the interfering effects of tinnitus on hearing ability (eg, "Tinnitus has caused a reduction in my speech understanding ability."). Finally, factor 3, which consists of four items, explores the patient's view of tinnitus (eg, "The general public does not know about the devastating nature of tinnitus.").

SCORING AND INTERPRETATION. For each item, the individual responds with a number between 0 and 100 indicating how much he or she disagrees (0 = strongly disagrees) or agrees (100 = strongly agrees) with the statement. Mean scores for the total and for each of the three factors are calculated, with higher scores indicating greater handicap. Prior to determining the average values, it is necessary to invert the responses obtained on items 25 and 26 by subtracting them from 100. Kuk and colleagues provided a method for determining the severity of an individual's handicap by comparing his or her average scores against the authors' published normative data.[29] This is nicely illustrated in Figure 2 in the Kuk and colleagues' article.[29] For example, a mean THQ score of 50% places the patient's overall tinnitus handicap at approximately the 70th percentile. This suggests that for the patient in this example, his or her perceived tinnitus handicap is more severe than 70% of the patients comprising the normative sample.

PSYCHOMETRIC ADEQUACY. The THQ demonstrated high internal consistency reliability for the total scale (Cronbach's α = .95), factor 1 (.95), and factor 2 (.88). Factor 3 yielded a low alpha (.47), which the investigators attributed to the small number of items comprising this subscale and the low correlations among the individual items. Henry and Wilson obtained similar factor structures in their Australian sample.[26] Adequate construct validity of the THQ was documented by the observation of moderately high ($r >$ .50) correlations with perceived tinnitus loudness judgments, life satisfaction, hearing threshold, depression, and general health status. Newman and colleagues, assessing test–retest stability over a 6-week period, found high test–retest correlations for the total score (r = .89), factor 1 (r = .89), and factor 2 (r = .90), whereas factor 3 yielded inadequate retest reliability (r = .50).[40]

STRENGTHS AND WEAKNESSES. The THQ is useful for potentially evaluating the effects of tinnitus on lifestyle, health, hearing, and emotional well-being. The percentile ranking for a given patient is helpful in determining severity on an individual basis relative to other patients with tinnitus. The authors caution, however, that this technique should not be the only criterion used to determine a particular type of management program. Further, based on reliability data (both internal consistency and test–retest), application of factor 3 (patient's view of tinnitus) as an independent measure is questionable. Moreover, scoring each of the items using a 100-point scale may be somewhat problematic. That is, using a response format between 0 and 100 that corresponds with subjective strength of belief may be unwieldy or too esoteric for some patients.

Tinnitus Handicap/Support Scale Description The 28-item Tinnitus Handicap/Support Scale (TH/SS) devised by Erlandsson and colleagues assesses the attitudes of family and friends toward the person with tinnitus.[41] Based on a principal component analysis, three factors with relatively equivalent weightings were identified. These included factor 1 (9 items), perceived attitudes or reactions of others (eg, "People get annoyed with me."); factor 2 (10 items), social support (eg, "Family shows me that they care."); and factor 3 (9 items), personal and social handicaps (eg, "Tinnitus affects functioning at home.").

SCORING AND INTERPRETATION. Each statement on the scale is scored from 1 (strongly disagree) to 5 (strongly agree). The authors provided no guidelines for interpretation.

PSYCHOMETRIC ADEQUACY. The reliability of the TH/SS has not been examined. Construct validity of the TH/SS was assessed using a 10-item Tinnitus Severity Questionnaire (TSQ). Significant relationships between tinnitus severity and perceived attitudes (factor 1) and between tinnitus severity and disability or handicap (factor 3) were found. No significant relationship was observed between tinnitus severity and social support (factor 2). Positive correlations were shown between perceived attitudes and reactions of others (factor 1) and items on the TSQ, including life quality, concentration difficulties, discomfort in quiet environments, ability to suppress tinnitus, anxiety or worry, and tense or irritable and depressed feelings.

STRENGTHS AND WEAKNESSES. This is the only questionnaire that has been designed to assess the influence of significant others in the overall management process. This information might prove useful for counseling purposes. Unfortunately, this scale is limited in its clinical use because of the lack of retest reliability data. Further, the authors attest to the fact that the social support factor of the scale is not sufficiently sensitive to quantify the complexity of social support in patients with tinnitus.

Tinnitus Reaction Questionnaire Description Wilson and colleagues developed the TRQ to quantify the psychological distress associated with tinnitus.[21] The 26 items comprising the TRQ stem from the four general symptom categories described by Tyler and Baker.[19] Items within the categories relate to distress consequences such as anger, confusion, annoyance, helplessness, activity avoidance, and panic.

SCORING AND INTERPRETATION. Each item on the TRQ is scored on a 5-point scale, with anchors from 0 points (not at all) to 4 points (almost all of the time). The scores are summed with the total score ranging from 0 to 104 points, with higher scores reflecting greater distress.

PSYCHOMETRIC ADEQUACY. Overall, the psychometric properties of the TRQ are robust. The scale was found to have high internal consistency reliability (Cronbach's $\alpha = .96$), as well as test–retest reliability ($r = .88$). The construct validity of the instrument is supported by moderate to high correlations between the TRQ and clinician ratings and self-reported measures of anxiety and depression. Low correlations with neuroticism were observed. Using a principal components analysis, four factors emerged: factor 1, general distress, which accounted for 50% of the variance ("My tinnitus has made me feel helpless."); factor 2, interference ("My tinnitus has interfered with my ability to work."); factor 3, severity, in which some items overlap with factor 2 ("My tinnitus has interfered with my sleep."); and factor 4, avoidance ("My tinnitus has led me to avoid noisy situations."). These factorial structures may assist in describing individual patterns of responses to tinnitus.

STRENGTHS AND WEAKNESSES. The TRQ provides the clinician with a global measure of tinnitus distress. The brevity and ease of scoring of this questionnaire make it appealing as a clinical tool. Yet the TRQ is limited by its lack of severity (eg, mild, moderate, severe) cutoff values. For example, is the score of 72 significantly (ie, statistically) more severe than the score of 66? High test–retest reliability data observed indicate that the TRQ is useful in quantifying treatment outcome; however, the authors do not report what is considered a statistically significant change on the measure. Without the latter information, it is difficult to interpret changes in TRQ total scores between pre- and postintervention administrations. For example, 95% critical difference scores (based on confidence interval data) allow clinicians to determine whether a true change in perceived handicap for a given individual occurs following treatment. Further, because the retest period ranged from 3 days to 3 weeks, the long-term stability of the TRQ cannot be assumed.

Tinnitus Severity Scale Description Sweetow and Levy designed the 15-item multiple-choice questionnaire named the Tinnitus Severity Scale (TSS) to help quantify individuals' cognitive and behavioral responses to tinnitus and to assist the clinician in establishing treatment goals and measuring therapeutic progress.[42] The scale items were derived primarily from factors identified by Tyler and Baker[19] and Jakes and colleagues.[2] The authors categorized each item under one of the following factors: intrusiveness (four items), distress (six items), hearing loss (three items), sleep disturbance (one item), and medication (one item).

SCORING AND INTERPRETATION. The multiple-choice response for each item ranges in score from 1 (no impact) to 4 (most impact). For example, the item "I am bothered by my tinnitus" has the choice options of "extremely" (4 points), "very much" (3 points), "slightly" (2 points), and "not at all" (1 point). The respondent indicates how he or she has felt for the past week. Further, each item is weighted from 1 to 3 points (total weight score = 39 points), with the greatest weighting for questions focusing on distress (16 points total) and the least weighting related to medication (3 points total). The weighting assignments were based on the amount of variance accounted for by each factor in the

Jakes and colleagues' study.[2] The total score is calculated by multiplying each item's score by its weighting and summing these products. Accordingly, the TSS score can range from 39 points (39 weighting points × 1-point item score) to 156 points (39 weighting points × 4-point item score).

PSYCHOMETRIC ADEQUACY. The TSS has acceptable test–retest reliability ($r = .86$). No other psychometric data are available.

STRENGTHS AND WEAKNESSES. An item analysis of the scale may be useful for clinicians in helping to establish treatment goals and for counseling patients. In light of the limited psychometric data, however, clinical and research applications are currently limited.

QUESTIONNAIRES FOR COGNITIVE REACTION AND COPING STYLE

In addition to the scales assessing distress and disability or handicap, another group of scales has recently been developed. These scales focus on the patient's reaction to tinnitus from a cognitive perspective. For example, has the patient developed maladaptive reactions or dysfunctional thoughts to tinnitus? What coping mechanisms are being used by the patient to deal with the stresses brought on by tinnitus? Quantifying the patient's cognitive response to tinnitus is especially important given the current emphasis on the psychological management of tinnitus.

Tinnitus Cognitions Questionnaire Description The 26-item Tinnitus Cognitions Questionnaire (TCQ) developed by Wilson and Henry assesses the positive and negative thoughts associated with tinnitus.[43] The rationale for undertaking the development of the TCQ was to explore the cognitive processes involved in coping with tinnitus, devise an instrument that could be used to monitor treatment effectiveness, and provide a means by which to select patients who might benefit from cognitive-behavioral therapy. Within the context of the questionnaire, the 13 negative items (eg, "What did I do to deserve this?") are clearly separated from the 13 positive items (eg, "I'm not the only person with tinnitus.").

SCORING AND INTERPRETATION. Each of the items is rated on a 5-point scale (0–4) with anchor descriptors of "never" and "very frequently." The negative items (1 to 13) are scored 0 to 4, whereas the positive items (14 to 26) are reverse-scored, 4 to 0. The scoring involves the simple addition of the negative items and the reverse-scored positive items. Accordingly, the total TCQ scores range from 0 to 104, with higher scores reflecting a greater tendency to engage in negative thoughts in response to tinnitus and low engagement in positive thoughts.[43]

PSYCHOMETRIC ADEQUACY. The TCQ yielded both good test–retest reliability ($r = .88$) and internal consistency reliability (Cronbach's $\alpha = .91$). A factor analysis revealed two independent subsets of questions, namely negative and positive cognitions. The TCQ-positive and TCQ-negative scales correlate similarly ($r = .77$ and .71, respectively) with the total score. As anticipated, the two subsets of questions are unrelated ($r = .09$). Construct and convergent validity was assessed between the TCQ-total, TCQ-positive, and TCQ-negative scores and other measures of tinnitus-specific symptomatology (eg, distress, handicap, complaint behavior), depression, automatic thoughts, and locus of control. Overall, the TCQ showed moderate correlations with other tinnitus-related measures (ie, TRQ, THQ, and TQ), with the TCQ-negative subscale demonstrating higher correlations with each of the tinnitus- and nontinnitus measures.

STRENGTHS AND WEAKNESSES. The TCQ is an excellent addition to the clinician's armamentarium, providing a useful index of the cognitive responses observed in individuals with tinnitus. In addition to its excellent psychometric performance, the information gleaned from the TCQ responses (eg, patients with high reported levels of negative thoughts with a low endorsement rate for positive thoughts) would be helpful to clinicians selecting candidates for cognitive therapy and developing cognitive-behavioral therapy strategies as well. The authors of the TCQ, however, caution that the scale is a self-assessment measure and does not evaluate the extent to which people actually engage in the reported cognitions or thoughts.

Tinnitus Coping Style Questionnaire Description The Tinnitus Coping Style Questionnaire (TCSQ) developed by Budd and Pugh is a 33-item scale developed to assess a broad range of adaptive and coping strategies, based on a model of coping with the symptom of chronic pain.[44,45] The 33 items comprise two factors:

the maladaptive coping subscale and the effective coping subscale. Eighteen items comprise the maladaptive coping factor and focus on, for example, individuals' attempts to avoid tinnitus, praying that tinnitus will go away, fantasizing about not having tinnitus, and dwelling on tinnitus. Fifteen items comprise the effective coping subscale and evaluate, for example, acceptance of tinnitus, use of positive talk, attention switching, and engaging in activities to help minimize the intrusiveness of the noises.

Scoring and Interpretation. For each item, the respondent indicates how frequently he or she employs each of the coping strategies on a 1 ("never") to 7 ("always") scale. Higher scores on the maladaptive coping subscale reflect poorer coping skills, characterized by greater catastrophic thinking about the consequences of tinnitus. In contrast, higher scores on the effective coping dimension are characterized by better acceptance of the tinnitus and use of a broad range of adaptive coping skills.

Psychometric Adequacy. The internal consistency reliability values for the maladaptive coping and effectiveness coping subscales were .90 and .89, respectively. It was anticipated that the two subscales were not significantly correlated ($r = .13$). In the standardization study, maladaptive coping strategies were significantly associated with measures of tinnitus severity, depression, and anxiety.[45] In contrast, effective coping was not correlated with any of the tinnitus adjustment measures.

Strengths and Weaknesses. This scale is only one of two questionnaires (the other being the TCQ) that attempts to quantify adaptive and coping strategies used by tinnitus sufferers. The TSCQ might be helpful to the clinician in identifying the behaviors and thought patterns affected by tinnitus, as well as the coping strategies currently used. This knowledge is fundamental in developing a cognitive-behavioral therapy program. For example, during cognitive-behavioral therapy, the clinician works to change the way the patient interprets, thinks, and feels about the tinnitus and to remove inappropriate beliefs, anxieties, and fears.[5] Further study of the test–retest reliability of the TSCQ would be necessary before it could be used as an assessment tool for monitoring changes following the provision of cognitive-behavioral therapy.

CLINICAL AND RESEARCH APPLICATIONS

In light of the fact that psychophysical measures are insufficient for describing the impact that tinnitus has on the individual's everyday life functioning, self-report tinnitus questionnaires take on several important roles in the clinical management process and in the research arena. One application is in determining treatment candidacy. Another use is in defining subject samples for investigational studies. A third application is for the purposes of accountability by demonstrating short- and long-term outcome for medical, surgical, and rehabilitative intervention. Finally, we propose the use of tinnitus questionnaires as a method for evaluating treatment cost-effectiveness. The following section addresses each of the aforementioned applications.

Determination of Treatment Candidacy and Management Approach

Candidacy Tinnitus questionnaires are instrumental in determining candidacy for treatment by evaluating the patient from a functional perspective. That is, there is often a mismatch between tinnitus impairment, as assessed by psychophysical measures, and the self-perceived disability or handicapping nature of the tinnitus. Individuals seek audiologic management because of the consequences of their tinnitus, not because it has a pitch match of 4,000 Hz and a sensation level of 10 dB, for example. In this connection, treatment candidacy may be linked to the severity of the scores on measures of self-perceived tinnitus disability or handicap. For example, a patient receiving a score of 18 points on the THI (mild category) might benefit from a single counseling session that provides information on such topics as the prevalence of tinnitus, causes of tinnitus, anatomy and physiology of the auditory system, associated symptoms, and coping strategies. Discussion of these topics alone may provide the patient with minimal severity with the information and reassurance that is needed to cope with the tinnitus. In contrast, an individual scoring a 72 on the THI (severe category) may require intensive management.

Management Approach The use of tinnitus questionnaires coupled with other nontinnitus measures may provide the clinician with some insight into the selection of a particular treatment option. A number of management approaches are available, ranging from the use of prescribed medications to the use of sound generators as part of the audiologic rehabilitation process to counseling-based approaches.

The following scenario illustrates the importance of using questionnaires when a sound therapy approach, for example, is considered for a patient presenting with a hearing loss. The question arises as to whether to fit the patient with a sound generator, a hearing aid, or a combination unit that incorporates a hearing aid and a sound generator within the same device. In this situation, the use of a companion scale, such as the HHIE or HHIA, will determine to what extent the hearing loss interferes with the patient's psychosocial and communication functioning and directs the clinician in the selection of the most appropriate instrumentation. For example, if the hearing loss has little to no impact on the patient's communication function, the use of a sound generator may be indicated. In contrast, if the hearing loss poses significant handicap, the use of a hearing aid or a combination unit may be warranted.

Coupling tinnitus questionnaires with measures that explore cognitive factors will also be of benefit when selecting the most appropriate management options. For instance, Newman and colleagues[46] suggested that patients who demonstrate high levels of self-focused and somatic attention, as assessed using the Private Self-Consciousness Subscale of the Self-Consciousness Scale[47] and the Somatization Subscale of the Symptoms Checklist-90-Revised,[48] may benefit from medication and rehabilitative (eg, cognitive-behavioral therapy) approaches directed toward a reduction in depression and somatic awareness. In contrast, those individuals demonstrating low levels of self-focused and somatic attention may benefit sufficiently from the provision of informational or educational counseling and maintaining a "sound-enriched" environment.

Subject Selection

A major problem in evaluating tinnitus research relates to subject selection in a research protocol. Using inappropriate inclusion and exclusion criteria may compromise the internal and the external validity of an investigation. Internal validity indicates the degree to which the experimental design accomplishes what it intended to accomplish, whereas external validity indicates the degree to which the results of the study can be generalized.[15] Subject responses to tinnitus questionnaires allow the researcher to define the sample and verify appropriate selection for a given research methodology.

Between-Subjects Research Design It is important that the researcher select subjects who exceed a preset level of perceived tinnitus disability and handicap prior to enrolment in a study with a between-subjects design. Unless this is accomplished, the threat to internal validity is substantial. For instance, an investigator may wish to study reductions in tinnitus handicap for two different treatment modalities: medical (eg, benzodiazepines) and rehabilitative (eg, tinnitus maskers). It is critical that the composition of each group, in terms of tinnitus handicap, is comparable at the time of enrolment into the study. Otherwise, differences following treatment may not be a factor of the treatment modality, and the study will be significantly flawed and of little value.

Within-Subjects Research Design For within-subjects studies, subject stratification or a more heterogeneous subject sample may be desirable. That is, subject recruitment may entail individuals representing the continuum from mild to severe on the defining tinnitus variable. For example, an investigator may be interested in evaluating the association between perceived tinnitus handicap and depression. The sample would need to consist of individuals whose scores on the THI would range from mild to severe. A correlational analysis would be conducted to reveal associations between the severity of the tinnitus handicap score and the degree of depression.

Outcome Measures

Evaluation of perceived psychological distress, disability, and handicap using quantitative tinnitus questionnaires provides an index for documenting the effectiveness of an intervention (eg, medical, surgical, or rehabilitative) when used in a pre- and post-treatment paradigm. That is, a reduction in self-perceived tinnitus disability and handicap (which may or may not be accompanied by a change in tinnitus impairment) may be reflective of the subjective benefit derived from a particular treatment approach. In contrast, no change or an increase in perceived disability and handicap may suggest that the treatment is not providing sufficient benefit, and additional or alternative options should be considered. Moreover, because the quality of clinical services may be indirectly evaluated using tinnitus questionnaires, these indices could serve as quality indicators for accrediting agencies such as the Joint Commission on the Accreditation of Healthcare Organizations.

As indicated earlier, to ensure that reductions in distress, disability, and handicap following intervention represent a true change in perceived benefit, it is necessary that the metric employed has adequate test–retest reliability. Currently, measures such as the THI, THQ, and TRQ possess good test–retest reliability and could be considered adequate for measuring outcome. It must be cautioned, however, that the available test–retest reliability data are for relatively short durations. Accordingly, these scales are more appropriate for evaluating short-term benefit from a treatment that may provide more immediate relief, such as tinnitus masking. Future study should include test–retest stability of the questionnaires so that judgments about treatment outcome requiring longer time intervals, such as habituation therapy and cognitive-behavioral therapy, may be assessed with greater precision in the long term.

The following studies illustrate how tinnitus questionnaires have been used for quantifying treatment outcome following various treatment modalities. More specifically, two studies illustrate the use of tinnitus questionnaires in the area of medical or surgical intervention, whereas two other studies illustrate the application in the rehabilitative arena. Finally, the potential application of using tinnitus questionnaires in cost-effectiveness models to document treatment efficacy is presented.

Medical or Surgical Intervention

Dobie and colleagues conducted one of the few drug studies using a standardized tinnitus scale to evaluate the effects of intervention.[49] They evaluated 92 patients with disabling tinnitus, as assessed by the THQ, in a double-blind randomized clinical trial comparing nortriptyline (a tricyclic antidepressant) with a placebo. To assess and document improvement, other questionnaires, such as the Beck Depression Inventory, Hamilton Anxiety Rating Scale, and Hamilton Depression Rating Scale, as well as psychoacoustic measures (tinnitus intensity match, loudness discomfort level), were used. Although 67% of the nortriptyline patients stated that the drug helped them, almost all of the patients demonstrated a reduction in tinnitus handicap, as documented by the THQ, with the placebo patients showing almost as much improvement as the patients receiving the nortriptyline.

Kinney and colleagues employed three companion handicap measures, namely, the HHIE or HHIA, DHI, and THI, to evaluate long-term effects in patients with Meniere's disease who were either medically (salt-restricted diet and diuretics, labyrinthine sedatives) or surgically (sac decompression, shunt, vestibular nerve section) treated.[50] On average, the duration between the initial treatment and post-treatment evaluation with the handicap measures was 8 years. No statistically significant differences were observed for any of the inventories; however, when the data were collapsed into one group, patients with Meniere's disease continued to demonstrate long-term symptoms. As shown in Figure 17-1, when the data were dichotomized into "no handicap" versus "handicap" (mild, moderate, and severe), over three-quarters of the patients reported that hearing, dizziness, and tinnitus handicap affected their quality of life. It is noteworthy that the impact of tinnitus was relatively equivalent to hearing and dizziness.

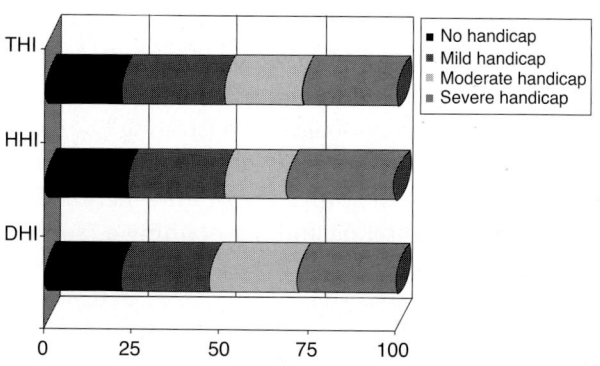

FIGURE 17-1. The level of handicap for the Tinnitus Handicap Inventory (THI), the Hearing Handicap Inventory for the Elderly and the Hearing Handicap Inventory for Adults (HHI), and the Dizziness Handicap Inventory (DHI). Note that more than 75% of patients in this sample with Meniere's disease had self-perceived handicap in all three areas. Adapted from Kinney SE et al.[50]

Rehabilitative Intervention

Hearing Aids Surr and colleagues at the Walter Reed Army Medical Center assessed the effects of hearing aids on the perception of tinnitus using the THI.[51] Hearing aids were fit on a sample of 34 men who were hearing impaired with reported tinnitus. There was a wide distribution across baseline THI handicap categories, with 9 subjects classified as no or minimal handicap, 11 classified as mild, 8 classified as moderate, and 6 classified as severe. The THI was then administered 6 weeks postfitting. Statistically significant differences were observed between the aided and unaided THI for total score and for functional and catastrophic subscales; however, only a few subjects exceeded the 95% critical difference, indicating a true and valid reduction in tinnitus handicap as a function of amplification. In fact, for some individuals, the hearing aids actually increased the self-perceived tinnitus handicap. The THI, therefore, may be a useful tool for alerting audiologists that the hearing aid's output characteristics may need modification.

Tinnitus Retraining Therapy Berry and colleagues employed the THI in a prospective study of TRT efficacy.[52] In their investigation, 32 patients seen at the University of Maryland Tinnitus and Hyperacusis Center were enrolled in a TRT protocol. The THI was administered before treatment and at the 6-month follow-up evaluation. Following 6 months of treatment, there was a statistically significant reduction in perceived handicap for the total score and for each of the three subscales.

Psychological Management In an interesting study conducted by Henry and Wilson, 60 subjects were assigned to one of three conditions: (1) cognitive coping skills training, including techniques such as attention diversion, imagery training, and thought management combined with education; (2) educational or informational counseling only covering such topics as the auditory system, causes of tinnitus, and treatments; and (3) a waiting list control.[53] Both treatment programs (conditions 1 and 2) involved one 90-minute session per week for 6 weeks. Several treatment outcome measures were employed, including the TRQ, THQ, TQ, TCQ, and TCSQ. These questionnaires were administered before and after treatment and at a 12-month follow-up appointment. Overall, subjects who received some form of treatment (combined cognitive and education or education alone) improved significantly more than those on the waiting list. On average, individuals receiving the combined cognitive and educational sessions yielded significant reductions in distress (TRQ and TQ-Emotional subscale), tinnitus handicap (THQ), and dysfunctional cognitions (TCQ) in comparison with the education-only group. These findings suggest that although education alone may be helpful in increasing a patient's knowledge about tinnitus, informational counseling does little to produce changes in perceived distress, handicap, and dysfunctional thinking. It is noteworthy that at 12 months posttreatment, there were no significant differences between the combined cognitive and education group and the education-only group. These observations highlight the need for ongoing or "refresher" cognitive therapy to ensure maintenance of treatment gains over time.

Cost-Effectiveness Models

Given the demand by the current health care climate that intervention results in a positive outcome, the systematic evaluation of the effectiveness of medical, surgical, and rehabilitative management should become a research priority. The latter is especially important in light of the increase in cost associated with the provision of health care and the need to demonstrate to third-party payers the clinical effectiveness of tinnitus treatment approaches. We propose the incorporation of tinnitus questionnaires as part of an economic analysis for evaluating cost-effectiveness.

Currently, several economic evaluation methods can be used to compare the costs of different treatment options and to determine costs as a function of benefit achieved. These techniques could be applied to examine the cost-effectiveness of one treatment option against the "cost" of another treatment option. For example, it may be possible to evaluate the cost-effectiveness of TRT against cognitive therapy or combined sound therapy approaches against an education program only. The following section provides two examples of how health economic analyses are computed using data discerned from psychometrically robust tinnitus instruments.

Cost-Effectiveness Analysis Cost-effectiveness analysis uses three separate incremental comparisons: cost (ie, of treatment), effectiveness (ie, benefit), and cost-effectiveness ratio (C:E) between two treatment alternatives (eg, TRT versus cognitive therapy alone).[54] In this example, benefit refers to the difference score derived from the pre- and postadministration of a tinnitus questionnaire. The calculation for each of the incremental comparisons is provided in Table 17-5. Based on the information provided in Table 17-5, the C:E ratio for comparing two tinnitus treatment options was the difference in their cost divided by the difference in their effectiveness. In this example, the C:E ratio is essentially the additional (incremental) cost (price) of an additional unit of benefit obtained from a particular tinnitus treatment approach when compared with another treatment option (eg, TRT versus cognitive-behavioral therapy). The C:E ratio indicates which intervention option produces the most benefit for a given expenditure. It would be beneficial if we knew, for example, that for a group of comparable patients, TRT produced an average reduction in tinnitus disability and handicap of 30% at a cost of $1,000, whereas cognitive-behavioral therapy achieved the same results but at a much lesser cost.

Cost-Utility Analysis Cost-utility analysis incorporates quality of outcome and survival information, resulting in quality-adjusted life-years (QALYs).[55] The analysis comprises three components: (1) cost of treatment for each alternative intervention, (2) change in scores on a measure of benefit as a function of treatment, and (3) estimated quality of life in years remaining that may be affected by the treatment. The following formula can be used to calculate QALYs[56]:

$$\text{Cost per QALY} = \frac{\text{Cost of treatment}}{\text{Obtained benefit (in \%)} \times \text{life expectancy (actuarial table)}}$$

Benefit is based on the reduction of tinnitus distress, disability, or handicap derived from quantitative tinnitus questionnaires. Using this approach, QALYs calculated for different tinnitus treatment options can be determined with direct comparison to other health care services, such as cochlea implantation or the provision of hearing aids.

CONCLUSION

This chapter highlights the role of tinnitus questionnaires in the evaluation process. Insight into the psychosocial impact of tinnitus on a person's everyday life is critical for planning intervention strategies and for quantifying outcome. Currently, several questionnaires have been standardized to document tinnitus distress, disability, handicap, and coping styles. Yet, at the present time, there is no consensus as to which instrument(s) should be used either singly or in combination as the primary measurement tools.

It is our recommendation that a panel of experts from national (eg, American Academy of Audiology, American Academy of Otolaryngology-Head and Neck Surgery, American Tinnitus Association, Association for Research in Otolaryngology) and international (eg, Australian Tinnitus Association, British Tinnitus Association, German Tinnitus League, Tinnitus Association of Canada) lay and professional organizations join forces to evaluate psychometrically robust instruments with the purpose of proposing a minimum consensus tinnitus questionnaire battery for clinical and research applications. Achieving this goal

TABLE 17-5. Incremental Comparison Calculations

Variable	Description
Let:	
TC_1 = total cost for treatment – X	Cost for treatment visits, devices, etc
TC_2 = total cost for treatment – Y	Cost for treatment visits, devices, etc
E_1 = total effectiveness	Benefit* from treatment–X
E_2 = total effectiveness	Benefit* from treatment–Y
IC = incremental cost $TC_1 - TC_2$	Difference in cost between treatments
IE = incremental effectiveness: $E_1 - E_2$	Difference in benefit between treatments
C:E = IC:IE	Cost divided by benefit

Adapted from Gold MR et al.[54]
*Benefit refers to a reduction in tinnitus distress, disability, or handicap as quantified by a difference score (pretreatment minus post-treatment) on a questionnaire.

would be beneficial in that it would permit (1) clinicians to compare the results of intervention for a given individual with a large stratified normative database and (2) researchers to make comparisons across studies, promoting the use of meta-analysis in tinnitus research.

REFERENCES

1. Meikle MB, Vernon J, Johnson RM. The perceived severity of tinnitus. Some observations concerning a large population of tinnitus patients. Otolaryngol Head Neck Surg 1984;92:689–96.
2. Jakes SC, Hallam RS, Chambers C, Hinchcliffe R. A factor analytical study of tinnitus complaint behavior. Audiology 1985;24:195–206.
3. Noble W. Tinnitus self-assessment scales: domains of coverage and psychometric properties. Hear J 2001;54:20–5.
4. Henry JL, Wilson PH. The psychological management of chronic tinnitus: a cognitive-behavioral approach. Needham Heights (MA): Allyn & Bacon; 2001.
5. Sweetow R. Cognitive behavior modification. In: Tyler R, editor. Tinnitus handbook. San Diego (CA): Singular Publishing Group; 2000. p. 297–312.
6. Erlandsson S. Psychological profiles of tinnitus in patients. In: Tyler R, editor. Tinnitus handbook. San Diego (CA): Singular Publishing Group; 2000. p. 25–58.
7. Dobie RA. A review of randomized clinical trials of tinnitus. Laryngoscope 1999;109:1202–11.
8. World Health Organization. International classification of impairments, disabilities and handicaps: a manual of classification relating to the consequences of disease. Geneva: World Health Organization; 1980.
9. World Health Organization. International classification of functioning, disability and health (ICIDH-2), pre final draft. Geneva: World Health Organization; 2002.
10. Tyler RS. Tinnitus disability and handicap questionnaires. Semin Hear 1993;14:377–84.
11. Tyler R. Psychoacoustical measurement. In: Tyler R, editor. Tinnitus handbook. San Diego (CA): Singular Publishing Group; 2000. p. 149–80.
12. Noble W. Self-assessment of hearing and related function. London: Whurr Publishers Ltd; 1998.
13. Hyde ML. Reasonable psychometric standards for self-report outcome measures in audiological rehabilitation. Ear Hear 2000;21(4 Suppl):24S–36S.
14. Demorest ME, DeHaven GP. Psychometric adequacy of self-assessment scales. Semin Hear 1993;14:314–25.
15. Ventry IM, Schiavetti N. Evaluating research in speech pathology and audiology. Reading (MA): Addison-Wesley Publishing Company; 1980.
16. Schechter MA, Henry JA. Assessment and treatment of tinnitus patients using a "masking approach." J Am Acad Audiol 2002;13:545–58.
17. Henry JA, Jastreboff MM, Jastreboff PJ, et al. Assessment of patients for treatment with tinnitus retraining therapy. J Am Acad Audiol 2002;13:523–44.
18. Stouffer JL, Tyler RS. Characterization of tinnitus by tinnitus patients. J Speech Hear Disord 1990;55:439–53.
19. Tyler RS, Baker LJ. Difficulties experienced by tinnitus sufferers. J Speech Hear Disord 1983;48:150–4.
20. Newman CW, Jacobson GP, Spitzer JB. Development of the Tinnitus Handicap Inventory. Arch Otolaryngol Head Neck Surg 1996;122:143–8.
21. Wilson PH, Henry J, Bowen M, Haralambous G. Tinnitus Reaction Questionnaire: psychometric properties of a measure of distress associated with tinnitus. J Speech Lang Hear Res 1991;34:197–201.
22. Sanchez L, Stephens D. A tinnitus problem questionnaire in a clinic population. Ear Hear 1997;18:210–7.
23. Halford JBS, Anderson SD. Tinnitus severity measured by a subjective scale, audiometry and clinical judgment. J Laryngol Otol 1991;105:89–93.
24. Hallam RS, Jakes SC, Hinchcliffe R. Cognitive variables in tinnitus annoyance. Br J Clin Psychol 1988;27:213–22.
25. Hallam RS. Manual of the tinnitus questionnaire. London: The Psychological Corporation/Harcourt Brace; 1996.
26. Henry JL, Wilson, PH. The psychometric properties of two measures of tinnitus complaint and handicap. Int Tinnitus J 1998;4:114–21.
27. Hiller W, Goebel G. A psychometric study of complaints of chronic tinnitus. J Psychosom Res 1992;36:337–48.
28. Hiller W, Goebel G, Rief W. Reliability of self-rated tinnitus distress and association with psychological symptom patterns. Br J Clin Psychol 1994;33:231–4.
29. Kuk FK, Tyler RS, Russell D, Jordan H. The psychometric properties of a tinnitus handicap questionnaire. Ear Hear 1990;11:434–42.
30. Newman CW, Sandridge SA, Jacobson GP. Psychometric adequacy of the Tinnitus Handicap Inventory (THI) for evaluating treatment outcome. J Am Acad Audiol 1998;9:153–60.
31. Beck AT, Ward CH, Mendelson M, et al. An inventory for measuring depression. Arch Gen Psychiatry 1961;4:561–71.

32. Main CJ. The Modified Somatic Perception Questionnaire (MSPQ). J Psychosom Res 1983;27:503–14.
33. Baguley DM, Humphriss RL, Hodgson CA. Convergent validity of the Tinnitus Handicap Questionnaire and the Tinnitus Questionnaire. J Laryngol Otol 2000;114:840–3.
34. Ventry IM, Weinstein BE. The Hearing Handicap Inventory for the Elderly: a new tool. Ear Hear 1982;3:128–34.
35. Newman CW, Weinstein BE, Jacobson, GP, Hug GP. The Hearing Handicap Inventory for Adults; psychometric adequacy and audiometric correlates. Ear Hear 1990;11:430–3.
36. Jacobson GP, Newman CW. The development of the Dizziness Handicap Inventory. Arch Otolaryngol Head Neck Surg 1990;116:424–7.
37. Zachariae R, Mirz F, Johansen LV, et al. Reliability and validity of a Danish adaptation of the Tinnitus Handicap Inventory. Scand Audiol 2000;29:37–43.
38. Baguley DM, Andersson G. Factor analysis of the Tinnitus Handicap Inventory. Am J Audiol 2003;12:31–4.
39. Herraiz C, Hernandez CJ, Plaza G, et al. Evaluacion de la incapacidad en los pacientes con acufenos. Acta Otorrinolaringol Esp 2001;52:534–8.
40. Newman CW, Wharton JA, Jacobson GP. Retest stability of the Tinnitus Handicap Questionnaire. Ann Otol Rhinol Laryngol 1995;104:718–23.
41. Erlandsson SI, Hallberg LRM, Axelsson A. Psychological and audiological correlates of perceived tinnitus severity. Audiology 1992;31:168–79.
42. Sweetow RW, Levy MC. Tinnitus severity scaling for diagnostic/therapeutic usage. Hear Instrum 1990;41:20–46.
43. Wilson PH, Henry JL. Tinnitus Cognitions Questionnaire: development and psychometric properties of a measure of dysfunctional cognitions associated with tinnitus. Int Tinnitus J 1998;4:23–30.
44. Budd RJ, Pugh R. The relationship between coping style, tinnitus severity and emotional distress in a group of sufferers. Br J Health Psychol 1996;1:219–29.
45. Budd RJ, Pugh R. Tinnitus coping style and its relationship to tinnitus severity and emotional distress. J Psychosom Res 1996;41:327–35.
46. Newman CW, Wharton JA, Jacobson GP. Self-focused and somatic attention in patients with tinnitus. J Am Acad Audiol 1997;8:143–9.
47. Fenigstein A, Scheier MD, Buss AH. Public and private self-consciousness: assessment and theory. J Consult Clin Psychol 1975;43:522–7.
48. Derogatis LR. SCL-90-R: administration, scoring and procedures manual I. Baltimore: Clinical Psychometrics Research; 1977.
49. Dobie RA, Sakai CS, Sullivan MD, et al. Antidepressant treatment of tinnitus patients: report of randomized clinical trial and clinical prediction of benefit. Am J Otol 1993;14:18–23.
50. Kinney SE, Sandridge, SA, Newman CW. Long-term effects of Meniere's disease on hearing and quality of life. Am J Otol 1997;18:67–73.
51. Surr RK, Kolb JA, Cord MT, Garrus NP. Tinnitus Handicap Inventory (THI) as a hearing aid outcome measure. J Am Acad Audiol 1999;10:489–95.
52. Berry JA, Gold SL, Frederick EA, et al. Patient-based outcomes in patients with primary tinnitus undergoing tinnitus retraining therapy. Arch Otolaryngol Head Neck Surg 2002;128:1153–7.
53. Henry JL, Wilson PH. The psychological management of tinnitus: comparison of a combined cognitive educational program, education alone and a waiting-list control. Int Tinnitus J 1996;2:9–20.
54. Gold MR, Siegel JE, Russell LB, Weinstein MC. Cost-effectiveness in health and medicine. New York: Oxford University Press; 1996.
55. Drummond M, O'Brien B, Stoddard G, Torrance G. Methods for economic evaluation of health care programs. 2nd ed. New York: Oxford University Press; 1997.
56. Abrams HB, Hnath-Chisolm T. Outcome measures. The audiologic difference. In: Hosford-Dunn J, Roeser RJ, Valente M, editors. Audiology practice management. New York: Thieme; 2000. p. 69–95.

CHAPTER 18

Imaging Tinnitus

Alan H. Lockwood, MD, Robert F. Burkard, PhD, Richard J. Salvi, PhD

Improvements in imaging technology have made it possible to evaluate the human auditory system in a manner that would have bewildered our predecessors. Conventional radiographs have been augmented by the development of computed tomography (CT) to provide highly detailed images of osseous and soft tissue structures in and about the ear. The same is true for magnetic resonance imaging (MRI), particularly when gadolinium contrast enhancement is used. Both of these technologies are evolving rapidly, and new MRI pulse sequences, stronger magnets, and improved image reconstruction techniques hold the promise for further improvements. Other imaging techniques, particularly positron emission tomography (PET) and single photon emission computed tomography, provide the clinician and investigator with critical data that have made it possible to attribute specific auditory tasks or sensations to discrete regions of the brain. This chapter is designed to provide a guide so that these resources can be used optimally.

ESTABLISHING A DIAGNOSTIC FRAMEWORK

To use imaging techniques efficiently, it is essential to establish a diagnostic framework for the patient with tinnitus. Two broad categories for these patients are (1) those who have subjective tinnitus, the false perception of sound in the absence of an environmental source, and (2) those who have objective tinnitus, in which the sounds are real but possibly not perceptible to an observer-clinician. Some causes of objective tinnitus are shown in Table 18-1.

TABLE 18-1. Objective Tinnitus

Pulsatile Tinnitus

Neoplasms (typically vascular in nature)
   Glomus tumors or paragangliomas (chemodectoma, paragangliomas)
      Glomus tympanicum, glomus jugulare, glomus jugulotympanicum
   Hemangioma
      Facial nerve hemangioma, cavernous hemangioma
   Other less vascular neoplasms
      Meningioma, adenoma
Vascular lesions
   Acquired arterial lesions
      Atherosclerotic plaque (carotid or intracranial)
      Vascular malformations (intracranial, dural; may be sequel to trauma)
      Aneurysm
      Carotid artery dissection (spontaneous or traumatic)
   Congenital arterial abnormalities
      Aberrant internal carotid artery
      Persistent stapedial artery
   Venous abnormalities
      Jugular bulb abnormality (high position, diverticulum, dehiscence, enlargement)
   Miscellaneous vascular abnormalities
      Fibromuscular dysplasia of carotid artery
      Vascular compression of cochlear or auditory nerve at root entry zone
Miscellaneous causes
   Valvular heart disease (aortic stenosis, insufficiency)
   Benign intracranial hypertension or pseudotumor cerebri
   Hyperdynamic state (eg, anemia, thyrotoxicosis)
   Otosclerosis with anastomoses between haversian bone and endochondral layer

Nonpulsatile Tinnitus

Palatal myoclonus
Spasm, fasciculations, or fibrillations of tensor tympani or stapedius muscles
Spontaneous otoacoustic emissions
Patulous eustachian tube

CLINICAL IMAGING IN PATIENTS WITH SUBJECTIVE TINNITUS

Most patients with subjective tinnitus have a partial or complete loss of hearing. This deficit may range from mild loss at high frequencies to total deafness. Although the literature describes a small portion of patients with tinnitus as having normal hearing, we raise the question as to whether this normal ability to perceive stimuli represents a decline from a prior level. A patient with a threshold of 20 dB HL at 4 kHz would be considered to have normal hearing. However, if this threshold represents a decline from 10 dB HL, this patient has lost hearing. The audiogram is typically measured from 125 to 8,000 Hz in octave steps. A patient could have normal thresholds at these discrete frequencies, but losses could go undetected between test frequencies or frequencies above 8,000 Hz. If hearing loss is an important factor in the pathogenesis of tinnitus owing to plastic changes in the central part of the auditory system caused by deafferentation, then these seemingly minor changes may be important.

Studies from our laboratory suggest strongly that subjective tinnitus is the consequence of plastic transformations in the central auditory pathways that arise as the result of auditory deafferentation.[1] We further suggest that the transformed centers and pathways that contain aberrant connections (including connections to nonauditory systems) perceive sound when, in fact, there is no source of sound. Restated, tinnitus may be the result of neural plasticity gone awry. Thus, tinnitus may be the auditory system analog to neuropathic pain syndromes in which the intensity of the pain is proportional to the degree to which somatosensory pathways have been transformed by an alteration in the afferent input to the somatosensory system. Therefore, imaging of patients with subjective tinnitus is largely the same as the imaging of hearing loss. This much broader topic, which is outside the scope of this chapter, has been well reviewed from an imaging perspective.[2]

Among patients with subjective tinnitus, the question "Does this patient have a vestibular schwannoma?" arises frequently, particularly among patients who complain of tinnitus confined to a single ear. The emphasis on the early diagnosis of these tumors has increased with the development of surgical techniques that preserve hearing and gamma knife radiation therapy, which may obviate the need for surgery. On the basis of the history, clinical examination, and audiologic assessment, it is usually possible to differentiate patients with retrocochlear lesions from those with cochlear pathology. In making this determination, the auditory brainstem response (ABR) is often particularly helpful. For those patients in whom the index of suspicion is particularly high, a stacked ABR should be performed.[3] This technique appears to be more sensitive than conventional ABR testing in the detection of small tumors. In patients with retrocochlear lesions or a high index of suspicion pointing to a tumor, MRI with gadolinium enhancement is the diagnostic test of choice.[4] A small intracanalicular vestibular schwannoma is shown in Figure 18-1. For those patients who are unable to undergo MRI, CT with air or positive contrast must suffice.

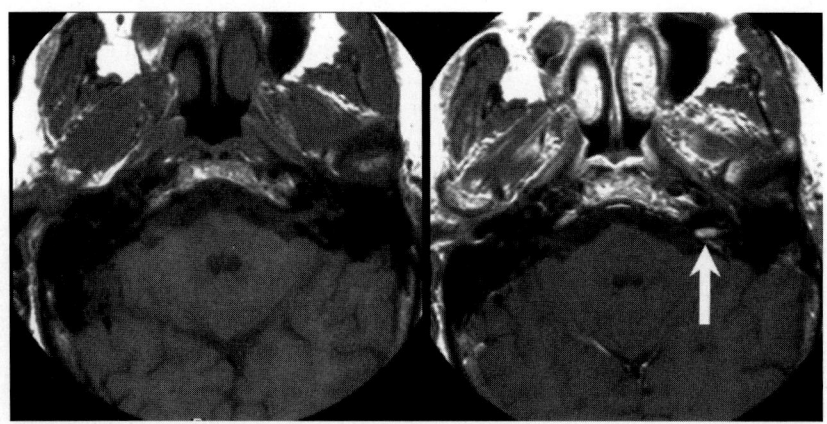

FIGURE 18-1. T_1-weighted magnetic resonance images of a small intracanalicular vestibular schwannoma before (*left*) and after (see *arrow, right*) the administration of gadolinium. Image courtesy of Rohit Bakshi, MD.

CLINICAL IMAGING OF PATIENTS WITH OBJECTIVE TINNITUS

In patients with objective tinnitus, the sounds are real. Therefore, it is important to clarify the mechanism that underlies the generation of the sound and to determine how these sounds are transmitted to the cochlea. When evaluating patients with objective tinnitus, it is important to differentiate those with pulsatile tinnitus from those whose tinnitus is not pulsatile. Bruits or other sounds emanating from arteriovenous malformations and tumors, for example, may be heard by the examiner under appropriate conditions. Every effort should be made to determine whether the bursts of sound coincide with cardiac systole.

Pulsatile Tinnitus For most patients with pulsatile tinnitus, the sounds are generated by turbulence in arteries or other vessels with rapid blood flow. The turbulence creates pressure waves in the vascular system that are transmitted through bone or blood to the cochlea. In the cochlea, these fluctuations in pressure are converted into neural impulses that are experienced as sound. Virtually any condition that creates intravascular turbulence can result in the symptom of objective tinnitus. During the physical examination of patients with pulsatile tinnitus, it is important to auscultate the portion of the head identified by the patient as the site of his or her sounds. The most common conditions causing objective tinnitus are listed in Table 18-1.

Because the prevalence of pulsatile tinnitus and the prevalence of atherosclerotic cardiovascular disease increase with age, many patients with pulsatile tinnitus will be found to have stenotic arteries. An example of this condition is illustrated in the angiogram shown in Figure 18-2. Stenosis of any of the intracranial arteries causes turbulence at and distal to the site of the stenosis. The mechanical energy created by the turbulence stimulates the cochlea. The bifurcation of the carotid artery is a particularly common site for these lesions. The intraosseous portion of the carotid artery is in close proximity to the cochlea. This facilitates transmission of vibrations from any carotid lesion to the cochlea. Carotid stenosis at other sites, particularly at the siphon, and other lesions of the carotid, such as fibromuscular dysplasia, may also cause pulsatile tinnitus. Stenotic lesions in other intracranial arteries, including the vertebrobasilar system and its branches, may be associated with pulsatile tinnitus. Other vascular lesions, such as dissections or aneurysms, may also be associated with audible pulsations.

Arteriovenous malformations are also a site where turbulent blood flow may give rise to audible pulsations. The malformation may be found at virtually any intracranial location. Intracerebral malformations and dural malformations are particularly common. Occasionally, a head injury will cause a traumatic arteriovenous malformation in which arteries communicate with dural or other venous structures.

In rare instances, an aberrant internal carotid artery, a persistent stapedial artery, or an abnormality of the jugular bulb will be responsible for pulsatile tinnitus.

Some highly vascular tumors, as exemplified by the glomus jugulare tumor shown in Figure 18-3, may be the source of pulsatile tinnitus. Again, flow turbulence produces the sound. These lesions may be seen during an otoscopic examination. Other tumors associated with pulsatile tinnitus are listed in Table 18-1.

Other conditions that may be associated with pulsatile conditions include valvular heart disease, particularly aortic stenosis and mitral regurgitation, and a hyperdynamic state associated with severe anemia or thyrotoxicosis. Patients with thyrotoxicosis may

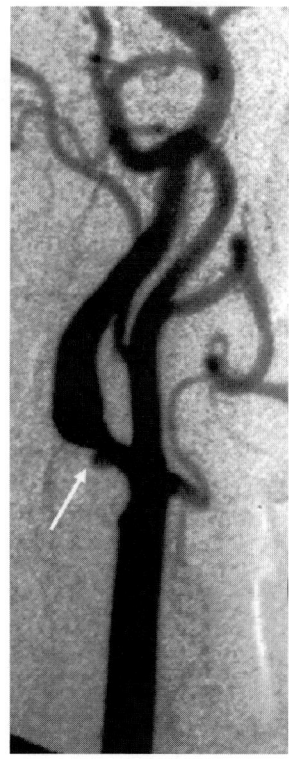

FIGURE 18-2. Carotid stenosis with an ulcerated plaque (*arrow*) as a cause of pulsatile tinnitus. Turbulent blood flow at the site of the stenotic internal carotid artery generates sound waves that are transmitted to the cochlea. A loud bruit may be heard, and a thrill may be palpable. Image courtesy of Rohit Bakshi, MD.

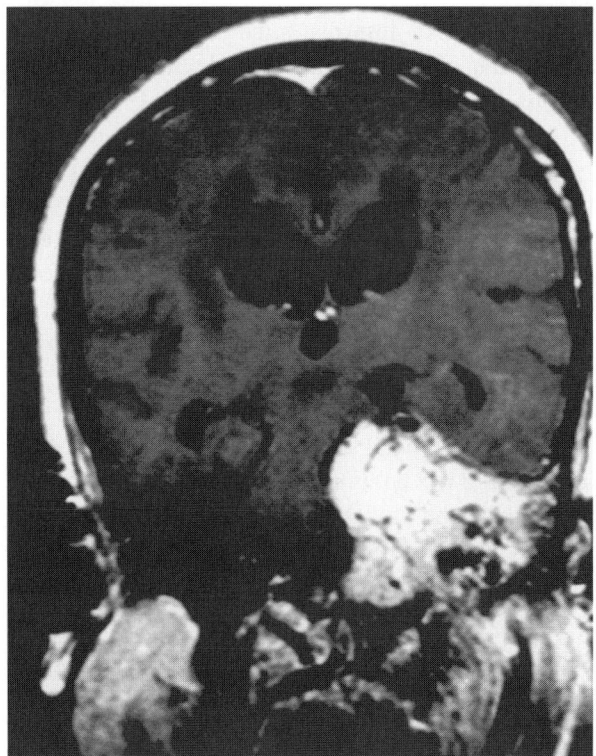

FIGURE 18-3. T$_1$-weighted magnetic resonance image of large glomus jugulare tumor after the administration of gadolinium. The characteristic salt and pepper appearance is caused by gadolinium enhancement (salt) with flow voids (pepper). Image courtesy of Rohit Bakshi, MD.

also have atrial fibrillation, making it more difficult to link the audible sounds to the pulse.

Patients with pulsatile tinnitus should have a radiologic evaluation to determine the site and severity of the lesion.[4] Because of the diversity of the lesions that may give rise to audible pulsations, no single procedure suffices for all patients. The results of the history and physical examination usually serve to orient the physician to the appropriate test. Diagnostic procedures designed to identify vascular lesions are changing rapidly with the advent of CT and magnetic resonance angiography. The degree of invasiveness, and hence the risk associated with these investigations, is substantially lower than that for catheter-based angiography, the gold standard for image quality. However, rapid improvements in software and the introduction of magnets with higher field strength into clinical practice are closing this quality gap. Unless one is familiar with the procedures performed by the imaging specialists, a personal contact to establish an appropriate plan is likely to lead to the best result for any given patient.

Nonpulsatile Tinnitus Nonpulsatile objective tinnitus is less common. The major causes are shown in Table 18-1. Palatal myoclonus is characterized by rapid rhythmic contractions of the muscles in the soft palate. These are often associated with similar time-locked contractions of other muscles in the pharynx, mouth, and lower face and, occasionally, other muscles subserving the neck and eyes and even muscles associated with respiration. These contractions result in the opening and closing of the eustachian tube, the source of the sound perceived by these patients. On examination, contractions of the affected muscles should be visible, and auscultation may allow the examiner to hear the sounds perceived by the patient. Infarcts of the pons or other lesions that interrupt the pathways connecting the inferior olivary nucleus and the red nucleus cause this rare disorder. MRIs may show the lesion and the characteristic combination of hypertrophy and degeneration of the inferior olivary nucleus.

FUNCTIONAL IMAGING OF THE AUDITORY SYSTEM

NORMAL CENTRAL PART OF THE AUDITORY SYSTEM

It is essential to understand the functional anatomy of the normal auditory system to understand the results of altering this complex system. Although there are numerous and detailed descriptions of the anatomic and physiologic features of the central part of the auditory system, few studies have sought to identify all of the human brain regions that are activated by simple stimuli.

We used PET to map the central auditory pathways in a group of normal young adults using methods specifically designed to minimize the impact of scanner and ambient noise.[5] This strategy uses water, labeled with radioactive oxygen, to measure cerebral blood flow, which is a surrogate measure of neural activity. By comparing cerebral blood flow images in two states, for example, scans done during auditory stimulation minus scans done in the absence of sound, it is possible to identify brain regions that respond to the stimulus. By superimposing these results on an anatomic representation of the brain, typically an averaged MRI, it is possible to deduce the anatomic sites activated by the stimulus. Thus, when we stimulated the right ear, we identified a network of sites in the left brainstem that extended from the level of the cochlear nuclei, superiorly to the level of the medial geniculate body, and bilaterally to both primary auditory cortices, as shown in Figure 18-4. By using stimuli of different frequencies (0.5 and 4.0 kHz), we found the expected tonotopic relationships in the primary auditory cortex with low-frequency sounds activating lateral sites and higher-frequency sounds activating the same lateral site but also a more medially located site, confirming and extending prior studies, including an earlier PET study confined to image planes that included only the superior temporal gyrus.[6]

These studies have served several important purposes. First, they identify the neural sites most active during the processing of simple auditory stimuli that are free of linguistic content. Second, they serve as a basis for understanding the effects of various conditions that have the potential to affect neural activity in the central part of the auditory system, most notably, hearing loss and tinnitus.

CENTRAL PART OF THE AUDITORY SYSTEM IN PATIENTS WITH HEARING LOSS AND TINNITUS

Our studies have focused on two groups of patients with tinnitus. The first involved patients with sensorineural hearing loss who localized their subjective tinnitus to the right ear.[7] In this investigation, we stimulated the tinnitus ear with 2 kHz tones and applied the same stimulus to control subjects, all of whom had normal hearing. The stimuli activated a larger region of the temporal lobe in the patients with hearing loss and tinnitus compared with the controls, as shown in Figure 18-5. The additional regions activated by the stimuli were observed in the anterior portion of the superior temporal gyrus and a second site slightly posterior and inferior to the primary auditory cortex. This confirmed numerous studies in experimental animals that have shown expansion of brain regions responding to auditory stimuli after partial deafferentation.[8]

In a second series of studies, we studied patients with gaze-evoked tinnitus (GET).[9] This unusual phenomenon is usually the consequence of surgery to treat a cerebellopontine angle tumor and is characterized by tinnitus that either appears or increases in loudness, pitch, or both with gaze directed away from the primary position.[10,11] These patients had all been treated for vestibular schwannomas, had tinnitus in the operated ear that was present in the primary gaze

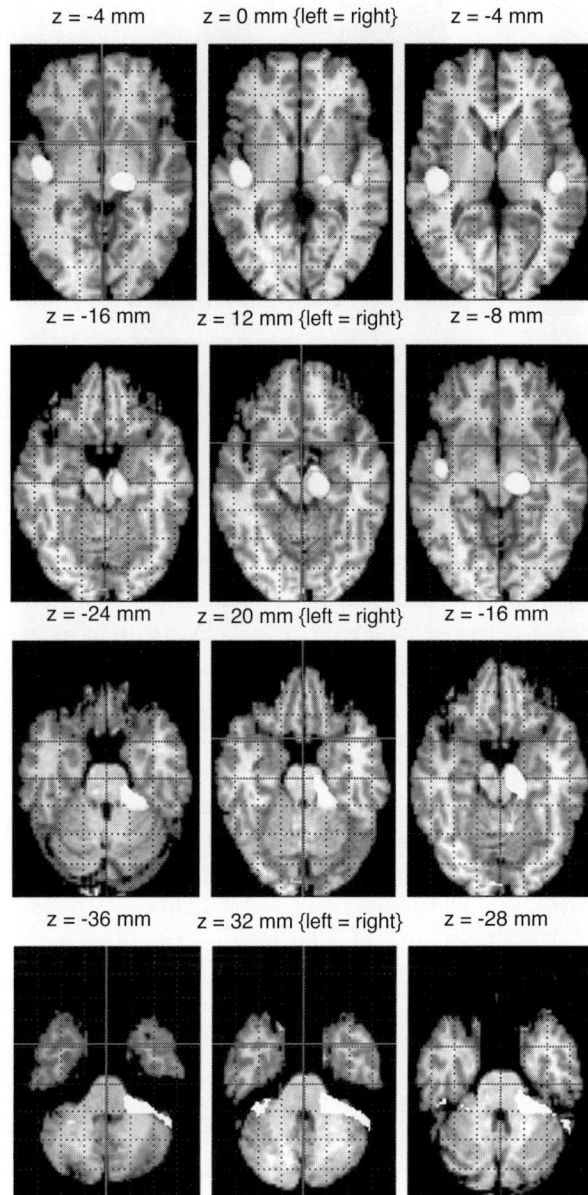

FIGURE 18-4. Sites of neural activation during right ear stimulation with a 4.0 kHz tone at 90 dB SPL. The results of the analysis of positron emission tomographic images (white "blobs" in the book, colored on the CD) are superimposed on idealized T_1-weighted magnetic resonance images in the transaxial plane. Numbers (z = mm) indicate distance above and below the commissural plane. Images are shown with the right side of the brain on the left side of the figure. See Lockwood and colleagues[5] for additional details.

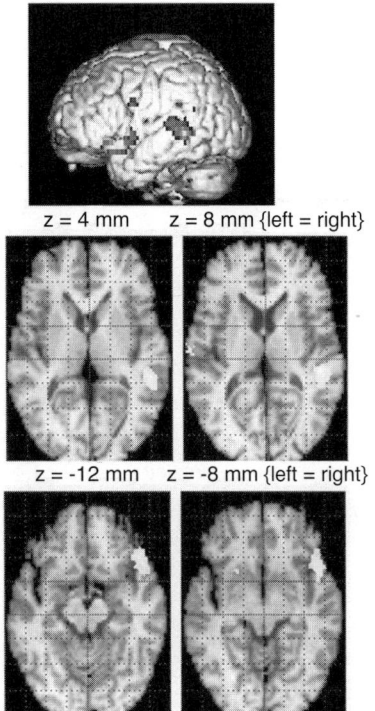

FIGURE 18-5. Expansion of neural sites activated by tonal stimuli delivered to the right ear in patients with subjective tinnitus reported in the right ear and sensorineural hearing loss. The data in this image set were produced by subtracting the sites activated by 2 kHz tones in normal controls from sites activated by the same stimulus delivered in an identical manner to the patients. Sites of additional activation in the patients are seen in the anterior portion of the superior temporal gyrus and a second site posterior and inferior to the primary auditory cortex. See Lockwood and colleagues[7] for additional details.

position, and reported an increase in subjective loudness with sustained horizontal gaze. Hearing in the unaffected ear was normal or nearly normal.[9] In this study, we stimulated either the right or the left ear and again observed the bilateral cortical activation in the control subjects and in the two patients with right vestibular schwannomas after stimulation of the left ear and in five patients with left vestibular schwannomas after stimulation of the right ear, as shown in parts A to C of Figure 18-6. Parts B and C suggest strongly that the volume of brain reactive to the stimuli is larger in the patients than in the controls, an impression that is confirmed by subtracting the control scan activations from those observed in the patients, as shown in parts D, E, and F of Figure 18-6. Thus, it is evident that deafferentation accompanying a deafened ear expands the locus of the sites of neural activity when the remaining normal ear is stimulated.

The results of these studies show that the combined effects of hearing loss and tinnitus have profound effects on the central part of the auditory system. We are unaware of any PET studies of patients with hearing loss without tinnitus. Hearing loss may be caused by a variety of disorders that can be diagnosed by appropriate radiologic examinations.[2]

RESEARCH IMAGING OF PATIENTS WITH TINNITUS

Research techniques, particularly PET and functional magnetic resonance imaging (fMRI), have made it possible to perform studies that have expanded our understanding of tinnitus. PET uses a measure of cerebral blood flow as an index of neural activity, and fMRI uses a change in the redox state of hemoglobin. Both allow a superimposition of a site of change on an anatomic reference, usually the participant's own structural MRI or a standard MRI obtained by averaging multiple, usually T_1-weighted, scans from normal individuals. PET has an advantage in that the imaging system is associated with almost no noise[12] and is relatively insensitive to small movements of participants. fMRI examinations are usually less expensive and yield functional images of a single subject with greater ease. However, MRI systems, particularly those with magnets with high field strength that are best suited to fMRI applications, are noisy and highly sensitive to movement, including small movements of the brainstem caused by arterial pulsations. Thus, it is appropriate to consider each of these approaches as complementing the other.

We have used PET to study three different groups of patients with tinnitus. In the first of these, we examined patients who had unilateral tinnitus that was reported to come from the right ear.[7] These patients were also able to alter the perceived loudness of their phantom sensation by voluntarily contracting the muscles of the jaw. In this study, we obtained multiple scans at rest (no jaw clench) and during the performance of a jaw clench. When we subtracted the tinnitus-soft from the tinnitus-loud scans and applied a correction for the jaw clench, obtained from scans in normal participants without tinnitus, we found a brain region in which neural activity increased and

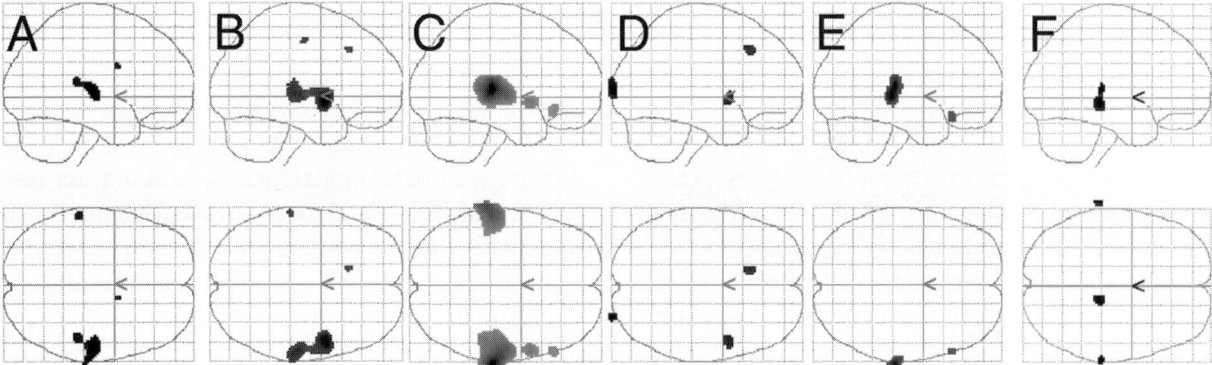

FIGURE 18-6. Expansion of neural sites activated by 0.5 kHz tonal stimuli to the unaffected ear of patients with gaze-evoked tinnitus. These "glass brain" statistical parametric maps are generated by projecting the three-dimensional data set onto two dimensions, in this case, in the transaxial plane. All sites portrayed are in and around the primary auditory cortex and depict sites of neural activity revealed by the various comparisons. For all images, the front of the brain is on the right side of the figure and the right hemisphere is on the top. *A* depicts the activations observed in the controls, right ear stimulation, compared with rest (no sound). *B* depicts the same stimulus minus rest condition for two patients treated for right-sided vestibular schwannomas and stimulated in the left ear. *C* shows the analogous comparison for the patients with left-sided tumors. *D* to *F* show the results of subtracting the expected activations in the normal group from the activations in the patients [contrast form = patient(active − rest) − control(active − rest)]. *D* and *E* show data from subjects with right and left vestibular schwannomas, respectively. *F* is similar to *E* (left vestibular schwannoma), except after omission of subject 3, the only patient in the group with preserved hearing. Reproduced with permission from Lockwood AH et al.[9] For additional details, see Lockwood and colleagues.[9]

decreased in parallel to changes in the reported loudness of tinnitus. This site, shown in Figure 18-7, was confined to a cortical region immediately adjacent to the primary auditory cortex. Because cochlear stimulation in patients with tinnitus and normal controls produced bilateral activation of auditory cortical sites, we interpreted the unilateral nature of this brain region as evidence to support a noncochlear, that is, central auditory, origin of tinnitus. This finding has been supported by data from two other studies, one involving patients with GET[9] and another in which we administered intravenous lidocaine.[13] In both studies, we found unilateral changes in neural activity associated with changes in tinnitus loudness.

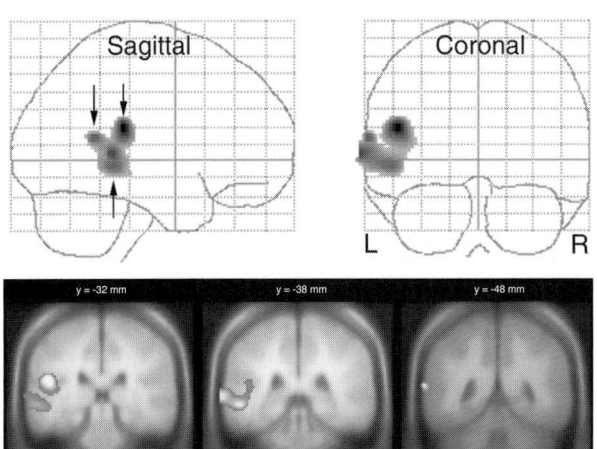

FIGURE 18-7. Sites of neural activity associated with tinnitus. Positron emission tomographic images of patients with tinnitus altered by jaw clenches were obtained. Tinnitus-soft images were subtracted from tinnitus-loud images as described in Lockwood and colleagues.[7] The sagittal and coronal statistical parametric maps were produced as described in Figure 18-6. The *arrows* shown on the sagittal projection identify the plane of the coronal plane images shown in the lower panel, where y distances in millimeters are referenced to the anterior commissural plane. Reproduced with permission from Massachusetts Medical Society, Lockwood AH et al.[1]

In the brainsteams of the patients with GET, we found evidence for abnormal activity during lateral gaze, as shown in Figure 18-8.[9] We interpreted this as evidence of an abnormal interaction between neural centers controlling eye movements and those mediating auditory perception. Neural firing rates increase as needed to execute a lateral eye movement. Apparently, some of this increased activity is transmitted through aberrant connections to neurons in the auditory system. This aberrant activity may explain the shifts in the apparent pitch and loudness of the tinnitus associated with eye movements that are experienced by many of these patients.

The study of patients with GET yielded the additional important result shown in Figure 18-9. When we scanned normal participants, who did not have GET, during full lateral gaze, we found a reduction of activity in auditory cortical areas. This appears to be a physiologic correlate of "crossmodal inhibition." Thus, during the execution of a visually based task, auditory sites are inhibited. There was no inhibition of neural activity in auditory cortical sites when the patients with GET executed the same visual task, that is, there was a failure of crossmodal inhibition in the patients with GET. This lack of inhibition may cause the increase in the loudness and possibly the pitch of the tinnitus that these patients report.

In a final study, we administered lidocaine intravenously to patients with tinnitus.[13] To our initial surprise, almost half of our patients reported an increase, rather than the expected decrease, in the perceived loudness of their tinnitus. This response is well described in the anesthesia literature. This fortuitous circumstance worked to our advantage by allowing us to separate the global effects of lidocaine on neural function from those associated with tinnitus. This ability to differentiate specific from nonspecific effects is particularly important in drug studies because drugs frequently have effects other than those that form the focus of the research. In the tinnitus-focused analysis of these data, we found a unilateral focus in the auditory cortex, similar in location to the site of activity

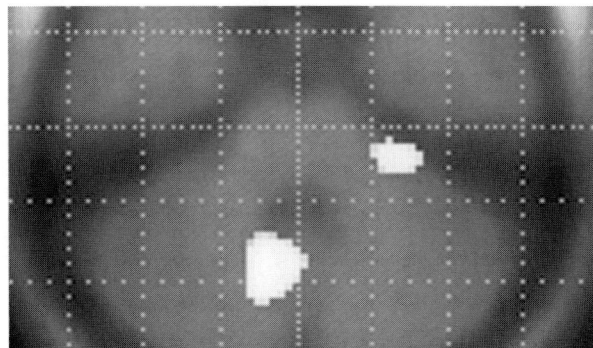

FIGURE 18-8. Sites of neural activation in the brainstem associated with gaze-evoked tinnitus (GET). Sites of neural activity associated with extreme lateral gaze in normal subjects were subtracted from sites in patients with GET. Crosstalk between sites controlling eye movements and auditory perception may cause this phenomonon. Reproduced with permission from Lockwood AH et al.[9] For additional details, see Lockwood and colleagues.[9]

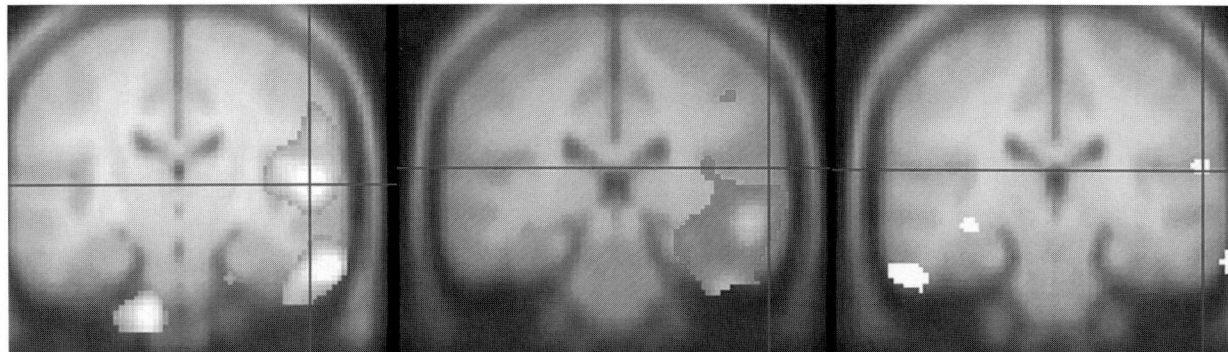

FIGURE 18-9. Crossmodal inhibition in patients with gaze-evoked tinnitus (GET). In the *left panel,* sites of reduced neural activity associated with extreme left lateral gaze are shown, including a prominent site in the auditory cortex. The *center panel* depicts the sites of reduced neural activity under exactly the same conditions in patients with GET. The *right panel* is the result of subtracting the center panel from the left panel and identifies a site in the auditory cortex where inhibition fails to occur in patients with GET. Reproduced with permission from Lockwood AH et al.[9] For additional details, see Lockwood and colleagues.[9]

EDITORIAL COMMENTARY

Wackym and Friedland describe the bedside neur-otologic examination essential in the evaluation of the patient with tinnitus. They call attention to the important role of vestibular tests in the examination, particularly cerebellar tests and the head thrust and shake, Valsalva's maneuvers, and hyperventilation, and they outline the findings that lead to the audiologic assessment, electrophysiologic tests, and imaging necessary for a definitive diagnosis. The importance of auscultation of the head and neck in pulsatile tinnitus and palatal myoclonus, stapedial or tensor tympani muscle spasm, and the patulous eustachian tube is noted, as well as the need for direct observation of the oropharynx and nasopharynx in myoclonic tinnitus.

Wackym and Friedland point out that although the combination of pulsatile tinnitus and conductive hearing loss is most commonly due to eustachian tube dysfunction, it may be due to a middle fossa encephalocele or dehiscence of the jugular bulb. They emphasize computed tomograpy for the diagnostic erosion of the jugular foramen caused by glomus jugulare tumors and magnetic resonance imaging for posterior fossa lesions.

Henry emphasizes that tinnitus does not share the same psychophysical characteristics as external acoustic stimuli. Most notably, masking of tinnitus differs from the masking of sound in that frequency dependence in tone-on-tone masking is usually not found in tinnitus. Interestingly, he points out that residual inhibition occurs in 80 to 90% of patients who receive appropriate acoustic stimulation.

Although great individual variation limits generalizations about the psychoacoustic profile of tinnitus, Henry calls attention to the fact that in large populations of patients with tinnitus, 75% have pitch matches above 4 kHz and 55% have pitch matches above 6 kHz. Patients with tinnitus can generally provide repeat loudness matches within a few decibels, but repeated pitch matching tends to produce variance over several octaves. He calls attention to the as yet unexplained merging and parallel categories of patients with tinnitus on the basis of their loudness match functions compared with their hearing levels across frequencies.

Henry has been working and continues to work on computer automation of tinnitus testing procedures, in part to achieve much needed standardization of tinnitus assessment.

Newman and Sandridge summarize the currently most used questionnaires for assessing the qualitative and quantitative nature of tinnitus and point out that qualitative questionnaires have formed the basis for items in the quantitative questionnaires. The effects of tinnitus on sleep and hearing are more frequently found through questionnaires than emotional problems and the effects on one's general health. Quantitative questionnaires are necessary because psychoacoustic measures do not fully characterize the impact of tinnitus on the individual. Quantitative questionnaires can serve as outcome measures in before and after treatment comparisons for an individual patient or in clinical trials. The Tinnitus Handicap Inventory, the Tinnitus Handicap Questionnaire, and the Tinnitus Reaction Questionnaire have the test–retest reliability over short time intervals to serve as outcome measures, at least for therapy requiring short intervals. Newman and Sandridge call attention to the need for an internationally recognized minimal outcome measure for clinical trials and other research on tinnitus. Indeed, such a standard would be very welcome.

Lockwood and colleagues review the progress with positron emission tomography (PET) and functional magnetic resonance imaging in imaging evidence of tinnitus in various parts of the brain. PET has the advantages of producing almost no noise and being relatively insensitive to small movements, such as those from arterial pulsations in the brainstem. They used subtraction techniques to good advantage in patients with tinnitus who can alter the tinnitus with jaw clenching and patients with gaze-evoked tinnitus and by administering intravenous lidocaine to subjects with tinnitus. They demonstrated unilateral changes in the neural activity associated with changes in tinnitus loudness.

Lockwood and colleagues point out that with magnetoencephalography, Muhlnickel and colleagues have demonstrated displacement of the site responsive to a tone, the frequency of which was matched to the frequency of the tinnitus, providing additional evidence of the reorganization of the central auditory pathways with tinnitus.

James B. Snow Jr

Clinical Trials and Drug Therapy for Tinnitus

Robert A. Dobie, MD

This chapter reviews randomized clinical trials (RCTs) that have been done to test treatments for tinnitus. As in my earlier review of this topic,[1] the articles selected for review were found by a *MEDLINE* search (1966–2003) for English-language articles matching both "tinnitus" and "randomized clinical trials," supplemented by reports found in personal files. Although some articles were not published in refereed journals, all are publicly available. I excluded studies in which

1. tinnitus was a side effect of treatment (eg, cisplatin for cancer),
2. there was inadequate detail for analysis,
3. another more detailed article described results from the same trial,
4. only a single otologic disorder (eg, Meniere's disease or acoustic trauma) was included, or
5. there was no contemporaneously treated control group (ie, there were only waiting list or historical controls).

Because it is still true that no treatment "has been shown to eliminate tinnitus more frequently than placebo, or even to provide replicable long-term reduction in the impact of tinnitus on everyday life, in excess of placebo effects,"[1] this chapter may be of more interest to tinnitus researchers than to practicing clinicians, and I have included many methodologic suggestions for their future studies. I hope that clinicians who want to be able to read the clinical trial literature critically will also find the discussion useful. The chapter concludes with some rather tentative and personal recommendations for drug therapy for patients with tinnitus. Many of the treatments that do not use drugs are discussed in more detail in Chapter 21, "Tinnitus Retraining Therapy," Chapter 22, "Role of Hearing Aids in Management of Tinnitus," Chapter 23, "Psychological Treatments for Tinnitus," and Chapter 24, "Electrical Suppression of Tinnitus."

WHAT IS AN RCT?

An RCT is an experiment in which patients with a particular condition receive one of two or more treatments, with the choice of treatment determined by a coin flip or some other random process. Frequently, one "treatment" is an active drug, whereas the other is a placebo, such as a sugar pill, which is not expected to have any specific effect on the disease or condition being studied. In other cases, one treatment (often new) is compared with another (often an older or better established treatment). In an RCT, neither the patient nor the physician can decide which treatment a patient will receive. If the number of patients in each treatment group is large enough and if the differences in outcome are large enough, it may be possible to conclude with some statistical confidence that one treatment is better than the other(s).

In most RCTs, each patient receives only one treatment. In contrast, "crossover" RCTs are particularly attractive for reversible, relatively brief treatments given to patients with stable disorders (ie, for most tinnitus treatments). In this type of study, each patient receives both treatments but in a randomly determined order with a "washout" period interposed between the active and placebo periods. Crossover RCTs require far fewer patients for two reasons. Obviously, the number of patients receiving each treatment is twice what it would be in an ordinary RCT. More importantly, each patient acts as his or her own control, so interindividual differences are much less important.

WHEN DO WE NEED RCTs?

Randomization in clinical trials increases the odds that the treatment groups will be similar and will have, on average, the same prognosis. Without randomization, physicians may consciously or unconsciously recommend different treatments for patients based on their clinical characteristics. For example, in a comparison of radiation versus surgery for tongue cancer, physicians might assign patients with larger tumors to surgery and those with smaller tumors to radiation. If patients are allowed to choose, younger and healthier patients might choose surgery more often than older and less vigorous patients. In either case, the final comparison would be flawed because the treatment groups would not have comparable prognoses. To the extent to which we can identify important prognostic factors (such as tumor size and general health), we may be able to correct for this imbalance after the data have been collected. Even better, as is discussed later (see the section on stratification), we can design the study to take known prognostic factors into account. Nevertheless, we can never know all of the prognostic factors for a particular condition; randomization is thus always desirable in clinical trials.

We do not always need RCTs. Consider conductive hearing loss caused by otosclerosis, a condition that does not improve spontaneously. When fenestration surgery was introduced, it was immediately apparent that almost all patients had considerable hearing improvements. Approximately 20 years later, stapes surgery was shown to improve hearing, in almost all cases, much more than fenestration. The large treatment effects, the relatively small variability in treatment outcomes, and the stability of the underlying condition made it possible to conclude that surgery helped patients with otosclerosis and that stapes surgery was better than fenestration, without the need for RCTs. To return to the tongue cancer example, we do not need RCTs to know that either radiation or surgery is better than no treatment: treatment effects for both are large (many patients survive) and relatively predictable compared to the natural history. We do need RCTs to determine whether, for a particular stage of cancer, surgery is preferable to radiation (because the differences between the two treatments are small compared with the variability in results).

We do not know a great deal about the natural history of tinnitus (see Chapter 1, "Overview: Suffering from Tinnitus"), but we can say that tinnitus that has been present for more than a year or two is very unlikely to disappear spontaneously. We also know that the disappearance of tinnitus is rare in patients enrolled in RCTs, whether they receive active or placebo treatment. If someone were to develop a treatment that frequently made chronic tinnitus disappear, and if this result were to be replicated in several centers, we would not need an RCT for this new treatment. Today, unfortunately, we have only tinnitus treatments that attempt to reduce tinnitus sensation or tinnitus suffering, and we cannot be sure that any of them are effective without RCTs. Thus, in this chapter, only RCTs are considered.

WHAT ARE THE CHARACTERISTICS OF A GOOD RCT?

Randomization alone does not ensure that an RCT gives valid and useful information to guide clinical management. A good RCT should minimize the chances of either a false-positive error (saying that a treatment works when it actually does not) or a false-negative error (saying that the treatment does not work when it actually does work). In this section, I discuss some of the features of good RCTs, relating each of them to the tinnitus literature, and make some recommendations for future tinnitus RCTs.

CHOICE OF CONTROL GROUP AND BLINDING

In one of the earliest RCTs for tinnitus, half of the patients received amobarbital (a barbiturate sleeping pill), whereas the other half received no treatment.[2] This type of control group is often referred to as a "waiting-list" control. Although the drug-treated patients did better than the untreated patients, it is impossible to know whether this was due to any specific effect of the drug or to other differences in the treatment of the two groups. For example, patients in the drug group had more contact with the physician and more time out of the house. The authors could have improved the study by giving the control group a placebo pill, thus making the treatment of the two groups more similar. But if the physician and the patient knew which pill was which, both would probably expect more benefit from the active drug. And because "the wish is father to the thought,"[3] the active drug would probably show better results than would the placebo. The solution is, of course, to "double-blind" the study so that neither physician nor patient knows whether the drug given is active or placebo. A double-blinded placebo-controlled RCT that shows superior results for the active drug is relatively easy to interpret, especially if patients cannot tell (from side effects) which pill they are taking. Almost all of the drug RCTs reviewed in this chapter were double-blinded; exceptions are noted.

Side effects pose a difficult problem. Many of the drugs that have been tried for tinnitus cause noticeable drowsiness, sleeplessness, dry mouth, sexual dysfunction, or other symptoms. If patients can tell that they are taking the active drug, they might expect, and then actually realize, greater benefit. Ideally, investigators should assess whether patients can identify which pill they are taking; in some cases, "active placebos"—drugs that cause similar or at least equally noticeable side effects—should then be used. If the two drugs turn out to work equally well, however, it may be because the "active placebo" actually helps the patient. For example, one study used diphenhydramine (Benadryl), an antihistamine, as a control for various tranquilizers being given to patients with tinnitus.[4] Because diphenhydramine causes drowsiness and is often prescribed for insomnia, we could expect it to be helpful to tinnitus patients, who often complain of trouble sleeping. In cases like this, it would be better to use both an "active placebo" and an inert placebo, unless both drugs under study have already been shown to be effective, so that the study can focus narrowly on the differences between them.

Problems with control groups and blinding are much more severe with nondrug treatments. Many psychological treatments (using methods such as cognitive or behavioral therapy) have been compared with waiting-list control groups. In general, these RCTs show that treated patients do better than do those on the waiting list, but it is impossible to tell whether the benefit is attributable to the particular type of treatment or simply to time spent with a sympathetic, knowledgeable clinician. One can imagine a "placebo" treatment in which the therapist spent the same amount of time with the patient but used methods believed to be ineffective. The problem with this approach is that the therapist's lack of faith in this "placebo" would be obvious to the patient, making blinding impossible. The same pitfall faces any nondrug RCT in which the control group is "doing it wrong" (eg, putting the acupuncture needles in the wrong places, using the wrong massage technique). Many nondrug RCTs have not even attempted to include a placebo group but have instead compared one treatment with another. The problem with this approach is that if no difference is found, we do not know if both treatments work or neither works.

Statistical Testing

Almost all tinnitus RCTs have reported some type of statistical testing. In general, the results of the trial are considered positive when the difference between active and control treatments is large enough that it would occur only rarely by chance (typically less than 5% of the time). The most common statistical error is using too many outcome variables, with each tested for statistical significance, as in one study comparing yoga to cognitive-behavioral therapy.[5] Investigators should usually select one or only a very few key outcome variables. The proper analysis of multiple outcome variables is a complex statistical task usually requiring expert consultation.

In many RCTs, dropouts are a significant problem, especially if the treatment is long and arduous and the patients are not highly motivated. There is general agreement among clinical trial experts that data from dropouts should be included in an analysis "by intention to treat" rather than limiting analysis to patients who complete treatment. For example, one study of oral ginkgo biloba began with 60 patients randomly assigned to receive either active drug or placebo.[6] Unfortunately, by the end of the 12-week treatment period, only 18 remained (6 in the placebo group, 12 in the ginkgo biloba group). Patients who dropped out after the initial 4-week or 8-week visit had those measurements "carried forward" to the 12-week visit as if they had stayed in the trial to the end—obviously an imperfect solution. Because the drug apparently had few, if any, side effects, it seems likely that many of the dropouts were patients with very mild tinnitus of recent onset (there were no severity or duration entry criteria, and 25% of patients had tinnitus of less than 3 months duration). Fortunately, very few tinnitus RCTs have had dropout problems that were this severe.

Long-Term Results

Clinically significant tinnitus is, by definition, a long-term problem, and clinically worthwhile treatment should confer long-term benefit. Unfortunately, very few studies have followed patients for more than a few months. For example, although there are now several studies showing that tricyclic antidepressants help some patients with tinnitus,[7-9] none of them has measured results beyond 6 months.

OUTCOME MEASURES

As argued in Chapter 1, tinnitus sensation is not well correlated with tinnitus suffering. Until we have a tinnitus treatment that can frequently eliminate tinnitus altogether, we should measure the effects of treatment on tinnitus suffering rather than on tinnitus sensation. This does not mean that treatments aimed at tinnitus sensation (such as masking) cannot work but rather that they cannot be helpful unless they reduce both tinnitus suffering and tinnitus sensation.

One of the best-known tinnitus RCTs tested alprazolam (Xanax, a benzodiazepine tranquilizer) against placebo. After treatment, tinnitus loudness was reduced in the alprazolam group but not in the placebo group.[10] Unfortunately, no measure of suffering (see Chapter 17, "Tinnitus Questionnaires") was reported, so we cannot tell whether patients were helped, even in the short term.

It is a shame that there is still no consensus in the research community regarding the outcome variable for tinnitus suffering. Until such a consensus emerges, it will be difficult to compare one treatment with another unless they have been tested together in the same RCT.

SAMPLE SIZE

Blinding, placebos, and proper statistical testing reduce the risk of false-positive errors but do nothing to control false-negative error. A negative study can never prove that the treatment in question is absolutely worthless; it can only prove that it is unlikely that a benefit of a certain magnitude has been missed. Large studies, if negative, are very unlikely to have missed even small treatment effects, but small studies can miss quite large effects. The statistical power of a study (in percent) is equal to 100 minus the risk of a false-negative; all other things being equal, power increases with sample size. Ideally, sample size should be determined during the design of a study by specifying the size of a clinically meaningful effect on a single key outcome variable (eg, a 10 or 20% reduction in average score on a questionnaire measuring tinnitus suffering), the variability in that measure, and the acceptable power (eg, 80 or 90% probability of detecting an effect of the specified size).

Even when a power analysis has not been done, or when sample size has been determined by practical considerations, such as patient availability, negative results should be accompanied by some retrospective estimate of the risk of false-negative error. The simplest way to do this is to state the 95% confidence interval for the difference between the treatment groups on the key outcome variable. For small negative studies, the confidence interval will, of course, include zero (no difference), but it will also include very large treatment effects. To give one example, melatonin in a crossover trial was given to 30 patients, 15 of whom had sleep disturbance blamed on their tinnitus.[11] Of these 15, 7 (47%) were helped by melatonin and 3 (20%) by placebo. The difference is not statistically different, given the small sample size, but this study could have missed a rather large effect: the 95% confidence interval for the percentage helped by melatonin extends from 22 to 73%. The confidence interval for the placebo extends from 4 to 45%. Obviously, a larger study would be needed to establish or exclude a clinically important effect of this drug for sleep-deprived patients with tinnitus. Unfortunately, most tinnitus RCTs have involved fewer than 30 patients and were only powerful enough to find large effects.

INCLUSION CRITERIA

The only negative RCT for a tricyclic antidepressant was not only a small study, it also failed to specify whether the patients had severe tinnitus.[12] If the authors believed that the drug would strongly reduce tinnitus sensation (tricyclics can directly reduce pain in some patients), this was not an unreasonable plan. If, on the other hand, the intent was to reduce tinnitus suffering as expressed in depressive symptoms, one would want to study tinnitus patients who were depressed or at least suffering.

When patients with mild and/or short-lived tinnitus are permitted into RCTs, one can expect more dropouts because patients will be less motivated. This can lead to statistical difficulties, as described earlier.

Because tinnitus can accompany any disorder that causes hearing loss, it seems likely that the pathophysiology, and thus the type of treatment that might help, could be very different for different types of patients. If a drug were thought likely to be effective in a particular type of tinnitus, we would want to test it in the subset of patients who had that type, not in a random sample of patients with tinnitus. Unfortunately, we do not yet have any good way to classify patients with tinnitus, so even large negative tinnitus RCTs fail to prove that the treatment would not be helpful for some subset of patients with tinnitus. One simple design solution for drug treatments has emerged: restrict the RCT to patients who have claimed benefit in a preliminary open trial of the drug. One group gave gingko biloba to 80 patients with tinnitus, 21 of whom claimed benefit.[13] Twenty of these 21 patients were then entered into a crossover RCT in which each patient received both ginkgo biloba and placebo but in a randomly selected order; there was no outcome difference between gingko biloba and placebo. This negative result was more compelling and much less expensive than a negative trial of all 80 patients would have been.

Several negative RCTs have offered tantalizing hints that the treatment being studied, although ineffective for the entire group, might have been helpful for a subgroup, typically one that was too small for meaningful statistical analysis. Some of these treatments and the tinnitus subgroups that may have been helped (but appear never to have been examined in follow-up studies) are listed below:
1. Flunarizine for Meniere's disease[14]
2. Lidocaine iontophoresis for noise-induced hearing loss[15]
3. Ginkgo biloba for cervical spondylosis[13]
4. Melatonin for sleep interference[11]
5. Tocainide for totally deaf ears[16]

PROGNOSIS AND STRATIFICATION

Factors that predict prognosis can be incorporated into the design of an RCT by stratification. If we knew, for example, that men had a worse prognosis than did women, then we would not want to rely on randomization to ensure that the percentage of men was the same in both treatment groups. Instead, we would first divide the patients by gender and then randomize men and women separately. We do not know the prognostic variables for tinnitus, so it is unfair to criticize existing studies for failure to stratify, but it is important to recognize this important gap in our knowledge. Failure of randomization to achieve a good prognostic balance between treatment groups can cause both false-positive and false-negative errors in RCTs. Crossover RCTs are much less susceptible to this problem.

Our inability to describe the prognostic features of a group of tinnitus patients also makes it difficult to compare the results from one RCT with those from another. A treatment that achieved only modest benefit in a very difficult to treat group of patients might be a lot better than one that achieved the same degree of benefit in an easy to treat group.

RECOMMENDATIONS FOR FUTURE RESEARCH

Guyatt and colleagues listed important minimal criteria for RCTs[17]:
1. Blinding when feasible
2. Complete follow-up to the extent possible
3. Analysis by intention to treat when there are dropouts
4. Group similarity postrandomization (not a problem in crossover designs)
5. Equal treatment other than the treatment under study
6. Testing for statistical significance

Most of these criteria have been met most of the time in the tinnitus RCT literature, yet the state of our therapeutic knowledge is still quite primitive. Future tinnitus RCTs can be improved in several ways:
1. Statistical consultation prior to an RCT will almost always result in a better study. In most cases, only one or a very few outcome variables should be selected.
2. Investigators should focus on tinnitus suffering, not tinnitus sensation, unless the treatment to be studied frequently abolishes tinnitus altogether.
3. The tinnitus research community should try to agree on a single key outcome measure of tinnitus suffering so that the benefits of different treatments can be compared across different studies.
4. Investigators should identify prognostic factors, both in natural history studies and in RCTs, so that future RCTs can use them as inclusion criteria and stratifying variables.
5. Until we know more about prognostic variables, tinnitus RCTs should be limited to patients who are unlikely to improve spontaneously: those with severe, long-standing tinnitus.
6. Treatments that appear to be promising should be tested in formal open trials before embarking on RCTs because
   a) large, well-designed RCTs are expensive and should be limited to really promising treatments;

b) open trials permit estimation of treatment effect size and variability, which is essential for power analysis and determination of sample size for a subsequent RCT;
c) open trials may identify subgroups that are more or less likely to respond, thus enabling better choices of inclusion and exclusion criteria;
d) open trials can determine whether patients have noticeable side effects that may require an active placebo group;
e) if the preliminary open trial shows strong reported benefits, but only for a few patients, without any obvious way to predict who will be a responder, investigators should consider an RCT design that begins with an open trial, followed by a blinded placebo-controlled RCT restricted to open-trial responders[13]; and
f) animal models (see Chapter 7, "Animal Models of Tinnitus") can elucidate pathophysiology and can test drugs that may reduce tinnitus sensation and may thus be candidates for clinical trials but cannot predict whether human tinnitus suffering will be ameliorated.

7. RCTs should be large enough to detect clinically important treatment effects; this requires a power analysis.
8. Even when power analysis has not been done, or when the desired sample size could not be achieved, investigators should report not only whether the treatment showed statistically significant benefit but also the confidence interval for the treatment effect.
9. Crossover designs should be considered for any treatment that is reversible, blindable, and not too time consuming.
10. Future RCTs need not be limited to new treatments. Many previous studies, both positive and negative, deserve replication (eg, alprazolam, melatonin), and hints of subgroup effects are worthy of follow-up study (eg, tocainide for totally deaf ears).
11. Treatments that show replicable, clinically meaningful short-term benefit in RCTs (such as antidepressant drugs for depressed patients with tinnitus) should be subjected to longer-term study to determine whether the benefits persist.
12. If and when we have both a consensus outcome measure for tinnitus suffering and a good prognostic staging system, it may be possible to use open trial data to compare treatments for which placebo design and blinding are difficult, including most nondrug treatments. Although RCTs will always be preferable, cost-effectiveness comparisons for prognostically similar groups of patients, across studies, could prove to be the best way to evaluate treatments such as tinnitus retraining therapy (TRT) and cognitive-behavioral therapy.[18]

DO NONDRUG TREATMENTS WORK?

MASKING DEVICES

External sounds often mask (render inaudible) tinnitus. Patients often discover by themselves that they can mask their tinnitus at home using a radio or fan. Anecdotally, many patients with tinnitus sleep better with some background noise in the bedroom. Many appliance and department stores sell electronic noise machines that allow the user to select from a variety of pleasant sounds, such as waves on a beach, rain on the roof, or wind in the trees. Since the 1980s, wearable masking devices that deliver sound (usually a narrow-band hissing noise) into the ear have been available. Masking devices are sometimes combined with hearing aids (they are then called "tinnitus instruments"). Of course, hearing aids can provide some masking by amplifying ambient sounds (see Chapter 22, "Role of Hearing Aids in Management of Tinnitus").

No one doubts that masking devices can often reduce or eliminate tinnitus sensation, at least while the devices are being worn. Indeed, some patients experience absence of tinnitus for minutes or even hours after the devices are removed. The important question is whether they reduce tinnitus suffering. After an initial period of enthusiasm in the 1980s, masking devices declined in popularity among clinicians because it became clear that most patients who agreed to try them were nonusers 6 months later. Nonuse need not be synonymous with absence of benefit; nonusers could be people who have

1. experienced some benefit but not enough to justify their own out-of-pocket expenses and, therefore, returned the devices during the trial period;
2. received substantial benefit but not enough to justify the inconvenience and discomfort of daily use (if such a patient keeps the device "for when [he or she] might need it" and thereby achieves the satisfaction of knowing that his or her tinnitus can be temporarily eliminated on demand, the device can hardly be considered a failure, even if it is used rarely); or
3. failed to be helped at all.

Some investigators have tried to determine the value of masking devices through RCTs. Placebo control and blinding are difficult for masking devices, as for most nondrug treatments; patients know when they are hearing masking noise. When maskers were compared with sham devices that did nothing (patients were told that they produced electrical stimulation of the ear), small but statistically significant differences in favor of maskers were found on an unvalidated tinnitus questionnaire.[19] Two studies of maskers versus hearing aids found that patients given maskers noted more improvement in sleep interference than did patients given hearing aids[20] but that the more hearing loss patients had, the more likely they were to prefer hearing aids to maskers.[21] Maskers have been compared with nonacoustic treatments (hypnosis, acupuncture, cognitive therapy), with no conclusive results.[22–24]

Electrical Stimulation

Electrical current delivered to electrodes in or near the cochlea can suppress tinnitus sensation (see Chapter 24, "Electrical Suppression of Tinnitus"); for some patients with deafness who have received cochlear implants, this is a welcome bonus. Electrical suppression of tinnitus is not simply a special case of masking because the electrical stimulus does not always produce a sound. For a few years in the 1980s, a wearable electrical stimulation device was marketed in the United States for tinnitus relief. RCTs were easy to perform because the device created neither sound nor any other perceptible sensation, such as tingling, and could be internally switched off, so patients could not tell whether the device was on (active) or off (placebo). The device failed to show significant benefit in groups of patients,[25,26] but two studies showed an intriguing result: each had a single patient who repeatedly and reliably showed strong tinnitus suppression when the device was on but not when it was off.[25,27] If and when wearable or surgically implantable electrical stimulation for tinnitus is again clinically available, it will be important to determine whether it reduces tinnitus suffering, especially in long-term use.

Magnetic, Electromagnetic, Laser, and Ultrasound Stimulation

Devices purporting to deliver magnetic, electromagnetic, laser, or ultrasound stimulation through the skin over the mastoid have either failed to show any benefit[28–32] or have been reported to show benefit in a brief proceedings paper, with no subsequent refereed report.[33]

Biofeedback and Musculoskeletal Treatments

As described in Chapters 1 and 9, jaw and neck muscle contraction can induce and modulate tinnitus, but there is no strong evidence that treatments of musculoskeletal conditions help tinnitus patients.

Biofeedback therapy attempts to teach patients to reduce muscle tension. Electrodes placed over muscles in the head and neck area can be connected to an amplifier and speaker to allow a patient to hear his or her own electromyographic (EMG) activity. As with so many nondrug treatments, placebo design is difficult. One group compared "real" biofeedback with a condition in which the patient heard another person's EMG recordings.[9,34] Although patients receiving feedback from their own EMG did better, it seems likely that those receiving sham biofeedback must have known that this was the case. In other words, they were not blinded to their treatment. Other studies of biofeedback produced negative results compared with baseline[35,36] or temporomandibular therapy (in a group of patients with both tinnitus and temporomandibular disorders).[37]

"Active" massage and stretching of the neck and jaw muscles were said to work better than "inactive" therapy ("doing it wrong") in one study.[38] As with all such control groups, it is hard to know whether patients were truly blinded to treatment.

Acupuncture

Acupuncture performed "the wrong way" works as well as acupuncture performed "correctly."[39–42]

Hypnosis

Two positive studies of hypnosis compared it with alternative treatments that were not comparable in important ways. In one study, the control group received only cursory counseling.[43] The other study, which included only patients preselected to be "susceptible" to hypnosis, compared hypnosis (by an expert) with masking (using a "Walkman" tape) or cursory counseling.[22] It seems likely that hypnosis, like almost any treatment offered with some enthusiasm by a caring, unhurried clinician, is better than nothing, but the data do not show that it is any better than other treatments of equal intensity and cost.

PSYCHOTHERAPY

In the context of this chapter, "psychotherapy" means any treatment that involves talking as opposed to the use of drugs, devices (including biofeedback), or application of physical energy (heat, light, electricity, magnetic field, mechanical manipulation). It encompasses the brief and informal counseling and education that are part of a routine office visit with a physician or audiologist, as well as more formal and time-consuming approaches, such as relaxation, cognitive, and behavioral therapy (see Chapter 23, "Psychological Treatments for Tinnitus"). TRT (see Chapter 21, "Tinnitus Retraining Therapy") can be thought of as psychotherapy plus a device (a sound generator set just below the level needed to mask tinnitus). It is also clear that the most enthusiastic proponents of masking devices dispense healthy doses of psychotherapy along with their devices.

There seems to be little doubt among clinicians that at least some education and counseling (psychotherapy) is helpful to patients, and RCTs with waiting-list controls have routinely shown that more formal approaches are better than no treatment at all. Thus, the most relevant questions about psychotherapy are the following:

1. Does it matter how the therapist spends time with the patient? Is one type of talking therapy better than another?
2. What is the relationship between cost and benefit for different types of patients? If a little bit (at low cost) is good, will a longer, more expensive course be better? For whom?

The long history of studies of psychotherapy for psychiatric disorders[44] suggests that the answer to question 1 is likely to be "No." Indeed, RCTs comparing different types of psychotherapy for tinnitus, when the duration and frequency of patient-therapist interaction are held constant, have failed to demonstrate meaningful and persistent differences in outcome.[45-52] TRT has not been included in any of these RCTs.

Question 2 is more difficult and will be tractable only when there is consensus in the research community on preferred outcome measures for tinnitus, so that comparisons can be made across studies. One could hazard a guess that the amount of therapy a patient needs is probably proportional to his or her degree of suffering.

DO DRUG TREATMENTS WORK?

ANTIARRHYTHMICS

The ability of systemic doses of lidocaine to eliminate temporarily or at least to change tinnitus sensation was probably discovered by accident but was later documented in well-controlled trials.[53,54] Because this drug cannot be taken by mouth, many investigators turned to tocainide, which, after oral administration, is converted to lidocaine in the liver. Several RCTs were done, and, as a group, they failed to show that this drug has any effect on tinnitus sensation or suffering.[16,55-60] A possible subgroup effect can be noted: some patients with totally deaf ears appeared to have been helped.[16] Some related oral antiarrhythmic drugs have also been tried and found wanting.[61,62] Topical lidocaine can be driven through the tympanic membrane by electrical current, but two RCTs failed to show significant relief of tinnitus with this treatment.[15,63]

ANTICONVULSANTS

Drugs such as carbamazepine have effects on neural tissue that are somewhat similar to those of the antiarrhythmics. In addition, some of them can help patients with chronic pain, a condition that is often compared with tinnitus, and anecdotal reports suggested that they could reduce tinnitus sensation. Unfortunately, RCTs using carbamazepine and amino-oxyacetic acid have failed to demonstrate any benefit at subtoxic doses.[64-68] Furthermore, these drugs have very serious side effects and require frequent medical monitoring.

BENZODIAZEPINES

This class of drugs includes diazepam (Valium) and alprazolam (Xanax); most have tranquilizing and anticonvulsant effects, with serious potential for dependency and abuse. As previously described, alprazolam has been shown in a single RCT to reduce tinnitus sensation but not to reduce tinnitus suffering.[10] Another weakness of this study is that the patients in the active drug group had their dosages adjusted until either side effects or benefits were observed or the maximum dose was reached. The placebo group was not treated in this way; they therefore had less interaction with clinicians and had no clues (from side effects) about the identity of their pills. Other studies with benzodiazepines[4,62,69] have failed to show statistically significant benefit and have suggested that tinnitus may rebound after these drugs are stopped.

Antidepressants

Three RCTs using tricyclic antidepressant drugs (nortriptyline and amitriptyline) for patients with severe tinnitus have shown benefit,[7–9] which may be greater for patients who complain of sleep disturbance.[8] The one negative tricyclic RCT, using trimipramine,[12] has been discussed; it was a small study that appeared not to limit entry to patients with severe tinnitus and thus does not refute the positive studies.

Newer antidepressants of the class of selective serotonin reuptake inhibitors (SSRIs), such as fluoxetine (Prozac) and paroxetine (Paxil), have not been studied in any of the RCTs published to date, but Chapter 20, "Antidepressant Therapy for Tinnitus," addresses antidepressant therapy for tinnitus, including SSRIs, in more detail.

Ginkgo Biloba

Extracts of the leaves of the ginkgo biloba tree have been used in Chinese herbal medicine for centuries and are frequently used in the United States and Europe as well. A recent meta-analysis of mostly European studies suggests that ginkgo biloba may have genuine benefit in treating cognitive impairment and dementia; it is also quite popular for treating both tinnitus and dizziness in France and Germany.[70] Most English-language publications of RCTs using ginkgo biloba for tinnitus, however, failed to prove any benefit compared with placebo.[31,71] One recent article purports to show a reduction in tinnitus "volume" in decibels (this was either a matching level or a masking level) after administration of oral ginkgo biloba, but the study had a 70% dropout rate (as discussed above under statistical testing).[6] In addition, the hypothesis testing appeared to be flawed: a one-tailed Mann-Whitney test was used, with a reported p value of .034; this is tantamount to assuming the efficacy of the drug in advance. The more appropriate two-tailed test would surely have failed to show significance at the 5% level. The article does not provide enough data to recalculate the Mann-Whitney statistic, but the normally more powerful Student's t-test, calculated from their Table 2, yielded a two-tailed p value of .1661 (not statistically significant).

Miscellaneous Drugs (and Zinc)

Many unrelated drugs have been tried in single RCTs (sometimes for no apparent reason). These include melatonin,[11] baclofen,[72] lamotrigine,[73] misoprostol,[74] nicotinamide,[75] betahistine,[62] cinnarizine,[34] cyclandelate,[76] flunarizine,[14] caroverine,[77] and eperisone[78] and a homeopathic preparation containing salicylate, quinine, coniine, and ascaridole.[79] None of these has been shown to reduce tinnitus suffering for patients with tinnitus, although both cyclandelate (Cyclospasmol) and eperisone slightly reduced tinnitus match levels. Zinc, a dietary supplement, was ineffective in one RCT[80] and was said to be helpful (using a locally developed tinnitus questionnaire) in another.[81] The latter study, from Turkey, included several patients with low blood zinc levels. It would be interesting to see whether these results can be replicated in other populations using more widely used outcome measures.

CAN ANY DRUGS BE RECOMMENDED?

The literature on RCTs does not even begin to establish a "standard of practice" for patients with tinnitus, especially with respect to drugs. Most patients with tinnitus need only a history and physical examination, an audiogram, and sympathetic, brief (but unhurried) counseling. Some need imaging studies or other tests to rule out dangerous disorders, such as vestibular schwannoma. Many need hearing aids and can be offered the hope that this will help their tinnitus and their hearing loss (see Chapter 22, "Role of Hearing Aids in Management of Tinnitus"). A few will be clinically depressed (see Chapter 20, "Antidepressant Therapy for Tinnitus"); most otolaryngologists will refer these patients to psychiatrists or to their primary care physicians for treatment, which will usually include an antidepressant drug. The tinnitus RCT literature does not prove that one antidepressant drug is better than another. An even smaller number of patients, although not clinically depressed, are suffering enough to merit referral to tinnitus centers that offer masking, TRT, or cognitive-behavioral therapy. The choice of referral will often depend on local availability and interest.

Sleep disturbance is an important component of tinnitus suffering that deserves direct attention. I suspect that any drug (or other regimen) that improves sleep will reduce tinnitus suffering; thus, I often suggest to referring physicians that judicious use of hypnotics may be of value. Because of the potential for abuse and the need for long-term supervision, I almost never prescribe hypnotics or other sedating drugs myself.

The only drug I prescribe with any frequency for tinnitus patients (about two or three times a year, for a nondepressed, otherwise healthy, patient suffering with tinnitus) is nortriptyline, 25 mg at bedtime, increasing the dose as needed every week up to a maximum of 100 mg at bedtime. This was the regimen my colleagues and I used in our 1993 study.[8] Patients who feel that the drug is helpful are encouraged to continue it for 3 to 6 months. Relative contraindications to nortriptyline include glaucoma, some cardiac arrhythmias, and severe prostatic hypertrophy.

The RCT literature does weakly suggest some other options. Two drugs available in the United States (alprazolam and cyclandelate) have been shown in single studies to slightly reduce tinnitus loudness. Neither of them has demonstrated benefit in terms of tinnitus suffering, and alprazolam carries the risk of abuse and dependence. Zinc may be helpful in people with zinc deficiency, which is not rare in vegetarians.

REFERENCES

1. Dobie RA. A review of randomized clinical trials in tinnitus. Laryngoscope 1999;109:1202–11.
2. Donaldson I. Tinnitus: a theoretical view and a therapeutic study using amylobarbitone. J Laryngol Otol 1978;92:123–30.
3. Henry IV Part 2: act 4, scene 5, line 91.
4. Lechtenberg R, Shulman A. Benzodiazepines in the treatment of tinnitus. J Laryngol Otol Suppl 1984;9:271–6.
5. Kroner-Herwig B, Hebing G, van Rijn-Kalkmann U, et al. The management of chronic tinnitus: comparison of a cognitive-behavioural group training with yoga. J Psychosom Res 1995;39:153–65.
6. Morgenstern C, Biermann E. The efficacy of ginkgo special extract EGb 761 in patients with tinnitus. Int J Clin Pharmacol Ther 2002;40:188–97.
7. Bayar N, Boke B, Turan E, Belgin E. Efficacy of amitriptyline in the treatment of subjective tinnitus. J Otolaryngol 2001;30:300–3.
8. Dobie RA, Sakai CS, Sullivan MD, et al. Antidepressant treatment of tinnitus patients: report of a randomized clinical trial and clinical prediction of benefit. Am J Otol 1993;14:18–23.
9. Podoshin L, Ben-David Y, Fradis M, et al. Idiopathic subjective tinnitus treated by amitriptyline hydrochloride/biofeedback. Int Tinnitus J 1995;1:54–60.
10. Johnson RM, Brummett R, Schleuning A. Use of alprazolam for relief of tinnitus: a double-blind study. Arch Otolaryngol Head Neck Surg 1993;119:842–5.
11. Rosenberg SI, Silverstein H, Rowan PT, Olds MJ. Effect of melatonin on tinnitus. Laryngoscope 1998;108:305–10.
12. Mihail RC, Crowley JM, Walden BE, et al. The tricyclic trimipramine in the treatment of subjective tinnitus. Ann Otol Rhinol Laryngol 1988;97(2 Pt 1):120–3.
13. Holgers KM, Axelsson A, Pringle I. Ginkgo biloba extract for the treatment of tinnitus. Audiology 1994;33:85–92.
14. Hulshof JH, Vermij P. The value of flunarizine in the treatment of tinnitus. ORL J Otorhinolaryngol Relat Spec 1986;48:33–6.
15. Willatt DJ, O'Sullivan G, Stoney PJ, Jackson SR. A sequential double blind crossover trial of iontophoresis. In: Feldmann H, editor. Proceedings of the Third International Tinnitus Seminar: Münster. Karlsruhe (Germany): Harsch Verlag; 1987. p. 316–9.
16. Hazell JWP, Wood SM. Drug therapy and tinnitus: the UK experience. J Laryngol Otol Suppl 1984;9:277–80.
17. Guyatt GH, Sackett DL, Cook DJ. Users' guides to the medical literature, II: how to use an article about therapy or prevention. Part A: are the results of the study valid? Evidence-Based Medicine Working Group. JAMA 1993;270:2598–601.
18. Dobie RA. Randomized clinical trials for tinnitus: not the last word? In: Patuzzi R, editor. Proceedings of the Seventh International Tinnitus Seminar. Perth: University of Western Australia; 2002. p. 3–6.
19. Erlandsson S, Ringdahl A, Hutchins T, Carlsson SG. Treatment of tinnitus: a controlled comparison of masking and placebo. Br J Audiol 1987;21:37–44.
20. Stephens SD, Corcoran AL. A controlled study of tinnitus masking. Br J Audiol 1985;19:159–67.
21. Mehlum D, Grasel G, Fankhauser C. Prospective crossover evaluation of four methods of clinical management of tinnitus. Otolaryngol Head Neck Surg 1984;92:448–53.
22. Attias J, Shemesh Z, Sohmer H, et al. Comparison between self-hypnosis, masking and attentiveness for alleviation of chronic tinnitus. Audiology 1993;32:205–12.

23. Jansson G, Warfvinge J, Edensvärd A, Wiberg A. The effects of acupuncture versus masker treatment in patients with tinnitus. In: Reich GE, Vernon JA, editors. Proceedings of the Fifth International Tinnitus Seminar. Portland (OR): American Tinnitus Association; 1996. p. 489–99.
24. Jakes SC, Hallam RS, McKenna L. Group cognitive therapy for medical patients: an application to tinnitus. Cognit Ther Res 1992;16:67–82.
25. Dobie RA, Hoberg KE, Rees TS. Electrical tinnitus suppression: a double-blind crossover study. Otolaryngol Head Neck Surg 1986;95(3 Pt 1):319–23.
26. Thedinger BS, Karlsen E, Schack SH. Treatment of tinnitus with electrical stimulation: an evaluation of the Audimax Theraband. Laryngoscope 1987;97:33–7.
27. Lyttkens L, Lindberg P, Scott B, Melin L. Treatment of tinnitus by external electrical stimulation. Scand Audiol 1986;15:157–64.
28. Coles R, Bradley P, Donaldson I, Dingle A. A trial of tinnitus therapy with ear-canal magnets. Clin Otolaryngol 1991;16:371–2.
29. Mirz F, Zachariae B, Andersen SE, et al. The low-power laser in the treatment of tinnitus. Clin Otolaryngol 1999;24:346–54.
30. Rendell RJ, Carrick DG, Fielder CP, et al. Low-powered ultrasound in the inhibition of tinnitus. Br J Audiol 1987;21:289–93.
31. von Wedel H, Calero L, Walger M, et al. Soft-laser/ginkgo therapy in chronic tinnitus: a placebo-controlled study. Adv Otorhinolaryngol 1995;49:105–8.
32. Nakashima T, Ueda H, Misawa H, et al. Transmeatal low-power laser irradiation for tinnitus. Otol Neurotol 2002;23:296–300.
33. Roland NJ, Hughes JB, Daley MB, et al. Electromagnetic stimulation as a treatment of tinnitus: a double blind placebo trial with cross-over. In: Reich GE, Vernon JA, editors. Proceedings of the Fifth International Tinnitus Seminar. Portland (OR): American Tinnitus Association; 1996. p. 341–50.
34. Podoshin L, Ben-David Y, Fradis M, et al. Idiopathic subjective tinnitus treated by biofeedback, acupuncture and drug therapy. Ear Nose Throat J 1991;70:284–9.
35. Borton TE, Clark SR. Electromyographic biofeedback for treatment of tinnitus. Am J Otol 1988;9:23–30.
36. Haralambous G, Wilson PH, Platt-Hepworth S, et al. EMG biofeedback in the treatment of tinnitus: an experimental evaluation. Behav Res Ther 1987;25:49–55.
37. Erlandsson SI, Rubinstein B, Carlsson SG. Tinnitus: evaluation of biofeedback and stomatognathic treatment. Br J Audiol 1991;25:151–61.
38. Eriksson M, Gustafsson S, Axelsson A. Tinnitus and trigger points: a randomized cross-over study. In: Reich GE, Vernon JA, editors. Proceedings of the Fifth International Tinnitus Seminar. Portland (OR): American Tinnitus Association; 1996. p. 81–3.
39. Marks NJ, Emery P, Onisiphorou C. A controlled trial of acupuncture in tinnitus. J Laryngol Otol 1984;98:1103–9.
40. Axelsson A, Andersson S, Gu LD. Acupuncture in the management of tinnitus: a placebo-controlled study. Audiology 1994;33:351–60.
41. Vilholm OJ, Moller K, Jorgensen K. Effect of traditional Chinese acupuncture on severe tinnitus: a double-blind, placebo-controlled clinical investigation with open therapeutic control. Br J Audiol 1998;32:197–204.
42. Hansen PE, Hansen JH, Bentzen O. Acupuncture treatment of chronic unilateral tinnitus: a double-blind cross-over trial. Clin Otolaryngol 1982;7:325–9.
43. Mason JD, Rogerson DR, Butler JD. Client centered hypnotherapy in the management of tinnitus: is it better than counseling? J Laryngol Otol 1996;110:117–20.
44. Luborsky L, Singer B, Luborsky L. Comparative studies of psychotherapies. Is it true that "everyone has won and all must have prizes"? Arch Gen Psychiatry 1975;32:995–1008.
45. Jakes SC, Hallam RS, Rachman S, Hinchcliffe R. The effects of reassurance, relaxation training and distraction on chronic tinnitus sufferers. Behav Res Ther 1986;24:497–507.
46. Lindberg P, Scott B, Melin L, Lyttkens L. The psychological treatment of tinnitus: an experimental evaluation. Behav Res Ther 1989;27:593–603.
47. Davies S, McKenna L, Hallam RS. Relaxation and cognitive therapy: a controlled trial in chronic tinnitus. Psychol Health 1995;10:129–43.
48. Henry J, Wilson PH. The psychological management of tinnitus: comparison of a combined cognitive educational program, education alone and a waiting-list control. Int Tinnitus J 1996;2:9–20.
49. Dineen R, Doyle J, Bench J. Managing tinnitus: a comparison of different approaches to tinnitus management training. Br J Audiol 1997;31:331–44.
50. Wise K, Rief W, Goebel G. Meeting the expectations of chronic tinnitus patients: comparison of a structured group therapy program for tinnitus management with a problem-solving group. J Psychosom Res 1998;44:681–5.
51. Ireland CE, Wilson PH, Tonkin JP, Platt-Hepworth S. An evaluation of relaxation training in the treatment of tinnitus. Behav Res Ther 1985;23:423–30.

52. Dineen R, Doyle J, Bench J, Perry A. The influence of training on tinnitus perception: an evaluation 12 months after tinnitus management training. Br J Audiol 1999;33:29–51.
53. Martin FW, Colman BH. Tinnitus: a double-blind crossover controlled trial to evaluate the use of lignocaine. Clin Otolaryngol 1980;5:3–11.
54. Duckert LG, Rees TS. Treatment of tinnitus with intravenous lidocaine: a double-blind randomized trial. Otolaryngol Head Neck Surg 1983;91:550–5.
55. Blayney AW, Phillips MS, Guy AM, Colman BH. A sequential double blind cross-over trial of tocainide hydrochloride in tinnitus. Clin Otolaryngol 1985;10:97–101.
56. Hulshof JH, Vermeij P. The value of tocainide in the treatment of tinnitus. A double-blind controlled study. Arch Otorhinolaryngol 1985;241:279–83.
57. Shea JJ, Emmett JR, Orchik DJ, et al. Medical treatment of tinnitus. Ann Otol Rhinol Laryngol 1981;90(6 Pt 1):601–9.
58. Emmett JR, Shea JJ. Medical treatment of tinnitus. J Laryngol Otol Suppl 1984;9:264–70.
59. Lenarz T. Treatment of tinnitus with lidocaine and tocainide. Scand Audiol Suppl 1986;26:49–51.
60. Cathcart JM. Assessment of the value of tocainide hydrochloride in the treatment of tinnitus. J Laryngol Otol 1982;96:981–4.
61. Harker LA, Tyler RS, Fredell PA, et al. Evaluation of flecainide acetate (Tambocor) as a treatment of tinnitus. In: Feldmann H, editor. Proceedings of the Third International Tinnitus Seminar: Münster. Karlsruhe (Germany): Harsch Verlag; 1987. p. 322–5.
62. Kay NJ. Oral chemotherapy in tinnitus. Br J Audiol 1981;15:123–4.
63. Laffree JB, Vermeij P, Hulshof JH. The effect of iontophoresis of lignocaine in the treatment of tinnitus. Clin Otolaryngol 1989;14:401–4.
64. Donaldson I. Tegretol: a double blind trial in tinnitus. J Laryngol Otol 1981;95:947–51.
65. Hulshof JH, Vermeij P. The value of carbamazepine in the treatment of tinnitus. ORL J Otorhinolaryngol Relat Spec 1985:47:262–6.
66. Marks NJ, Onisiphorou C, Trounce JR. The effect of single doses of amylobarbitone sodium and carbamazepine in tinnitus. J Laryngol Otol 1981;95:941–5.
67. Reed HT, Meltzer J, Crews P, et al. Amino-oxyacetic acid as a palliative in tinnitus. Arch Otolaryngol 1985;111:803–5.
68. Guth PS, Risey J, Briner W, et al. Evaluation of amino-oxyacetic acid as a palliative in tinnitus. Ann Otol Rhinol Laryngol 1990;99:74–9.
69. Busto U, Fornazzari L, Naranjo CA. Protracted tinnitus after discontinuation of long-term therapeutic use of benzodiazepines. J Clin Psychopharmacol 1988;8:359–62.
70. Birks J, Grimley EV, Van Dongen M. Ginkgo biloba for cognitive impairment and dementia. Cochrane Database Syst Rev 2002;(4):CD003120.
71. Drew S, Davies E. Effectiveness of gingko biloba in treating tinnitus: double-blind, placebo-controlled trial. BMJ 2001;322:73.
72. Westerberg BD, Roberson JB, Stach BA. A double-blind placebo-controlled trial of baclofen in the treatment of tinnitus. Am J Otol 1996;17:896–903.
73. Simpson JJ, Gilbert AM, Weiner GM, Davies WE. The assessment of lamotrigine, an anti-epileptic drug, in the treatment of tinnitus. Am J Otol 1999;20:627–31.
74. Briner W, House J, O'Leary M. Synthetic prostaglandin El misoprostol as a treatment for tinnitus. Arch Otolaryngol Head Neck Surg 1993;119:652–4.
75. Hulshof JH, Vermeij P. The effect of nicotinamide on tinnitus: a double-blind controlled study. Clin Otolaryngol 1987;12:211–4.
76. Hester TO, Theilinan G, Green W, Jones RO. Cyclandelate in the management of tinnitus: a randomized, placebo-controlled study. Otolaryngol Head Neck Surg 1998;118(3 Pt 1):329–32.
77. Domeisen H, Hotz MA, Häuser R. Caroverine in tinnitus treatment. Acta Otolaryngol (Stockh) 1998;118:606–8.
78. Kitano H, Kitahara M, Uchida K, Kitajima K. Treatment of tinnitus with muscle relaxant. In: Feldmann H, editor. Proceedings of the Third International Tinnitus Seminar: Münster. Karlsruhe (Germany): Harsch Verlag; 1987. p. 326–30.
79. Simpson JJ, Donaldson I, Davies WE. Use of homeopathy in the treatment of tinnitus. Br J Audiol 1998;32:227–33.
80. Paaske PB, Pedersen CB, Kjems G, Sam IL. Zinc in the management of tinnitus: placebo-controlled trial. Ann Otol Rhinol Laryngol 1991;100:647–9.
81. Arda HN, Tuncel U, Akdogan O, et al. The role of zinc in the treatment of tinnitus. Otol Neurotol 2003;24:86–9.

CHAPTER 20

Antidepressant Therapy for Tinnitus

Shannon K. Robinson, MD, Erik S. Viirre, MD, PhD, Murray B. Stein, MD

Several chapters in this book have dealt with the evidence supporting the cortical nature of chronic tinnitus. Along with the recent accumulation of basic scientific data supporting such claims, tinnitus has for years been associated with other cortical phenomena, such as depression and anxiety. The data on the relationship between depression and anxiety and tinnitus are reviewed before discussing the use of antidepressants to treat patients with tinnitus.

TINNITUS AND DEPRESSION AND ANXIETY

The literature linking depression and anxiety to tinnitus dates back to the late 1970s and early 1980s.[1-3] However, most of the studies examining the relationship between depression and anxiety and tinnitus have used self-report measures designed to describe personality variables, such as the Minnesota Multiphasic Personality Inventory (MMPI), Eysneck Personality Questionnaire (EPQ), and Crown Crisp Experimental Inventory (CCEI). Additionally, some studies have used self-report psychiatric symptom measures, such as the Beck Depression Inventory (BDI), State Trait Anxiety Inventory (STAI), Symptom Checklist-90-Revised (SCL-90-R), and General Health Questionnaire (GHQ). Fewer studies have used interviews to diagnose participants with psychiatric disorders and judge the severity of their depressive symptoms. These studies are reviewed below.

Six studies have used the MMPI. House reported on 150 patients who accepted referral to a psychologist for biofeedback training because their tinnitus was a serious problem.[3] Of the 150 subjects referred for evaluation, 132 were interviewed and were given the MMPI. Based on the author's protocols, the 132 patients were classified into three groups: 48 patients in the depressive group (this group responded best to biofeedback), 54 patients in the neurotic conversion group (although treatment was successful, they did not report as much improvement as the depressed group), and 30 patients in the borderline group (many of whom did not complete treatment). T scores (a standardized score for the MMPI) and exact MMPI profiles were not given for this study; the patients were grouped only as mentioned above, and the determinants of these groups were not described. The above patients were compared to 24 patients who described their tinnitus as something they could live with. All the patients who described their tinnitus as something they could live with had normal MMPI profiles.

Reich and Johnson used the short-form MMPI (168-question version[4]) with patients with tinnitus and noted statistically significant elevations on the Schizophrenia, Paranoia, Depression, and Hysteria scales for those who suffered from a primary complaint of tinnitus ($n = 87$) compared with those who suffered from a primary complaint of hearing loss ($n = 59$).[5] However, only the Schizophrenia scale had a mean greater than 2 standard deviations (SD) above 50, which is the usual cutoff for indicating psychopathology. Gerber and colleagues reported on 45 subjects referred to the Long Beach Veterans Affairs audiology clinic with tinnitus as their primary complaint.[6] Only six subjects had typical psychosomatic or hysterical profiles, and the results did not indicate repression of affect, neurotic or psychotic character structures, increased hostility, obsessiveness, or somatizing. Collet and colleagues reported on 100 subjects with tinnitus who were given the Mini-Mult MMPI.[7] The Mini-Mult MMPI is a 71-question version of the 500-question MMPI that maintains good reliability.[8] Collet and colleagues found that the overall profile was normal. Meric and colleagues reported on 281 French patients with tinnitus who were administered the Mini-Mult MMPI, which revealed that the population as a whole had a normal MMPI profile.[9]

In a separate study, Meric and colleagues reported on 173 patients with either acute or chronic tinnitus who were given the French version of the Mini-Mult MMPI.[10] Elevations (greater than 2 SD above the mean) were seen on the Depression scale in 12% of this group, Psychasthenia scale in 21%, and Anxiety index in 3.5%. The mean scores and SD were 55.82 (11.2), 57.36 (10.55), and 63.22 (12.06), respectively. Two of the above six studies indicate normal profiles.[7,9] Only one of the above studies gives any comparative or normative data of what percentage of abnormality would be found in another population of patients[5]; therefore, it is difficult to assess if there is a higher percentage of elevated scores in the tinnitus population.

Three studies have been reported that used the EPQ. The results of these studies are mostly inconsistent with each other. Wood and colleagues reported on 13 patients with chronic disturbing tinnitus.[11] The group of patients who did not respond as well to treatment had higher levels of extroversion. Both groups scored within the normal range on the neuroticism scale. Hallam and colleagues used the EPQ to evaluate complainers and noncomplainers and found both to be slightly introverted compared with the general population.[12] O'Connor and colleagues found that neuroticism scores on the EPQ were significantly elevated in cases versus noncases.[13] Cases were defined by an interview with the Clinical Interview Schedule (CIS), a semistructured standardized psychiatric interview.[14]

Four studies have been reported that used the CCEI. One of these studies used the CCEI to assess improvement associated with treatment.[15] The other three studies present data on tinnitus patients compared with normative data or control groups. Hallam and Stephens reported on 62 subjects enrolling in a masking versus counseling trial.[16] The sample fell between normal populations and psychoneurotic outpatients. Stephens and Hallam reported on 472 patients whose main complaint was tinnitus with and without comorbid dizziness.[17] Anxiety and depression scales were consistently elevated for tinnitus patients compared with published norms. McKee and Stephens' report revealed that somatic anxiety was greater in female patients with tinnitus than in female controls and that somatic anxiety, free-floating anxiety, and obsessionality were more common in males with tinnitus than in male controls.[18] Eighteen patients with chronic tinnitus were compared with 19 age-matched controls in this trial.

In contrast to the personality measures used in the studies described above, the following studies used standard measures that are used in depression and anxiety treatment trials. Fourteen studies have reported means for the BDI, a self-report measure of depressive symptoms with 22 questions, and 2 studies used an abbreviated Beck Depression Inventory (aBDI) with 13 questions. Additionally, three studies used the Hamilton Rating Scale for Depression (HRSD), an interviewer-based measure of depressive symptoms. Mean results on the HRSD were not given in the Sullivan and colleagues trial,[19] were 12.20 in the Robinson and colleagues trial[20] and were 4.4 (within the normal range) in the Robinson and colleagues trial.[21] The Sullivan and colleagues and Robinson and colleagues trials are described in the next section of this chapter because they are both double-blind randomized trials of antidepressants for tinnitus.[19,21] In the trial conducted by Robinson and colleagues, patients on antidepressants and benzodiazepines were excluded, but these are not mentioned as exclusionary criteria in the Sullivan and colleagues trial. The importance of this is that the HRSD scores from the Robinson and colleagues trial are not representative of the tinnitus population because many people already being treated for comorbid psychiatric conditions were excluded from participating; this likely yielded a lower and attenuated range of HRSD scores in that study.[21] However, the Robinson and colleagues trial reports baseline HRSD scores for patients entering a treatment trial comparing cognitive-behavioral therapy immediately compared with a randomized group assigned to a waiting-list condition before receiving cognitive-behavioral therapy.[20]

Wood and colleagues were the first to publish on the use of the BDI in 13 patients with chronic tinnitus.[11] The more depressed patients responded better to treatment. Ireland and colleagues reported on 30 patients referred for treatment of tinnitus because traditional treatments were not recommended or had failed.[22] Subjects were assigned to receive relaxation training with counterdemand instruction, neutral demand instructions, or no treatment. Pretreatment BDI scores ranged from 8.7 to 16.1 depending on the group. Haralambous and colleagues reported on 26 patients (who were referred by otolaryngologists or responded to an article in the newspaper) assigned to receive biofeedback with counterdemand instructions, neutral demand instructions, or no treatment.[23] Pretreatment mean BDI scores ranged, on average, from 6.2 to 12.4 depending on group assignment. Andersson and McKenna reported on 30 patients who were referred to an audiology clinic for tinnitus, and they had mean BDI scores of 10.5 (SD = 7.5).[24] Kirsch and colleagues reported on 77 adults who acknowledged having acute or chronic tinnitus during a visit with an otolaryngologist.[25] Based on their responses to a coping scale, the subjects were divided into low and high copers. Overall BDI scores were not given, but low copers had significantly higher scores (9.3, SD = 6.6 vs 5.5, SD = 5.4) on the BDI than did high copers. Wilson and colleagues reported on 69 subjects referred to an audiology unit of a Veterans Affairs hospital who had a mean BDI of 11.57 (SD = 7.44), and 50 participants responded to a radio advertisement for psychological treatment of tinnitus who had a mean BDI of 9.35 (SD = 8.71).[26] Davies and colleagues reported on a trial that randomized patients with chronic tinnitus with no major psychiatric illness and no prior psychiatric treatment for tinnitus to three forms of cognitive therapy.[27] Pretreatment BDI means were 14.10 (SD = 8.7). Henry and Wilson reported on 81 tinnitus sufferers who responded to an advertisement.[28] The high-distress sample (as defined by Tinnitus Reaction Questionnaire scores of ≥ 17) scored higher on depression measures. Overall BDI scores were not given, but high-distress patients had a mean of 10.18 (SD = 5.65), and low-distress patients had a mean of 4.70 (SD = 3.68). Newman and colleagues reported on 66 subjects from a Veterans Affairs hospital and the Henry Ford Medical Center who reported tinnitus as a primary or secondary complaint and had mean BDI scores of 5.9 (SD = 5.7).[29] In another study, Newman and colleagues reported on 51 outpatients being seen in the Division of Audiology at the Henry Ford Medical Center with tinnitus as their primary or secondary complaint (secondary to hearing loss) who had a mean BDI score of 5.3 (SD = 4.4).[30] These two studies, reported closely in time, appear to be based on separate populations of patients. Erlandsson and Persson reported on 104 subjects with chronic tinnitus who had a mean BDI of 13.3 (SD = 8.0).[31] Henry and Wilson reported on 60 patients with chronic tinnitus who were seeking treatment and were randomly assigned to cognitive coping skills plus education, education only, or waiting-list control.[32] Mean BDI scores were as follows for the above groups, respectively: 13.2 (SD = 7.84), 10.32 (SD = 9.02), and 10.85 (SD = 6.29). Henry and Wilson reported on a different study of 54 participants with chronic distressing tinnitus who were randomly assigned to attention control and imagery training; cognitive restructuring, attention control, and imagery training; cognitive restructuring; or a waiting-list control condition.[33] Baseline BDI scores were as follows for the above groups, respectively: 11.3 (SD = 6.3), 10.5 (SD = 4.3), 9.6 (SD = 6.9), and 8.4 (SD = 3.9). Wilson and Henry reported on 200 subjects drawn from a Veterans Affairs audiology unit and subjects who responded to a media advertisement.[34] The mean BDI score for this combined group was 11.01 (SD = 7.36). Mean BDI scores of 15.01 (SD = 9.69) were obtained at baseline in a group of 65 patients with tinnitus who enrolled in a cognitive-behavioral therapy versus waiting-list control condition trial.[20]

In summary, scores on the BDI ranged from 4.7 to 16.1, depending at least in part on the inclusion and exclusion criteria employed in each study. This indicates that some tinnitus patients do not endorse symptoms of depression when compared with standard cutoff scores of < 10. However, clearly, many patients with tinnitus do endorse depressive symptoms in the mild range, based on standard cutoff scores of 10 to 18.[35] Some patients with tinnitus endorse moderate or severe levels of depressive symptoms; however, this does not appear to be the majority of patients who have been enrolled in the above trials. The vast majority of patients with tinnitus are endorsing few or no depressive symptoms.

Regarding the use of the aBDI, Folmer and colleagues reported on 160 patients who were mailed questionnaire packets before their initial appointment with a tinnitus clinic.[36] Self-rated tinnitus loudness was highly correlated with sleep disturbance, STAI, aBDI, and tinnitus severity. Mean scores of the aBDI were 5.0 (SD = 5.4) for males and 5.7 (SD = 5.8) for females. Folmer also reported on a group of 190 patients (patients were sent questionnaires before their first clinic appointment and 6 to 36 months later).[37] Mean scores on the aBDI for the total population were 5.2 (SD = 5.3) at baseline and 5.9 (SD = 6.6) at follow-up. A score of 5 to 7 on this version can indicate mild depressive symptoms, 8 to 15 moderate depressive symptoms, and 0 to 4 no depressive symptoms.[38]

Four measures of anxiety have been reported on in different studies with people with tinnitus: the

STAI, Anxiety Sensitivity Index (ASI), Beck Anxiety Inventory (BAI), and Hamilton Rating Scale for Anxiety (HRSA). Nine studies have used the STAI. Parenthetically, state anxiety refers to anxiety that may be present at one time but not at other times. Specifically, state anxiety is present when a person becomes anxious about a given situation. Trait anxiety refers to anxiety that is present throughout the patient's life, reflecting what has been called a personality characteristic, and is thought to be a fairly permanent way of interacting with others and viewing the world. Ireland and colleagues reported on 30 patients with tinnitus referred for treatment because traditional treatments were not recommended or had failed.[22] Subjects were assigned to receive relaxation training with counterdemand instruction, no demand instructions, or no treatment. The state anxiety scores of the STAI were 36.3 to 47.1, depending on the group. Haralambous and colleagues reported on 26 patients (who were referred by otolaryngologists or responded to an article in the newspaper) who were assigned to receive biofeedback with counterdemand instructions, neutral demand instructions, or no treatment.[23] Pretreatment STAI mean scores ranged from 38.6 to 41.0 depending on group assignment. Kirsch and colleagues reported on 77 adults who complained of acute or chronic tinnitus during a visit with an otolaryngologist.[25] Low copers were significantly more distressed on the STAI compared with high copers (state anxiety portion of the STAI: 44.4, SD = 12.9 vs 8, SD = 10.4; trait anxiety portion of the STAI: 42.7, SD = 13.3 vs 32.3, SD = 9.4). Wilson and colleagues reported on two samples of patients with tinnitus.[26] Sample 1 consisted of referrals to an audiology unit in a Veterans Affairs hospital and had a state anxiety mean of 38.07 (SD = 14.01) and a trait anxiety mean of 40.23 (SD = 12.75). Sample 2 consisted of subjects who responded to a radio advertisement for psychological treatment of tinnitus. This group showed a state anxiety mean of 35.85 (SD = 10.91) and a trait anxiety mean of 38.73 (SD = 12.18). Erlandsson and colleagues reported on 36 patients with tinnitus being evaluated for entry into a study of biofeedback and relaxation training.[39] Anxiety scores on the STAI were not correlated with the intensity and severity of the tinnitus, based on self-ratings. Mean STAI scores were 46.4 (SD = 13.0). Halford and Anderson reported on 112 members of the British Tinnitus Association with acute and chronic tinnitus.[40] Although anxiety trait and depression were significantly correlated with tinnitus severity, the correlations were low (0.28). The trait anxiety portion of the STAI was used, and significant differences were found in mean scores (46.3 vs 39.9) for patients high and low on the Tinnitus Severity Scale. Davies and colleagues reported on three forms of cognitive therapy in patients with chronic tinnitus as their main problem and no major psychiatric illness and no previous psychiatric help for tinnitus.[27] Pretreatment STAI scores were 45.48 (SD = 14.4). Erlandsson and Persson reported on 104 subjects with chronic tinnitus who were examined with the STAI (state anxiety mean 44.2, SD = 13; trait anxiety mean 47, SD = 13).[31] Folmer and colleagues found in 160 subjects that tinnitus severity was highly correlated with sleep disturbance, STAI, and aBDI. State anxiety means were 36.73 (SD = 14.84) for males and 39.71 (SD = 15.11) for females.[36] Trait anxiety means were 36.90 (SD = 12.46) for males and 41.19 (SD = 12.33) for females. No significant differences between males and females were found.

Four of the above studies provide total STAI scores. Five of the above studies provide state anxiety scores, and three of those studies also provide trait anxiety scores. Total scores ranged from 38.6 to 46.4, providing fairly consistent results across studies. State anxiety means ranged from 8.0 to 47.1; however, all except one study had means of 35.85 to 47.1. Trait means ranged from 32.3 to 42.7. For comparison, total scores in a group of working adults aged 50 to 69 were 42.4 (SD = 13.8), and in general medical and surgical patients were 44.6 (SD = 14.1).[41] Therefore, the results obtained from these tinnitus populations do not appear to be dramatically different, if different at all, from the general healthy or medically compromised adult population.

Andersson and Vretblad reported on the use of the ASI in 127 patients with tinnitus seen at the Department of Audiology, University Hospital, Uppsala University in Uppsala, Sweden.[42] All participants were referrals for tinnitus complaints. Anxiety sensitivity (defined as a trait tendency to fear anxiety–related situations) correlated significantly with tinnitus distress. The association was significantly stronger in female participants. Female participants also displayed more signs of anxiety sensitivity. Regression analysis revealed anxiety sensitivity and minimal masking level to be significant in a multiple regression model as predictors of the Tinnitus Reaction Questionnaire. Mean ASI scores were 17.5

(SD = 12.4). No other studies have used this measure to assess anxiety-related traits in this population. Normal college students score 15 to 20 on average on this scale compared with anxiety-disordered patients, who scored 23 to 38 on average, indicating that this sample of tinnitus patients did not have significant anxiety symptoms.[43]

In psychiatric populations, the most common anxiety measures are the BAI and the HRSA. Robinson and colleagues reported on BAI scores in a population of 120 subjects enrolling in a tinnitus treatment trial of paroxetine versus placebo.[21] The mean for the BAI was 4.07 (SD = 4.86), which falls in the range of no anxiety symptoms. Additionally, this study reports the only results of the use of an interview-rated questionnaire for anxiety symptoms. The mean for the HRSA was 8.44, which indicates no anxious symptoms. However, it must be kept in mind that this study excluded people who were currently receiving antidepressants or other antianxiety agents and, therefore, is not a good representation of anxiety symptoms in a general tinnitus population.

Two measures of general psychiatric symptoms have been used in the tinnitus population: the SCL-90 (and more recently the SCL-90-Revised) and the GHQ. Five studies reported the use of the SCL-90 or the SCL-90-R. Harrop-Griffiths and colleagues' results appear to be included in a larger sample presented by Sullivan and colleagues[44,45] resulting in four populations of patients. None of these four articles reported subscale scores and total mean scores. Sullivan and colleagues wrote about 40 patients with disabling tinnitus (defined as causing social or vocational impairment) who were given the SCL-90 and the National Institute of Mental Health Diagnostic Interview Schedule (DIS) to diagnose major depressive disorder (MDD).[45] Patients with current MDD and tinnitus had significantly higher scores on all SCL-90 scales compared with patients with tinnitus without current depression and with the controls. Patients without depression were not significantly different from controls. Goebel and colleagues reported on 155 inpatients suffering from chronic tinnitus who participated in behavioral psychotherapy.[46] All means on the SCL-90-R were pathologic before treatment. Hiller and colleagues reported that the correlations between the Tinnitus Questionnaire (devised by Hallam and colleagues) and the SCL-90-R total were 0.34 to 0.37.[47] Many of the subscales were correlated, including the obsessive-compulsive, depression, paranoid ideation, psychoticism, and general psychopathology subscales. This population consisted of adult inpatients admitted to a psychosomatic inpatient unit in Germany for chronic tinnitus. Attias and colleagues reported on help-seeking (HS) versus non–help-seeking (NHS) patients with tinnitus.[48] Group 1 consisted of 100 male active military personnel with chronic tinnitus, group 2 consisted of 50 HS tinnitus sufferers and 50 NHS sufferers, and group 3 consisted of 73 age-matched controls (active military). HS subjects scored significantly higher on total scores and all subscales (somatization, obsessive-compulsive disorders, interpersonal insecurity, overt anxiety, hostility, depression, phobic anxiety, paranoid thoughts, and psychoticism), as well as on the positive symptom subscale and positive symptom distress index, than did the NHS subjects. The NHS subjects scored significantly higher than did controls on total score, positive symptom subscale, and positive symptom distress index. The most severe symptoms were on the obsessive-compulsive disorders and hostility subscales.

Berrios and colleagues completed a prospective assessment of psychiatric symptoms in an otolaryngology clinic population based on the administration of the GHQ (60-item version).[49] Cases were defined as having a score of greater than 11 or 12 (which was not specified). Of the patients with tinnitus in this group of patients attending an otolaryngology clinic, 47% showed caseness based on the GHQ, and they had a mean GHQ score of 11.5 (SD = 10.3). McKenna and colleagues used the GHQ (60-item version) and compared it with a structured interview conducted by a psychologist to obtain the sensitivity and specificity of the GHQ in neurotology patients (including tinnitus sufferers).[50] Mean GHQ scores were not given, but the GHQ (using a cutoff score of 11) had a sensitivity of 87% and a specificity of 82% in this population when compared with the interview. Loumidis and colleagues reported on 36 patients with a primary complaint of tinnitus in a neurotology clinic.[51] These subjects were administered the 30-item version of the GHQ. Total GHQ scores were not given. Using the recommended cutoff score, subjects were divided into low and high GHQ scores. Those subjects who scored high on the GHQ tended to score high on the subscales of the Tinnitus Questionnaire (devised by Hallam and colleagues) (see Chapter 17, "Tinnitus Questionnaires"). Based on these studies, it does not seem that the GHQ provides us with additional information above and beyond any of the other scales described here.

In the mental health field, diagnoses are made based on interviewing the patient. These interviews can be done in a very structured fashion, such as the Structured Clinical Interview for Diagnosis (SCID), or in a less structured fashion, similar to the way in which a physician might routinely elicit a medical history from a patient. At times, questionnaires are used to analyze progress in treatment, and the gold standards of these questionnaires are the HRSD, HRSA, BDI, and BAI (the first two are interviewer rated, and the second two are self-report measures). However, it is important to consider that diagnoses are only made based on interviews and not based on questionnaires.

O'Connor and colleagues published the first report of use of a psychiatric interview for the tinnitus population.[13] They used the Clinical Interview Schedule (CIS)[14] in a population of "patients who were considered by the [ear, nose, and throat] surgeon to have reported tinnitus severity unaccounted for by organic etiology and patients with no clear organic cause of tinnitus" (group 1) and compared this population with a group of whom the otolaryngologist thought that the reported tinnitus severity matched the organic etiology and that the participants were without evidence of psychiatric morbidity (group 2). The CIS was administered by a psychiatrist trained in its use in a three to one fashion, that is, for every three patients in group 1 who participated in the interview, one person in group 2 participated in the interview. Of this total population, 41% were identified as having a psychiatric disorder with the CIS. The two otolaryngologists who referred participants to this study missed 11 of the 43 (25.6%) persons who were diagnosed as cases (definite psychiatric morbidity based on the CIS): "There was a significant relationship between caseness and high scores on the seven point linear scale of subjective tinnitus annoyance."[13]

Harrop-Griffiths and colleagues reported on the first 21 patients attending a tinnitus clinic who were interviewed by a physician using the DIS and compared them with 14 patients with hearing impairment.[44] Patients with tinnitus had a significantly higher prevalence of current major depression (48% vs 7%) and lifetime prevalence of major depression (62% vs 21%) than did controls. Although in the group of patients with tinnitus, a higher percentage had phobic anxiety, panic attacks, sexual problems, and lifetime alcohol abuse or alcohol dependence than did the control group, these were not significantly different.

Simpson and colleagues used the SCID of the *Diagnostic and Statistical Manual of Mental Disorders, Third Edition-Revised* (*DSM-IIIR*)[52] to evaluate both axis I (mood, anxiety, psychotic, and somatoform disorders) and axis II disorders (personality disorders).[53] This was given by a psychiatrist to 24 patients with severe tinnitus that was defined as "ear or head sound that dominates the person's life and is perceived to be responsible for a change in lifestyle or sleep pattern." Of these, 63% had at least one *DSM-IIIR* diagnosis, 46% had a current mood disorder (33% major depression; 21% dysthymia), 29% had a current anxiety disorder (8% panic disorder [with or without agoraphobia] or agoraphobia without panic disorder; 8% other phobias; 8% generalized anxiety disorder; 8% somatoform disorder), and 33% had a past psychiatric disorder (mostly mood disorders). Patients with tinnitus with no hearing loss had "more psychiatric disorders per patient (1.33 vs. 0.86) and more anxiety disorders (56 vs. 14%)" compared with patients with tinnitus with hearing loss. No results were given regarding any axis II disorders.

Sullivan and colleagues reported on 40 patients with disabling tinnitus (defined as causing social or vocational impairment) who were interviewed with the DIS by one of two physicians and compared with 14 controls.[45] Lifetime prevalence of MDD was found in 78% of patients compared with 21% of controls, and current MDD was found in 60% of patients compared with 7% of controls. Panic attacks, sexual problems, and lifetime alcohol abuse or alcohol dependence were numerically but not significantly higher in patients with tinnitus than in controls, and current alcohol abuse or dependence and phobic anxiety were not even numerically higher. This appears to be a larger sample but may include the 21 patients reported on by Harrop-Griffiths and colleagues.[44]

Sullivan and colleagues reported that prior to enrolment in a nortriptyline versus placebo trial, all patients were interviewed with the DIS, and they found that 33% met the criteria for MDD, and the remaining patients were all labeled as having depression not otherwise specified, that is, some symptoms of depression that impair their life but do not meet the full criteria for MDD.[19]

Erlandsson and Persson evaluated 104 chronic tinnitus patients with the BDI (mean 13.3, SD = 8).[31] Thirty-four (20%) of these patients were characterized as having a psychologically vulnerable profile (BDI at or above the sample mean). The subjects with the psychologically vulnerable profile were asked to engage in a SCID interview for axis II disorders, and 17 did. The results are as follows: borderline personality disorder and histrionic personality disorder, one male; obsessive-compulsive personality disorder, one male and one female; and borderline personality disorder, phobic personality disorder, and passive aggressive personality disorder, two males and one female. Ten of these patients (59%) reported suicidal ideation versus 20% of the entire original sample. The patients with suicidal thoughts were significantly more depressed and anxious than those who did not report suicidal thoughts, based on the BDI and STAI. Additionally, the group without suicidal thoughts was significantly more hearing impaired than the group with suicidal thoughts. The patients with personality disorders were not significantly more depressed or anxious than the group without personality disorders.

McKenna and colleagues reported on 120 outpatients attending the neurotology clinic at the Royal National Throat, Nose and Ear Hospital who were assessed with interviews conducted by clinical psychologists.[50] Medicolegal cases were excluded from the study. Of those with tinnitus, 45% were categorized as psychologically disturbed and were offered psychological help. Psychologically disturbed was defined as the patient who reported and was judged to have severe behavioral and/or mood disturbance.

Attias and colleagues reported on enrolling subjects in a study comparing self-hypnosis, masking, and attention with patient complaints.[54] Forty-seven male career army personnel with chronic tinnitus were referred for diagnosis and treatment of tinnitus and were evaluated with a psychiatric interview. Two of 47 (4%) were excluded because of MDD. This study was seeking subjects with suicidal ideation, depression, severe anxiety, and risk of developing a dissociative disorder.

Andersson and colleagues reported the results of 216 patients with tinnitus seeking treatment in a department of audiology who were given a structured interview, which was performed by a psychologist.[55] This interview consisted of 30 questions. The interviewer asked only two psychological questions: Do you have any psychological consequences of your tinnitus: irritation, depression, anxiety, concentration difficulties? and Have you or are you currently seeing a mental health professional? Of these, 91% answered yes to the first question: irritation, 69%; depression, 58%; anxiety, 27%; and concentration difficulties, 70%. Only 28% said yes to the second question. Additionally, 71% complained of sleep problems in another question.

Zoger and colleagues reported on the use of the SCID-P (performed by a psychiatrist) to diagnose axis I and II disorders.[56] These interviews were conducted on patients with tinnitus without severe hearing loss who were referred to an audiology clinic and occurred 24 months after initial intake in the clinic. Lifetime depressive disorder (*DSM-IIIR* dysthymia, mild depression, moderate depression, severe depression, bipolar depression) occurred in 62% of this population, and lifetime anxiety disorders (social phobia, panic disorder, generalized anxiety disorder, somatoform disorder, obsessive-compulsive disorder) occurred in 45% of this population. Thirty-nine percent had current depressive disorder, and 45% had current anxiety disorder. Additionally, one of their subjects had schizophrenia, three subjects had alcohol dependence, and one had benzodiazepine dependence. Of these individuals, 34% had had contact with the mental health field during their lifetime, but only 5 of 82 (6%) had had contact in the last 3 years. Seven percent reported the onset of their tinnitus prior to the onset of their depression and anxiety. No personality disorders were diagnosed.

Robinson and colleagues reported on a group of 120 participants enrolling in an antidepressant treatment trial for tinnitus.[21] Patients already on antidepressants or benzodiazepines were excluded from enrolling in the trial. Only three subjects (2.5%) met the criteria for a current depressive disorder (MDD, one patient; depression not otherwise specified, two patients), and only eight subjects (6.7%) met the criteria for a current anxiety disorder (public speaking phobia, two patients; generalized anxiety disorder, two patients; anxiety disorder not otherwise specified, two patients; social phobia, one patient; and specific phobia, one patient). Thirty-three percent met the criteria for lifetime depressive disorder (major depression, 29 patients; depression not otherwise specified, nine patients; and adjustment disorder with depressed mood, two patients) and 17.5% for lifetime anxiety disorder (posttraumatic stress disorder, five patients; public speaking phobia, three patients; anxiety disorder not otherwise specified, five patients; panic disorder, two patients; social phobia, five patients; and specific phobia, one patient).

Of the studies reviewed above, listing either current depressive disorders, current anxiety disorders, lifetime depressive disorders, or lifetime anxiety disorders, there appear to be somewhat inconsistent results (Table 20-1). In five of six studies in Table 20-1, tinnitus was consistently associated with a higher current and lifetime prevalence of depressive and anxiety disorders than is found in the general population (or control groups). In the Attias and colleagues study, the prevalence of depression was similar to that in general population studies.[54] The Robinson and colleagues trial was not included in this table because this research group excluded potential subjects who were on antidepressants or antianxiety agents from the trial; therefore, those results are not comparable to the other results.[21] Additionally, insomnia and inability to concentrate (often seen as symptoms of anxiety or depression) are commonly reported to accompany tinnitus.[57] Wells and colleagues found disability resulting from depression to equal that associated with chronic medical illnesses such as diabetes and arthritis.[58] Broadhead and colleagues and Johnson and colleagues found that MDD and subsyndromal forms of depression, when found concomitantly with medical illness, tend to be additive with regard to disability.[59,60] These observations suggest strongly that the co-occurrence of depressive or anxiety disorders in patients with tinnitus may magnify their level of impairment and, accordingly, that treatment directed toward these conditions may lead to an improvement in functioning and quality of life. The data do not, however, provide support for the notion that tinnitus, even in patients with comorbid mood or anxiety disorders, is a forme fruste of these conditions, nor do they suggest that depression or anxiety can magnify awareness (or complaints) of tinnitus. Rather, they point to an association between tinnitus and affective or anxiety disorders that is still poorly understood with regard to etiology and should be further studied.

TINNITUS AND ANTIDEPRESSANTS

There are numerous case reports about antidepressants being associated with the onset of tinnitus. This has been described for the monoamine oxidase inhibitor phenelzine, tricyclic antidepressants (although not nortriptyline), trazodone, fluoxetine, venlafaxine, and bupropion. Tinnitus has also been associated with withdrawal syndromes for bupropion and sertraline. However, there is also some evidence that tinnitus may improve with the use of antidepressants. The reports of tinnitus as a side effect, as a withdrawal symptom, and the improvement of tinnitus with antidepressant therapy are reviewed below.

TABLE 20-1. Comparison of Prevalence of Depression and Anxiety Disorders in Tinnitus Studies and General Populations

Disorder	Harrop-Griffiths et al[44]	Simpson et al[53]*	Sullivan et al[45]*	Sullivan et al[19]*	Attias et al[54]	Zoger et al[56]*	General Population[90–93]
Current depression	48% MDD	46% depression; 33% MDD; 21% dysthymia	60% MDD	100% depression; 33% MDD; 67% depression NOS	4% MDD	39% depression	2–4.9% MDD
Lifetime depression	62% MDD		78% MDD			62% depression	6–25% MDD
Current anxiety disorder		29% anxiety				45% anxiety	18% anxiety
Lifetime anxiety disorder						45% anxiety	25% anxiety

*Where depression is listed, that indicates that the category includes major depressive disorder, dysthymia, and, at times, depression not otherwise specified and minor depression.

Glass reported on a patient who had dysthymia, had been unresponsive to and had had a side effect from amitriptyline, and had been started on phenelzine.[61] The patient developed tinnitus after 5 weeks of treatment, at which time he was taking a dose of 75 mg/d. The following week, he developed inhibition of orgasm, and his phenelzine was stopped because of this new side effect. He was then started on imipramine but again had sexual dysfunction, stopped taking the medication, and dropped out of treatment. He did not have tinnitus with either amitriptyline or imipramine, nor did his mood improve on these medications. However, he had improvement of his mood on phenelzine but had tinnitus.

TINNITUS AND TRICYCLIC ANTIDEPRESSANTS

Tinnitus has been reported to occur with the following tricyclic antidepressants: amitriptyline, protriptyline, doxepin, and imipramine. Despite this, there is some evidence to suggest that tricyclic antidepressants may help alleviate tinnitus or tinnitus-related distress. The data for tinnitus as a side effect of tricyclic antidepressants and for tricyclic antidepressants as a possible treatment for tinnitus are reviewed below.

Amitriptyline Miles reported that amitriptyline 150 mg/d was prescribed for a patient with MDD, and the patient developed a constellation of symptoms (including tinnitus), which occurred approximately 30 minutes after taking the medication and lasted for 2 to 3 hours.[62] However, when the dosage was changed to 50 mg three times per day, the side effects resolved.

Feder reported that amitriptyline was initiated for a patient with MDD, and the dose was gradually increased.[63] Two days after amitriptyline was increased to 150 mg/d, the patient noticed tinnitus. The patient had an amitriptyline level of 32 µg/L and a nortriptyline level of 23 µg/L, which are relatively low levels. One week later, the tinnitus continued, and the medication was discontinued. One week after cessation of medication, the tinnitus resolved, and 3 weeks later, the amitriptyline was restarted. The tinnitus recurred. When the medication was discontinued, the tinnitus resolved again.

Despite the above reports of tinnitus as a side effect of amitriptyline, Koshes reported that, 6 months after the onset of tinnitus, a patient developed MDD that she related to fear of activities causing a worsening of the ringing in her ears.[64] She was started on amitriptyline, and 1 month later, she noted that she was less bothered by the noise. Her depression resolved with continued treatment (medication and psychotherapy) despite no notable change in the loudness of her tinnitus.

The use of amitriptyline for tinnitus was also described by Podoshin and colleagues.[65] This study used amitriptyline 10 mg three times per day for 10 weeks compared with biofeedback for 10 weeks. Subjects were randomly assigned to one of four groups: biofeedback, amitriptyline, sham biofeedback, and placebo control. The biofeedback group reported greater improvement than did the amitriptyline group, but the amitriptyline group reported greater improvement than did either control group.

Bayar and colleagues reported a single-blind randomized trial (37 patients) of amitriptyline 100 mg versus placebo for the treatment of tinnitus that revealed a significant decrease in subjective complaints of tinnitus, as assessed by a modified version of the Tinnitus Patient Survey of the American Tinnitus Association.[66] The right ear revealed a 17 dB decrease in tinnitus intensity from before to after treatment and the left ear a 13 dB decrease compared with 2 and 4 dB increases for the placebo group; this difference was significant in the amitriptyline group but not in the placebo group.

Protriptyline Antidepressants other than amitriptyline have also been associated with the onset of tinnitus. Protriptyline was prescribed for MDD and gradually increased to 45 mg/d in divided doses.[67] Twelve days after initiation of treatment, the patient began to complain of tinnitus. This and other side effects persisted over the next 21 days of treatment; therefore, the medication was discontinued and replaced with desipramine. This change in medication initially resulted in occasional tinnitus that resolved after 3 weeks of treatment.

Doxepin Doxepin was prescribed for MDD in a person who had electrocardiographic abnormalities while on imipramine.[68] Tinnitus developed when her dose was increased to 175 mg/d. Her doxepin and desmethyl doxepin level was 35 ng/dL; it had been 32 ng/dL on 150 mg/d, and she did not have tinnitus at that time. The dose was decreased to 100 mg/d and the tinnitus resolved, but when she was rechallenged at 150 mg/d, the tinnitus recurred. It was then decreased and remained at 100 mg/d for 2 months of follow-up. At that time, the patient was free of tinnitus.

Imipramine Racy and Ward-Racy noted that doses ranged from 50 to 150 mg/d on imipramine when tinnitus occurred.[69] Imipramine 50 mg was started for a patient with depression, and after 1 week, the patient reported tinnitus. Her dose was decreased to 25 mg/d, and her tinnitus and depression resolved. Another patient was started on imipramine for depression, and the dose was increased to 150 mg/d, at which time she complained of tinnitus. Her dose of imipramine was decreased to 125 mg/d, and her tinnitus and depression improved. A third patient was started on imipramine for anxiety and depression; when the dose was increased to 150 mg/d, tinnitus occurred. The dose was decreased, and at 110 mg/d, her depression and tinnitus improved. A fourth patient was started on imipramine for anxiety and depression. At 150 mg/d, the patient complained of tinnitus, and the dose was decreased to 75 mg/d. However, the tinnitus continued, and there was no clinical benefit, so the medication was discontinued. Desipramine was started, which alleviated his psychiatric symptoms, and no further tinnitus occurred. When tinnitus developed, decreasing the dose was an effective intervention for three of the four patients, allowing them to have improvement of their psychiatric symptoms and resolution of their tinnitus.

In a double-blind comparison of trazodone and imipramine, tinnitus was reported as a side effect of imipramine in 1 of 29 patients taking imipramine and no patients taking trazodone.[70]

Tandon and colleagues conducted a retrospective chart review of 475 patients on tricyclic antidepressants and found that tinnitus started in 1% of this population within 2 to 3 weeks of starting imipramine.[71] Patients who developed tinnitus were on doses between 150 and 250 mg/d and had combined plasma imipramine-desipramine levels between 200 and 450 ng/dL. Each patient's tinnitus resolved within 2 to 4 weeks of onset, despite no changes in treatment with imipramine. Two of the five patients were started on antipsychotics (thiothixene and chlorpromazine) after development of tinnitus but before its resolution. The authors were unable to identify any "clinical profiles or constellation of adverse events" within these patients.

Laird and Lydiard reported that a patient in a double-blind placebo-controlled trial was given imipramine 100 mg for recurrent major depression, and the patient experienced the onset of tinnitus within 1 week.[72] The imipramine was increased to 150 mg without an apparent change in tinnitus. The tinnitus remained for 6 weeks and then diminished and ceased. Despite the patient receiving open-label imipramine (at the same dose) after completion of the study, the tinnitus did not recur.

Trimipramine Despite multiple reports of tricyclic antidepressants causing tinnitus, Mihail and colleagues enrolled 26 patients (19 completed) in a double-blind crossover trial for the treatment of tinnitus with trimipramine.[73] They reported that 37% of patients improved (based on self-report) with trimipramine, and 37% improved with placebo. After trimipramine administration, seven participants reported that their tinnitus got worse, eight reported improvement, and three were unchanged. After placebo administration, four participants reported that their tinnitus got worse, eight reported improvement, and seven were unchanged. The order in which the drug and placebo were administered had no effect on the outcome. There were significant changes in the frequency of the tinnitus, starting with a mean of 4,300 Hz and ending with 4,800 Hz for trimipramine and starting with 5,800 Hz and ending with 6,000 Hz in the placebo portion of the study. The mean intensity of the tinnitus increased from 46 to 58 dB during trimipramine treatment and remained constant during placebo treatment, at 52 dB. This finding was statistically significant. These results do not support the use of trimipramine in the treatment of tinnitus.

Nortriptyline Sullivan and colleagues also performed a trial using tricyclic antidepressants in the treatment of tinnitus.[74] They reported that nortriptyline showed promise when tried in a single-blind, placebo, nonrandomized controlled trial with 19 patients and found a 63% mean reduction in depressive symptoms as measured by the HDRS, decreased tinnitus loudness by a mean of 10 dB, and decreased tinnitus severity, psychological symptoms, and psychosocial disability.[74]

Following this single-blind trial, their group performed a double-blind placebo-controlled trial of nortriptyline in tinnitus patients. In the only double-blind placebo-controlled trial of nortriptyline, it was found to reduce loudness in the worst ear at the tinnitus frequency when adjusted for baseline levels.[19] No other effects were seen on other measures of tinnitus, such as the question of whether the patient's tinnitus has improved, or on the 27-item Tinnitus Handicap Questionnaire.[75] Nortriptyline was found to be superior to placebo in decreasing depression levels, as measured by the HRSD, and in reducing functional disability, as measured by the Multidimensional Pain Inventory modified for tinnitus.[19] These results did not include the intention-to-treat sample but only the completers, raising the possibility that the effects would have been less impressive in the former. Additionally, the improvement that occurred in tinnitus intensity was a modest 6 dB.

In summary, after reviewing the data surrounding the association between antidepressants and tinnitus, although some tricyclic antidepressants seem to cause tinnitus as an adverse effect, there are also reports of these medications (eg, nortriptyline in a double-blind study) resulting in some improvement in tinnitus.

TINNITUS AND THE NEXT GENERATION OF ANTIDEPRESSANTS

Tinnitus has been reported in association with the next generation of antidepressants. This group of medication as a whole was reported on in a retrospective analysis of a group of 37 patients who started taking selective serotonin reuptake inhibitors (SSRIs) after the onset of their tinnitus.[76] Thirty of these patients returned follow-up questionnaires a mean of 20 months later. Their results show a significant improvement in total Tinnitus Severity Scale, a 15-question scale, for those patients who began taking an antidepressant after the onset of their tinnitus. Each specific medication (fluoxetine, trazodone, mianserin, bupropion, venlafaxine, sertraline, and paroxetine) with reports of tinnitus as a side effect or withdrawal symptom or its beneficial effect on tinnitus is described below.

Fluoxetine The first case of tinnitus in the next generation of antidepressants was reported by Feighner in 1985.[77] Tinnitus occurred during an MDD trial in one fluoxetine patient and no amitriptyline patients of 22 people in each group. However, Shemen reported the abolishment of tinnitus in three patients with fluoxetine, 10 mg/d, within 1 week of beginning treatment.[78]

Trazodone Tinnitus has also been reported to occur with trazodone.[79] The details of this case were not reported—only that this side effect occurred.

Mianserin Marais reported on a case of tinnitus occurring after mianserin (a tetracyclic antidepressant).[80] This drug has not been released in the United States, where it is still under investigation, but it is used in other countries. Marais also reviewed a number of previously reported cases of tinnitus associated with this drug. Tinnitus appears to be a common side effect of this medication.

Bupropion Settle reported that tinnitus occurred in two patients who were taking bupropion for MDD.[81] The first patient was started on bupropion, which was gradually increased to 450 mg/d. Tinnitus started after 3 weeks of treatment and was still present at 12 weeks. The tinnitus resolved after 9 months of treatment, but then the patient's depression worsened. Bupropion was stopped but eventually restarted, and the tinnitus recurred within 3 weeks. Tinnitus remained at a follow-up appointment 3 months later. The second patient was started on bupropion, and after 3 weeks, the dosage was 100 mg tid, and tinnitus was noted. When the dosage was decreased, the tinnitus persisted, and the depression worsened. After increasing the bupropion, the tinnitus worsened, but the depression improved. After 12 weeks of treatment, the tinnitus remained; therefore, bupropion was discontinued. Fluoxetine was started, and the tinnitus ceased. Humma and Swims reported on a patient with tinnitus occurring in association with paresthesia, dizziness, gait impairment, and confusion that occurred 1 week after starting to take bupropion 100 mg tid for smoking cessation.[82] The side effects resolved after the medication was discontinued but recurred when the patient resumed the medication. All three of these patients had the onset of tinnitus after 3 weeks of gradually increasing the dose of bupropion, with the dose ranging from 300 to 450 mg/d.

Venlafaxine A patient had been taking venlafaxine 37.5 mg/d for 3 weeks when tinnitus developed.[83] Eventually, the venlafaxine was discontinued, and over the next 7 days, the tinnitus resolved. When rechallenged with 75 mg/d of venlafaxine, the tinnitus recurred. The patient then again stopped taking the antidepressant, and again the tinnitus resolved.

In contrast to the above reports of tinnitus as a side effect of antidepressants, tinnitus has also been associated with the cessation of antidepressants (venlafaxine and sertraline). Tinnitus was reported as a symptom of venlafaxine withdrawal by Farah and Lauer in 1996.[84]

Sertraline Leiter and colleagues reported on a patient with tinnitus developing in association with discontinuation of sertraline.[85] The patient decreased his sertraline from 150 to 50 mg for 5 days and then stopped his medication, without the input of his psychiatrist. Leiter and colleagues reported a number of withdrawal symptoms, including whooshing in the ears. The patient's symptoms began to resolve 7 days later and were completely resolved within 14 days of discontinuing his sertraline.

Paroxetine Paroxetine has been described as helpful in tinnitus in both case reports and in a double-blind placebo-controlled trial reviewed below. Christensen described a patient with chronic depression and panic disorder whose tinnitus responded to paroxetine 30 mg/d after 8 weeks of treatment.[86]

To our knowledge, the only double-blind placebo-controlled trial of an SSRI in tinnitus was recently completed by our research group.[21] We randomly assigned patients with chronic tinnitus to paroxetine or placebo and gradually increased the dose. Patients stayed on their maximally tolerated dose of medication (up to 50 mg/d) for an average of 31 days. This study showed that, overall, there was improvement only on the question "How aggravated are you by your tinnitus?" but on no other subjective or objective (matching) measure of tinnitus. However, in those patients who received the maximal dose of 50 mg of paroxetine, there is evidence of improvement in numerous subjective and objective measures of tinnitus, which include the percentage of patients with a 10 dB decrease in tinnitus intensity, the answers to the following questions: How severe is your tinnitus? How bothered are you by your tinnitus? and How aggravated are you by your tinnitus? and the Tinnitus Handicap Questionnaire subscale 2 (hearing ability). This study was not designed as a dose-finding study, and, as such, the above analysis was done post hoc. However, these results bear repeating. They suggest that some patients, if able to tolerate higher doses of paroxetine, may benefit, even though the majority of patients in the study did not derive antitinnitus benefits from paroxetine.

In summary, based on the above reports, there is a growing body of evidence to suggest that the SSRIs might be helpful in tinnitus. This must be balanced with reports that some people have had a worsening of tinnitus with the SSRIs and with bupropion and venlafaxine. Furthermore, the recent findings from our double-blind placebo-controlled trial suggest that most nondepressed patients with tinnitus are unlikely to benefit from paroxetine, although its efficacy at the higher end of the dosage range should be further studied. Additionally, the possibility that tinnitus represents a withdrawal symptom from discontinuing these medications too quickly should now be considered in the differential diagnosis of new-onset tinnitus.

POSSIBLE MECHANISMS OF ANTIDEPRESSANT EFFECTS ON TINNITUS

Few studies in the literature help us infer mechanisms either for tinnitus as an adverse effect of antidepressants or for the improvement in tinnitus that is sometimes seen with antidepressants. A possible origin of tinnitus with antidepressants may be associated with the anticholinergic properties of the medication because switching to a less anticholinergic medication resulted in no tinnitus in the same patient.[69] However, tinnitus has been reported with trazodone, which is thought to be devoid of anticholinergic side effects.[79] In 1988, Mihail and colleagues postulated that anticholinergic (and other properties of antidepressants) medications might be helpful for patients with tinnitus by leading to a decreased production of endolymph.[73] Mihail and colleagues went on to postulate that the antihistaminic effect of antidepressants might be beneficial by producing a vasoconstriction of the cochlear artery, and the adrenergic effects might lead to a decrease in cochlear potential. Shea and colleagues theorized that inhibiting the serotonin reuptake inhibits the transmission of the tinnitus impulse.[73,87] This idea is supported by an increasing amount of literature demonstrating that the auditory pathway is rich in serotonin receptors[88] and that alteration of these receptors can alter auditory evoked potentials.[89] In addition to the direct effect on serotonin receptors in the auditory cortex and this possibly having a direct effect on the perception of tinnitus, the data on the comorbidity of tinnitus and depression and anxiety disorders were reviewed in this chapter. Treatment of depression and anxiety (even in subsyndromal forms) is one possible cause of improvements in tinnitus with antidepressant therapy. However, the Robinson and colleagues trial, in which there were very few patients with even mild forms of depression and anxiety, suggests that something other than treatment of subsyndromal forms of depression and anxiety led to improvements in tinnitus (among responders to paroxetine in the 50 mg/d group, which was superior to placebo).[21]

FUTURE DIRECTIONS

Adequate power in clinical trials is always an important issue and does not seem to have always been appreciated in the tinnitus literature. Use of valid and reliable questionnaires is also an important issue. There has been a discussion in some literature in this area that individual questions, such as How severe is your tinnitus? How bothered are you by your tinnitus? and How aggravated are you by your tinnitus? may be more sensitive to change than multi-item questionnaires, such as the Tinnitus Handicap Questionnaire, Tinnitus Reaction Questionnaire, Tinnitus (Effects) Questionnaire, and the Tinnitus Handicap Inventory. The subjective nature of tinnitus brings to mind the question of the importance of changes in tinnitus intensity compared with changes that may be more meaningful to the patient (such as being less aggravated by their tinnitus). The lack of follow-up on promising initial results is also a problem that has plagued this field. This is best demonstrated when the literature for benzodiazepines and tinnitus is reviewed. Despite the suggestion from small trials that certain benzodiazepines may be effective, no attempts at replication have been published.

In the area of antidepressants in tinnitus, the suggestive single-blind placebo-controlled results with amitriptyline, double-blind placebo-controlled results with nortriptyline, and double-blind placebo-controlled results with paroxetine all bear repeating and being expanded. For example, a dose-finding study is suggested based on the results that paroxetine appears to be effective in both subjective and objective measures of tinnitus at 50 mg/d when compared with patients on placebo. At the present time, the evidence base for the use of antidepressants in tinnitus is small and inconclusive. Much additional work remains to be done to determine for whom, at what doses, and for how long antidepressant (eg, SSRI) medication will be useful to treat patients with tinnitus.

REFERENCES

1. House JW, Miller L, House PR. Severe tinnitus: treatment with biofeedback training (results of 41 cases). Trans Am Acad Ophthalmol Otolaryngol 1977;84:697–703.
2. Singerman B, Riedner E, Folstein M. Emotional disturbance in hearing clinic patients. Br J Psychiatry 1980;137:58–62.
3. House PR. Personality of the tinnitus patient. Ciba Found Symp 1981;85:193–203.
4. Overall JE, Hunter S. Factor structure of the MMPI-168 in a psychiatric population. J Consult Clin Psychol 1973;41:284–6.
5. Reich GE, Johnson RM. Personality characteristics of tinnitus patients. J Laryngol Otol Suppl 1984;9:228–32.
6. Gerber KE, Nehemkis AM, Charter RA, Jones HC. Is tinnitus a psychological disorder? Int J Psychiatry Med 1985–86;15:81–7.
7. Collet L, Moussu MF, Disant F et al. Minnesota Multiphasic Personality inventory in tinnitus disorders. Audiology 1990;29:101–6.
8. Hathaway SR, McKinley JC. A multiphasic personality schedule (Minnesota). Construction of the schedule. J Psychol 1940;10:249–54.
9. Meric C, Gartner M, Collet L, Chery-Croze S. Psychopathological profile of tinnitus sufferers: evidence concerning the relationship between tinnitus features and impact on life. Audiol Neurootol 1998;3:240–52.
10. Meric C, Pham E, Chery-Croze S. Validation assessment of a French version of the Tinnitus Reaction Questionnaire: a comparison between data from English and French versions. J Speech Lang Hear Res 2000;43:184–90.
11. Wood K, Webb W, Orchik D, Shea J. Intractable tinnitus: psychiatric aspects of treatment. Psychosomatics 1983;24:559–61, 565.
12. Hallam R, Rachman S, Hinchcliffe R. Psychological aspects of tinnitus. In: Rachman S, editor. Contributions to medical psychology. Oxford (UK): Pergamon Press; 1984. pp. 31–50.
13. O'Connor S, Hawthorne M, Britten S, Webber P. Part II. Identification of psychiatric morbidity in a population of tinnitus sufferers. J Laryngol Otol 1987;101:791–4.
14. Goldberg DP, Cooper B, Eastwood MR, et al. A standardized psychiatric interview for use in community surveys. Br J Prev Soc Med 1970;24:18–23.

15. Jakes SC, Hallam RS, McKenna L, Hinchcliffe R. Group cognitive therapy for medical patients: an application to tinnitus. Cognit Ther Res 1992;16:67–82.
16. Hallam RS, Stephens SD. Vestibular disorder and emotional distress. J Psychosom Res 1985;29:407–13.
17. Stephens SD, Hallam RS. The Crown-Crisp Experiential Index in patients complaining of tinnitus. Br J Audiol 1985;19:151–8.
18. McKee GJ, Stephens SD. An investigation of normally hearing subjects with tinnitus. Audiology 1992;31:313–7.
19. Sullivan M, Katon W, Russo J, et al. A randomized trial of nortriptyline for severe chronic tinnitus: effects on depression, disability, and tinnitus symptoms. Arch Intern Med 1993;153:2251–9.
20. Robinson SK, McQuaid JR, Viirre ES, et al. Relationship of tinnitus questionnaires to depressive symptoms, quality of well-being and internal focus. Int Tinnitus J 2003;9:97–103.
21. Robinson SK, Viirre ES, Bailey KA, et al. Randomized placebo controlled trial of a selective serotonin reuptake inhibitor in the treatment of tinnitus. [In preparation].
22. Ireland CE, Wilson PH, Tonkin JP, Platt-Hepworth S. An evaluation of relaxation training in the treatment of tinnitus. Scand Audiol 1985;16:167–72.
23. Haralambous G, Wilson PH, Platt-Hepworth S, et al. EMG biofeedback in the treatment of tinnitus: an experimental evaluation. Behav Res Ther 1987;25:49–55.
24. Andersson G, McKenna L. Tinnitus masking and depression. Audiology 1998;37:174–82.
25. Kirsch CA, Blanchard EB, Parnes SM. Psychological characteristics of individuals high and low in their ability to cope with tinnitus. Psychosom Med 1989;51:209–217.
26. Wilson PH, Henry JL, Bowen M, Haralambous G. Tinnitus Reaction Questionnaire: psychometric properties of a measure of distress associated with tinnitus. J Speech Hear Res 1991;34:197–201.
27. Davies S, McKenna L, Hallam RS. Relaxation and cognitive therapy: a controlled trial in chronic tinnitus. Psychol Health 1995;10:129–43.
28. Henry JL, Wilson PH. Coping with tinnitus: two studies of psychological and audiological characteristics of patients with high and low tinnitus-related distress. Int Tinnitus J 1995;1:85–92.
29. Newman CW, Jacobson GP, Spitzer JB. Development of the Tinnitus Handicap Inventory. Arch Otolaryngol Head Neck Surg 1996;122:143–8.
30. Newman CW, Wharton JA, Jacobson GB. Self-focused and somatic attention in patients with tinnitus. J Am Acad Audiol 1997;8:143–9.
31. Erlandsson SI, Persson ML. Clinical implications of tinnitus and affective disorders. In: Reich GE, Vernon JA, editors. Proceedings of the Fifth International Tinnitus Seminar 1995. Portland (OR): American Tinnitus Association; 1996. p. 557–62.
32. Henry JL, Wilson PH. The psychological management of tinnitus: comparison of a combined cognitive educational program, education alone and a waiting-list control. Int Tinnitus J 1996;2:9–20.
33. Henry JL, Wilson PH. An evaluation of two types of cognitive intervention in the management of chronic tinnitus. Scand J Behav Ther 1998;27:156–66.
34. Wilson P, Henry JL. Tinnitus Cognitions Questionnaire: development and psychometric properties of a measure of dysfunctional cognitions associated with tinnitus. Int Tinnitus J 1998;4:23–30.
35. Beck AT, Steer RA, Garbin MG. Psychometric properties of the Beck Depression Inventory: twenty-five years of evaluation. Clin Psychol Rev 1988;8:77–100.
36. Folmer RL, Griest SE, Martin WH. Chronic tinnitus as phantom auditory pain. Otolaryngol Head Neck Surg 2001;124:394–400.
37. Folmer RL. Long-term reductions in tinnitus severity. BMC Ear, Nose and Throat Disord 2002;2:3–11.
38. Beck AT, Beck RW. Screening depressed patients in family practice. Postgrad Med 1972;52:81–5.
39. Erlandsson SI, Rubinstein B, Axelsson A, Carlsson SG. Psychological dimensions in patients with disabling tinnitus and craniomandibular disorders. Br J Audiol 1991;25:15–24.
40. Halford JB, Anderson SD. Anxiety and depression in tinnitus sufferers. J Psychosom Res 1991;35:383–90.
41. Speilberger CD. Manual for the State-Trait Anxiety Inventory. Palo Alto (CA): Consulting Psychologists Press; 1983.
42. Andersson G, Vretblad P. Anxiety sensitivity in patients with chronic tinnitus. Scand J Behav Ther 2000;29:57–64.
43. Reiss S, Peterson RA, Gurksy DM, McNally RJ. Anxiety sensitivity, anxiety frequency and the prediction of fearfulness. Behav Res Ther 1986;34:1–8.
44. Harrop-Griffiths J, Katon W, Dobie R, et al. Chronic tinnitus: association with psychiatric diagnoses. J Psychosom Res 1987;31:613–21.
45. Sullivan MD, Katon W, Dobie R, et al. Disabling tinnitus: association with affective disorder. Gen Hosp Psychiatry 1988;10:285–91.
46. Goebel G, Hiller W, Fruhauf K, Fichter MM. Effects of in-patient multimodal behavioral treatment on complex chronic tinnitus. In: Aran JM, Dauman R, editors. Tinnitus 91: proceedings of the Fourth

International Tinnitus Seminar. Amsterdam: Kugler Publications; 1992. p. 465–70.
47. Hiller W, Goebel G, Rief W. Reliability of self-rated tinnitus distress and association with psychological symptom patterns. Br J Clin Psychol 1994;33:231–9.
48. Attias J, Shemesh Z, Belich A, et al. Psychological profile of help-seeking and nonhelp-seeking tinnitus patients. Scand Audiol 1995;24:13–8.
49. Berrios GE, Ryley JP, Garvey TP, Moffat DA. Psychiatric morbidity in subjects with inner ear disease. Clin Otolaryngol 1988;13:259–66.
50. McKenna L, Hallam RS, Hinchcliffe R. The prevalence of psychological disturbance in neurotology outpatients. Clin Otolaryngol 1991;16:452–6.
51. Loumidis KS, Hallam RS, Cadge B. The effect of written reassuring information on out-patients complaining of tinnitus. Br J Audiol 1991;25:105–9.
52. Spitzer RL, Williams JB, Gibbon M, First MB. The structured clinical interview for DSM-III-R (SCID). History, rationale, and description. Arch Gen Psychiatry 1992;49: 624–9.
53. Simpson RB, Nedzelski JM, Barber OH, Thomas MR. Psychiatric diagnosis in patients with psychogenic dizziness or severe tinnitus. J Otolaryngol 1988; 17:325–30.
54. Attias J, Shemesh Z, Gold S, et al. Comparison between self hypnosis, masking and attentiveness for alleviation of chronic tinnitus. Audiology 1993;32:205–12.
55. Andersson G, Lyttkens L, Larsen HC. Distinguising levels of tinnitus distress. Clin Otalaryngol 1999; 24:404–10.
56. Zoger S, Svedlund J, Holgers KM. Psychiatric disorders in tinnitus patients without severe hearing impairment: 24 month follow-up of patients at an audiological clinic. Audiology 2001;40:133–40.
57. Simpson JJ, Davies WE. Recent advances in the pharmacological treatment of tinnitus. Trends Pharmacol Sci 1999;20:12–8.
58. Wells KB, Stewart AL, Hays RD, et al. The functioning and well-being of depressed patients. JAMA 1989; 262:914–9.
59. Broadhead WE, Blazer DG, George LK, Tse CK. Depression, disability days and days lost from work in a prospective epidemiologic survey. JAMA 1990; 264:2524–8.
60. Johnson J, Weissman MN, Klerman GL. Service utilization and social morbidity associated with depressive symptoms in the community. JAMA 1992; 267:1478–83.
61. Glass R. Ejaculatory impairment from both phenelzine and imipramine with tinnitus from phenelzine. J Clin Psychopharmacol 1981;1:152–3.
62. Miles SW. Amitriptyline side effect. N Z Med J 1980; 92:66–7.
63. Feder R. Tinnitus associated with amitriptyline. J Clin Psychiatry 1990;51:85–6.
64. Koshes R. Use of amitriptyline in a patient with tinnitus. Psychosomatics 1992;33:341–3.
65. Podoshin L, Ben-David Y, Fardis M, et al. Idiopathic subjective tinnitus treated by amitryptyline hydrochloride/biofeedback. Int Tinnitus J 1995;1: 54–60.
66. Bayar N, Boke B, Turan E, Belgin E. Efficacy of amitriptyline in the treatment of subjective tinnitus. J Otolaryngol 2001;30:300–3.
67. Evans D, Golden R. Protriptyline and tinnitus. J Clin Psychopharmacol 1981;1:404–6.
68. Golden RN, Evans DL, Nau CH. Doxepin and tinnitus. South Med J 1983;76:1204–5.
69. Racy J, Ward-Racy E. Tinnitus in imipramine therapy. Am J Psychiatry 1980;137:854–5.
70. Feighner JP, Merideth CH, Hendrickson MA. Maintenance antidepressant therapy: a double-blind comparison of trazodone and imipramine. J Clin Psychopharmacol 1981;1(6 Suppl):45S–8S.
71. Tandon R, Grunhaus L, Greden JF. Imiprimine and tinnitus. J Clin Psychiatry 1987;48:109–11.
72. Laird L, Lydiard R. Imipramine-related tinnitus. J Clin Psychiatry 1989;50:146.
73. Mihail RC, Crowley JM, Walden BE, et al. The tricyclic trimipramine in the treatment of subjective tinnitus. Ann Otol Rhinol Laryngol 1988;97:120–3.
74. Sullivan MD, Dobie RA, Sakai CS, Katon WJ. Treatment of depressed tinnitus patients with nortriptyline. Ann Otol Rhinol Laryngol 1989;98:867–72.
75. Dobie RA, Sakai CS, Sullivan MD, et al. Antidepressant treatment of tinnitus patients: report of a randomized clinical trial and clinical prediction of benefit. Am J Otol 1993;14:18–23.
76. Folmer RL, Griest SE, Bonaduce A, et al. Use of selective serotonin reuptake inhibitors (SSRIs) by patients with chornic tinnitus. In: Patuzzi R, editor. Proceedings of the Seventh International Tinnitus Seminar. Perth: University of Western Australia; 2002. p. 81–5.
77. Feighner JP. A comparative trial of fluoxetine and amitriptyline in patients with a major depressive disorder. J Clin Psychiatry 1985;46:369–72.

78. Shemen L. Fluoxetine for treatment of tinnitus. Otolaryngol Head Neck Surg 1998;118:421.
79. Golden R, Evans D. Imipramine and tinnitus. J Clin Psychiatry 1987;48:496–7.
80. Marais J. Cochleotoxicity due to mianserin hydrocholride. J Laryngol Otol 1991;105:475–6.
81. Settle EC. Tinnitus related to bupropion treatment. J Clin Psychiatry 1991;52:352.
82. Humma LM, Swims MP. Bupropion mimics a transient ischemic attack. Ann Pharmacother 1999;33:305–7.
83. Ahmad S. Venlafaxine and severe tinnitus. Am Fam Physician 1995;51:1830.
84. Farah A, Lauer TE. Possible venlafaxine withdrawal syndrome. Am J Psychiatry 1996;153:576.
85. Leiter FL, Neirenberg AA, Sanders KM, Stern TA. Discontinuation reactions following sertraline. Biol Psychiatry 1995;38:694–5.
86. Christensen RC. Paroxetine in the treatment of tinnitus. Otolaryngol Head Neck Surg 2001; 125:436–7.
87. Shea JJ, Emmett JR, Orchik DJ, et al. Medical treatment of tinnitus. Ann Otol Rhino Laryngol 1981;90:601–9.
88. Simpson JJ, Davies WE. A review of evidence in support of a role for 5-HT in the perception of tinnitus. Hear Res 2000;145:1–7.
89. Gallinat J, Senkowski D, Wernicke C, et al. Allelic variants of the functional promoter polymorphism of the human serotonin transporter gene is associated with auditory cortical stimulus processing. Neuropsychopharmacology 2003;28:530–2.
90. Weissman MM, Bruce ML, Leaf PJ, et al, editors. Psychiatric disorders in America. New York: Free Press; 1991.
91. Lewinsohn PM, Allen NB, Seeley JR, Gotlib IH. First onset versus recurrence of depression: differential processes of psychosocial risk. J Abnorm Psychol 1999;108:483–9.
92. Kessler RC, McGonagle KA, Zhao S, et al. Lifetime and 12-month prevalence of DSM-III-R psychiatric disorders in the United States. Results from the National Comorbidity Survey. Arch Gen Psychiatry 1994;51:8–19.
93. Spitzer RL, Kroenke K, Linzer M, et al. Health-related quality of life in primary care patients with mental disorders. JAMA 1995;274:1511–7.

EDITORIAL COMMENTARY

Dobie calls attention to the need for consensus on the measurement of outcome variables for tinnitus suffering so that the various treatments for tinnitus can be more effectively compared across studies.

There is variability in the pathophysiology of patients with tinnitus, and the possibility exists that different forms of treatment may benefit subgroups of patients with tinnitus. Dobie points out that one strategy to deal with this situation is to use open trials of new or promising drugs to identify individuals who might be responders and to restrict randomized clinical trials to subjects who appear to benefit from the drug in question in an open trial.

Several randomized clinical trials of tricyclic antidepressants have shown benefit for patients with severe tinnitus, and Dobie indicates that the benefit may be greater for patients with sleep disturbance. He also favors the judicious use of hypnotics for patients with tinnitus with insomnia.

Robinson and colleagues point out that although the majority of patients with tinnitus have few or no symptoms of depression, many patients with tinnitus do have mild symptoms of depression. They emphasize that depression and anxiety are more prevalent in patients with tinnitus than in the general population. The occurrence of depression and anxiety in patients with tinnitus may increase their level of impairment, and treatment directed toward depression and anxiety may lead to improvement in their functioning and quality of life.

In the double-masked placebo-controlled study of Robinson and colleagues, patients with tinnitus who tolerated 50 mg of paroxetine per day improved in several subjective and objective parameters of tinnitus, including the percentage of patients with a 10 dB decrease in tinnitus intensity; answers to questions such as How severe is your tinnitus? How bothered are you by your tinnitus? and How aggravated are you by your tinnitus? and subscale 2 (hearing ability) of the Tinnitus Handicap Questionnaire.

Robinson and colleagues conclude that the single-masked placebo-controlled clinical trial of amitriptyline and the double-masked placebo-controlled clinical trials of nortriptyline and paroxetine should be replicated and expanded.

James B. Snow Jr

CHAPTER 21

Tinnitus Retraining Therapy

Pawel J. Jastreboff, PhD, ScD, Margaret M. Jastreboff, PhD

Tinnitus retraining therapy (TRT) is a specific clinical implementation of the neurophysiological model of tinnitus,[1] discussed in detail in Chapter 8, "The Neurophysiological Model of Tinnitus." TRT aims to habituate the tinnitus signal and relieve decreased sound tolerance (see Chapter 2, "Decreased Sound Tolerance"), which frequently accompanies tinnitus. After successful TRT, patients can still hear their tinnitus when they focus attention on it, but the tinnitus does not affect their quality of life. They tolerate sound as well as other people around them. Although the goal of relieving tinnitus and decreased sound tolerance as problems is not always achievable, we strive to induce a positive improvement by decreasing anxiety and annoyance and helping with sleep problems, social interactions, and other affected activities. Hearing difficulties can frequently be addressed concurrently with tinnitus and decreased sound tolerance, offering dramatic changes in the quality of life for many patients.

There are two main components to TRT: retraining counseling, which can be described as teaching session(s) aimed at reclassification of the tinnitus signal to a category of nonsignificant signals, and sound therapy, which is aimed at consistent and prolonged weakening of the tinnitus signal.

OUTLINE OF THE NEUROPHYSIOLOGICAL MODEL OF TINNITUS

The elements of the neurophysiological model of tinnitus are particularly important in TRT and can be summarized as follows:
- Tinnitus is a phantom auditory perception, that is, a perception of an activity generated within the nervous system without a corresponding acoustic stimulus.
- The prominence of the generated neuronal activity is related to its difference from background neuronal activity.
- The auditory system adjusts its sensitivity (gain) to the average level of environmental signals, that is, the principle of automatic gain control.
- In the case of individuals experiencing but not suffering from tinnitus, the tinnitus-related neuronal activity is constrained within the auditory system, and there is no activation of other systems.
- In the case of clinically significant tinnitus, neuronal activity within the auditory system plays a secondary role, and the activation of other systems is dominant in determining tinnitus severity.

Observable behavioral reactions induced by tinnitus result from the overactivation of the limbic and autonomic nervous systems and are governed by principles of conditioned reflexes. It is important to remember that conditioned reflexes can be created just by temporal association, without the need for a causal relation between the sensory stimulus and the reinforcement. They cannot be changed by cognitive modifications, but they can be extinguished even when the stimulus is repeated if there is no reinforcement provided. This process is called "passive extinction of the conditioned reflexes"[2] or "habituation of reactions."

Plasticity is one of the crucial brain properties involved in learning, memory, and processes leading to habituation. Because it is possible to perform only one task requiring full attention at a given time, the vast majority of sensory stimuli undergo habituation, and actually all nonsignificant signals are habituated automatically. This principle provides justification for the need to reclassify tinnitus into a category of neutral stimuli and is the basis for achieving habituation of tinnitus.

It is recognized that the strength of the reaction to sound is not determined by the sound intensity but by its significance based on past experience. The significance of a signal is relative and depends on other signals present at the same time. Signals can be involved in overactivation of the limbic and autonomic nervous systems, automatically evoking the suppression of the ability to enjoy life activities. Anxiety, nervousness, and sleep problems evoke an attempt at medical intervention frequently involving the use of medications. A precaution should be taken to avoid drugs, such as benzodiazepines, which are known to impair brain plasticity, reduce or even prevent the ability to learn, and thus hinder habituation.

The neurophysiological principles also apply to decreased sound tolerance. Overamplification within the auditory pathways can result not only in tinnitus but also in hyperacusis. A decrease in the auditory input, caused by overprotection of hearing or hearing loss, triggers increased amplification in the auditory pathways.

The brain's systems involved in tinnitus and decreased sound tolerance are interconnected and act in the dynamic balance scenario. Consequently, when applying treatment properly, both problems can be helped simultaneously, even while focusing on the primary complaint. When appropriate, hearing loss has to be addressed as well. With the progress of the treatment, the focus of attention changes from one problem, for example, hyperacusis, to another, for example, hearing loss, and adjustments have to be made in the protocol used for an individual patient.

A rapid and positive outcome with TRT is strongly related to the patient's attitude and determination to follow the appropriate protocol. The patient should be emotionally engaged and interested in the treatment. TRT requires some modification of everyday life for several months, and if the patient is not sufficiently motivated, the compliance and, consequently, the outcome are reduced. Patients have to understand the basic physiologic mechanisms related to the neurophysiological model of tinnitus and the basis for sound therapy. They have to accept these concepts as "making sense." This is a crucial aspect because patients make decisions and modifications based on these principles in everyday implementation of the method. Although contacts with TRT providers are important in monitoring outcome and addressing questions and concerns, interaction that is too close and too frequent, particularly in the later stage of the treatment, is not recommended. It might promote continuous monitoring of tinnitus and attract the patient's attention instead of transferring tinnitus to the category of nonsignificant signals and inducing the gradual habituation of the tinnitus. It takes time to achieve a positive, sustained outcome and substantial improvement. The process of habituation involves changing the weight of neuronal connections in pathways between the auditory system and the limbic and autonomic nervous systems to yield extinction of conditioned reflexes involved in the reaction to the tinnitus signal. Once it happens, habituation of tinnitus perception will follow, inappropriate functional links will diminish, tinnitus-related neuronal activity will be constrained to the subconscious level of the auditory pathways, and clinically significant tinnitus will change to become part of familiar background, which is typically not perceived and not bothersome.

INITIAL EVALUATION AND DIAGNOSIS

INITIAL INTERVIEW

Proper recognition of the chief complaint is crucial for the efficient and successful implementation of TRT. The initial interview, medical evaluation, and audiologic assessment are helpful in achieving this goal. A send-home medical questionnaire, reviewing general health problems, medical history, medications used, and hearing, tinnitus, and decreased sound tolerance issues, allows the patient to compile useful information in the comfort of his or her home. During the first appointment, this information can be carefully reviewed and verified in direct discussion with patients. The structured interview following specific questions is very useful in this respect and ensures consistency in collecting answers related to tinnitus, decreased sound tolerance, and hearing loss, problems that are distinctively different and well defined but frequently confused by patients. For example, fear of progressive hearing loss, based on the false belief that tinnitus is its indicator, leads some patients to hearing overprotection under normal sound conditions and claims of having hyperacusis. Actually, these patients rarely have hyperacusis but frequently develop misophonia (see Chapter 2, "Decreased Sound Tolerance"). Patient interviews help not only in identifying their problems and main complaint but also facilitate the determination of the impact that these problems have on the patients' lives and the degree of distress that they cause. Numeric scales of selected parameters and lists of affected activities are helpful in monitoring the progress of the treatment.

The initial interaction with a patient is very important. It creates an atmosphere of trust, supporting future interactions, setting the stage for the counseling session, and helping during medical and audiologic evaluations.

AUDIOLOGIC ASSESSMENT

The audiologic assessment consists of pure-tone audiometry up to 12 kHz because, in many patients, the tinnitus pitch is above 8 kHz, and speech discrimination scores to assess the patient's hearing and to create the basis for the subsequent audiologic tinnitus characterization. Tinnitus and decreased sound tolerance measurements include pitch and intensity matching of the most troublesome tinnitus, minimal suppression ("masking") levels, and pure-tone loudness discomfort levels (LDLs). LDLs allow the estimate of the patient's tolerance to sound and assess the presence and extent of hyperacusis and misophonia.[3] Additional tests include distortion-product otoacoustic emission (DPOAE), which is performed with high-frequency resolution and acoustic immittance. Acoustic reflexes are performed only when there is an indication of possible retrocochlear pathology and decreased sound tolerance is not present. The results of audiologic testing also provide an indication of possible medical problems linked to the function of the auditory system, which should be further evaluated and treated, for example, conductive hearing loss, vestibular schwannoma, and Meniere's disease.

MEDICAL EVALUATION

The main role of the medical evaluation is diagnosis of problems that might require medical or surgical intervention. This includes vestibular schwannoma; Meniere's disease; otosclerosis; various somatosounds, mainly of vascular origin; and severe and obvious psychological or psychiatric conditions requiring immediate attention, for example, the threat of suicide. A definite diagnosis does not preclude the use of TRT. Actually, once it is firmly established that there is no health risk involved, TRT can be employed successfully. It is crucial to make a full attempt to diagnose all potential tinnitus-related medical conditions because one of the key points of discussion during the retraining counseling is a statement that tinnitus is not an indicator of further problems; this is an important and very common concern of patients. Additionally, many patients with tinnitus are taking medications for other health disorders or because of problems that they have developed in response to tinnitus, for example, anxiety and insomnia. Although immediate modification or discontinuance of their use is not recommended or expected, the full recognition of medications, interfering with brain plasticity, (eg, benzodiazepines), inducing tinnitus (eg, cisplatin), and having other associations with tinnitus (eg, worsening of tinnitus as a withdrawal effect of alprazolam [Xanax]), is very important. It helps in developing the counseling, encouraging realistic expectations, and planning the treatment.

DIAGNOSIS AND CATEGORIZATION OF PATIENTS

On the basis of information gathered during the initial interview, medical evaluation, and audiologic assessment, patients are diagnosed and assigned to one of five categories (Table 21-1).[4] The factors used for categorization are based on potential mechanisms indicated by the neurophysiological model of tinnitus combined with practical considerations and follow (1) the severity of the tinnitus or hyperacusis and their duration, (2) the presence of a subjectively significant hearing loss, (3) the presence of clinically significant hyperacusis, and (4) the presence of prolonged worsening of hyperacusis or tinnitus after sound exposure. Note that the other component of decreased sound tolerance, misophonia, is not included in the classification because it can be present in all categories and requires separate, specific treatment that can be implemented concurrently with treatment of tinnitus, hyperacusis, and hearing loss.[3]

The severity of tinnitus indirectly indicates the extent of neuronal modifications that should be retrained. If tinnitus is severe but emerged only a few weeks previously, the neuronal connections might not be strong and can be relatively easily retrained compared with those associated with chronic, severe tinnitus. Patients who do not have strong negative associations with tinnitus, even though they have noticed it for quite some time, or whose tinnitus does not significantly affect their life or is of very recent onset (less than 1 month) should be classified in category 0. This category of patients is the most common in audiology and otolaryngology practices, and if these patients are approached properly from the beginning, they do not require extensive treatment. Patients with severe, established tinnitus as the

TABLE 21-1. Categories of Patients with Tinnitus and Hyperacusis

Category	Impact on Life	Tinnitus	Subjective Hearing Loss	Hyperacusis	Prolonged Sound-Induced Exacerbation	Treatment (always involves counseling and use of enriched background sound)
0	Low	Present	—	—	—	Abbreviated counseling, no wearable instruments
1	High	Present	—	—	—	Sound generators set at a mixing point
2	High	Present	Present	—	—	Hearing aids or combination instruments with stress on enrichment of the auditory background
3	High	Not relevant	Not relevant	Present	—	Sound generators set below annoyance level (or combination instruments when subjective hearing loss is present)
4	High	Not relevant	Not relevant	Present	Present	Sound generators set at the threshold; very slow increase of the sound level

predominant complaint with no hyperacusis or subjectively significant hearing loss should be classified in category 1.

Hearing loss is an important factor in treating patients for tinnitus and hyperacusis. A decrease in the input to the auditory system results in increased gain, causing an enhancement of the tinnitus signal, and increases the difference between the tinnitus signal and the background neuronal activity. Additionally, the presence of the strain-to-hear phenomenon results in enhancement of tinnitus and the general level of stress. Any factor that increases the general level of anxiety and discomfort, particularly if linked to some aspect of hearing, will tend to promote and sustain the conditioned reflexes responsible for tinnitus-evoked reactions. High-frequency hearing loss can easily be overlooked yet can have a profound impact on one's life. Frequently, patients do not link problems with understanding speech in a noisy situation with hearing loss because they know that in a quiet environment, they do not experience problems. Consequently, they tend to avoid restaurants, decrease their social interaction, and experience problems at work. All of these problems are responsible for an increased level of stress and discomfort. Tinnitus is commonly blamed for problems with understanding speech, which, in turn, enhance tinnitus-related conditioned reflexes. Many patients worsen their situation by the use of ear protection, under the false assumption that sounds are too loud for them. This, in turn, tends to induce hyperacusis and misophonia.

Therefore, for patients with hearing loss, it is important to increase the auditory input, remove or at least decrease the strain-to-hear phenomenon, and reduce other factors inducing negative reactions linked to hearing. Careful analysis of available information, particularly the initial interview and audiologic assessment, is needed to determine if hearing loss is an important problem to the individual patient.

Therefore, the hearing needs have to be considered in the context of the patient's work, hobbies, and cultural and social background. Hearing loss can be unimportant to patients whose work and social interaction use hearing in a limited manner. On the other hand, patients whose work requires good understanding of speech in noisy situations or full appreciation of small differences in sound (eg, musicians) can be functionally disabled. Therefore, hearing loss is considered to be significant when it affects the patient's life in a negative manner, considering the broad aspect of potential problems not limited only to communication. Patients with significant hearing loss are placed in category 2.

The presence of clinically significant hyperacusis indicates abnormally high gain within the auditory system. This increased gain might enhance the tinnitus-related neuronal activity and yield enhanced activation of the limbic and autonomic nervous systems. The presence of significant hyperacusis has a more profound effect on the patient's life and general level of anxiety and should be addressed first.

There is no objective method to determine the presence and extent of hyperacusis. Typically, hyperacusis is confounded by coexisting misophonia. Low values of LDLs might reflect pure misophonia, pure hyperacusis, or a combination of both. Decreased LDLs are characteristic of hyperacusis, and when LDLs are normal (about 100 dB HL), hyperacusis is not present. Decreased LDLs can also be due to misophonia. Only by combining the information from the audiogram, LDLs, and the initial interview is it possible to estimate the presence and extent of hyperacusis and misophonia (see Chapter 2, "Decreased Sound Tolerance").[5] Patients with hyperacusis are classified in category 3 even if they have tinnitus and/or subjectively important hearing loss.

The final factor used to determine the category of the patient is prolonged worsening of tinnitus or hyperacusis after sound exposure. Whereas the majority of patients report that their tinnitus or hyperacusis is worse for minutes or hours after exposure to loud sound, some patients report worsening lasting days or weeks, even after exposure to moderate- or low-level sound. If this effect persists after a full night's sleep, it must be considered seriously.

The mechanisms for this effect are uncertain, and it is most commonly associated with hyperacusis. It tends to be more prevalent in patients with neurologic problems (head injury, Lyme disease) or strong hormonal changes (menopause). This effect also occurs in patients with severe misophonia.

Two types of situations associated with worsening after sound exposure can be differentiated: (1) after each exposure to a sound that has been preceded by multiple exposures to similar sounds and (2) after prolonged exposure to a sound when exposure for a shorter time does not evoke this effect. The effects described resemble "kindling" and "winding-up" phenomena observed in epilepsy and chronic pain.[6] These most difficult to treat patients belong to category 4.

Patients exhibit a continuum of problems, and categories provide only a general guidance for a specific approach. Each patient should be treated individually. Furthermore, during treatment, patients can move from one category to the other. Nevertheless, assigning the patient to the correct category is essential for successful management.

TREATMENT IMPLEMENTATION

All patients undergo counseling and receive recommendations to avoid silence and to enrich their sound background. Counseling and sound therapy are tailored to the specific needs of patients in each category.

COMMON ELEMENTS OF COUNSELING

Certain elements of counseling are common for patients in all categories. The goal of the initial session of counseling is to neutralize tinnitus, at least partially, by providing patients with coherent, valid information and showing that the perception of tinnitus is common and is not associated with threatening pathology. It is not the tinnitus signal but reactions induced by it that cause the problem. These reactions just happened to be linked to tinnitus owing to a certain situation, frequently negative counseling, or a very important, stressful situation in life. There is no attempt to detect and argue with patients' specific beliefs about their tinnitus, for example, tinnitus is responsible for hearing loss, but to present patients with a new view on tinnitus by explaining what tinnitus is, why they most probably got it, mechanisms through which tinnitus evokes negative reactions, and how to use this knowledge to achieve control over tinnitus. This process is labeled as demystification of tinnitus. The same general principles are applied to discuss issues of hyperacusis and misophonia.

All of the main principles that are discussed are illustrated with everyday examples and parables. These examples are general and are aimed at a wide variety of patients; nevertheless, they should be adjusted to age (eg, children), education, and cultural and social environment.

TRT counseling is based on the principles of the neurophysiological model of tinnitus (presented in Chapter 8, The Neurophysiological Model of Tinnitus") addressing tinnitus, hyperacusis, misophonia, and hearing loss. Counseling related to tinnitus encompasses all aspects of the model. In the case of hyperacusis, stress is on the consequences of increased gain in the auditory pathways, including secondary activation of the limbic and autonomic nervous systems owing to overamplification of signals evoked by external sounds. Application of the model to misophonia is basically the same as for tinnitus; the difference is in the initial signal: the tinnitus-related neuronal activity versus activity evoked by external sounds. Finally, hearing loss plays a role in generating the tinnitus-related neuronal activity, enhancing the tinnitus signal in the auditory pathways, and directly enhancing activation of the limbic and autonomic nervous systems.

Problems discussed during the initial counseling include the following:
1. Tinnitus signal as a phantom auditory perception
2. The role of the limbic and autonomic nervous systems
3. Conditioned reflexes
4. Habituation

Tinnitus Signal as a Phantom Auditory Perception
Tinnitus is a phantom auditory perception, the perception of which does not follow the same rules as external sounds. It is a real perception, but there is no corresponding physical stimulus. An example of a phantom limb is always presented to patients. The concept that phantom perception reflects exclusively neuronal activity is helpful in the introduction of the tinnitus-related neuronal activity in the auditory system, makes tinnitus more concrete and real for patients, and makes visualization of its propagation to other systems easier, particularly to the limbic and autonomic nervous systems.

Possible Mechanism of the Origin of the Tinnitus Signal In the neurophysiological model of tinnitus, the specific origin of the tinnitus-related neuronal activity is irrelevant. The model and TRT are not dependent on the mechanism responsible for emergence of the tinnitus signal. It is helpful to explain to patients a hypothesis aligned with their specific problem. The discordant dysfunction theory is most useful and easy to discuss with patients; this theory has been outlined in Chapter 8, "The Neurophysiological Model of Tinnitus," and is presented in detail elsewhere.[1,7] Commonly, it is sufficient to present only the final conclusion of this theory, that is, that the tinnitus signal is linked to missing or dysfunctional outer hair cells (OHCs) in the cochlea. It is pointed out that manipulations known to induce tinnitus reliably in humans (or animals) have the common feature of disabling active properties of OHCs without affecting inner hair cells, for example, high doses of aspirin and quinine and high levels of sound.

To introduce OHCs during the first part of counseling, the basic mechanisms involved in transduction of sound are presented. OHCs are presented as serving the role of a mechanical amplifier; in other words, they are biologic hearing aids. Although OHCs are very useful, they are not essential for our hearing, and their function can be replaced by hearing aids, which are not as good as OHCs, but they still can provide a reasonable functional substitute. Therefore, once patients accept that OHCs are linked to their tinnitus, it provides them with a reasonable explanation as to the source of their tinnitus while simultaneously showing that hearing tinnitus is basically benign and reflects a dysfunction of OHCs. In the case of coexistent significant hearing loss, when hearing aids or combination instruments are going to be recommended, the concept of OHCs acting as "biological hearing aids" prepares the patient for instrumentation using the concept of replacement of missing OHCs with hearing aids, not as perfect but performing basically the same function as OHCs.

The concept of linking tinnitus to OHCs is also very helpful to patients with tinnitus with normal hearing. It is argued that up to 30% of OHCs may be damaged without inducing hearing loss,[8] and dysfunction of OHCs can be documented by high-frequency resolution DPOAE. The results from obtaining DPOAE show the patient, in an objective manner, that there are some areas of dysfunctioning OHCs.

Obviously, when patients clearly have the central type of tinnitus, such as after transection of the auditory nerve or if they experience auditory imagery, the OHC concept is not used, and alternative mechanisms are discussed.

Role of the Limbic and Autonomic Nervous Systems
The normal function of the limbic and autonomic nervous systems is briefly described to all patients, with the focus on the behavioral effects of activation of the sympathetic part of the autonomic nervous system. These consequences are described in detail in Chapter 8, "The Neurophysiological Model of Tinnitus." Common elements of counseling involve presentation of the concept that tinnitus-related problems result from prolonged activation of the autonomic nervous system, causing various physiologic and behavioral consequences. One of these conse-

quences related to high activation of the sympathetic part of the autonomic nervous system automatically evoking suppression of the ability to enjoy things in life is of particular clinical importance. Because it is one of the basic subconscious reflexes and a very powerful defensive reaction, it is not possible to modify this reaction by cognitive processes. Consequently, the quality of life decreases dramatically. Indeed, it is postulated that this phenomenon may be the crucial force evoking depression, which may explain why depression is so prevalent among patients with tinnitus. Other consequences, for example, problems with sleep, disturbed concentration, and increased general stress and anxiety, are also discussed.

The counseling stresses physiologic mechanisms underlying behavioral reactions in an attempt to enhance the concept that tinnitus-related problems have a physiologic basis and should be analyzed and treated by modifying the way in which information is processed in the brain. The concept that tinnitus is "in the brain (as the biologic structure) but not in the mind" is commonly invoked.

The goal of this part of counseling is to provide sufficient information to reach the conclusion that the source of tinnitus-induced problems is not in the tinnitus signal but in functional connections governing the spread of this signal to the limbic and autonomic nervous systems. Therefore, removing stimulation of the limbic and autonomic nervous systems by the tinnitus-related neuronal activity can eliminate these problems. To achieve this goal, it is necessary first to understand mechanisms governing processing of the tinnitus-related neuronal activity.

Conditioned Reflexes It is argued that the link between tinnitus-related neuronal activity in the auditory system and overstimulation of the limbic and autonomic nervous systems is governed by principles of conditioned reflexes (see Chapter 8, "The Neurophysiological Model of Tinnitus," for details). Because reactions evoked by the autonomic nervous system act as negative self-reinforcement, if tinnitus is constant, this link will not be extinguished but will become stronger.

To create a conditioned reflex, it is sufficient that a sensory stimulus occurs at the same time as reinforcement, without causal relation. This observation explains why clinically significant tinnitus emerges typically without any associated problems with the auditory system. For many patients, understanding that temporal association is sufficient to create a conditioned reflex shifts tinnitus toward a category of nonsignificant stimuli, which, by accident, got linked to a negative reinforcement and started to evoke strong negative reactions (the concept of "correct response but to a wrong signal").

The concept of conditioned reflexes provides the explanation why, contrary to intuitive assumption and in agreement with clinical data, the intensity of tinnitus as determined by tinnitus loudness matching is not associated with tinnitus severity. The strength of the reaction to a sound is determined by its significance and past experience, and sound intensity is secondary. At the same time, the perceived loudness of tinnitus is not linked directly to the result of loudness matching and can fluctuate dramatically, whereas the loudness matching can remain constant.

A principle crucial for potential treatment is that conditioned reflexes cannot be modified by cognition, for example, it is impossible to learn to drive a car on the left side of the road by talking, thinking, or arguing about it. However, any reflex can be extinguished by a specific procedure. The method used in TRT is based on the principle that all conditioned reflexes can be extinguished when the stimulus is repeated, but no reinforcement is provided. This process is called "passive extinction of the conditioned reflexes"[2] or "habituation of reactions."[9] A consequence of this phenomenon is that all nonsignificant signals are automatically habituated. To allow habituation to occur, it is necessary to make tinnitus as neutral as possible (by counseling) and weaken it consistently over a period of months (by sound therapy).

Habituation There are two types of habituation: habituation of reactions and habituation of perception. Because reactions of the limbic and autonomic nervous systems are responsible for tinnitus-induced problems, habituation of reactions is necessary and sufficient to provide improvement (Figure 21-1). Habituation of reactions and perception to all nonsignificant signals is absolutely necessary for normal life because it is possible to perform only one task requiring full attention at a given time. This limitation necessitates habituation of both reactions to and perception of the vast majority of sensory stimuli. Otherwise, sensory overload would cause paralysis and prevent function. Therefore, once habituation of the tinnitus-induced reaction occurs, the habituation of perception automatically follows (see

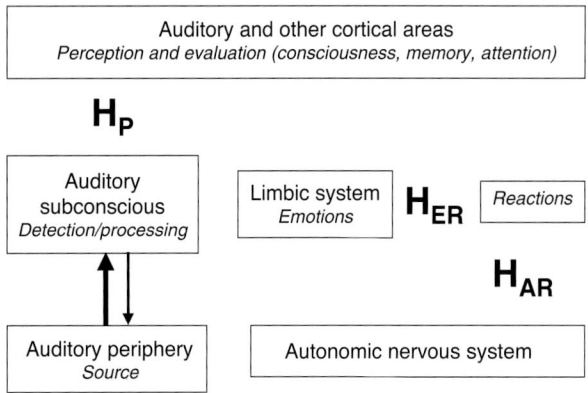

FIGURE 21-1. Habituation of reactions induced by tinnitus and of the perception of tinnitus. HAR = habituation of autonomic reactions; HER = habituation of emotional reactions; HP = habituation of perception. Republished with permission from Jastreboff PJ and Jastreboff MM.4

Figure 21-1). To be effective, habituation must occur at a subconscious level. Indeed, the majority of relevant connections occur at a subconscious level. One of the important aspects discussed with patients is that conditioned reflexes can be created, sustained, and modified at a subconscious level and that habituation of perception has to occur subconsciously (see Chapter 8, "The Neurophysiological Model of Tinnitus").

The final conclusion is that even if we cannot change the conditioned link directly by creating a situation promoting emergence of habituation, it is possible to break the conditioned reflex arcs responsible for tinnitus-induced reactions. The first stage involves removing or at least decreasing input from high-level cognitive centers by demystifying tinnitus and presenting an alternative model explaining its existence and why it evokes such strong reactions. The remaining processes of weakening and finally removing conditioned reflex connections occur at a subconscious level, and weakening of the tinnitus signal using sound therapy facilitates retraining.

Counseling related to hyperacusis focuses on the peripheral and central mechanisms of gain modulation within the auditory pathways. The principle of desensitization is discussed, as well as the need to avoid ear overprotection.

For misophonia, the systems and principles of their connection are the same as those described for tinnitus. The difference is the source of the signal; consequently, counseling closely follows the one used for tinnitus. Because, however, it is possible to control external sounds, a more powerful technique, based on the association of sound with positive reinforcement (active extinction of conditioned reflexes), is used for treatment. The basis of this technique is explained during the counseling session, and specific instructions are given to the patient.[3]

SOUND THERAPY

The role of sound therapy is to decrease in a consistent and systematic manner the strength of the tinnitus-related neuronal activity within the auditory system

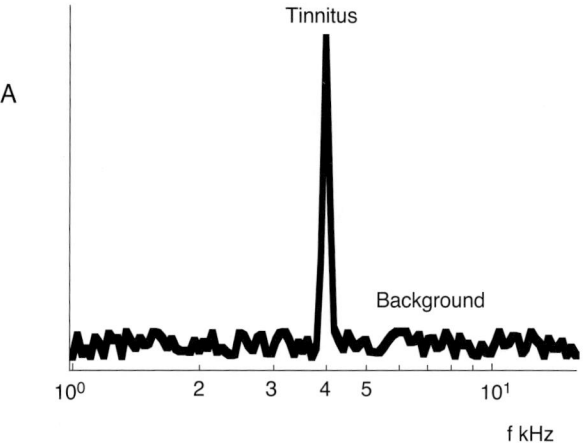

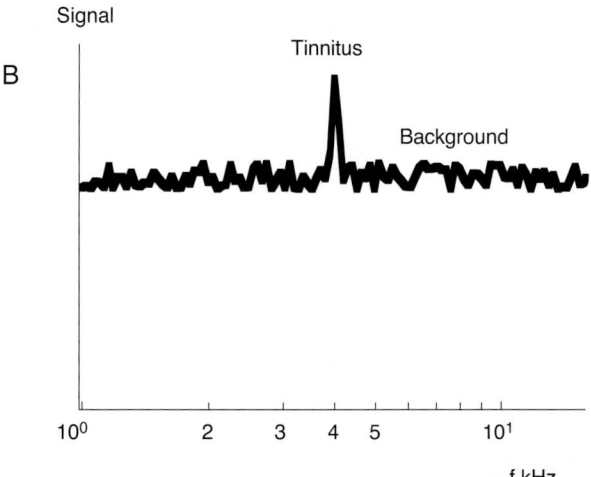

FIGURE 21-2. The strength of a signal depends on its difference from activity evoked by background sound. A, Tinnitus signal in silence; B, tinnitus with enriched background sound.

and, consequently, to decrease the stimulus activating the limbic and autonomic nervous systems. This is achieved by an increase in background neuronal activity in the auditory system by exposing the patient to a low-level, continuous, neutral sound (Figure 21-2).

Mechanisms of Sound Perception Relevant to Tinnitus and Decreased Sound Tolerance All sensory systems adjust their sensitivity (gain) to the average level of environmental signals (automatic gain control principle). The Heller and Bergman experiment with transient tinnitus induced by a few minutes presence in an anechoic chamber[10] is discussed with all patients with tinnitus to make them realize that it is possible to induce tinnitus in practically anyone by simply decreasing the ambient background sound level. The results of this experiment support the postulate that patients should avoid silence and enrich their sound environment. It is suggested that overamplification within the auditory pathways could result in both tinnitus and hyperacusis.[1] Therefore, by decreasing this overamplification, for example, treating hyperacusis, improvement in tinnitus is observed as well. This, in fact, is a common clinical observation.

The Heller and Bergman experiment has implications for patients with hearing loss by pointing out that a decrease in the auditory input, caused by the hearing loss or overprotection of hearing, triggers increased amplification in the auditory pathways, resulting in enhancement of tinnitus. For these patients, increased problems with speech perception frequently result from high-frequency hearing loss, which increases the auditory gain and the tinnitus.

Unilateral deafness, or unilateral profound hearing loss, must be addressed separately. It has been shown that, using the principle of multisensory integration, it is possible to treat phantom limb perception by integrating somatosensory and visual information and that this treatment results in partial restoration of abnormal cortical activity evoked by deafferentation.[11-13] These results yield a specific approach to patients with unilateral hearing impairment: sound is transmitted from the impaired side to the other by artificial means, such as contralateral routing of signal (CROS), bilateral contralateral routing of signal (BICROS), or transcranial stimulation, and patients are instructed to perform exercises aimed at recalibration of the localization in space of auditory stimuli. The expectation is that through this process, a part of the auditory pathways that was less active owing to decreased auditory input from one side will be partially reactivated. This hypothesis remains to be proven, but patients improve very well. This approach is aimed at another effect: improved localization in space of stimuli that further yields some increase in understanding speech in noise. This decreases the strain-to-hear phenomenon and the general level of stress and anxiety.

The majority of patients with tinnitus experience problems with sleeping. In this respect, two mechanisms are worth consideration. First, the increased level of activation of the autonomic nervous system results in difficulty falling asleep; second, the mechanisms responsible for problems with sleep continue through the night. Sleep is cyclic in nature, and approximately every 90 minutes, awakening occurs for a short time, and then sleep resumes. Patients with tinnitus, when awakened during the night, perceive tinnitus that seems to be particularly loud in a quiet surrounding and makes falling asleep more difficult. By providing increased sound background throughout the night, for example, the sound of nature from tabletop sound machines, the tinnitus signal is weakened, and the probability of falling asleep increases. Because the auditory pathways are fully active up to the level of inferior colliculi during sleep, it is possible to expect some additional benefit from using sound during the night even for individuals who do not have a problem with sleep.

Common Elements of Sound Therapy All patients are advised to avoid silence and enrich the sound background by a variety of means, for example, use of tabletop sound machines and compact disc players. The sounds used, however, have to fulfill several general requirements:

1. Sounds used as part of sound therapy should never evoke annoyance or discomfort of any kind owing to their loudness, quality, or type. Otherwise, they would activate the limbic and autonomic nervous systems and actually enhance the reflex arc that is to be extinguished.
2. Sounds used should minimize the strength of the tinnitus signal.
3. These sounds should not suppress ("mask") tinnitus, even partially. Total suppression of tinnitus will prevent habituation by definition because it is impossible to retrain an individual to a stimulus that the brain cannot detect. Note that detection is not equivalent to perception because it is possible to achieve training at a subconscious

level. Partial suppression would not prevent habituation, but it would hinder it because retraining would occur to a stimulus different from the original. Only owing to the generalization principle would the habituation to the original stimulus still occur, but it would be weaker. Thus, sound should not change the characteristic features of the tinnitus signal, that is, the pattern of neuronal activity or the perceived spectrum of the signal, to ensure the most effective habituation.

4. The sounds should not be close to the threshold of hearing. If sound is close to the threshold of hearing, it will induce only a small increase in background neuronal activity and consequently result in only a mild decrease of the tinnitus signal strength. Furthermore, owing to stochastic resonance, it might enhance the tinnitus signal.[14,15] Indeed, a significant increase with tinnitus loudness matching is observed when patients are exposed to noise with an intensity lower than 6 dB SL.

5. Sounds used for sound enrichment should be easily habituated and preferably induce some relaxation.

These five rules provide guidance for selecting the type of sound and an optimal sound level. For tinnitus alone, attempts to minimize the tinnitus signal would promote the use of high levels of sound; however, avoidance of annoyance and tinnitus suppression impose restrictions on the highest sound levels that can be used for TRT. Therefore, the highest level that could be used is the beginning of partial suppression ("partial masking"), described by patients as a "mixing" or "blending" point. At this point, patients can still perceive separately the sound of tinnitus and the external sound, but they perceive them as starting to mix, blend, and intertwine with each other. Patients should aim to be at or below this level provided that the sound used is below the level inducing annoyance or discomfort.

On the other hand, avoidance of sounds close to the threshold of hearing imposes a restriction on the lowest recommended sound levels. The final outcome resulting from the combination of the above rules is presented in Figure 21-3. To achieve habituation, it is not necessary to be at the mixing point, which frequently cannot be reached owing to the limitation imposed by being below the sound level inducing annoyance, and there is a range of effective sound levels.

Two categories of sound are used to ensure easy habituation. For tabletop sound machines and compact discs, the use of sounds of nature, particularly gently flowing water (eg, a stream, rain), is favored. These sounds should be stable and not overwhelming; thus, the sound of waves or waterfalls is not rec-

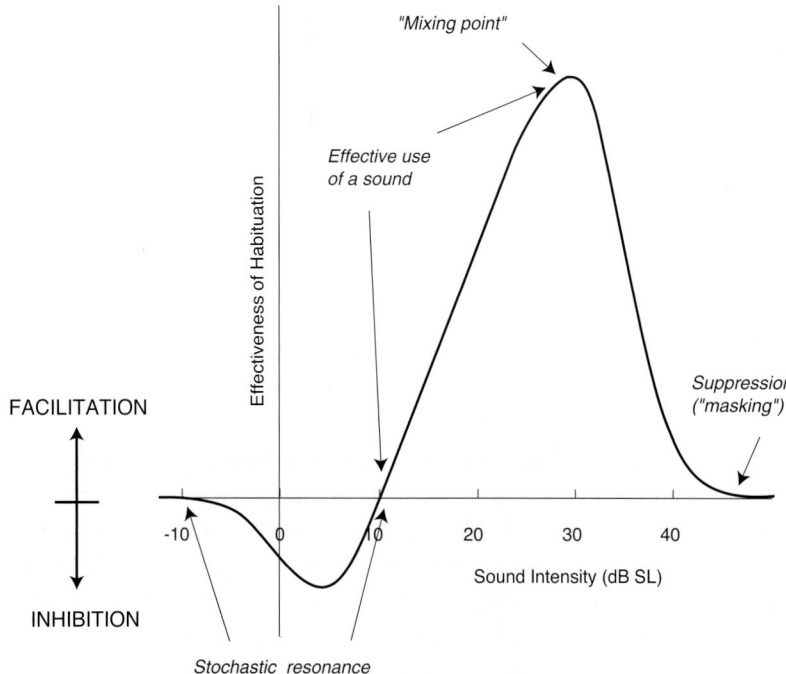

FIGURE 21-3. The effectiveness of habituation depends on sound intensity. Republished with permission from Jastreboff PJ and Jastreboff MM.[4]

ommended. For wearable sound generators, a broadband noise with a frequency range from about 1 to 4 kHz is typically used. An optimal sound type depends on the patient's past experience and personal preferences and should be discussed and selected with the active participation of the patient.

For hyperacusis without secondary tinnitus, the sound should be as loud as it is allowed by the principle of sound use below the level of inducing annoyance or discomfort. For coexisting tinnitus and hyperacusis, the stress for the initial stage of treatment is on hyperacusis (trying not to suppress tinnitus but being more lax on this point) and later resetting the sound level optimal for tinnitus.

Precise setting of the sound level is impossible while using sound sources that are not attached to the head because any movement of the body and head will change the sound levels reaching the ears. Therefore, to achieve stable and well-controlled sound levels, it is necessary to use wearable sound generators. For these instruments, that is, sound generators, hearing aids, and combination instruments, specific fitting and programming are necessary. All instruments are fitted with as open a mold as is possible. Sound generators should not change the threshold of hearing by mechanical obstruction of the ear canal.

A more complex situation exists when amplification by hearing aids or combination instruments is needed. Even the best hearing aids are unable to transmit sound below 200 Hz. If a hearing aid is used that blocks the ear canal, it can act as an earplug for low frequencies. This phenomenon may explain the clinical observation that some patients experience enhancement of tinnitus when wearing hearing aids. Therefore, hearing aids completely in the canal or occluding the ear canal typically are not recommended in TRT, except if the patient has significant hearing loss for low frequencies. However, hearing aids with a large vent might be acceptable.

Many modern hearing aids have special programs attenuating background environmental noise. Although such programs are helpful under usual circumstances, they act against the sound enrichment goal of TRT by suppressing purposefully introduced low-level sounds. These programs should be disabled for the duration of TRT or at least activated only when communication is the main requirement.

Patients with tinnitus who have decreased sound tolerance (hyperacusis and/or misophonia) will be particularly sensitive to overstimulation with sound. Therefore, the initial gain should be set lower than typically used, and compression should be set higher. Only after significant improvement or elimination of decreased sound tolerance should amplification be set at parameters appropriate for people with hearing loss only.

Category-Specific Variations of Treatment

For category 0 patients, counseling is abbreviated with particular attention to avoid presenting tinnitus as a worse problem than what the patient is experiencing. Encouragement, reassurance, and the advice to avoid silence are commonly what these patients need. Sound therapy is based on using enrichment of background sound delivered by tabletop sound machines, compact discs, or tapes with the sounds of nature or other things such as indoor or outdoor fountains or waterfalls. Sound enrichment should be carefully chosen not to induce annoyance. The sound should be pleasant, easy to ignore, and relaxing. Wearable instrumentation is not recommended. If a patient is very insistent on using sound generators, a clear explanation should be provided pointing out the danger of unnecessarily bringing attention to the tinnitus.

Category 1 patients receive full tinnitus-oriented counseling following the path presented in general counseling and focusing on issues that are particularly important to the individual patient. Sound therapy uses all of the elements as for category 0 (sound enrichment), and sound generators are recommended as well. Setting of the sound level is aimed at the mixing point but is always set at the level that does not induce annoyance or discomfort of any type.

For category 2 patients, counseling is similar as for category 1, with a strong focus on the concept of OHCs as biologic hearing aids. All issues related to hearing loss also have to be addressed. All patients in this category receive the recommendation for amplification in the form of hearing aids or, when appropriate, combination instruments. Sound generators alone are not used for these patients. They would contribute to problems with speech understanding and increase the strain-to-hear phenomenon. In the use of hearing aids, special stress is placed on maximal use of enrichment of background sound and explanation to patients that hearing aids alone will not work to help with tinnitus because they act only as amplifiers of sound that is present in the environment. Stress is placed on continuous use of hearing aids, not only for communication purposes.

Patients with unilateral hearing impairment are a separate challenge. On the bases of multisensory integration and the possibility of influencing activity within the auditory system with visual information, CROS or BICROS systems are recommended, and exercises improving localization of sound in space are suggested.

Counseling of category 3 patients focuses on issues related to hyperacusis, with stress on tinnitus only when hyperacusis is successfully treated. If hyperacusis is a great and dominant problem, counseling regarding tinnitus is abbreviated. Frequently, after improvement in hyperacusis, tinnitus improves to such an extent that it does not require specific treatment. All patients in this category receive the recommendation for sound generators used alone or as part of combination instruments (in patients with accompanying hearing loss). Sound generators are set at a comfortable level, gradually increasing with time up to the mixing point if tinnitus is present. General sound enrichment is important as well.

Category 4 patients are the most difficult group, and they should be treated in a case-by-case manner with careful attention to any medical issues that might be linked to altered brain activity. Counseling must be very sensible, and the appropriate expectation should be discussed very carefully. Sound generators or combination instruments are always recommended. Because many of the patients in category 4 exhibit oversensitivity to other sensory modalities, including somatosensory stimulation, as a standard precaution, they are instructed to wear instruments for a few days without any sound. The sound level is gradually increased under constant supervision to ensure that additional sounds do not induce prolonged worsening of their problems.

FITTING INSTRUMENTATION WHEN APPROPRIATE

Although, in theory, TRT can be practiced with sound therapy based exclusively on enrichment of background sound, it is not practical. Wearable devices (sound generators, hearing aids, or combination instruments) provide important help, improve compliance, facilitate the process of habituation by exposing the patient to better controlled sound levels, and, therefore, increase the probability of success. Consequently, for a substantial proportion of patients, wearable instruments are recommended.

Bilateral devices are always recommended when physically possible to preserve or restore symmetry of stimulation of the auditory pathways. The obvious exception is unilateral hearing impairment when CROS, BICROS, or transcranial stimulation is used.

Providing sound through wearable devices has an additional advantage. All external sounds evoke correlated activity in left and right auditory nerves, and the activity changes with movement of the body and head in space. This changing activity occurs through all of the auditory pathways. Tinnitus is very different in this respect because it does not exhibit a specific, side-related relationship, and the tinnitus-related neuronal activity does not change when the subject moves or turns the head. Sound from wearable sound generators shares this unique property with tinnitus. The brain learns to habituate more easily to this unusual signal delivered by sound generators over which patients have full control. The sound does not evoke negative reinforcement (annoyance or discomfort) and is gradually habituated. This ability is later passed to the habituation of tinnitus, which, consequently, is easier to achieve.

During the fitting appointment, the basis of sound therapy is reiterated, and detailed instructions are provided regarding setting sound generators, daily use, and expectations. The level of sound set by the patient is checked with real-ear measurements to ensure an appropriate range of sound intensity and symmetric sound setting.

It is important to remember that hearing aids and combination instruments are used primarily for tinnitus and/or hyperacusis, and the improvement of speech understanding is a secondary goal. Careful gradual adjustment of gain and compression settings and checking for compliance of sound enrichment are crucial.

FOLLOW-UP VISITS

Follow-up contacts are important. Their primary role is to continue with counseling, answering questions, addressing concerns, checking compliance, helping the patient understand the treatment protocol, and evaluating the patient's progress. Potential unsolved concerns can provide further stimulation of the limbic and autonomic nervous systems, making it much more difficult for habituation to occur. During follow-up visits, selected audiologic tests are performed. Evaluation of LDLs is repeated when they were previously lower than 100 dB HL. Real-ear measurements are also a standard part of follow-up evaluations in patients using sound generators or combination instruments.

EVALUATION OF TREATMENT PROGRESS AND OUTCOME

The evaluation of tinnitus offers a substantial challenge because there is no objective method for detecting the presence of tinnitus and measuring its severity. Determining the LDLs is helpful in the evaluation of decreased sound tolerance but is not sufficient to differentiate hyperacusis and misophonia, and normal LDL values can be observed in some misophonia patients. Careful questioning of patients is crucial to collect the information needed to evaluate treatment outcome.

Usually, the first important effects of TRT in patients with tinnitus can be detected 3 months from the initial visit, with progressive improvement in 6 months. Many patients achieve high levels of tinnitus habituation by 9 to 12 months. Patients with hyperacusis usually improve faster, and the success rate exceeds tinnitus treatment outcome. To prevent a relapse, patients are advised to follow the TRT protocol for at least 12 to 18 months. At the end of this time, they gradually relinquish the use of instruments and are more relaxed in continuing environmental sound enrichment. Some patients notice continuous, although proportionally smaller, improvement with time and are reluctant to cease the treatment, wanting to get even better. The use of sounds of nature during the night is usually the last aspect of therapy that they stop. These sounds provide the feeling of security and relaxation that helps sleeping in general.

RESULTS

A substantial proportion of reported results in the tinnitus field describe data expressed as a percentage of patients who reached preset criteria of a "significant improvement" based on the usual clinical practice, and limited data are from purposefully designed studies. There is also no agreement with respect to specific criteria of improvement. A frequently used criterion is the requirement that at least two recorded scores on tinnitus questionnaires improve by at least 20 to 40%, with different specific percentages used by various centers. This criterion resembles the standard criterion used in the field of chronic pain, in which improvement of 30 to 50% is considered significant.

The results reported by independent clinical centers using TRT are promising, showing a consistent success rate of about 80% or higher. Sheldrake and colleagues (United Kingdom) presented the results from 483 patients using the criterion of at least 40% improvement in at least two measures and showed an 84% success rate.[16] A success rate greater than 80% has been reported by Lux-Wellenhof (Germany) in 122 patients.[17] Bartnik and colleagues (Poland) presented the results on 556 patients with a success rate of 80%.[18] Heitzmann and colleagues (Spain) had an 84% success rate in 56 patients,[19] and Herraiz and colleagues (Spain) had an 88% success rate in 172 patients.[20]

Several centers reported the results from studies specifically aimed at the evaluation of patients during TRT. A stratified trial involving 169 patients in the United Kingdom demonstrated a significant improvement in 83.3% of 36 patients treated with TRT compared with only 6% spontaneous recovery in the nontreated group (113 subjects).[21]

An interesting study was performed in Germany, in which the authors contacted 84 former patients at least 5 years after beginning TRT, that is, at least 3.5 to 4 years after formal treatment was ended.[22] The results showed that patients remained in very good status, with 85% reporting improvement.

Statistically significant improvement on the Tinnitus Handicap Inventory scores of 32 patients treated with TRT was reported by Berry and colleagues.[23] Perhaps the most interesting results are coming from a recently finished study performed on veterans. The results were presented during the 2003 annual meeting of the American Academy of Audiology, and an outline of main the results was published recently.[24] Subjects were randomly assigned to TRT or the "masking" group, treated by one of these methods, and were evaluated in an identical manner (structured interviews and various questionnaires, including the Tinnitus Handicap Inventory). The results revealed significant improvement with the treatment and consistently better results with TRT than with "masking" for all of the parameters studied (see Chapter 25, "Veterans and Tinnitus").

Our results from the University of Maryland and Emory University show significant improvement in over 80% of patients.[5,25–28] Further carefully designed studies are needed to validate the efficacy of TRT.

CONCLUSIONS

TRT has a number of positive attributes: it can be effectively used to treat patients with tinnitus and decreased sound tolerance, requires only limited time for treatment, and does not have side effects. Although TRT does not offer elimination of the perception of tinnitus, it does offer the possibility of achieving relief for clinically significant tinnitus, that is, of tinnitus-induced negative reactions. Note that tinnitus perception is decreased significantly as well. The patient can still hear the tinnitus when attention is focused on it, but even then the tinnitus causes mild or no annoyance.

Interestingly, 19.6% of 149 patients reported that for some time (from a few hours to months, on average 10.5 days), they could not hear their tinnitus, even when focusing attention on it.[29] Although it is not our clinical goal, it shows that TRT can lead to a state close to a cure for tinnitus perception.

One of the negative aspects of TRT is the required time commitment, particularly for the first visit. Although the total time of interaction during a 2-year period is about 15 to 20 hours, a large portion of this time is spent during the first visit.

TRT is not a stagnant method. It undergoes constant modifications aimed at decreasing the time needed for treatment and increasing its effectiveness. Although the neurophysiological model of tinnitus has remained basically the same since its introduction in 1990, certain elements of the original model are still not incorporated in TRT, for example, the role of the prefrontal cortex in task switching and multisensory integration performed by the cerebellum. A number of changes have been made in recent years in the practical implementation of TRT, for example, modification of counseling with stress on conditioned reflexes, introduction of strict control of sound levels used by patients (real-ear measurements), relaxed rules for setting the sound level for patients in category 3, and incorporation of combination instruments into the sound therapy, resulting in facilitation of the process of habituation and decreasing of the time needed for improvement.

REFERENCES

1. Jastreboff PJ. Phantom auditory perception (tinnitus): mechanisms of generation and perception. Neurosci Res 1990;8:221–54.
2. Konorski J. Conditioned reflexes and neuronal organization. Cambridge (UK): Cambridge University Press; 1948.
3. Jastreboff MM, Jastreboff PJ. Decreased sound tolerance and tinnitus retraining therapy (TRT). Aust N Z J Audiol 2002;21:74–81.
4. Jastreboff PJ, Jastreboff MM. Tinnitus and hyperacusis. In: Snow JB, Ballenger JJ, editors. Ballenger's otorhinolaryngology head and neck surgery. Hamilton (ON): BC Decker; 2003. p. 456–75.
5. Jastreboff PJ, Jastreboff MM. Tinnitus retraining therapy (TRT) as a method for treatment of tinnitus and hyperacusis patients. J Am Acad Audiol 2000;11:156–61.
6. Jastreboff PJ, Jastreboff MM. Tinnitus retraining therapy for patients with tinnitus and decreased sound tolerance. Otolaryngol Clin North Am 2003;36:321–36.
7. Jastreboff PJ. Tinnitus as a phantom perception: theories and clinical implications. In: Vernon J, Møller AR, editors. Mechanisms of tinnitus. Boston: Allyn & Bacon; 1995. p. 73–94.
8. Chen GD, Fechter LD. The relationship between noise-induced hearing loss and hair cell loss in rats. Hear Res 2003;177:81–90.
9. The American heritage dictionary. 3rd ed. Boston: SoftKey International; 1994.
10. Heller MF, Bergman M. Tinnitus in normally hearing persons. Ann Otol Rhinol Laryngol 1953;62:73–93.
11. Borsook D, Becerra L, Fishman S, et al. Acute plasticity in the human somatosensory cortex following amputation. Neuroreport 1998;9:1013–7.
12. Ramachandran VS, Rogers-Ramachandran D. Phantom limbs and neural plasticity. Arch Neurol 2000;57:317–20.
13. Ramachandran VS, Rogers-Ramachandran D. Synaesthesia in phantom limbs induced with mirrors. Proc R Soc Lond B Biol Sci 1996;263:377–86.
14. Jastreboff PJ, Jastreboff MM. Potential impact of stochastic resonance on tinnitus and its treatment [abstract]. In: Popelka GR, editor. Abstracts of the Twenty-Third Annual Midwinter Research Meeting of the Association for Research in Otolaryngology. Mt. Royal (NJ): Association for Research in Otolaryngology; 2000. p. 216.
15. Morse RP, Evans EF. Enhancement of vowel coding for cochlear implants by addition of noise. Nat Med 1996;2:928–32.
16. Sheldrake JB, Hazell JWP, Graham RL. Results of tinnitus retraining therapy. In: Hazell J, editor. Proceedings of the Sixth International Tinnitus Seminar. London: The Tinnitus and Hyperacusis Centre; 1999. p. 292–6.

17. Lux-Wellenhof G. Treatment history of incoming patients to the Tinnitus & Hyperacusis Centre in Frankfurt/Main. In: Hazell J, editor. Proceedings of the Sixth International Tinnitus Seminar. London: The Tinnitus and Hyperacusis Centre; 1999. p. 502–6.
18. Bartnik G, Fabijanska A, Rogowski M. Our experience in treatment of patients with tinnitus and/or hyperacusis using the habituation method. In: Hazell J, editor. Proceedings of the Sixth International Tinnitus Seminar. London: The Tinnitus and Hyperacusis Centre; 1999. p. 415–7.
19. Heitzmann T, Rubio L, Cardenas MR, Zofio E. The importance of continuity in TRT patients: results at 18 months. In: Hazell J, editor. Proceedings of the Sixth International Tinnitus Seminar. London: The Tinnitus and Hyperacusis Centre; 1999. p. 509–11.
20. Herraiz C, Hernandez FJ, Machado A, et al. Tinnitus retraining therapy: our experience. In: Hazell J, editor. Proceedings of the Sixth International Tinnitus Seminar. London: The Tinnitus and Hyperacusis Centre; 1999. p. 483–4.
21. McKinney CJ, Hazell JWP, Graham RL. An evaluation of the TRT method. In: Hazell J, editor. Proceedings of the Sixth International Tinnitus Seminar. London: The Tinnitus and Hyperacusis Centre; 1999. p. 99–105.
22. Lux-Wellenhof G, Hellweg FC. Long term follow up study of TRT in Frankfurt. In: Patuzzi R, editor. Proceedings of the Seventh International Tinnitus Seminar. Perth: The University of Western Australia; 2002. p. 277–9.
23. Berry JA, Gold SL, Frederick EA, et al. Patient-based outcomes in patients with primary tinnitus undergoing tinnitus retraining therapy. Arch Otolaryngol Head Neck Surg 2002;128:1153–7.
24. Henry JA. Tinnitus retraining therapy: description and clinical efficacy. ENT News 2004;13:48–50.
25. Henry JA, Jastreboff MM, Jastreboff PJ, et al. Assessment of patients for treatment with tinnitus retraining therapy. J Am Acad Audiol 2002;13:523–44.
26. Jastreboff PJ, Jastreboff MM, Mattox DE. Statistical analysis of the progress of tinnitus treatment during tinnitus retraining therapy (TRT) [abstract]. In: Santi PA, editor. Abstracts of the Twenty-Fourth Annual Midwinter Research Meeting of the Association for Research in Otolaryngology. Mt. Royal (NJ): Association for Research in Otolaryngology; 2001. p. 15.
27. Jastreboff PJ. Categories of the patients in TRT and the treatment outcome. In: Hazell J, editor. Proceedings of the Sixth International Tinnitus Seminar. London: The Tinnitus and Hyperacusis Centre; 1999. p. 394–8.
28. Jastreboff PJ, Gray WC, Gold SL. Neurophysiological approach to tinnitus patients. Am J Otol 1996;17:236–40.
29. Sheldrake JB, Jastreboff PJ, Hazell JWP. Perspectives for total elimination of tinnitus perception. In: Vernon JA, Reich GE, editors. Proceedings of the Fifth International Tinnitus Seminar. Portland (OR): American Tinnitus Association; 1996. p. 531–6.

CHAPTER 22

Role of Hearing Aids in Management of Tinnitus

Jacqueline B. Sheldrake, RHAD, BSHAA, Margaret M. Jastreboff, PhD

Tinnitus is a symptom reflecting disorder in the auditory system, and even though many patients with tinnitus have hearing within normal limits, the majority of people complaining about tinnitus have some changes in their hearing. It is estimated that close to 70% of individuals with hearing impairment have tinnitus as well.[1] For this reason, it seems fully justifiable to consider hearing aids for tinnitus relief. Actually, it is fair to say that the use of hearing aids to help tinnitus sufferers is the most common attempt to treat tinnitus in audiology and hearing aid dispensing clinics. This practice potentially achieves a double benefit: better speech communication and help with the tinnitus.

HEARING AIDS AND THE NEUROPHYSIOLOGICAL MODEL OF TINNITUS

There is no consensus with respect to the mechanisms involved in the successful outcome of hearing aid use in providing tinnitus relief. One potential explanation, based on the neurophysiological model of tinnitus,[2,3] could be that hearing aids provide amplification of an ambient sound, which helps to increase the stimulation of the auditory pathways. This, in turn, decreases the difference between the tinnitus signal and the background neuronal activity, decreasing the strength of the tinnitus signal and causing the tinnitus to be less intrusive and less noticeable. Consequently, less attention is placed on the tinnitus signal, which will gradually be placed in the category of unimportant, nonsignificant stimuli and to which gradual habituation will occur. Amplification offered by hearing aids decreases the "strain to hear" and so reduces the stress and anxiety caused by tinnitus. Through this mechanism, hearing aids further diminish the perception of tinnitus and its impact on the patient's life.

The study of Surr and colleagues assessed the effects of hearing aids on tinnitus.[4] The authors used the Tinnitus Handicap Inventory (THI)[5] and examined scores of aided versus unaided subjects and separately the benefits provided by hearing aids measured with the Abbreviated Profile of Hearing Aid Benefit inventory and speech subscales. The results showed the significant effect of hearing aid use on THI scores; however, the effect was small. It is not clear if the conclusion can be made with respect to tinnitus significance in patients' lives. The results from the Emory Tinnitus and Hyperacusis Center indicate that it is possible to observe a highly statistically significant improvement in THI scores when using hearing aids or combination instruments, even though patients still perceive considerable problems with their tinnitus.[6]

MASKING HYPOTHESIS OF THE EFFECTS OF HEARING AIDS

Many people experiencing tinnitus notice that its perception can be diminished by environmental sound. They use this observation to get relief by enriching the background sound. In psychoacoustics, suppression of tinnitus perception by external sound is labeled "masking," which reflects the common meaning of this word, namely "covering up." Masking is, however, a peripheral phenomenon of interacting traveling waves in the cochlea. It exhibits a V-type frequency dependency of effectiveness and requires that the masking sound be within a certain frequency range (critical band).[7] Tinnitus "masking" does not fulfill these requirements. Its behavior is consistent, however, with neuronal suppression occurring within the higher levels of the auditory pathway. Although the term "tinnitus masking" is not correct, it is commonly used in the tinnitus literature related to hearing aids, and to facilitate presentation, the term is, therefore, used in this chapter.

The article from 1947 by Saltzman and Ersner is the earliest report on the beneficial effects of hearing aids in patients with tinnitus[8] and was later followed by other articles that describe hearing aids reducing or eliminating the perception of tinnitus.[9–11] They indicate that hearing aids cause tinnitus to be substantially reduced in loudness or even make it inaudible, most probably owing to the increase in an ability to hear the ambient noise (environmental or produced by hearing aids), which effectively masks tinnitus.

Follow-up studies of 598 patients who could successfully mask their tinnitus revealed that hearing aids were effective for 16% of these patients.[12] The success rate is even lower (7% of 192 patients) when patients are simply told that their tinnitus could be relieved just by using hearing aids.[13] It was speculated that the low success rate, when attempting to use hearing aids for tinnitus treatment, reflects the fact that most patients with tinnitus match their tinnitus in the high-frequency range in which hearing aids have limited ability to provide amplification of background sound, which, in turn, could mask tinnitus. The results obtained by Feldmann, which showed that tinnitus can be easily masked by sounds with frequencies distant from the tinnitus pitch,[7] argue against this hypothesis.

Von Wedel and colleagues reported studies comparing the benefits of hearing aids and tinnitus maskers to relieve tinnitus and discussed masking effects during the use of instruments, residual inhibition (reduction of tinnitus for a period after masking ceased), and a subjective scaling of therapeutic efficiency.[14] After 4 to 6 weeks of the trial period, 88 of 472 patients (18.6%) purchased hearing aids, and 80% of these continued wearing them, achieving successful tinnitus relief. Thus, the effective success rate was 14.9% of the initial population of subjects trying hearing aids for masking. Reported results over a period of at least 1 year of hearing aid use showed a stable benefit for these patients.

Sheldrake and Hazell studied the records of 131 patients followed for as long as 10 years for their continuing rehabilitation for tinnitus.[15] These patients were using maskers or hearing aids according to their main problem. If there was a substantial hearing problem, the focus was on hearing aid fitting and auditory rehabilitation, stressing the beneficial effect that this will have on the patient's tinnitus. The fitting was binaural wherever possible, with an effort to preserve symmetry of stimulation and with the earmold as open as possible to avoid occlusion of the ear canal. Equally good results were obtained with hearing aids or maskers. Patients showed improvement within 6 months of the beginning of this management, with continuous positive changes over a period of 2 to 8 years.

According to Vernon, patients with low-frequency tinnitus, particularly when the hearing impairment includes the areas of low frequency, obtain the greatest benefit from the use of hearing aids.[16] He postulated that amplified background sound efficiently masked tinnitus even when hearing aids did not produce residual inhibition. Clinical observations indicate that it is worth trying to use hearing aids even in patients with high-pitched tinnitus. Vernon and Meikle suggest that hearing aids provide a masking stimulus to cover or reduce the level of tinnitus regardless of the tinnitus pitch[13] because some individuals can experience effective masking by any sound regardless of its frequency.[7] Similarly, in some patients with severe hearing loss for whom hearing aids are unable to provide benefits in speech understanding, hearing aids can help with tinnitus.

Continuing with the idea of masking and the issue of the potential benefits of residual inhibition, von Wedel and colleagues found that 94.7% of hearing aids users reported partial or complete residual inhibition lasting less than 30 seconds and 0.3% lasting about 60 seconds.[14] Unfortunately, longer-lasting residual inhibition in hearing aid users was not shown.

TINNITUS INSTRUMENTS

In response to the needs of patients with high-frequency hearing loss and tinnitus, the tinnitus instrument, a hearing aid combined with a tinnitus masker, was developed. Until then, according to Hazell, a surprising number of patients ended up wearing a masker in one ear and a hearing aid in the other ear because hearing aids alone or a masker alone did not provide satisfactory benefits.[17] Schleuning and colleagues reported that 63% of patients wearing the combination instrument could successfully mask tinnitus, whereas when a masker or hearing aid alone was used, only 21% and 16% of patients, respectively, benefited.[12]

At the time when the first tinnitus instruments were developed, it was a common belief that frequency-specific maskers would offer the most benefit to patients with tinnitus. Tinnitus instruments offered selectable frequency bands so that the masker frequency could be adjusted to obtain the optimal masking effect for a given patient. Unfortunately, in spite of masking advantages, low quality of the hearing aid part, poor cosmetic appearance of the devices, and difficulties with their control and handling caused their use to be limited. Only recently, as hearing aid technology has advanced, new tinnitus combination instruments have been developed, offering a programmable, digital hearing aid portion of the instrument and a multiband sound generator. In most instances, they are used successfully following the protocol of tinnitus retraining therapy (TRT) (see Chapter 21, "Tinnitus Retraining Therapy").

PRACTICAL CONSIDERATIONS

For some patients, hearing aids provide complete suppression of tinnitus perception when they are worn. Even though this complete relief is much welcomed by patients, they might be severely affected by their tinnitus when they remove the hearing aids temporally during the day or during the night. These patients are advised to spend some time during the day with the hearing aids turned down so that the tinnitus is audible or switched off while exposed to an enriched background sound to initiate the process of habituation.

Modern hearing aids typically have advanced programs to suppress background sounds. Because they decrease the contribution of ambient sound, they can enhance the tinnitus. It is recommended that these programs be disabled while patients are not involved in communication. Continuous exposure to low levels of background sound results in a decrease in gain within the auditory pathways that is useful for the treatment of tinnitus and essential for the treatment of hyperacusis.

Modern hearing aids also have a low level of internal noise; therefore, without a proper level of external sound, they do not provide any stimulation and benefit for patients with tinnitus. Therefore, it is important to discuss with patients the need for sound enrichment, to pay attention to the details of their lifestyle, and to plan individual requirements for each patient.

Proper fitting of hearing aids is crucial. Too much occlusion can be responsible for the exacerbation of tinnitus. It is important to increase the gain of hearing aids in patients with tinnitus in a very gradual manner. Sudden overamplification can induce strong reactions and lead to the development of misophonia (see Chapter 2, "Decreased Sound Tolerance").

Patients frequently have many misconceptions regarding tinnitus and hearing. High-frequency hearing loss results in rapid deterioration of ability to understand speech in noise. Patients tend to blame the tinnitus for masking speech and preventing them from understanding. Removal of the strain-to-hear phenomenon with hearing aids substantially improves the general life situation, thereby decreasing the negative associations linked to tinnitus. Consequently, tinnitus becomes much less of a problem. In this respect, improved spatial localization and speech understanding in noise observed with a binaural fitting offer additional support to fitting hearing aids binaurally when physically possible.

For patients with unilateral hearing impairment, the contralateral routing of signal (CROS) system is recommended. The rationale for this approach is based on multisensory integration and is presented in Chapter 21, "Tinnitus Retraining Therapy." The technical limitations of CROS systems (noisy FM-based system, inconvenience with a hard-wired unit) should be taken into account and may hinder successful implementation of this approach.

All elements that could attract patients' attentional focus to their tinnitus and hearing should be minimized. Therefore, care is taken to use comfortable, personal molds rather than a standard fitting. Another consequence of this issue is the tendency to use hearing aids with one program rather than with different programs for various situations to decrease the potential temptation of patients to fiddle continuously with the instruments in an attempt to find the optimal program or setting for each situation.

For all discussed above, proper education of the patient is crucial to successful use of hearing aids for tinnitus. For many patients, it is not necessary to embark into full TRT counseling, and a shorter session, with use only of selected elements of the neurophysiological model of tinnitus, can provide substantial benefit alongside amplification.

REFERENCES

1. Office of Population Censuses and Surveys. 1983 general household survey. The prevalence of tinnitus 1981. London: GHS 83/1, Office of Population Censuses and Surveys; 1983.
2. Jastreboff PJ. Phantom auditory perception (tinnitus): mechanisms of generation and perception. Neurosci Res 1990;8:221–54.
3. Jastreboff PJ, Jastreboff MM. Tinnitus and hyperacusis. In: Snow JB, Ballenger JJ, editors. Ballenger's otorhinolaryngology head and neck surgery. Hamilton (ON): BC Decker; 2003. p. 456–75.
4. Surr RK, Kolb JA, Cord MT, Garrus NP. Tinnitus Handicap Inventory (THI) as a hearing aid outcome measure. J Am Acad Audiol 1999;10:489–95.
5. Newman CW, Wharton JA, Jacobson GP. Retest stability of the tinnitus handicap questionnaire. Ann Otol Rhinol Laryngol 1995;104:718–23.
6. Jastreboff PJ, Jastreboff MM, Mattox DE. Statistical analysis of the progress of tinnitus treatment during Tinnitus Retraining Therapy (TRT) [abstract]. In: Santi PA, editor. Abstracts of the Twenty-Fourth Annual Midwinter Research Meeting of the Association for Research in Otolaryngology. Mt. Royal (NJ): Association for Research in Otolaryngology; 2001. p. 15.
7. Feldmann H. Homolateral and contralateral masking of tinnitus by noisebands and by pure tones. Audiology (Basel) 1971;10:138–44.
8. Saltzman M, Ersner MS. A hearing aid for the relief of tinnitus aurium. Laryngoscope 1947;57:358–66.
9. Surr RK, Montgomery AA, Mueller HG. Effect of amplification on tinnitus among new hearing aid users. Ear Hear 1985;6:71–5.
10. Melin L, Scott B, Lindberg P, Lyttkens L. Hearing aids and tinnitus—an experimental group study. Br J Audiol 1987;21:91–7.
11. Vernon J. Attempts to relieve tinnitus. J Am Audiol Soc 1977;2:124–31.
12. Schleuning AJ, Johnson RM, Vernon JA. Evaluation of a tinnitus masking program: a follow-up study of 598 patients. Ear Hear 1980;1:71–4.
13. Vernon JA, Meikle MB. Tinnitus masking. In: Tyler RS, editor. Tinnitus handbook. San Diego (CA): Singular, Thomson Learning; 2000. p. 313–56.
14. von Wedel H, von Wedel U, Walger M. Tinnitus masking with tinnitus-maskers and hearing aids. In: Vernon J, Møller AR, editors. Mechanisms of tinnitus. Boston: Allyn & Bacon; 1995. p. 187–92.
15. Sheldrake JB, Hazell JWP. Maskers versus hearing aids in the prosthetic management of tinnitus. In: Aran J-M, Dauman R, editors. Tinnitus 91. Proceedings of the Fourth International Tinnitus Seminar. Amsterdam: Kugler Publications; 1992. p. 395–9.
16. Vernon JA. Current use of masking for the relief of tinnitus. In: Kitahara M, editor. Tinnitus: pathophysiology and management. Tokyo: Igaku-Shoin; 1988. p. 96–106.
17. Hazell JWP. Tinnitus masking therapy. In: Hazell JWP, editor. Tinnitus. Edinburgh: Churchill Livingstone; 1987. p. 96–117.

CHAPTER 23

Psychological Treatments for Tinnitus

Richard S. Tyler, PhD, William Noble, PhD, John P. Preece, PhD, Camille C. Dunn, PhD, Shelley A. Witt, MA

It may be decades before a magic pill is found to eliminate tinnitus, and, for the present, the most helpful treatment is appropriate psychological counseling. Millions of people have tinnitus and are not bothered by it, so it is logical to focus on moving tinnitus sufferers from the "bothered by" to the "not bothered by" group. In this chapter, we provide a general account of common psychological approaches to help patients with tinnitus.

NURTURING PATIENT EXPECTATIONS

Patient expectations can have a positive or negative effect on treatment outcomes in many clinical interventions.[1] Patient-clinician interactions seem to be most important with patients who exhibit high levels of stress or who are suffering from depression[2] or anxiety.[3] It has also been noted that the effect of nurturing is larger for subjective sensations than for sensations that are under autonomic control.[4] These observations suggest that to nurture patients' expectations could be useful in tinnitus management.

Tyler and colleagues have presented a protocol for maximizing the possible effects of patient expectation on outcomes of treatment for tinnitus.[5]

BEING PERCEIVED AS A KNOWLEDGEABLE PROFESSIONAL

Patients need to perceive the clinician as respected, well educated, and responsible. Professional attire and organized office arrangements can contribute to this. The clinician should demonstrate a deep knowledge of tinnitus and related problems and be able to express this in ways that are understandable to the patient.

BEING SYMPATHETIC TO THE PATIENT

It is axiomatic that a clinician needs to listen, but it is especially important for tinnitus sufferers, who, all too often, feel that they have not been heard. Also, the tinnitus patient may have felt that tinnitus was dismissed as a minor symptom. It is important for the clinician to acknowledge that the problems are real and important.

DEMONSTRATING AN UNDERSTANDING OF THE PROBLEM

Discussing tinnitus well is part of informational counseling. The clinician can discuss the prevalence, possible causes, related problems, common issues, and treatment options.

PROVIDING A CLEAR THERAPY PLAN

The patient needs a therapy plan. The specific plan may be developed from discussions of the specifics of the patient's situation, but it should be a concrete plan that is fully described. Patients need to know what is expected of them. The plan itself must be reasonable and achievable. Written procedures and patient diaries are helpful. These foster the feeling that "something is being done." The expected outcomes of the plan should be discussed. It is desirable that the patient partakes in designing the plan. Patients should not be left feeling that the clinician is necessary for their long-term well-being.

SHOWING THAT YOU SINCERELY CARE

Sincere caring will probably flow from the previous points. Plans for follow-up care can contribute to a positive feeling. The patient needs to feel welcome as an important part of the plan.

PROVIDING FEELINGS OF MASTERY

Many patients with tinnitus feel powerless. When given a plan to be carried out, they may begin to see that they are on the road to improvement, thus providing them with a better sense of control over the problem. This feeling is helped by involving the patient in at least some details of creating the therapy plan.

PROVIDING HOPE

The patient needs to believe that there is at least some likelihood of improvement. The patient may well have been previously told "There's nothing we can do" or "You'll just have to learn to live with it." Statements such as "Many patients benefit from this treatment" are helpful. In this regard, groups that include patients at different stages of treatment can be useful, as can meetings with patients who have experienced improvement. Confidence will be built up from all of the previous features, particularly the specific plan. It is equally important for the clinician to believe that the treatment protocol will be successful.

Flasher and Fogle have provided several excellent guidelines for audiologists and otolaryngologists interested in counseling.[6]

PROVIDING INFORMATION

Probably one of the oldest ways of trying to help patients with tinnitus is by providing information.[7] Helping people understand their disorder allows them to correct misconceptions and make informed decisions. Many people can have very inaccurate concepts about the disorder and can develop very maladaptive behaviors based on these misunderstandings. This is the basis of cognitive therapy (see below). Several clinicians have found that providing information is a critical part of treatment.[8-15] Patients with tinnitus are often concerned that they are going to become deaf, their tinnitus is a sign of a more significant disease, they are experiencing an hallucination or delusion as a symptom of a mental disorder, and there is nothing that can be done about their tinnitus.

Information that addresses these topics, and others, is listed in the following examples of areas usually covered when providing information:
- How we hear and what hearing loss is
- The causes and prevalence of tinnitus
- The difficulties caused by tinnitus
- Treatments available for tinnitus
- Things other people with tinnitus have done and found successful, such as playing soft sounds in the background

COUNSELING FOR SOUND THERAPIES

Many patients spontaneously report that the presence of a low-level background sound makes their tinnitus easier to tolerate at times.[16] Patients often devise ways of surrounding themselves with sound, and several management approaches include sound therapy.[8,17] Counseling is an integral part of all sound therapies.

Table 23-1 reviews four general categories of sound therapies. Environmental sounds, music, or broadband noise can be used. Tinnitus retraining therapy uses a noise set to "mix" with the tinnitus, but with the tinnitus still audible.[18] Masking therapy uses a noise that either fully masks the tinnitus or results in partial masking.[19] In all cases, when the sound is

TABLE 23-1. Rationale and Counseling for Different Types of Sound Therapy

Different Types of Sound Therapy	Type of Sound	Rationale	Counseling
Everyday sounds	Background environmental	Attention	Not attend to tinnitus
Music	Background music	Attention	Not attend to tinnitus
Retraining therapy	Noise at mixing point	Habituation	Do not fear tinnitus
Masking therapy	Low level or masking noise	Perception	Not attend to tinnitus; provide control

removed, the tinnitus is present. However, the temporary relief experienced in all of these procedures by some patients may have useful consequences. It arguably gives patients some control and demonstrates that they can "escape" from their tinnitus, even if only while they are exposed to the sound. In addition, the relief provided may be sufficient to change their attitude to a more positive approach toward their tinnitus and its management. The counterargument has been made by Budd and Pugh that use of masking sounds is a form of "passive coping," an avoidance or postponement of the time when materially different strategies for improved coping will be attempted (see the following sections of this chapter).[20]

The rationale and, therefore, the form of counseling accompanying each of the sound therapies are different (see Table 23-1). Counseling for the use of environmental sounds and music is expressed in terms of shifting attention away from the tinnitus. The sound can be seen as a "distracter." Counseling about the "mixing point" in retraining therapy is explained as eliminating the fear of tinnitus so that habituation can occur. Counseling for masking therapy is couched in terms of reducing or eliminating the prominence of the tinnitus, not attending to it, and providing the patient with control.[21]

DIRECTIVE COUNSELING FOR RETRAINING THERAPY

A tinnitus management procedure that has enjoyed considerable clinical support recently is tinnitus retraining therapy.[22] The components of this approach include a combination of partial masking at a "mixing point" and "directive counseling." The nature of the counseling component was not spelled out in detail by the original authors but generally involved teaching patients to adopt a different attitude to the tinnitus, to be less fearful of or threatened by it. At least four directive counseling sessions, of 1 to 2 hours each, were said to be needed.

Bartnik and Skarzynski recently made a comprehensive description of directive counseling.[23] According to these authors, directive counseling comprises, first, information about the auditory pathway and how noise and other injurious agents affect outer hair cells and thus the tuning properties of the basilar membrane. Next, patients are advised about random spontaneous neural activity that does not normally register cortically as an audible event but that injury at the cochlear level or higher may somehow be transformed into a phantom perception and experienced as akin to an audible sound. Patients are next taken through the results of the audiometric tests that they have undergone, including auditory brainstem responses and distortion-product otoacoustic emissions. They are reassured that abnormal test results are evident because this provides a tangible reason for the source of their tinnitus. This is combined with measurements of tinnitus pitch and loudness matches to indicate that their tinnitus originates as a peripheral disorder. Patients are advised that listeners naturally attend to audible events that are salient and hence cannot help focusing on tinnitus just because they believe that it must indicate something more serious.

The goal of directive counseling is explained to patients as training (or retraining) the auditory and associated systems to reduce the salience, hence the annoying quality, of the tinnitus. The point is made that even a low-energy signal such as tinnitus is highly detectable in very low-level backgrounds; hence, it is essential, as part of this (re)training, to ensure constant competing noise partly to "mix with" the tinnitus to promote long-term habituation, that is, reduced noticeability and audibility. Mixing is said to be achieved by the use of personally worn noise generators, in some cases in combination with hearing aids.

Several features of directive counseling deserve careful reflection.[24] For one, insistence that tinnitus is a "phantom perception" on the part of the person who experiences it lays some responsibility for its very presence on that person as against an approach that recognizes tinnitus as a consequence of cochlear injury, hence as something that happens to people. For another, the proposal that neurons in the auditory or limbic systems can be (re)trained may be puzzling for some patients. Training implies acquisition of a skill, and some patients might have difficulty with the concept that neurons can be "trained." Further, the argument that silence must always be avoided offers a less than appealing future to many patients. For some, even low-level noise makes their tinnitus worse, and others find it more difficult to communicate in noise. Finally, other patients report that they can get used to listening to the tinnitus and the noise, but when the noise is removed, the tinnitus regains its prominence.

It may be that modifications to directive counseling might improve its effectiveness.[25] For example, Goebel and colleagues modified and expanded the counseling for retraining therapy to encompass four weekly sessions of 4.5 hours each.[26] These authors state that they modified the counseling procedure to conform more with professional psychological standards for delivery of such programs. The results from the study by Goebel and colleagues suggest that their expanded counseling component is what achieved any traction in reducing tinnitus annoyance and distress.

COGNITIVE THERAPY

Cognitive therapy was developed as a treatment for depression, anxiety, pain, and related emotional problems[27] and was eventually applied to tinnitus.[14,28–30]

The basis of cognitive therapy is that the tinnitus is a stimulus that cannot be changed, but how one evaluates the tinnitus can be changed. It is how one evaluates or thinks about the tinnitus that influences the resulting anxiety and depression. A set of negative beliefs about tinnitus ("This noise means that I have a brain tumor," "This proves that I am seriously flawed," "This means that I'm a failure," "This stops me from enjoying things") causes negative evaluations of the self and its possibilities.

The cognitive restructuring approach for tinnitus was described in great detail by Henry and Wilson.[14,31] They propose sessions that include the following:
- The effect of thoughts on feelings and behavior
- The relationship among the situation (or events), our thoughts (or beliefs), and our emotions (or behaviors)
- Thinking and tinnitus: challenging and questioning negative automatic thoughts
- Identifying styles of negative thinking
- Controlling negative thoughts: thought management techniques
- Using self-instructional statements

Two extensive and well-written books by Henry and Wilson (one for clinicians and one for patients) have combined a tested cognitive therapy and behavior therapy (see below) and represent a landmark in tinnitus treatment.[14,31]

BEHAVIORAL THERAPY

Behavior can be modified, maintained, or shaped by events in our environment. If the consequences of tinnitus can be defined by a specific behavior, then conditioning principles can be applied to these behaviors. This includes systematic desensitization, which has been successfully applied to many phobias. Other applications of behavioral therapy to tinnitus can be found in the discussion of tinnitus treatment based on activities (see below).

Henry and Wilson have developed a detailed protocol for tinnitus management that combines some aspects of cognitive therapy and behavioral therapy.[14] Their protocol includes (1) information and education about the nature of the treatment program and about tinnitus; (2) cognitive restructuring, which is aimed at self-identifying and challenging of negative thoughts, as well as training in multiple skills to achieve this; and (3) a set of three behavior modification techniques: (a) imagery techniques: imagining tinnitus noises as positive signifiers; (b) attention control: training in refocusing of attention to nontinnitus events; and (c) relaxation training: progressive muscular relaxation and tension reduction techniques. The protocol occupies eight weekly sessions, together with intensive homework exercises.

IMAGERY TRAINING

Imagery involves focusing thoughts on something specific (usually pleasant) and therefore diverting thoughts away from something undesirable, such as tinnitus. One approach for tinnitus is to begin with an attractive visual image, such as lying on a beach in the Caribbean or in a cornfield in Iowa. Next, it might be useful to include auditory images, such as the sound of waves or wind through the leaves. It can also be possible to include the sound of the individual's tinnitus in the background, maintaining a pleasant image. These skills are intended to provide relief from tinnitus when it is particularly troublesome. Henry and Wilson provide specific protocols to accomplish imagery for tinnitus.[14]

ATTENTION CONTROL

Attention control can be used to switch attention away from the tinnitus when the tinnitus is bothersome. Patients are taught that they can control the focus of their attention. Practice sessions include bringing one of a pair of stimuli into the foreground while the other member of the pair is in the background. This could begin with two pictures placed side by side and then progresses to two acoustic stimuli, such as a fan noise and talking in an adjacent room. One of the acoustic stimuli can be replaced with the patient's tinnitus. Next, a picture and the tinnitus are paired, and then a thought and the tinnitus can be paired. The goal is to enable tinnitus sufferers to apply this to their tinnitus in stressful situations during the day. Ten minutes of daily home practice are prescribed in the protocol by Henry and Wilson.[14]

RELAXATION TRAINING

Relaxation can be helpful for everyone. Tinnitus sufferers can be tense and anxious, and relaxation therapy can be helpful.[14,32] The most common approach is progressive muscle relaxation, which involves tensing and relaxing different muscle groups (arms, face, neck, shoulders/abdomen, and legs/feet) using a guided protocol. Learning relaxation techniques is a skill, takes time (sometimes several months), and should be accompanied by home practice. Although self-help tapes are available, the results are often better with professional training. It is important to be able to recognize the tense states in everyday situations when tinnitus is bothersome and then to apply relaxation techniques.

COUNSELING FOR THE WHOLE PATIENT

Although we can focus on tinnitus and changing the way patients think and act regarding their tinnitus, it can be even more important to consider the patient in the broader context of his or her life situation. Such beliefs are incorporated into humanistic therapy and existential therapy.[6] Thus, it is important that the patient has a good self-image and finds meaning in life. The patient may be experiencing many traumas, tinnitus being only one. Understanding the person in his or her social environment and being generally supportive can be as helpful as dealing with the tinnitus.

TINNITUS TREATMENT BASED ON ACTIVITIES AND IMPAIRMENTS

In general, the problems created by tinnitus can be grouped as difficulties with emotional well-being, sleep, hearing, and concentration. Not everyone experiences problems in each area, and the magnitude of difficulties within each area varies across patients. These areas are also interrelated. We have been developing a new treatment procedure based on these activities and impairments. The exact procedure selected depends on the needs of the individual patient.

EMOTIONAL WELL-BEING

Tinnitus is often accompanied by anxiety and depression. These can be fed by difficulties in sleep, hearing, and concentration. Improvements in these and other areas often improve emotional well-being. Several approaches can help in improving the effects of tinnitus on the patient's emotional well-being. We characterize our approach into the following categories:
- Listening to the patient
- Providing information about hearing loss and tinnitus
- Ways to make tinnitus less important
- Changing things to manage better

Listening to the Patient It is critical to determine what is important for the individual patient. Why are they there? What do they expect? Are they alone, or do they have support? Are other important things going on in their life in addition to tinnitus? Probing questions can help obtain such information. The answers to these questions can influence the direction of counseling. Having the patient describe how tinnitus has affected his or her life can be a useful way to begin.

Providing Information about Hearing Loss and Tinnitus Providing information (see above) about hearing loss and tinnitus helps patients understand their disorder and its effects on their life, including the stress and intrusiveness. Figure 23-1 shows a picture that is used to help patients understand the effect of hearing loss on the number of nerve fibers and on spontaneous activity. These pictures, which are used in all aspects of our counseling, facilitate understanding and provide structure. Various causal models of tinnitus are explained. Specific issues are addressed (see cognitive restructuring above), for example, "Am I going to become deaf?" and "Do I have a tumor?" The importance of attention is emphasized. For example, Hallam notes that we normally attend to only one thing at a time.[9] He notes that our attention can be diverted to things that are unusual or surprising. He gives the example of a refrigerator hum being repetitive and meaningless, so our brain automatically tunes it out. Another example provided by Hallam is

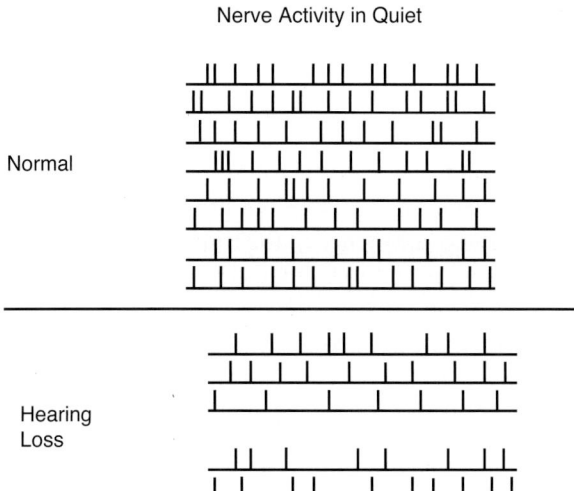

FIGURE 23-1. Picture shown to patients to help describe the effect of hearing loss on nerve survival and spontaneous activity. Earlier pictures, not shown here, are used to introduce the concepts of nerve fibers and spontaneous activity.

that we "cannot decide not to pay attention" to items because our brain subconsciously monitors the sensory environment for significant events. This is normal. If the patient decides that tinnitus is important to monitor, then he or she will not be able to habituate to it. Hallam suggests that most people can learn to ignore tinnitus in about 18 months.

Ways to Make Tinnitus Less Important Hopefully, providing information about tinnitus helps the patient understand that the tinnitus need not be threatening. It is helpful to know that others no longer attend to or substantially worry about their tinnitus. Sometimes this can be facilitated in group counseling. Other stress factors in the patient's life may also make the tinnitus more important than it would be otherwise.

Changing Things to Manage Better If appropriate, helping patients sleep, hear, and concentrate will help their emotional status too. Other approaches are to have the patient refocus on other activities, such as joining new clubs and learning new tasks. Support from others can be important. We ask some patients to make a list (sometimes keeping a diary for a few weeks) of situations in which their tinnitus is worse and situations in which their tinnitus is better. It is then possible to discuss these situations and determine if the patient's environment can be modified to increase the good situations and decrease the bad situations.

Sleep

Sleep disturbances are among the most commonly reported problems associated with tinnitus[16,32–34] and are even frequent in children with tinnitus.[35] Hallam and colleagues reported insomnia as the largest single factor in an analysis of tinnitus annoyance.[29] The nature of the sleep disturbance is quite variable and may include difficulty falling asleep, waking during the night, early awakening, or related factors, such as chronic fatigue.[32] An unclear issue is whether insomnia is directly the result of tinnitus or is caused by an emotional reaction to the tinnitus. It is conceivable that, at least for some patients, it is a combination of both. Sometimes helping people divert their attention away from tinnitus and improving their emotional well-being will improve sleep. Many people have misconceptions about normal sleep patterns and benefit from knowledge of the diverse common patterns. We suggest that they make their bedroom primarily a place for sleeping. They should avoid alcohol, smoking, and eating before bedtime and go to bed only when tired. Background sound, for example, soothing music, can be very helpful to tinnitus patients trying to sleep. Figure 23-2 shows an example of a picture shown to patients. In some cases, relaxation therapy might be appropriate.[36]

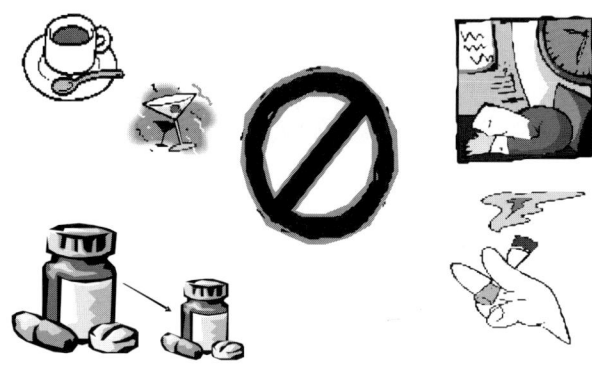

FIGURE 23-2. Picture shown to patients to facilitate discussion of factors influencing sleep.

IMPROVING HEARING

Improving hearing includes providing information about hearing, hearing loss, and tinnitus and implementing specific strategies to enhance hearing.

Information about Hearing, Hearing Loss, and Tinnitus In our procedure, we review with the patient the basic anatomy and physiology of the auditory system and how it is affected by hearing loss. We then discuss various difficulties that result from hearing impairment. We explain to the patient that hearing loss will make some sounds they hear seem distorted, whereas other sounds may be completely inaudible. We explain that tinnitus can cause difficulties in distinguishing one sound from another because it can be confused with other sounds.

Strategies to Improve Hearing The three main areas are using amplification, improving the listening environment, and enhancing communication. Patients who should benefit from hearing aids should obtain and use them. Patients are often unaware of how the environment influences their hearing performance. We advise them about good lighting, positioning, minimizing visual distractions, and minimizing noise. We teach the concepts involved in using an effective communication style. This includes the use of repair strategies for communication breakdowns and anticipatory strategies prior to communication interactions, how to disclose hearing loss to others when appropriate, and speech-reading strategies.

CONCENTRATION

We focus on three activities to improve concentration in patients with tinnitus: providing information, decreasing the prominence of the tinnitus, and increasing attention to the task at hand.

Providing Information about Concentration Difficulties We discuss with patients the fact that everyone can be distracted by visual and auditory stimuli. Stimuli that are distracting are often annoying, fearful, competing with the desired target, loud, unpredictable, and uncontrollable.

Reducing the annoying and fearful interpretation of tinnitus can reduce its influence on concentration. We review the differences among people in their ability to concentrate. Some people cannot read in a noisy café, whereas others are not bothered by the surrounding noise. Some people have also learned ways to focus their attention away from chronic pain. Many people find that they can perform some tasks without being distracted by tinnitus. We discuss reasons for these individual differences. We ask the patient if there are situations in which they are not distracted by their tinnitus. What is it about these tasks, and can some of their characteristics be transposed to other situations?

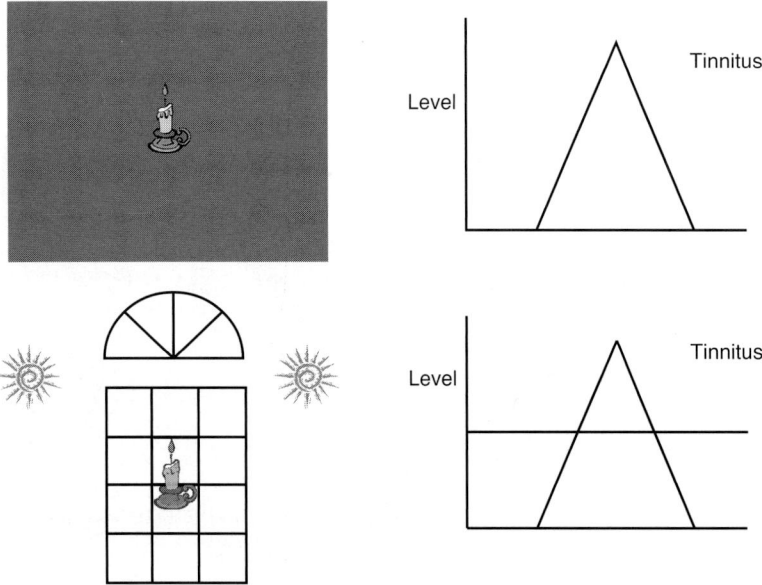

FIGURE 23-3. Picture shown to patients to discuss the potential advantage of introducing low-level background sound with the tinnitus still audible (partial masking). The candle appears bright in a dark room, but the same candle is not as prominent when other light sources are in the background. The prominence of the tinnitus depends on the contrast.

Decreasing the Intrusiveness of the Distracter
Decreasing the prominence of tinnitus can reduce its distracting nature. This can be accomplished by various kinds of sound therapy, including the use of background music, broadband noise, or inconsequential everyday sounds. Figure 23-3 shows a picture that is used to discuss the concept of decreasing the prominence of the tinnitus. A candle in a dark room appears to be brighter than the same candle in a light room. In some patients, introducing another sound could make attending more difficult. However, many prefer a broadband rushing-water sound compared with their screeching tinnitus. In addition, being able to tolerate external sounds reduces the intrusiveness of the tinnitus.

Facilitating Focusing Attention on the Task
Treatments to divert attention away from pain and onto other features have been studied for some time,[37] and analogies have been made between chronic pain and tinnitus.[30] One approach to attention diversion for tinnitus is described in detail by Henry and Wilson.[14] Patients practice alternately bringing stimuli into the foreground and background, such as the sensation of clothes on the skin. Similar practice occurs directing their attention to and from their tinnitus. They learn that there are some aspects of their attention that they can control and that they can divert attention away from their tinnitus and onto the task at hand, at least sometimes.

A different strategy is to manipulate the environment so that the patient can experience successful attention in the presence of their tinnitus. One approach is to make the task easier by reducing the complexity or duration of the task. For example, reading can be segmented into shorter intervals. It can also be helpful if a patient feels more confident about his or her ability to concentrate. This can be achieved by successfully learning a new task. The patient must be motivated and must want to learn the task. Examples might include learning to play a musical instrument or to use new computer software. A new task is necessarily more engaging,[38] which makes it easier to focus attention and disregard the tinnitus.

RESEARCH ON PSYCHOLOGICAL THERAPY EFFECTIVENESS

A recent meta-analysis has allowed direct comparison of various psychological treatments for tinnitus. Andersson and Lyttkens considered (1) differences in critical variables between treatment and no-treatment control groups, (2) differences between pre- and post-treatment scores in treatment groups, and (3) differences in pretreatment and follow-up scores in treatment groups.[39] To express in uniform fashion a range of different outcomes, involving different metrics, they used the effect size approach. In this statistic, the two values of interest (treatment vs control, post-treatment vs pretreatment, follow-up vs pretreatment) are compared. The difference between these two scores is divided by the (shared) standard deviation. A positive effect size reflects the reduction in the variable of interest (for the present purposes, reduction in tinnitus annoyance, reduction in negative affect, reduction in sleep disturbance). An effect size approaching 1.0 is considered large to very large for clinical research; an effect size approaching zero means that the distributions of the two sets of values are very similar.

The analysis performed by Andersson and Lyttkens demonstrates, first, the quantity and type of evidence of treatment effects across the range of psychological interventions. These interventions are (1) biofeedback, (2) cognitive-behavioral therapy, (3) education or information, (4) hypnosis, (5) relaxation, and (6) stress management or problem solving. Second, it showed that there is a better evidence base (randomized controlled

Table 23-2. Average Effect Sizes between Pretreatment and ≥ 3 Months Post-treatment owing to Various Psychological Tinnitus Management Procedures on Three Variables: Subjective Tinnitus Annoyance Level, Negative Affect (Depression/Anxiety), and Effect on Sleep

Treatment Type	Tinnitus Annoyance	Negative Affect	Sleep
Cognitive-behavioral therapy	0.5 (8)	0.29 (5)	0.26 (3)
Relaxation	0.45 (3)	—	−0.05 (2)
Education/information	0.29 (2)	−0.28 (1)	—

Values in parentheses indicate the number of studies contributing to this effect size value. Negative values indicate an increase in the problem.

treatments) for cognitive-behavioral therapy than for other psychological treatments. The authors concluded that cognitive-behavioral therapy emerges as more consistently effective than treatments based on hypnosis, biofeedback training, or relaxation. Table 23-2 shows a subset of their data comparing only studies with pretrial and post-trial data with at least 3 months of follow-up that used randomized controls. Note that the sleep effect size for relaxation (−0.05) was an average from two studies with quite different results. The procedure in one study was helpful in aiding sleep (effect size of 0.71), but a different procedure in another study had the opposite effect (effect size of −0.8). There are limitations on the use of effect sizes as summary measures across studies, and different implementations of any of the types of treatment might yield alternative results.

SUMMARY

No treatment is available to cure tinnitus. Until such a treatment is available, management must focus on helping people find ways to cope better with their tinnitus. Some commonly used psychological strategies have been reviewed here, and it is likely that other psychological principles could be helpful.[40] Generally, efforts to nurture the patient's expectations can create a more positive attitude toward his or her tinnitus. Providing information about tinnitus is a helpful first step. Various forms of sound therapy, which generally provide some background sound to compete with the tinnitus, are widely available. If used, each requires complementary counseling. Various combinations of cognitive and behavioral therapy are commonly applied. In addition, it is important to consider the patient in the broader context of his or her life problems and support. We describe a new procedure based on the common impairments of tinnitus: emotional well-being, sleep, hearing, and concentration.

Very few controlled studies have been reported to test the effectiveness of these strategies. Well-designed studies are needed. Preliminary results suggest that a combination of cognitive and behavioral therapy could be the best approach. All of these treatments will require further modification and adaptation to individual needs and verification of their effectiveness. Nonetheless, these psychological management strategies form the foundation of current tinnitus management.

ACKNOWLEDGMENTS

We wish to acknowledge grant support provided by the Obermann Center for Advanced Studies at The University of Iowa and the American Tinnitus Association. Anne-Mette Mohr, Cynthia Bergan, and Diana Kain made valuable contributions to the development of our ideas.

REFERENCES

1. Bootzin RR. The role of expectancy in behavior change. In: White L, Schwartz B, editors. Placebo: theory, research, and mechanisms. New York: Guilford Press; 1985. p. 196–201.
2. Frank JD, Frank JB. Persuasion and healing, a comparative study of psychotherapy. Baltimore (MD): Johns Hopkins University Press; 1991.
3. Shapiro AK. Factors contributing to the placebo effect, their implications for psychotherapy. Am J Psychother 1964;25:145–56.
4. Bourne HR. The rational use of the placebo. In: Melmon KL, Morelli HF, editors. Clinical pharmacology. 2nd ed. New York: Macmillan; 1978. p. 1052–62.
5. Tyler RS, Haskell G, Preece J, Bergan C. Nurturing patient expectations to enhance the treatment of tinnitus. Semin Hear 2001;22:15–21.
6. Flasher LV, Fogle T. Counseling skills for speech-language pathologists and audiologists. Albany (NY): Thomson/Delmar Learning; 2004.
7. Fowler EP, Fowler EP Jr. Somatopsychic and psychosomatic factors in tinnitus, deafness, and vertigo. Ann Otol Rhinol Laryngol 1955;64:29–37.
8. Tyler RS, Babin RW. Tinnitus. In: Cummings CW, Fredrickson JM, Harker L, et al, editors. Otolaryngology—head and neck surgery. St. Louis (MO): Mosby; 1986. p. 3201–17.
9. Hallam RS. Tinnitus—living with the ringing in your ears. San Francisco (CA): Harper Collins Publishing; 1989.
10. Tyler RS, Stouffer JL, Schum R. Audiological rehabilitation of the tinnitus client. J Acad Rehabil Audiol 1989;22:30–42.
11. Stouffer JL, Tyler RS. Characterization of tinnitus by tinnitus patients. J Speech Hear Disord 1990;55:439–53.
12. Dobie RA, Sullivan MD. Antidepressant drugs and tinnitus. In: Vernon JA, editor. Tinnitus: treatment and relief. Boston: Allyn & Bacon; 1998. p. 43–51.

13. Tyler R S, Erlandsson S. Management of the tinnitus patient. In: Luxon LM, Furman JM, Martini A, Stephens D, editors. Textbook of audiological medicine. Oxford (UK): Isis Publications; 2000. p. 571–8.
14. Henry JL, Wilson PH. The psychological management of chronic tinnitus: a cognitive-behavioral approach. Boston: Allyn & Bacon Publishers; 2001.
15. Tyler RS, Smith RJ. Management of tinnitus in children. In: Newton VE, editor. Paediatric audiological medicine. Philadelphia: Whurr Publishers Ltd; 2002. p. 397.
16. Tyler RS, Baker LJ. Difficulties experienced by tinnitus sufferers. J Speech Hear Disord 1983;48:150–4.
17. Vernon J, Schleuning A. Tinnitus: a new management. Laryngoscope 1978;88:413–9.
18. Jastreboff PJ. Tinnitus habituation therapy (THT) and tinnitus retraining therapy (TRT). In: Tyler RS, editor. Handbook of tinnitus. San Diego (CA): Singular Publications; 2000. p. 357–76.
19. Vernon J, Meikle M. Tinnitus masking: theory and practice. In: Tyler RS, editor. Handbook of tinnitus. San Diego (CA): Singular Publications; 2000. p. 313–56.
20. Budd RJ, Pugh R. The relationship between coping style, tinnitus severity and emotional distress in a group of tinnitus sufferers. Br J Health Psychol 1996;1:219–29.
21. Preece JP, Tyler RS, Noble W. The management of tinnitus. Geriatr Aging 2003;6:22–8.
22. Jastreboff PJ, Hazell JW. A neurophysiological approach to tinnitus: clinical implications. Br J Audiol 1993;27:7–17.
23. Bartnik G, Skarzynski H. In: Tyler RS, editor. Tinnitus treatment protocols.[In preparation]
24. Wilson PH, Henry JL, Andersson G, et al. A critical analysis of directive counseling as a component of tinnitus retraining therapy. Br J Audiol 1998;32:273–86.
25. Kroener-Herwig B, Biesinger E, Gerhards F, et al. Retraining therapy for chronic tinnitus. A critical analysis of its status. Scand Audiol 2000;29:67–78.
26. Goebel G, Rübler D, Stepputat F, et al. Controlled prospective study of tinnitus retraining therapy compared to tinnitus coping therapy and broad-band noise generator therapy. In Hazell J, editor. Proceedings of the Sixth International Tinnitus Seminar. London: The Tinnitus and Hyperacusis Centre; 1999. p. 302–6.
27. Beck AT, Rush AJ, Shaw BF, Emery G. Cognitive therapy for depression. New York: Guilford Press; 1979.
28. Sweetow RW. Cognitive-behavioral modification in tinnitus management. Hear Instrum 1984;35:14–52.
29. Hallam RS, Jakes SC, Hinchcliffe R. Cognitive variables in tinnitus annoyance. Br J Clin Psychol 1988;27:213–22.
30. Wilson PH, Henry JL, Nicholas M. Cognitive methods in management of chronic pain and tinnitus. Aust Psychol 1993;28:172–80.
31. Henry JL, Wilson PH. Tinnitus: a self-management guide for the ringing in your ears. Boston: Allyn & Bacon Publishers; 2002.
32. McKenna L. Tinnitus and insomnia. In: Tyler RS, editor. Handbook of tinnitus. San Diego (CA): Singular Publications; 2000. p 59–84.
33. Alster J, Shemesh Z, Ornan M, Attias J. Sleep disturbance associated with chronic tinnitus. Biol Psychiatry 1993;34:84–90.
34. Axelsson A, Ringdahl A. Tinnitus: a study of its prevalence and characteristics. Br J Audiol 1989;23:53–62.
35. Kentish RC, Crocker SR, McKenna L. Children's experience of tinnitus: a preliminary survey of children presenting to a psychology department. Br J Audiol 2000;34:335–40.
36. Hallam R, Rachman S, Hinchcliffe R. Psychological aspects of tinnitus. In: Rachman S, editor. Contributions to medical psychology. Vol 3. Oxford (UK): Pergamon Press; 1984. p. 31–53.
37. Turk DC, Genest M. Regulation of pain: the application of cognitive and behavioral techniques for prevention and remediation. In: Kendall P, Hollon S, editors. Cognitive-behavioral interventions: theory, research and prevention. New York: Academic Press; 1979.
38. Logan G. Automaticity and cognitive control. In: Uleman J, Bargh J, editors. Unintended thought. New York: Guilford; 1989.
39. Andersson G, Lyttkens L. A meta-analytic review of psychological treatments for tinnitus. Br J Audiol 1999;33:201–10.
40. Tyler RS. Perspectives on tinnitus. Br J Audiol 1997;31:381–16.

EDITORIAL COMMENTARY

Establishment of a conditioned reflex involving tinnitus that results in adverse physiologic and behavioral reactions is discussed in Chapter 8, "The Neurophysiological Model of Tinnitus." Chapter 21, "Tinnitus Retraining Therapy," is perhaps Jastreboff and Jastreboff's most comprehensive exposition of tinnitus retraining therapy (TRT).

Jastreboff and Jastreboff point out that TRT addresses the established conditioned reflex in which tinnitus-related neuronal activity in the auditory system activates the limbic and autonomic nervous systems to produce physiologic and behavioral reactions to the tinnitus. Two strategies are employed for the extinction of the conditioned reflex: counseling to help the patient reclassify the tinnitus signal as a neutral stimulus that weakens the connection between the auditory system and the limbic and autonomic nervous systems and thereby decreases the activation of these systems and sound stimulation to reduce the strength of the tinnitus signal in the auditory system, which further lessens the stimulus activating the limbic and autonomic nervous systems.

Jastreboff and Jastreboff advocate TRT for the treatment of decreased sound tolerance and clinically significant tinnitus. Variations in counseling and sound therapy for the two problems should be considered. In the management of the patient with tinnitus, counseling is directed at reclassifying the tinnitus signal as nonthreatening by discussing tinnitus as a phantom auditory perception, the role of the limbic and autonomic nervous systems, conditioned reflexes, and habituation. In hyperacusis, the counseling stresses the consequences of increased gain in the auditory pathway and secondary activation of the limbic and autonomic nervous systems owing to over-amplification of the signal evoked by external sounds. In misophonia, the initial signal is the activity evoked by external sounds. Sound therapy increases the background neuronal activity in the auditory system and thereby decreases the prominence of the tinnitus signal. Although there is an intensity range of effective sound for tinnitus therapy, in hyperacusis, the sound must be below the level inducing annoyance or discomfort.

Jastreboff and Jastreboff emphasize that the reactions of the limbic and autonomic nervous systems and not the percept of tinnitus are responsible for the suffering from tinnitus. Conditioned reflexes cannot be modified by cognition. Habituation of the reactions to tinnitus, not the perception of tinnitus, is sufficient to relieve clinically significant tinnitus. Habituation occurs at a subconscious level and is facilitated by decreasing negative input from cognitive centers and presenting an alternative view explaining how tinnitus occurs and why it evokes adverse reactions. The process of retraining involves changing the importance of neuronal connections in pathways between the auditory system and the limbic and autonomic nervous systems to minimize the reinforcement of the conditioned reflex. Extinction of a conditioned reflex occurs at a subconscious level and takes place when its reinforcement subsides, even though the stimulus, in this case the tinnitus signal, persists. Once extinction of the reflex occurs, counterproductive functional links will diminish, tinnitus-related neuronal activity will be constrained to the subconscious level of the auditory pathways, and the tinnitus will become part of the familiar background.

Sheldrake and Jastreboff point out that for some patients with tinnitus, hearing aids can provide complete suppression of the perception of tinnitus while they are worn. A hearing aid amplifies ambient sound, which increases the stimulation of the auditory pathways and thereby decreases the relative strength of the tinnitus signal. Hearing aids also reduce the strain to hear, thus lowering the stress and anxiety brought on by tinnitus. Furthermore, amplification of ambient sound masks the tinnitus for many individuals. Approximately 15% of initial hearing aid users experience effective and stable masking.

Sheldrake and Jastreboff emphasize that binaural hearing aid fitting is preferable whenever possible and that open earmolds should be used. Too much occlusion can make tinnitus worse. Care should be taken to minimize the patient's attention to tinnitus, and proper education of the patient is crucial for successful use of hearing aids for the management of tinnitus.

Regarding psychological methods of therapy, Tyler and colleagues point out that cognitive therapy is focused on how one thinks about tinnitus and avoidance of negative ideation, whereas behavioral therapy focuses on imagery techniques, attention control, and relaxation training.

They emphasize the beneficial roles of providing information and nurturing a positive attitude toward tinnitus and its management. Patients who should benefit from hearing aids should use them. The use of sound therapy requires individualized complementary counseling. They also emphasize the importance of considering the whole context of the patient's life situation.

Tyler and colleagues advocate combining cognitive and behavioral therapy to improve emotional well-being, sleep, hearing, and concentration according to the specific needs of the patient. Indeed, they point out that cognitive and behavioral therapy are the foundation of the current management of tinnitus.

James B. Snow Jr

CHAPTER 24

Electrical Suppression of Tinnitus

Jay T. Rubinstein, MD, PhD, Richard S. Tyler, PhD

HISTORY

Tinnitus is sufficiently common and distressing that it has been described in medical texts for more than three millennia. According to Feldmann, the first mention of tinnitus in archival materials derived from Egyptian papyri dates to the second or third century BCE.[1,2] It is not unexpected that efforts to treat tinnitus would be comparably ancient and would attempt to use all available technologies of a given era. Thus, the topical herbal treatments of ancient Egypt made way for the application of the battery at the dawn of the nineteenth century.[3] Volta first determined that current flowed from his battery by touching it to his tongue; it is not surprising that he subsequently applied it to his own external auditory canals.[3] The 50-volt shock he applied to himself reportedly knocked him down, plausibly owing to vestibular stimulation, and produced a loud and persistent tinnitus-like auditory percept. Volta's experiment arguably heralded the twin birth of cochlear implantation and electrical manipulation of tinnitus, but, apparently, he chose not to repeat the experience himself.

Within 1 year of Volta's publication describing the battery, the first reliable source of ongoing electrical current, a subsequent paper detailed a complex apparatus for electrical stimulation of the external ears (Figure 24-1).[4] Throughout the nineteenth century, various authors described multiple methods for such

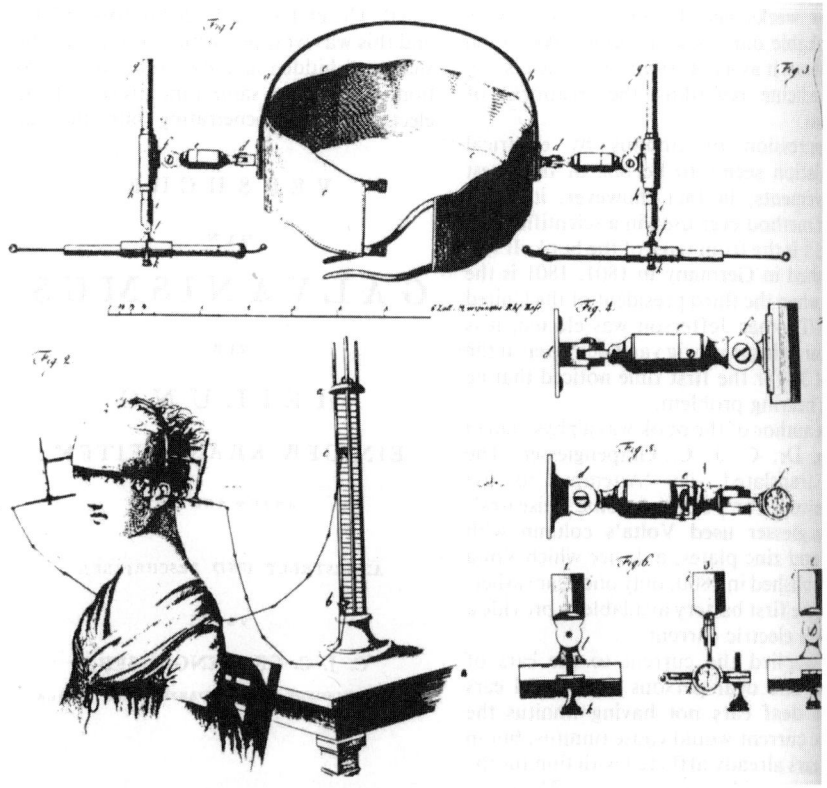

FIGURE 24-1. Apparatus for electrical stimulation of external auditory canals for treatment of deafness and tinnitus. Reproduced with permission from Grapengiesser CJC.[4]

stimulation as a treatment for deafness and tinnitus. Stimulation sites included the external auditory canal, auricle, zygoma, tragus, mastoid, and eustachian tube orifice. Electrodes included balls, wicks, and, in one case, needle electrodes applied simultaneously to the eustachian tube transnasally and the promontory transtympanically. Although, in the first half of the nineteenth century, all such stimulation used direct current, known as galvanization, the invention of the induction coil spawned the use of alternating current, or faradization. Such treatments were apparently so widespread that an entire book by Brenner was devoted to electrical stimulation of the ears: *Investigations and Observations on the Effect of Electric Current on the Hearing Organ in the Healthy and Ill.*[5] The subtitle of the book, *Attempts to Create a Rational Electro-Otology*, suggests a response to the appropriate skepticism with which claims of cures of deafness and tinnitus were met. By the early twentieth century, therapeutic electrical stimulation of the ears had fallen out of favor.

Despite the uncontrolled nature of the experiments reported during the nineteenth century, multiple authors noted a number of consistent observations. They frequently observed that anodal direct current applied to the ipsilateral mastoid or zygoma could temporarily suppress or eliminate tinnitus in some patients, whereas cathodal stimulation more commonly caused auditory percepts and an increased intensity of tinnitus. In this century, Hatton and colleagues replicated these findings using electrodes placed on the zygomatic arches bilaterally.[6] Similar findings were also noted in multiple publications from Bordeaux, France.[7–10] The latter group applied electrical stimuli via a transtympanic electrode to the round window and promontory.

The 200-year-old finding that anodal direct current can suppress tinnitus in some cases has, unfortunately, not resulted in a useful clinical intervention. This is due to limitations in the ability to stimulate biologic tissue with direct current chronically. Such stimulation leads to tissue necrosis from multiple mechanisms, including hydrolysis and other toxic electrochemical reactions.[11] Only specific frequencies and intensities of alternating current, such as those used in cochlear implants, are safe for chronic stimulation.

With the increasing use of cochlear implantation as a treatment for profound hearing impairment, a substantial literature documented that tinnitus suppression is a common beneficial side effect of this modern form of electrical stimulation.[12–20] Although the reported efficacy rate varies from 28 to 79%, it is quite unusual, even in a large cochlear implant center, to have implant recipients complain of disabling tinnitus. This is in contrast to individuals with moderate to severe hearing impairment using hearing aids, for whom marked and bothersome tinnitus is quite common. One might expect that patients with implants would suffer similarly if they were deprived of their speech processors for a period of time.

The promising early results with anodic direct current stimuli, the knowledge that direct current cannot be applied continuously without causing tissue injury, and the success with cochlear implants have led to numerous studies of alternating current stimulation for suppression of tinnitus.[21–27] These studies have used external and middle ear electrodes and a variety of stimulus waveforms and again suggest that in some patients, tinnitus can be suppressed and occasionally eliminated. The results of these studies are variable and confusing, however, and none of them were placebo controlled, limiting the conclusions that can legitimately be drawn. A tinnitus suppression device, the Audimax Theraband, initially produced considerable enthusiasm[28] but was relegated to historical interest by a carefully designed, double-blind, placebo-controlled trial.[29] It is of note, however, that this device produced a verifiable, repeatable, and clinically relevant tinnitus suppression in one subject using electrodes located on the mastoid.

PHYSIOLOGIC MECHANISMS

As described in the previous section, a wide variety of stimulus waveforms, electrode locations, and patients with tinnitus have been tested in an empiric and uncontrolled manner. Our current understanding of tinnitus pathophysiology is not much more advanced than it was in Volta's era, and well-executed empiric studies are still important and potentially powerful tools. It is, however, important to understand the possible mechanisms by which electrical stimulation can suppress tinnitus. It should be noted that although all of the mechanisms to be discussed presume a peripheral cause of tinnitus, none of them exclude the possibility of secondary central dysfunction, such as an increase in central auditory "gain" in response to loss of peripheral input. Many recent data point to such central dysfunction as an important physiologic correlate of tinnitus.[30–34]

An electrical stimulus to a normally functioning cochlea can evoke a variety of possible responses, including electrophonic activation of the basilar membrane, direct polarization of hair cells with modulation of transmitter release, and direct polarization of spiral ganglion cells with modulation of spontaneous firing or induction of spike activity.[35] Thus, if tinnitus were due to some abnormal increase in peripheral activity, a stimulus that decreased this activity could potentially suppress tinnitus without producing audible percepts. Alternatively, a stimulus that increased peripheral activity could potentially "mask" the tinnitus but would presumably also be audible, offering little advantage over acoustic masking.

Because tinnitus is most commonly associated with sensorineural hearing loss, the most plausible hypothesis is that tinnitus is due, at least initially, to a pathologic decrease in peripheral spontaneous activity.[36,37] If this is the case, an electrical stimulus could potentially suppress tinnitus without producing audible percepts through the restoration of normal levels of peripheral spontaneous activity. This intriguing concept is explored further in this chapter.

SITE OF EXCITATION

It is clear from work with galvanic stimulation of the vestibular system that small (~ 1 mA) currents applied to the external ear can excite the labyrinth.[38–40] Such stimuli can, however, also excite the somatosensory system. Stimuli on the zygoma will evoke trigeminal activity, whereas those posterior to the auricle will stimulate the cervical roots. Recent clinical work documents craniocervical somatosensory modulation of tinnitus,[41] and neurophysiological studies have documented the mechanisms by which such modulation can occur.[42] It seems likely that at least some of the electrical stimulations in studies discussed earlier, particularly those that demonstrate differences between anodal and cathodal stimuli applied to the skin around the ear, achieved their effects through modulating the somatosensory system and its connections to the cochlear nuclei. It is known that anodal electrical stimulation of fiber terminals hyperpolarizes the terminal but depolarizes the fiber more centrally. This would lead to increased excitability of a somatosensory axon[43] and possible tinnitus suppression via somatosensory modulation. A similar mechanism would lead to decreased excitability with cathodal stimuli. These effects are precisely the opposite of what is seen in auditory nerve fibers with intracochlear electrical stimulation.[44]

The previous discussion indicates that "electrical stimulation of the ear" implies only inner ear stimulation when the electrodes are intracochlear, and thresholds for auditory nerve fibers are typically well below those of other cranial nerves. Electrical stimulation in the middle ear allows the potential for stimulation of Jacobson's nerve or of somatic afferents from the tympanic membrane or external auditory canal. All have the theoretic potential to modulate tinnitus without altering firing in the auditory nerve directly. Thus, "middle ear stimulation," including round window and promontory electrode placements, suffers from similar ambiguity as "external ear stimulation" with regard to the neurons affected by the stimulus.

The possibility of multiple sites of excitation with both external and middle ear electrodes may be partly responsible for the variety of outcomes observed both within and across studies of electrical stimulation for tinnitus. This possibility is strengthened by contrasting this extraordinary variability with the far more consistent observation of tinnitus suppression in patients with cochlear implants. Studies in recipients of cochlear implants are complicated only by the variability of tinnitus and its perception, not by ambiguity as to the site of excitation. Although the variability of tinnitus perception is itself a significant experimental problem, psychoacoustic studies demonstrate that it is a tractable one.[45,46]

PLACEBO CONTROL

It is unclear to what degree placebo responses have played a role in earlier trials of electrical stimulation for tinnitus. Some investigators report minimal placebo effects,[22] whereas in other studies, placebo was more frequently effective than the treatment.[29] It should be noted, however, that even in the latter study, placebo effects were rare enough that 75% of subjects had no tinnitus improvement with the placebo or the test condition. Owing to substantial placebo effects in drug trials for tinnitus,[47,48] any potential therapy for tinnitus, including electrical stimulation, should undergo a rigorous placebo-controlled trial prior to widespread clinical use. Depending on the relationship between any percepts produced and the tinnitus suppression achieved by a given electrical stimulation paradigm, adequate placebo control may or may not be possible. If the stimulation is perceived by the subject, it is necessary to devise some sort of placebo stimulus that is identically perceived but has a different effect or no effect on the tinnitus. If this is not possible, other procedures can be used to minimize the likelihood of placebo responses. The time course of tinnitus suppression and recovery can be monitored and repeatedly measured. Repeatable tinnitus suppression with a consistent time course argues against placebo effects. The stimulus waveform, frequency, and intensity can be modified to search for some "optimal" parameter. If, for example, a "best intensity" exists, this argues against placebo effects.[22] Lastly, false trials without a stimulus presented can be implemented randomly without feedback to the subject.

"RATIONAL ELECTRO-OTOLOGY?"

As discussed earlier, one possible mechanism for tinnitus associated with sensorineural hearing loss is the loss of normal spontaneous activity that occurs with damage to inner hair cells.[36,37] Normally, the peripheral auditory nerve fibers are spontaneously active in quiet.[49] This spontaneous firing of the auditory nerve is due to continuous, undriven release of neurotransmitter at the inner hair cell synapse.[50] This release process and the resulting firing patterns of the spiral ganglion have been extensively observed, modeled, and analyzed in multiple species. For durations on the order of seconds, transmitter release reflects a Poisson process, a specific pattern of random vesicle release.[51] Refractory properties of the auditory neurons modify the transmitter release process, resulting in spike times reflecting what is known as a renewal process or a Poisson process with dead time. Early theories for the peripheral origin of tinnitus suggest that loss of this normal pattern of spontaneous activity can lead to abnormal central auditory activity perceived as sound.[36,37] In this light, spontaneous activity may be viewed as the "code for silence." This theory is consistent with the fact that most tinnitus is associated with hearing loss and most hearing loss is associated with loss or alteration of spontaneous activity.[52] It also explains why cochlear nerve section is usually ineffective and, not uncommonly, makes tinnitus worse.[12] Although investigators using animal models associate tinnitus with increased spontaneous activity in the dorsal cochlear nucleus, the presence of lateral inhibition in the cochlear nuclei could produce this finding in response to decreased spontaneous activity in the periphery.[53,54] The efficacy of acoustic masking with white noise can then be explained through the effect of such noise on the periphery; it evokes spike intervals similar to those of spontaneous activity. The primary difference between spontaneous activity and noise-evoked responses is the across-fiber correlation that acoustic noise produces in neurons innervating adjacent locations on the basilar membrane.

It has been demonstrated with a computational model that an appropriate electrical stimulus may produce a spontaneous-like renewal process in the auditory nerve, a process that is uncorrelated across fibers.[55] Much of the underlying theory has been confirmed in animal studies,[56-58] which demonstrate uncorrelated, Poisson-like activity across a population of auditory nerve fibers activated by an unmodulated 5,000 pulse/s stimulus. A rational hypothesis is that such stimuli can suppress tinnitus without producing an auditory percept by restoring the "code for silence." No prior studies have effectively examined such stimuli for tinnitus suppression owing to the engineering difficulties of delivering such high rates; these rates have become available only in cochlear implant stimulators recently.[59] Because most tinnitus sufferers do not have severe to profound hearing loss, such a hypothesis should be tested, at least initially, with stimuli applied outside the cochlea. As mentioned earlier, this then leads to ambiguity as to exactly what is stimulated, so a parallel test of the hypothesis should involve patients with severe to profound hearing impairment managed with cochlear implants. The recent advent of "hybrid" or "electroacoustic" cochlear implantation allows partial intracochlear insertion of an electrode array with preservation of residual low-frequency hearing.[60] If the hypothesis is correct, such technology creates the future potential for intracochlear stimulation for tinnitus suppression even in patients with mild hearing loss.

RESULTS

The hypothesis that unmodulated high-rate pulse trains can suppress tinnitus without producing a percept has now been tested using transtympanic stimulation in 13 subjects with mild to moderate hearing loss and intracochlear stimulation in four subjects with profound hearing loss who were managed with cochlear implants.[27]

No Response or Limited by Pain (Four Transtympanic Subjects, One Cochlear Implant Subject)

In two transtympanic subjects, no perception of the stimulus, pain, or effect on tinnitus could be elicited up to the maximal current output of the stimulator (> 1.1 mA at 80 μs/phase). In two other subjects, stimulation above approximately 400 μA evoked pain. No significant sound percept or tinnitus effect was noted below this pain threshold. Jacobson's nerve was found to be posteriorly displaced in one of these subjects. It was resting on the anterior lip of the round window niche and was likely responsible for the atypical pain percept in this subject. Multiple electrode placements were attempted to avoid pain perception without success. The cochlear implant subject noted no change in her tinnitus with current levels up to most comfortable loudness on multiple electrodes.

Electrical Tinnitus "Masking" (Three Transtympanic Subjects, One Cochlear Implant Subject)

Three transtympanic subjects showed tinnitus suppression only in the presence of a stimulus percept. All noted that the stimulus percept sounded similar to their underlying tinnitus. Figure 24-2 illustrates the tinnitus and stimulus percepts over time, along with the stimulus current presented for one of the subjects. The response pattern was similar for all three subjects and did not demonstrate any significant residual inhibition. No particular subject preference for the stimulus percept over the underlying tinnitus was noted in response to questioning. Figure 24-3 demonstrates a similar "masking" pattern in the cochlear implant subject. Tinnitus is suppressed only during perception of the stimulus and virtually mirrors this perception. There was no residual inhibition. Although this phenomenon is clearly different from acoustic masking, we call it a "masking" pattern to differentiate it from tinnitus suppression in the absence of a percept. It is virtually identical to the results reported by Dauman.[61]

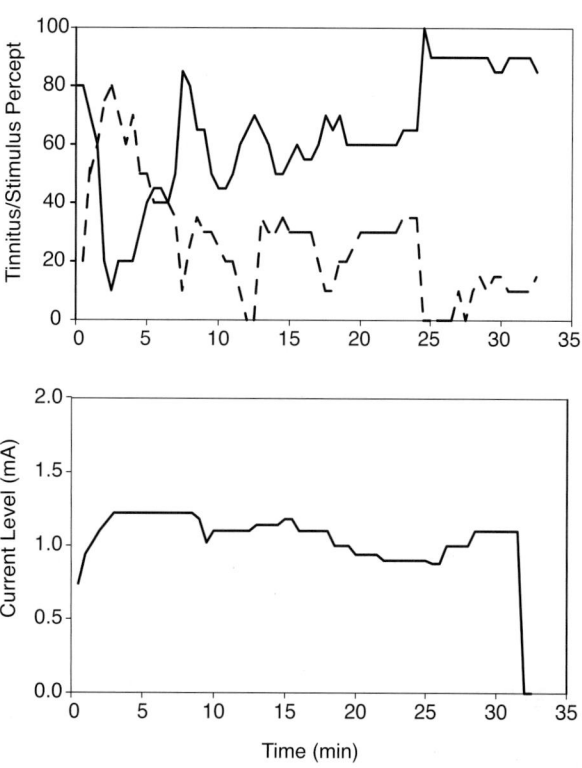

FIGURE 24-2. Tinnitus and stimulus perceptions of subject with transtympanic electrical stimulation of the round window. Stimulus frequency 4,800 Hz, 80 μs/phase. *Dashed line* is stimulus percept; *solid line* is tinnitus percept. The perception of the stimulus appeared to produce a masking effect on the perception of tinnitus in this subject.

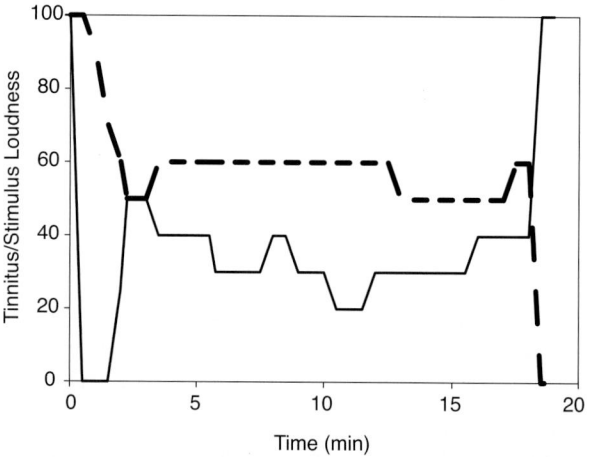

FIGURE 24-3. Tinnitus and stimulus perceptions of a subject with activation of his Cochlear Corporation CI-24M cochlear implant. Stimulus frequency 4,800 Hz, 25 μs/phase using electrode 14 in monopolar mode. Stimulus onset at time 0, offset at 18 minutes. *Dashed line* is stimulus percept; *solid line* is tinnitus percept. The perception of the stimulus appeared to produce a masking effect on the perception of tinnitus in this subject.

ELECTRICAL TINNITUS SUPPRESSION (SIX TRANSTYMPANIC SUBJECTS, TWO COCHLEAR IMPLANT SUBJECTS)

Six subjects showed suppression of tinnitus in the absence of a stimulus percept or after complete or nearly complete adaptation to the stimulus percept. In the development of speech processing strategies for cochlear implants, we noted that there is a dramatic degree of adaptation to the unmodulated high-rate pulse trains used in this study.[62] Round window stimulation demonstrated this phenomenon in four of the subjects, who initially perceived loud tinnitus-like sounds when the stimulus was ramped up. After several minutes, a time course comparable to that observed in our cochlear implant subjects, the stimulus perception adapted to zero or near-zero followed shortly after by a decrement in the perceived tinnitus. There was a residual inhibition lasting from 45 minutes to 72 hours in five of the subjects. Five of the six patients who suppressed in this manner found clinically significant relief from the annoyance of their tinnitus and were very pleased with the result. Figure 24-4 demonstrates the tinnitus and stimulus percepts from one of these subjects. In all of these individuals, stimulation at lower pulse rates and/or at lower current levels did not evoke tinnitus suppression.

Figure 24-5 demonstrates tinnitus suppression in one of the four cochlear implant subjects. It verifies that tinnitus suppression in this subject was repeatable. There appeared to be a level-dependent effect, with higher currents evoking more rapid and complete tinnitus suppression. The perceptions produced by the two stimuli were identical, and the tinnitus suppression was therefore effectively single-blinded because no feedback was given to the subject. Residual inhibition lasted approximately 45 minutes.

CASE STUDY

R. H. is a 63-year-old woman with a past history of Meniere's disease in the left ear. She underwent an endolymphatic shunt 10 years previously, which eliminated her incapacitating vertigo but was complicated by profound deafness and bothersome tinnitus in the involved ear. After informed consent was obtained, she underwent transtympanic round window stimulation following the protocol above,[27] and nearly complete tinnitus suppression was obtained for a period of

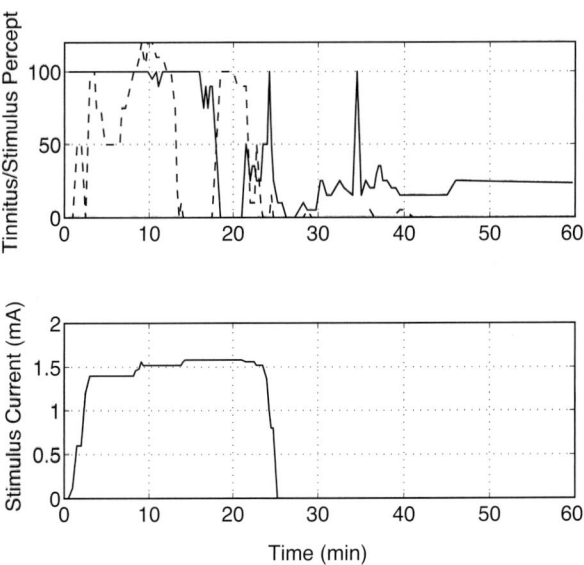

FIGURE 24-4. Tinnitus and stimulus perceptions of subject T. S. with transtympanic electrical stimulation of the round window. Stimulus frequency 4,800 Hz, 80 μs/phase. *Dashed line* is stimulus percept; *solid line* is tinnitus percept. The perception of the stimulus was followed by rapid adaptation and subsequent suppression of tinnitus.

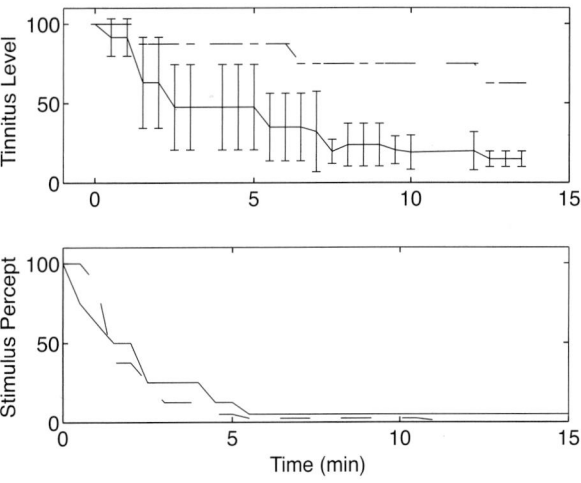

FIGURE 24-5. Tinnitus and stimulus perceptions of a subject with activation of her Cochlear Corporation CI-24M cochlear implant. Stimulus frequency 4,800 Hz, 25 μs/phase using electrode 7 in monopolar mode. The *dashed line* represents a stimulus intensity of 134 clinical units; the *solid line* represents 142 clinical units. Error bars represent the range of three repetitions on three separate days.

about 45 minutes. After further informed consent was obtained, she elected to undergo cochlear implantation in the deaf ear with the intention of determining whether chronic tinnitus suppression could be achieved with the same stimulus protocol. Surgical implantation of a CI-24 contour (Cochlear Corporation, Lane Cove, Australia) was uneventful.

One month postoperatively, her device was activated, and an apical electrode was pitch-matched to her low-frequency tinnitus. This electrode was then stimulated with a 4,800 pps unmodulated pulse train that was slowly increased while tinnitus and stimulus percepts were noted. Her transtympanic suppression was replicated with intracochlear stimulation, but, unfortunately, the effect was not long lasting. Although the tinnitus was nearly completely suppressed without any lasting percept of the stimulus, it would slowly rise back to prestimulation levels after approximately 45 minutes of continuous stimulation. After many sessions, we demonstrated that tinnitus suppression without a stimulus percept can be maintained over at least a 5-hour period by turning the stimulus on and off at several different levels every few minutes. Our current studies are focused on development of a placebo-controlled paradigm that produces similar transient percepts but does not suppress the tinnitus. R. H. is extremely gratified that she is able to exercise some level of control over her tinnitus. Her subsequent artwork provides her depiction of the distress caused by her tinnitus (Figure 24-6).

DISCUSSION

At this time, the only clinically effective treatment that decreases the loudness of tinnitus is acoustic masking. Although this is helpful for some patients, for others it simply replaces one undesirable sound with another. An ideal therapy for tinnitus would create the perception of silence or at least decrease the loudness of tinnitus without introducing any new sounds. We demonstrated in 6 of 13 subjects that this is possible, at least temporarily. Although placebo control in the current experimental paradigm is not ideal, we doubt that these six subjects are demonstrating significant placebo effects given the similarity of their responses to those of the cochlear implant subjects, for whom single-blinded placebo control was possible. In addition, multiple stimulus frequencies and intensities failed to suppress tinnitus in the process of data ac-

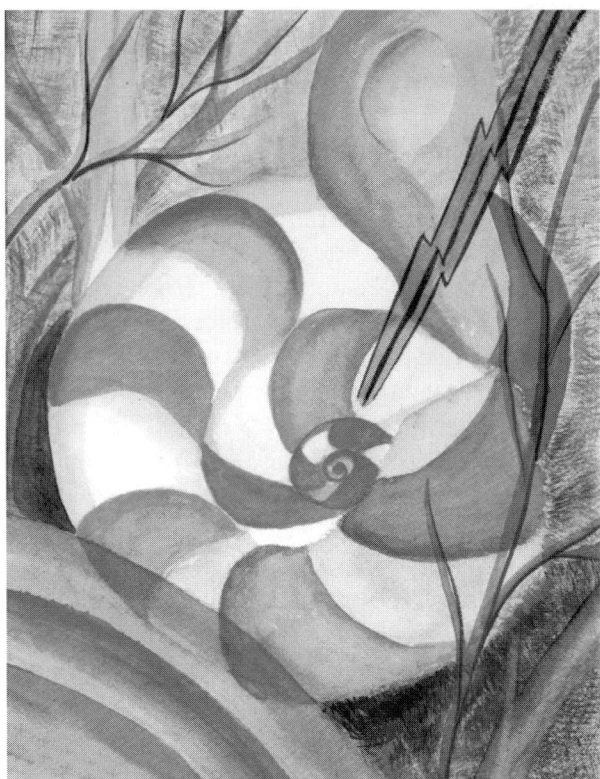

FIGURE 24-6. Painting by chronically implanted subject R. H. depicting her perception of the impact of tinnitus on her life. She performed this work after undergoing the studies described in the text.

quisition for these subjects. Because of the prolonged residual inhibition of tinnitus produced by the stimulus, test–retest variability could not be assessed in the transtympanic subjects because this would have required a second myringotomy at a later testing session.

Although the theory underlying the hypothesis tested would suggest rapid (< 20 milliseconds) onset and offset of spontaneous-like activity in the auditory nerve, tinnitus suppression as induced in the seven subjects appears to be a slow process. Onset of tinnitus suppression typically required between 5 and 15 minutes of stimulation, and residual inhibition lasted from minutes to days. This suggests involvement of an unknown central process and is in contrast to the immediate "masking" effects in four subjects. The prolonged residual inhibition is puzzling but must also represent some central effect and does not support or refute the underlying theory. Gibson reported that 8% of 27 cochlear implant patients with tinnitus note residual inhibition lasting from 30 to 60 minutes.[15]

One of our cochlear implant patients, who is not in this study, reported that his tinnitus returns only when his implant is turned off for more than 24 hours. Although unusually long relative to residual inhibition with acoustic masking,[63] the residual inhibition reported here may, in fact, make clinical application of a tinnitus suppression device easier.

Our findings support the hypothesis that high-rate electrical pulse trains applied to the round window can result in tinnitus suppression without an ongoing stimulus percept. Two problems must be addressed before a clinical device becomes feasible. First, with the notable exception of two cochlear implant subjects, it is still not clear whether the effects we describe are repeatable within a subject. Repeatability is critical for the long-term use of a tinnitus suppression device and for placebo control during a clinical trial. Second, it is not clear whether the stimulation has an effect on acoustic thresholds. On questioning, none of our subjects noted decreased hearing during stimulation. In fact, one subject spontaneously noted improved clarity of speech perception during the stimulation. Nevertheless, increased hearing thresholds and/or decreased speech recognition are a possibility owing to either a mechanical effect of the round window electrode or interaction between electrical stimulation and acoustically evoked hair cell activity.[35] Answering these questions will require that more human subjects undergo surgical implantation of a modern, cochlear implant–like device in the cochlea or at the round window that can be tested repeatedly and used chronically. Although electrical stimulation is clearly not a panacea, it will likely play a future role in the management of some patients with severe tinnitus.

REFERENCES

1. Feldmann H. History of tinnitus research. In: Shulman A, editor. Tinnitus diagnosis/treatment. San Diego (CA): Singular Publishing Group, Inc.; 1997. p. 3–37.
2. Feldmann H. Suppression of tinnitus by electrical stimulaton: a contribution to the history of medicine. J Laryngol Otol Suppl 1984;9:123–4.
3. Volta A. On the electricity excited by the mere contact of conduction substances of different kinds. Philos Trans R Soc Lond B Biol Sci 1800;90:403–31.
4. Grapengiesser CJC. Versuche den Galvanismus zur heilung einiger Krankheiten anzuwenden. Berlin: 1801.
5. Brenner R. Untersuchungen und Beobachtungen uber die Wirkung elektrischer Strome auf das Gehororgan im gesunden und kranken Zustande. Leipzig: 1868.
6. Hatton DS, Erulkar SD, Rosenberg PE. Some preliminary observations on the effect of galvanic current on tinnitus aurium. Laryngoscope 1960;70:123–30.
7. Aran JM. Neural correlates of electrically induced cochlear dysfunction. Clin Otolaryngol 1977;2:305–10.
8. Aran JM. Electrical stimulation of the auditory system and tinnitus control. J Laryngol Otol Suppl 1981;4:153–62.
9. Aran JM, de Sauvage R, Cazals Y. Observation of an electrically evoked whole-nerve response using the same stimulating and recording electrode. Hear Res 1980;2:343–6.
10. Aran JM, Cazals Y. Electrical suppression of tinnitus. Ciba Found Symp 1981;85:217–31.
11. Agnew WF, McCreery DB, Bullara LA, Yuen TGH. Effects of prolonged electrical stimulation of peripheral nerve. In: Agnew WF, McCreery DB, editors. Neural prostheses: fundamental studies. Englewood Cliffs (NJ): Prentice Hall; 1990.
12. House JW, Brackmann DE. Tinnitus: surgical treatment. Ciba Found Symp 1981;85:204–16.
13. House JW. Effects of electrical stimulation on tinnitus. J Laryngol Otol Suppl 1984;9:139–40.
14. Tyler RS, Kelsey D. Advantages and disadvantages reported by some of the better cochlear-implant patients. Am J Otol 1990;11:282–9.
15. Gibson WPR. The effects of electrical stimulation and cochlear implantation on tinnitus. In: Aran JM, Dauman R, editors. Tinnitus 91: proceedings of the Fourth International Tinnitus Seminar. Amsterdam: Kugler; 1992. p. 403–8.
16. Zwolan TA, Kileny PR, Souliere CR, Kemink JL. Tinnitus suppression following cochlear implantation. In: Aran JM, Dauman R, editors. Tinnitus 91: proceedings of the Fourth International Tinnitus Seminar. Amsterdam: Kugler; 1992. p. 423–6.
17. Bredburg G, Walden J, Lindstrom B. Tinnitus after cochlear implantation. In: Aran JM, Dauman R, editors. Tinnitus 91: proceedings of the Fourth International Tinnitus Seminar. Amsterdam: Kugler; 1992. p. 417–22.
18. Dauman R, Tyler RS, Aran JM. Intracochlear electrical tinnitus reduction. Acta Otolaryngol (Stockh) 1993;113:291–5.

19. Tyler RS. Tinnitus in the profoundly hearing-impaired and the effects of cochlear implants. Ann Otol Rhinol Laryngol Suppl 1995;165:25–30.
20. Ruckenstein MJ, Hedgepeth C, Rafter KO, et al. Tinnitus suppression in patients with cochlear implants. Otol Neurotol 2001;22:200–4.
21. Vernon JA, Fenwick JA. Attempts to suppress tinnitus with transcutaneous electrical stimulation. Otolaryngol Head Neck Surg 1985;93:385–9.
22. Kuk FK, Tyler RS, Rustad N, et al. Alternating current at the eardrum for tinnitus reduction. J Speech Hear Res 1989;32:393–400.
23. Hazell JWP, Jastreboff PJ, Meerton LE, Conway MJ. Electrical tinnitus suppression: frequency dependence of effects. Audiology 1993;32:68–77.
24. Okusa M, Shiraishi T, Kubo T, Matsunaga T. Tinnitus suppression by electrical promontory stimulation in sensorineural deaf patients. Acta Otolaryngol Suppl (Stockh) 1993;501:54–8.
25. Ito J, Sakakihara J. Tinnitus suppression by electrical stimulation of the cochlear wall and by cochlear implantation. Laryngoscope 1994;104:752–4.
26. Matsushima JI, Sakai N, Uemi N, et al. Evaluation of implanted tinnitus suppressor based on tinnitus stress test. Int Tinnitus J 1997;3:123–31.
27. Rubinstein JT, Tyler RS, Johnson A, Brown CJ. Electrical suppression of tinnitus with high-rate pulse trains. Otol Neurotol 2003;24:478–85.
28. Shulman A. External electrical stimulation in tinnitus control. Am J Otol 1985;6:110–5.
29. Dobie RA, Hoberg KE, Rees TS. Electrical tinnitus suppression: a double-blind crossover study. Otolaryngol Head Neck Surg 1986;95:319–23.
30. Salvi RJ, Lockwood A, Burkard R. Neural plasticity and tinnitus. In: Tyler RS, editor. Tinnitus handbook. San Diego (CA): Singular Publishing Group, Inc.; 2000. p. 1–24.
31. Lockwood AH, Salvi RJ, Coad ML, et al. The functional neuroanatomy of tinnitus: evidence for limbic system links and neural plasticity. Neurology 1998;50:114–20.
32. Lockwood AH, Wack DS, Burkard RF, et al. The functional anatomy of gaze-evoked tinnitus and sustained lateral gaze. Neurology 2001;56:472–80.
33. Melcher JR, Sigalovsky IS, Guinan JJ Jr, Levine RA. Lateralized tinnitus studied with functional magnetic resonance imaging: abnormal inferior colliculus activation. J Neurophysiol 2000;83:1058–72.
34. Plewnia C, Bartels M, Gerloff C. Transient suppression of tinnitus by transcranial magnetic stimulation. Ann Neurol 2003;53:263–6.
35. Miller CA, Abbas PJ, Rubinstein JT, et al. Effects of remaining hair cells on cochlear implant function. Fifth quarterly progress report NO1-DC-9-2106. Neural Prosthesis Program. Bethesda (MD): National Institutes of Health; 2000.
36. Kiang NYS, Moxon EC, Levine RA. Auditory-nerve activity in cats with normal and abnormal cochleas. In: Wolstenhome GEW, Knight J, editors. Sensorineural hearing loss. London: JEA Churchill; 1970. p. 241–73.
37. Kiang NYS, Liberman MC, Levine RA. Auditory nerve activity in cats exposed to ototoxic drugs and high-intensity sounds. Ann Otol Rhinol Laryngol 1976;75:752–68.
38. Jahn K, Naessl A, Schneider E, et al. Inverse U-shaped curve for age dependency of torsional eye movement responses to galvanic vestibular stimulation. Brain 2003;126:1579–89.
39. MacDougall HG, Brizuela AE, Curthoys IS, Halmagyi GM. Three-dimensional eye-movement responses to surface galvanic vestibular stimulation in normal subjects and in patients: a comparison. Ann N Y Acad Sci 2002;956:546–50.
40. Watson SR, Welgampola MS, Colebatch JG. EMG responses evoked by the termination of galvanic (DC) vestibular stimulation: 'off-responses.' Clin Neurophysiol 2003;114:1456–61.
41. Levine RA. Somatic (craniocervical) tinnitus and the dorsal cochlear nucleus hypothesis. Am J Otolaryngol 1999;20:351–62.
42. Shore SE, El Kashlan H, Lu J. Effects of trigeminal ganglion stimulation on unit activity of ventral cochlear nucleus neurons. Neuroscience 2003;119:1085–101.
43. Rubinstein JT. Axon termination conditions for electrical stimulation. IEEE Trans Biomed Eng 1993;40:654–63.
44. Miller CA, Robinson BK, Rubinstein JT, et al. Auditory nerve response to monophasic and biphasic electric stimuli. Hear Res 2001;151:79–94.
45. Tyler RS, Conrad-Armes D. Masking of tinnitus compared to masking of pure tones. J Speech Hear Res 1984;27:106–11.
46. Tyler RS. Psychoacoustical measurement. In: Tyler RS, editor. Tinnitus handbook. San Diego (CA): Singular Publishing Group, Inc.; 2000. p. 149–80.

47. Duckert LG, Rees TS. Placebo effect in tinnitus management. Laryngoscope 1984;92:697–9.
48. Dobie RA, Sakai CS, Sullivan MD. Antidepressant treatment of tinnitus patients: report of a randomized clinical trial and clinical prediction of benefit. Am J Otol 1993;14:18–23.
49. Liberman MC. Auditory nerve responses from cats raised in a low-noise environment. J Acoust Soc Am 1978;75:442–55.
50. Sewell WF. The relation between the endocochlear potential and spontaneous activity in auditory nerve fibers of the cat. J Physiol 1984;347:685–96.
51. Johnson DH. Point process models of single-neuron discharges. J Comput Neurosci 1996;3:275–99.
52. Liberman MC, Dodds LW. Single-neuron labeling and chronic cochlear pathology. II. Stereocilia damage and alterations of spontaneous discharge rates. Hear Res 1984;16:43–53.
53. Kaltenbach JA, Godfrey DA, Neumann JB, et al. Changes in spontaneous neural activity in the dorsal cochlear nucleus following exposure to intense sound: relation to threshold shift. Hear Res 1998;124:78–84.
54. Zhang JS, Kaltenbach JA. Increases in spontaneous activity in the dorsal cochlear nucleus of the rat following exposure to high-intensity sound. Neurosci Lett 1998;250:197–200.
55. Rubinstein JT, Wilson BS, Finley C, Abbas PJ. Pseudospontaneous activity: stochastic independence of auditory nerve fibers with electrical stimulation. Hear Res 1999;127:108–18.
56. Runge-Samuelson C. Response of the auditory nerve to sinusoidal electrical stimulation: effects of high-rate pulse trains [thesis]. Iowa City (IA): University of Iowa; 2002.
57. Litvak L, Delgutte B, Eddington D. Auditory nerve fiber responses to electric stimulation: modulated and unmodulated pulse trains. J Acoust Soc Am 2001;110:368–79.
58. Litvak L. Towards a better speech processor for cochlear implants: auditory nerve responses to high rate electric pulse trains [thesis]. Boston (MA): Massachusetts Institute of Technology; 2002.
59. Rubinstein JT, Hong RS. Signal coding in cochlear implants: exploiting stochastic effects of electrical stimulation. Ann Otol Rhinol Laryngol Suppl 2003;191:14–9.
60. Gantz BJ, Turner CW. Combining acoustic and electrical hearing. Laryngoscope 2003;113:1726–30.
61. Dauman R. Electrical stimulation for tinnitus suppression. In: Tyler RS, editor. Tinnitus handbook. San Diego (CA): Singular Publishing Group, Inc.; 2000. p. 377–98.
62. Hong RS, Rubinstein JT, Wehner D, Horn D. Dynamic range enhancement for cochlear implants. Otol Neurotol 2003;24:590–5.
63. Tyler RS, Conrad-Armes D, Smith PA. Postmasking effects of sensorineural tinnitus: a preliminary investigation. J Speech Hear Res 1984;27:466–74.

EDITORIAL COMMENTARY

Rubinstein and Tyler review the evidence that tinnitus is initially due to decreased spontaneous activity in the auditory nerve. They point out the ambiguity that exists in electrical stimulation of the middle ear as to whether the effect is due to auditory nerve stimulation or somatosensory stimulation that is known to be capable of modulating tinnitus.

In stimulating the inner ear, that ambiguity is avoided. A high rate of electrical pulses (5,000/s) restores spontaneous-like activity in the auditory nerve, and this may be the way in which it suppresses tinnitus.

Rubinstein and Tyler demonstrated that high-rate electrical pulse trains can suppress tinnitus without producing an audible percept. The remaining problems of repeatability, placebo control, and hearing effect require further research with surgical implantation of advanced cochlear implant–like devices in the cochlea to determine the future role of electrical suppression in the management of tinnitus.

James B. Snow Jr

CHAPTER 25

Veterans and Tinnitus

James A. Henry, PhD, Martin A. Schechter, PhD, Raymond T. Regelein, Kyle C. Dennis, PhD

There are presently over 26.6 million US military veterans.[1] Tinnitus has always been a concern for veterans because of their common history of noise exposure during military service. Through a claims process, veterans can apply for a "service-connected" disability for their tinnitus that, if successful, generally results in monthly compensation benefits and access to Veterans Affairs (VA) clinical services. In recent years, service-connected disabilities for tinnitus have been awarded at an accelerating rate. These claims are particularly problematic because there is no objective clinical method to verify a report of subjective tinnitus.

This chapter has the following objectives: (1) to bring awareness to the increasing problem of tinnitus as a health concern for veterans; (2) to bring awareness to the economic cost of a preventable health condition to the American taxpayers through the Department of Veterans Affairs (DVA) and its component administrations, the Veterans Health Administration (VHA) and the Veterans Benefits Administration (VBA); and (3) to provide suggestions for implementing short- and long-term solutions to meeting the needs of veterans with tinnitus and of the VHA for managing tinnitus as a clinical issue.

A MULTIFACETED PROBLEM

The problem of veterans and tinnitus is multifaceted. From the veteran's perspective, affliction with intractable tinnitus has a detrimental effect on quality of life, which can range from mild to severe. If a veteran believes that the tinnitus was caused by noise exposure during military service, he or she would reasonably expect to receive clinical management for the condition. Most VA medical centers, however, do not provide comprehensive clinical services for veterans suffering from tinnitus. Even when such services are offered, only veterans who have received an award for service-connected disability are usually eligible to receive the services. The claims process to apply for service connection can be lengthy and arduous, and military records often lack evidence to substantiate tinnitus claims.

In keeping with the mission of the VHA, the VA Healthcare System is accountable to meet the needs of veterans with all kinds of health concerns, including tinnitus. Incorporating any new form of clinical management into standard VA practice, however, requires research evidence.[2] To date, unequivocal evidence supporting the efficacy of any model of tinnitus treatment does not exist, although different methods of tinnitus treatment have been in clinical use for many years. The present challenge for the VA Healthcare System is to fulfill its obligation to meet the needs of veterans requiring tinnitus services without the proof of efficacy that is usually required.

As already mentioned, claims for tinnitus disability are being submitted and awarded at an ever-increasing rate. The total compensation amount for veterans with service-connected tinnitus, exceeding a quarter of a billion dollars yearly, is a revelation to most people. The VHA must address the escalating cost of providing compensation benefits, which points to the need to evaluate tinnitus claims more effectively to ensure that the claimed tinnitus is real and that the asserted cause is correct.[3]

TINNITUS PROGRAMS AT THE PORTLAND, OREGON, VA MEDICAL CENTER

The Portland VA Medical Center (PVAMC) has been atypical of VA medical centers with respect to the provision of tinnitus programs. For a number of years, the PVAMC has offered comprehensive clinical care for veterans with tinnitus who reside in the Portland, OR, vicinity. In addition, numerous clinical research projects have been conducted and are presently under way that focus on providing evidence for tinnitus treatment methods and developing standardized tinnitus assessment procedures.

In the audiology clinic at the PVAMC, tinnitus rehabilitation has been provided to veterans for over 20 years using a "tinnitus masking" approach.[4] This clinical program has been generally successful in meeting the needs of eligible veterans requiring tinnitus services in the Portland area. In addition, a tinnitus "support group" has been offered at the PVAMC since 1999. The consistently well-attended group has provided an educational outreach to all veterans with tinnitus, regardless of their eligibility for clinical services.

Tinnitus research has been conducted at the PVAMC since 1995 under the auspices of the VA National Center for Rehabilitative Auditory Research (NCRAR) since 1997. The longest-running tinnitus project has been the development of techniques for acoustically matching loudness, pitch, and other tinnitus characteristics using a computer-automated testing format.[5–7] The present phase of this work will develop a clinic-ready system that will include the capability to test for "tinnitus malingering." For treatment of tinnitus, a controlled clinical trial was recently completed (described briefly at the end of this chapter) that compared the clinical effectiveness of tinnitus masking and tinnitus retraining therapy (TRT).[8] A second clinical trial is under way to evaluate the efficacy of providing group education for veterans with tinnitus (outcome data are currently being collected at the VA Puget Sound Health Care System). Conclusions and insights drawn from these outcome studies will bear directly on future efforts to ameliorate problematic tinnitus in veterans.

Additional information about these various tinnitus programs is provided below. These programs have provided important insights concerning the needs of veterans with tinnitus and the avenues of pursuit to meet those needs.

ESTIMATED PREVALENCE OF TINNITUS IN VETERANS

Tinnitus prevalence in veterans can be estimated on the basis of its prevalence in the general population. Numerous epidemiologic studies are in general agreement that tinnitus is a chronic condition for 10 to 15% of adults.[9–13] If the prevalence of tinnitus in veterans is the same as in the general population, the estimates from these studies would suggest that 2.7 to 4 million of the 26.6 million veterans experience tinnitus as a chronic condition. The actual number of veterans with tinnitus may be higher because the veteran population tends to be older than the general population, and tinnitus prevalence is believed to increase with age.[14] Although 17% of the general population is at least 65 years of age, 36% of veterans are in this age category.[15] The oldest cohort of veterans is actually increasing and will increase over 500% in the next 15 years.[16] This is also the group most likely to complain of tinnitus.

Incidence data for diseases are obtained as a result of physicians reporting new cases to government agencies.[17] Tinnitus, however, is not a "reportable" disease; in fact, tinnitus is only a symptom and not a disease entity. Thus, incidence data are limited for tinnitus, either within or outside the VA (see Chapter 3, "Epidemiology of Tinnitus"). Nonetheless, two factors that will undoubtedly increase the incidence of tinnitus in the VA population are military noise exposure and the predominance of males, which increases the likelihood of nonmilitary noise exposure.

VETERANS BENEFITS ACT OF 2002

On December 6, 2002, President George W. Bush signed Public Law 107-330, the Veterans Benefits Act. Among other things, the law mandates that the DVA contract with the National Academy of Sciences to conduct an investigation of (1) noise exposure in the military and how noise can be the cause of hearing loss and tinnitus in veterans; (2) additional factors that could contribute to auditory disorders in veterans, including age and occupational history; (3) hearing conservation programs within the Armed Forces; and (4) accounting of claims submitted for hearing loss and tinnitus and the outcomes of those claims. The Academy's report is expected to be a landmark account of the problem of tinnitus in veterans.

In its original form, the Senate bill (S.2237) designated hearing loss and tinnitus as "presumptive" service-connected conditions for veterans who served in military occupations that involved hazardous levels of noise. Designating hearing loss and tinnitus as presumptive for certain noise-hazardous occupations would have benefited primarily those veterans who served before there were calibrated audiometric measurements or effective hearing conservation programs (before about 1980). Veterans who served later, however, would also have realized a significant advantage with respect to their eligibility to be awarded a service connection for their tinnitus. One can imagine how designating tinnitus as a presumptive service-connected condition could result in a flood of new claims that would practically be ensured of receiving approval.

Congress recognized the importance of a study on hearing loss and tinnitus in the military as the basis for possible future legislation related to hearing loss and tinnitus compensation. Congress therefore eliminated the language authorizing hearing loss and tinnitus as presumptive conditions and required the comprehensive report by the National Academy of Sciences. The Academy's study is presently under way.

DISABILITY COMPENSATION

The DVA regards tinnitus as a disabling condition. Veterans with service-connected disabilities may receive monetary benefits as compensation for this disability.

Service Connection for Disabilities

The term "service connected" refers to a disability resulting from "disease or injury incurred or aggravated during active military service."[18] Disability is based on the effect of the condition on the functioning of the whole person. The amount of disability compensation corresponds to the degree of disability on a scale of 0 to 100% (in 10% increments). Many veterans are rated at 0%, which awards an entitlement for VA health care services but without monetary compensation benefits. Forty-eight percent of original claims (all disabilities) in 2001 were rated at 0%.[19] For the same year, 40% of original claims were rated at 10%.

The payment amount for service-connected disability is based on a fixed scale assigned to the degree of disability, and the compensation amounts increase disproportionately for the higher percentage awards. For example, the current (2004) basic monthly award for a disability rated at 100% is $2,239, whereas the monthly award for a disability rated at 10% is $106.

Service Connection for Tinnitus

Current law allows the DVA to grant only a 10% disability rating for service-connected tinnitus, regardless of its severity or bilaterality. A 10% tinnitus disability presently pays $1,272 per year (based on $106 per month). Veterans groups have submitted initiatives to attempt to raise the 10% level in certain instances.

Figure 25-1 shows the numbers of veterans receiving compensation benefits for their tinnitus for 1994 to 2003.[20] Figure 25-2 shows the corresponding tinnitus disability compensation for these veterans. It is apparent that these numbers are increasing in an exponential fashion. By September 2003, 242,610 veterans had received a service connection for their tinnitus, including 18,367 rated at 0%, 224,195 rated at 10%, and 48 rated between 20 and 100%. There were, therefore, 224,243 veterans rated 10% or greater who received compensation for their tinnitus disability. The total yearly compensation amount for these veterans is $285,449,640 (based on

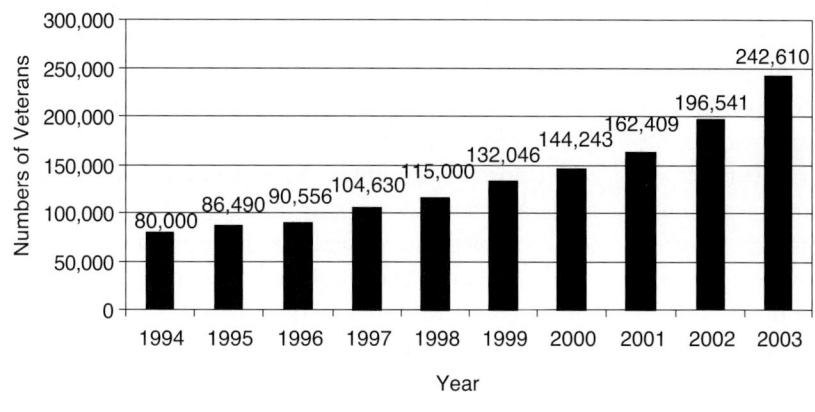

FIGURE 25-1. Numbers of veterans with a service-connected tinnitus disability, during years 1994 to 2003.

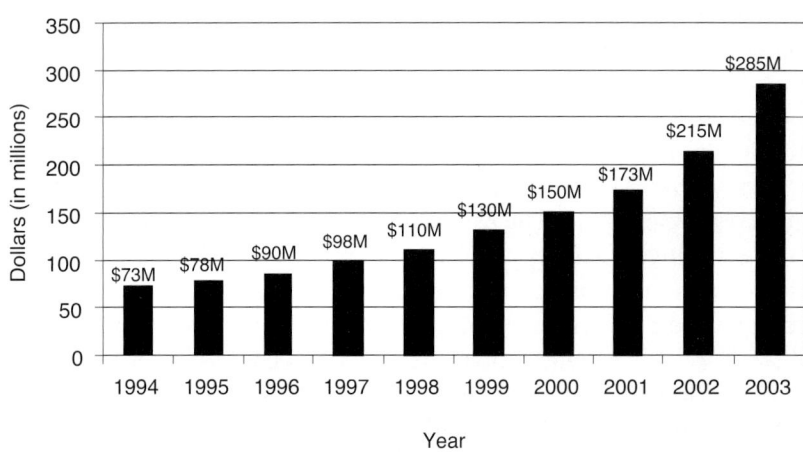

FIGURE 25-2. Yearly compensation dollars (in millions) to veterans for their service-connected tinnitus disability (corresponds directly with numbers shown in Figure 25-1).

tinnitus as the only service-connected disability; tinnitus combined with other disabilities requires formulae to determine precise compensation amounts; these data are not available). Tinnitus is now the most common service-related disability in veterans who first received disability compensation beginning in 2001.[19]

There are a number of reasons for the accelerated growth in tinnitus claims. Before 1999, the DVA awarded a tinnitus disability when tinnitus was a "persistent" symptom of one of three conditions: head injury, concussion, or acoustic trauma (noise exposure). In 1999, regulations in Title 38 of the Code of Federal Regulations were changed to award disability for "recurrent" tinnitus regardless of the cause. In other words, tinnitus caused by any condition that may have been incurred in or aggravated by military service can now be rated as a compensable service-connected disability, whereas before 1999, tinnitus was a compensable service-connected disability only when it was caused by one or more of the three conditions. Because tinnitus can now be related to so many medical conditions, there has consequently been a significant growth in tinnitus-related claims. Additional reasons for the increase in tinnitus claims have to do with improved separation and transition counseling for individuals leaving the military and increased awareness among veterans and veterans groups of the importance of claiming service-related injuries. The main reason for this increase, however, is increased eligibility for specialized audiologic services, primarily the dispensing of hearing aids (as explained further below).

Procedures for Evaluating Tinnitus Claims

Any veteran can claim tinnitus. The DVA must adjudicate the claim and find reasonable evidence to support it. Because tinnitus can be related to many medical conditions and, in most cases, can be perceived only by the veteran, the diagnosis of tinnitus is difficult and based predominantly on subjective report. There must be a reasonable likelihood ("at least as likely as not") that the condition was incurred in or aggravated by military service, which is the basis of all VA disability claims. Adjudication of tinnitus claims is much more difficult for veterans whose active duty occurred many years prior to the claim, which usually means that there is no formal hearing testing in the military record and a history that is confounded by aging, poor health, and occupational noise exposure.

Currently, regulations do not provide guidelines for evaluating tinnitus on the basis of the frequency, duration, or severity of symptoms, as in other subjective conditions (vertigo, pain, fatigue, migraine headaches, Meniere's disease). In contrast to the guidelines for rating tinnitus, Meniere's disease, for example, is rated as 100% when there is hearing loss with attacks of vertigo and cerebellar gait disturbance more than once a week with or without tinnitus, 60% for hearing loss with vertigo and cerebellar gait disturbance one to four times a month with or without tinnitus, and 30% for hearing loss with vertigo less than once a month with or without tinnitus. Meniere's disease can also be rated for each condition separately (hearing loss, vertigo, and tinnitus), whichever results in a higher rating. Unlike other subjective conditions that have graded levels of disability, tinnitus has a single level of compensable disability (10%).

A veteran claiming service connection for compensation and treatment starts the process by making a claim to his or her VBA Veterans Service Center. The claim is reviewed by a veterans service representative and a ratings specialist at the Veterans Service Center. If the claim is for tinnitus, the veteran is scheduled for a compensation and pension examination by a VA or contract audiologist.

In deciding a disability claim, the VBA considers the diagnosis and level of disability. To provide the required evidence to the VBA, audiologists must use the official VBA Worksheet 1305.[21] The worksheet ensures performance of an adequate examination and requires audiologists to comment on tinnitus, if present, by stating (1) the reported date and circumstances of onset; (2) the location of tinnitus (bilateral or unilateral); (3) whether it is recurrent and its frequency and duration; and (4) the most likely cause, and, specifically, if hearing loss is present, whether the tinnitus is due to the same cause as the hearing loss. In determining the most likely cause, the examiner must consider all causes of tinnitus. After taking a medical history and reviewing the medical record, the examiner must give an opinion on the most likely cause of the tinnitus. In those instances in which the record indicates the possibility of medical causes outside the audiologist's scope of practice, the audiologist refers the case to a physician for an opinion.

The basis for awarding a tinnitus disability is (1) that tinnitus is at least recurrent (intermittent) and (2) that it is related to military service. The audiologist provides an opinion as to the cause of the tinnitus and its connection (nexus) to military service or other causal factors. If the VBA determines that the tinnitus is related to military service or the tinnitus is due to the same cause or causal factor as a hearing loss that is related to military service, the veteran has sustained the required burden of proof.

For many veterans, it is difficult to prove that tinnitus was caused or aggravated by military service because of a lack of substantive evidence in their service or medical records that would link their tinnitus to their military experience. Veterans are no more likely to report tinnitus as a medical problem or seek treatment than the general population. For many veterans, there is no evidence that tinnitus has been a chronic or continuous symptom, or there exist the confounding factors of nonmilitary noise exposure, medication use, medical conditions, aging, or other causal factors that occurred after military service.

DIFFERENTIATING TINNITUS DISTRESS FROM MENTAL DISORDERS

The synergy between tinnitus and psychological status poses a kind of "chicken or egg" conundrum. Does tinnitus cause psychological distress, or does psychological instability aggravate an otherwise benign otologic condition? Psychological studies suggest that both occur. The questions have important implications for disability compensation. Should the DVA compensate veterans for tinnitus or for the underlying psychological condition (eg, anxiety, stress, or depression)? Although the psychological manifestations of tinnitus have been well described, few studies have looked at tinnitus in veterans. Studies using scales or questionnaires suggest that veterans have higher distress, anxiety, and depression than nonveterans and are similar to patients who cope poorly with stress.[22–25]

VETERANS WITH TINNITUS WHO DO NOT APPLY FOR BENEFITS

Given the accepted prevalence of tinnitus in the general population and the well-established association between noise exposure and tinnitus,[26,27] it is reasonable to assume that many veterans have tinnitus but do not seek compensation or treatment for the condition. For many of these veterans, the claim process is either too daunting and/or they feel that they lack the necessary evidence to link their tinnitus to their service experience. In many instances, especially in the case of older veterans, they feel that the condition, not being directly related to an injury, does not merit filing a claim. In spite of efforts by the DVA to inform veterans of the potential eligibility for benefits, many veterans are still intimidated by the process and never file a claim. The DVA continues its many outreach programs urging veterans to file claims and making every effort to provide the necessary assistance.

TINNITUS TREATMENT IN VA MEDICAL CENTERS

INCREASED DEMAND FOR GENERAL VA SERVICES

Demand is increasing at VA medical centers nationwide for both basic primary care and specialty care services. The numbers of veterans using these services increased from 2.7 million in 1995 to nearly 4.3 million in 2002.[28] In 2002, approximately 800,000 additional veterans were enrolled, bringing the enrolment in the VA health care system to nearly 6.5 million veterans. Several factors are driving demand for VA services: rising costs of private health insurance and prescription drugs, changes in demographics (aging, socioeconomic factors), changes in eligibility criteria, and the increasing reputation of VA health care for quality.

INCREASED DEMAND FOR TINNITUS SERVICES

The unprecedented rise in demand that is occurring for VA services will naturally cause an increase in the numbers of veterans seeking tinnitus services. The demand for tinnitus services may grow disproportionately, however, because tinnitus has become the most common new service-connected disability.[19] Demand for hearing loss services is also rapidly increasing, in part because hearing aids are not covered by Medicare or most other insurance and are too expensive for many veterans. Veterans are therefore increasingly applying for a service-connected disability as a means to obtain access to the VA hearing aid program. As more veterans seek evaluation, audiologists are finding more hearing loss and tinnitus.

Another important factor that may influence the increase in tinnitus disability and demand for services is awareness. The 2001 VBA Annual Report showed that 28% of disability claims were from veterans aged 35 years or less.[19] Eighty-six percent of claims were from veterans less than 65 years of age. Sixty-seven percent of initial claims were from veterans who served in the Gulf War I period. These data suggest that increased awareness of tinnitus and hearing loss as potentially significant health conditions, rather than aging of the veteran population, is the driving force behind the increase in claims for tinnitus and hearing loss disabilities. This increased awareness is due to better transition counseling provided by the DVA at the time of discharge, greater access to patient education, and awareness efforts on the part of veterans groups and other national organizations (eg, American Speech-Language-Hearing Association, American Academy of Audiology, and Self-Help for Hard of Hearing People, aka SHHH).

SURVEY OF VA AUDIOLOGISTS TO ASSESS LEVEL OF TINNITUS SERVICES

In an attempt to determine the level of tinnitus services provided at the different VA medical centers around the country, we distributed a questionnaire to VA clinical audiologists via the VA audiologist electronic mail (e-mail) group. Survey responses were received from audiologists representing 48 of the 132 VA audiology clinics. The responding clinics represented 29 states and were distributed fairly evenly across major population areas. Most of the largest VA medical centers were represented. The low response rate (36%) probably reflects (1) lack of interest on the part of clinics that did not respond (at least one audiologist from each VA audiology clinic subscribes to this e-mail group) and (2) the likelihood that many VA audiologists are not involved in tinnitus management.

The results of the survey are shown in Tables 25-1 and 25-2. Table 25-1 shows the results from the questions that required only a yes or no response. About 80% of the clinics that responded to the survey provide some kind of tinnitus information to their patients, but only about one-third have "any sort of a tinnitus treatment program." One-third reported that they use specific tinnitus questionnaires. Psychoacoustic tinnitus evaluations are performed in approximately half of the clinics. Approximately two-thirds of the clinics refer their tinnitus patients to other VA specialty clinics, but only a few refer their patients outside the DVA. Equally few clinics use criteria to determine the need for treatment.

Table 25-2 summarizes responses to questions concerning the numbers of different ear-level and sound-conditioning devices that have been used to treat patients with tinnitus. (Ear-level devices would be used for treatment with either tinnitus masking or TRT.) Only about 20% of the clinics reported dispensing more than 10 tinnitus maskers in the previous 5 years, and only one clinic dispensed more than 10 during the previous year. The numbers for combination devices (masker combined with hearing aid) were even lower, with approximately half of the clinics reporting that no combination devices were dispensed during the previous year. Various types of tabletop sound-conditioning units have been issued

TABLE 25-1. Responses of VA Audiology Clinics to Various Questions from the VA Tinnitus Survey*

Question	Response Choice		
	Yes	No	No Response
Does your audiology program have any sort of a tinnitus treatment program?	14	34	0
Do any audiologists in your program perform tinnitus evaluations (tinnitus matching, masking, test for residual inhibition)?	25	23	0
Does your program use a specific tinnitus questionnaire (or specific questions about tinnitus) for your patients?	15	33	0
Do you provide patients with tinnitus information/counseling materials?	39	9	0
Do you have criteria to determine whether or not a veteran qualifies for tinnitus treatment?	3	41	4
Do you refer patients to any other specialty services for tinnitus treatment (eg, psychology, dentistry)?	31	17	0
Are any of your patients referred outside of the VA to receive tinnitus treatment, eg, to receive masking devices, counseling, or tinnitus retraining therapy (TRT)?	3	45	0

VA = Veterans Affairs.
*For questions requiring yes or no answers.

TABLE 25-2. Responses of VA Audiology Clinics to Various Questions from the VA Tinnitus Survey*

Question	None	1–10	More than 10	Unknown
How many patients would you estimate have received tinnitus maskers in your audiology program in the last 5 years?	8	22	9	9
The past 1 year?	16	28	1	3
How many patients have received combination tinnitus masker/hearing aids over the past 5 years?	12	20	6	10
The last 1 year?	23	23	0	2
How many sound-conditioning units (ie, tabletop devices with preprogrammed noises such as surf, rainfall, etc) would you estimate have been issued by your audiology program?	29	10	8	1
How many tinnitus CD packages (eg, Petroff CD system, etc)?	42	2	0	4

CD = compact disc; VA = Veterans Affairs.
*For questions requiring numeric answers.

by less than half of the clinics, and 42 of the 48 clinics have never issued special compact disc packages for tinnitus treatment. In summary, the results of this survey suggest that VA audiology clinics provide minimal services for veterans with tinnitus.

The results of the survey were disseminated back to the audiologists via the e-mail group. An additional question was asked at that time: "At the NCRAR, we have been developing curricula to train VA audiologists to provide tinnitus management for veterans with bothersome tinnitus. …Would you be interested in such a program?" Of the 51 responses to this question, all indicated interest in a continuing education program. Thus, it appears that a substantial number of VA audiologists are interested in providing a higher level of service to veterans with tinnitus.

For veterans with clinically significant tinnitus, access to a high level of clinical management is clearly limited in VA facilities at this time. This situation is not, however, unique to the VA Healthcare System. In the private sector, tinnitus management is neither uniform nor ubiquitous. Only a handful of specialized tinnitus centers exist that provide comprehensive assessment and treatment. Also, audiologists typically do not receive training specific to tinnitus management, and many of them have little or no experience in this area. The following suggestions for improving the situation within VA medical centers might, therefore, also be appropriate for the private sector.

FUTURE VA NEEDS AND DIRECTIONS

Long-term solutions to the problem of veterans with tinnitus will require a commitment at all levels of the VHA to develop and to support effective clinical management strategies throughout the VA Healthcare System. Obtaining such consensual commitment will first require an awareness of the problem by VA administrators and staff. Second, key personnel should establish priorities and enact an action plan. The following sections offer suggestions for developing such a plan.

"Progressive Intervention" Model of Tinnitus Management

It is important for clinicians to be aware that tinnitus is a clinically significant problem for only approximately 20% of individuals who have permanent tinnitus.[14,29] The findings from our clinical trial evaluating tinnitus masking and TRT indicate that about this same percentage of veterans may require clinical intervention (see next paragraph). It is therefore necessary to assess accurately whether clinical intervention is necessary and, if so, to determine the level of service required. This approach to treatment has been used to treat other conditions and has been referred to as "progressive intervention" (by H. Abrams, Bay Pines, FL, VA Medical Center).

To provide tinnitus treatment according to each veteran's specific need, we are developing a hierarchy of services, that is, a tiered approach based on severity. Such a hierarchy, progressing from least to most need, is envisioned as (1) telephone screening and information, (2) group educational sessions, (3) clinical evaluation and counseling, and (4) comprehensive individualized management. Audiologists could provide this hierarchy of services with appropriate referrals to otolaryngologists, neurologists, psychologists, psychiatrists, or other clinicians who have specialized tinnitus expertise.

Telephone Screening and Information Recruitment of veterans for the masking versus TRT clinical trial demonstrated the effectiveness of providing telephone screening and information to veterans concerned about their tinnitus. During the recruitment phase of the study, over 800 veterans expressed interest in study participation, usually by telephone inquiry. The Tinnitus-Impact Screening Questionnaire (TISQ) in Appendix A was developed to select veterans with clinically significant tinnitus. This questionnaire uses selected questions from the TRT Initial Interview[30–32] and from the Tinnitus Severity Index.[33] Of the 800 veterans who called about the clinical trial, the TISQ identified 172 (22%) who felt that their tinnitus was sufficiently problematic to warrant a full evaluation for treatment. These results are consistent with estimates that only about 20% of individuals with tinnitus require clinical intervention.[14,29]

Many of the veterans who called about the clinical trial at the PVAMC reported that they experienced hearing difficulties that they felt were caused by their tinnitus. Studies have shown that ascribing hearing problems to tinnitus is a common misconception on the part of patients.[34] These veterans required education to dispel this misconception and to address their other tinnitus concerns. The telephone screening thus doubled as a brief educational session that provided sufficient information for about 80% of the callers to feel comfortable that they did not require clinical intervention for their tinnitus.

Group Educational Sessions Patients with tinnitus often receive counseling as their sole form of intervention. Most tinnitus counseling methods include basic information about the structure and function of the auditory system, effective coping strategies for making tinnitus less bothersome, and other information that would be useful to most patients. This kind of general counseling information can be packaged and presented to groups of veterans with tinnitus.

For the past 5 years, the first and second authors have facilitated a support or education group for veterans with tinnitus. The group, usually consisting of 10 to 20 veterans, has met approximately monthly at the PVAMC. The objectives of these meetings are to provide information that would be helpful to veterans in managing their tinnitus and to serve as a forum for veterans and their families to express any concerns or questions related to tinnitus. For some meetings, one of the moderators gives a formal presentation on a specific tinnitus topic followed by a question and answer period. For other meetings, outside speakers are invited, including tinnitus specialists from Oregon Health and Science University, staff from the American Tinnitus Association, professionals in the community who offer various forms of tinnitus treatment, and representatives of different veterans organizations. This type of support group could be replicated at other VA medical centers, minimally requiring the commitment of one individual who ideally possesses tinnitus expertise and would be willing to coordinate the meetings and arrange for guest speakers.

The success of the tinnitus support group spawned the idea for a research project to determine the efficacy of providing group tinnitus treatment to veterans via a series of educational sessions. A study was designed to test the hypothesis that structured group education, using the directive-counseling principles of TRT,[35] would provide effective intervention for the majority of veterans seeking treatment for their tinnitus. This study is presently being conducted at the two VA medical centers (American Lake and Seattle) that comprise the VA Puget Sound Health Care System. Veterans with clinically significant tinnitus are randomized into (1) the education group, (2) a traditional support group, or (3) a 1-year waiting-list group. Those randomized to the education and support groups attend four weekly sessions lasting 1.5 hours each. The education group receives education or counseling information in a *PowerPoint* presentation format. The support group is facilitated by a moderator who does not have tinnitus expertise but is trained to guide the veterans to discuss various methods of coping with their tinnitus. As a result of their involvement with this study, the participating audiology staff at the Seattle and American Lake VA medical centers have begun a tinnitus management program for veteran patients that uses a similar group education format.

Clinical Screening and Education The masking versus TRT clinical trial has also demonstrated the clinical value of providing an initial hearing and tinnitus assessment that includes some basic education. As described above, 800 veterans were screened initially by telephone. Of these callers, 172 were scheduled for an initial evaluation that involved a comprehensive hearing and tinnitus assessment, written questionnaires that were filled out in advance of the initial evaluation, and the TRT Initial Interview,[31–33] which was administered by the research audiologist during the appointment. In the process of performing the assessment and interview, the research audiologist provided some basic hearing and tinnitus education to these individuals. Following the initial evaluation, 48 of these 172 veterans decided that no further services were required, indicating that the information received during the appointment was sufficient. Thus, of the original 800 veterans who called about treatment, only 124 (16%) decided that they required further treatment after the two-stage screening process. Based on these findings, about 84% of veterans with the complaint of tinnitus may require only some minimal information to reach the conclusion that their tinnitus does not pose a significant problem.

Comprehensive Individualized Management The delivery of comprehensive individualized programs for veterans with tinnitus should be conducted only when medically treatable tinnitus has been ruled out and when patients have demonstrated that basic educational counseling is insufficient in meeting their needs. Of the many known methods purported to provide relief from tinnitus symptoms,[36] TRT and tinnitus masking may offer the best potential for widespread application by VA audiologists.[4,8,37] These methods have been refined through long-term clinical application, and the protocols are well defined. Because of the potential of these techniques to be efficiently implemented into VA audiology clinics, we conducted a controlled clinical trial to assess the relative efficacies of masking and TRT in veterans. (See the description of this study at the end of this chapter.) Other treatment options also have potential for VA use, including various forms of psychological management.[38,39] Further forms of tinnitus treatment are less well developed or require pharmacologic intervention.

EDUCATION OF VA AUDIOLOGISTS AND OTHER POTENTIAL TINNITUS CLINICIANS

Professional Training Although severe tinnitus can be treated successfully in the majority of cases, only a handful of tinnitus specialists exist at VA medical centers who have the expertise to provide a high level of treatment. This shortage is due primarily to the fact that tinnitus treatment methodology has not received global acceptance, nor has it received standardization, and few professionals have access to adequate training. There is a VA-wide network of audiologists, otolaryngologists, otologists, primary care providers, psychiatrists, and psychologists who all encounter tinnitus sufferers on a regular basis. Of these professionals, the hearing health specialists have received extensive education and training to classify, describe, and ameliorate most auditory problems. The treatment of severe tinnitus, however, is not specifically addressed in most professional training programs. There is a need for standardized training curricula for health care professionals who are most likely to encounter tinnitus sufferers in the clinic environment and who are expected to provide some level of amelioration.

For VA professionals who are the point of contact for most veterans who would present with tinnitus, information should be developed in a variety of formats, as suggested below and summarized in Table 25-3. First, a simple brochure could be developed that would present the basic message that noise causes tinnitus and that effective treatment is available (although presently on a limited basis). Such a brochure would enable the medical professional to provide simple and clear information to the veteran, including a list of factors that can cause or exacerbate tinnitus, a brief description of the kind of help that is available, and references to Web sites and telephone numbers to obtain further information.

Second, brief-training materials could be developed for professionals to provide a minimum of effective intervention for veterans with tinnitus. These materials would be specifically targeted to busy professionals, who have minimal time to spend with patients. Thus, the materials would include only the basics of what a practitioner would need to convey to the patient to understand the essentials of treatment, to make appropriate lifestyle changes, and to initiate activities that would be therapeutic. These materials could be developed as a brief-training booklet and a short Web site training course.

Third, a comprehensive training program should be developed for professionals who are interested in providing full treatment and who have the time necessary to do so. This program would be targeted primarily to audiologists, who would be in the best position to provide such treatment.[37] The program should also be accessible to physicians or counselors who might have an interest in providing comprehensive tinnitus treatment. Two formats could be developed: live seminars and a Web site that would provide step-by-step training instructions. The training seminar would be the most effective training vehicle for future tinnitus practitioners, but attending such a seminar would not be possible for many professionals. The next best training medium would be a carefully designed on-line training Web site that would cover all of the basic elements of the seminar. The Web site would provide a high level of training for VA professionals anywhere in the country who want to add or improve services to their patients with tinnitus.

Fourth, most audiologists and other professionals do not usually receive a significant amount of graduate-level training in tinnitus management. Graduate course curricula should therefore be developed for this purpose. Such curricula would be suitable as a lecture class for audiology students and could

TABLE 25-3. Suggested Elements of Professional Training to Equip VA Professionals for Treatment of Veterans with Tinnitus

Element	Purpose	Clinician Training Required
Brochure	Provide clinician with a handout for patients that contains basic tinnitus information, including self-help items and resources to receive further help	None
Brief training materials	Provide clinician with basic information to convey to patient: what can be done about tinnitus, beneficial lifestyle changes, and where to receive further help	Complete a short course given via booklet and/or Web site
Comprehensive training program	Provide practitioner with full training to conduct tinnitus treatment	Live seminar, Web site training course
Training for graduate students	Provide audiology graduate students with training needed to treat future patients with tinnitus	Complete course work

VA = Veterans Affairs.

be offered as such to university audiology programs. Shortened versions of the course could be developed to provide training lectures to medical students and residents and instructional courses for national otolaryngology and audiology conventions.

EDUCATING VETERANS ABOUT TINNITUS

Veterans with tinnitus need ready access to accurate and comprehensive information about tinnitus. As the VA system adds services and resources to help these veterans, they need to be made aware of the help that is available. The following suggestions are summarized more succinctly in Table 25-4.

Veterans Tinnitus Web Site The first need in this regard is for a comprehensive repository of accurate tinnitus information that is readily accessible to veterans and to VA professionals. With current technology, a single Web site could be developed as the most accessible single source of such information. Such a Web site could, for example, educate veterans regarding lifestyle changes to improve their condition, how to prevent tinnitus exacerbation, and where to obtain services. The VA professional could also benefit from a Web site that contained information relevant to answering their patients' questions and for guiding their patients to obtain adequate care. It is possible that an array of tinnitus publications, both lay and professional, could be presented in their entirety on such a Web site.

The DVA has recently developed a new health management Web site called MyHealth*e*Vet (<www.myhealthevet.va.gov>). This Web site addresses veterans' health issues and (1) assists veterans in managing their own health; (2) provides a single location for health information, VA programs, and services; (3) serves as a patient educational tool; (4) provides a single touch-point to reach the entire veteran population; (5) broadcasts health tips and health bulletins; and (6) serves as an interactive outreach to veterans for health education, VA-specific programs, and opportunities to participate in research. These features make the MyHealth*e*Vet Web site an ideal medium to present tinnitus information to veterans.

Public Service Announcements There is a general lack of awareness, both within and outside the VA Healthcare System, that noise causes tinnitus and that problematic tinnitus can often be treated successfully. For the purposes of prevention and rehabilitation, this rudimentary information should become common knowledge to veterans and to VA clinicians. The most efficient mechanism to disseminate this message on a national scale would be a television and radio campaign, in the form of public service announcements. As a further prevention effort, data should be made available to the Department of Defense urging stronger enforcement of regulations regarding the use of devices for hearing protection and comprehensive hearing conservation programs. Hearing protection should also be integrated into basic military safety education.

Veteran Service Organization for Tinnitus There are veteran service organizations (VSOs) for practically every conceivable condition experienced by veterans. Surprisingly, there is no VSO for veterans with tinnitus. It would seem that thousands of veterans with tinnitus could benefit from a national VSO with a mission statement that focuses exclusively on tinnitus. Such a VSO would serve as a national organization of veterans dedi-

Table 25-4. Potential Resources that Could Provide Tinnitus Information to Veterans

Resource	Purpose	Information Provided
Veterans tinnitus Web site	Repository of up-to-date information about tinnitus that can be accessed from any networked computer	Self-help information; articles about tinnitus; listings of available clinical services
Public service announcements	Outreach to veterans to inform them that tinnitus can be prevented and that treatment is available	Noise causes tinnitus; tinnitus is a treatable condition; telephone number and Web site for further information
Veteran service organization	Advocacy organization to promote programs that would benefit veterans with tinnitus	Resources to obtain help; advice from fellow veterans; advocacy information

cated to the promotion of programs that would improve the condition of veterans with tinnitus. A VSO for tinnitus would have far-reaching impact into areas of research, prevention, treatment, and training of tinnitus treatment professionals within the VA Healthcare System.

PREVENTION OF TINNITUS

It is well documented that tinnitus is associated with noise-induced hearing loss more than with any other cause.[26,40–43] It is also common knowledge that many veterans have been exposed to acoustic trauma and excessive levels of noise with little or no hearing protection. VA audiologists are intimately familiar with veterans' accounts of exposure to gunfire, artillery fire, explosions, jet noise, helicopter noise, etc. The key to the prevention of tinnitus incurred during military service is to implement and enforce effective hearing conservation programs in the military. Fortunately, military hearing conservation programs have made significant progress in the prevention of noise-induced hearing loss of military troops.[44] The positive news is tempered, however, by recent reports that implementation of effective hearing conservation is inconsistent across military units.[45–47] Although noise exposure continues to be a problem in the military, it is clear that a concerted effort is under way to minimize its impact.

For veterans, prevention of tinnitus is primarily a matter of educating them that exposure to loud noise is the main cause of tinnitus onset and exacerbation. Veterans will generally have received this information during their active military service, but because they will likely be exposed to hazardous occupational and/or recreational noise throughout their lives, the message bears repeating. In this regard, formation of a VSO that is dedicated to veterans with tinnitus could serve as a resource of veterans who could make themselves available to military units to educate them about the long-term consequences of unprotected noise exposure.

DEVELOPMENT OF OBJECTIVE EVALUATION METHODS

Evaluation Methods for Diagnosis Tinnitus diagnosis mainly involves determining if the tinnitus is surgically correctable and, if so, establishing the cause.[48] "Somatosounds" are sounds that are mechanically generated by the body. Although only a small number of individuals who complain of tinnitus actually experience somatosounds, it is important to make this distinction to determine if the tinnitus might be surgically correctable. Thus, patients complaining of tinnitus should receive a thorough evaluation from a physician who is qualified to make such a diagnosis. It is unknown how many otolaryngology physicians within the VA system have such expertise. Considering that the majority of non-VA otolaryngologists do not specialize in tinnitus diagnosis and surgery, it is likely that the same is true for VA otolaryngologists. Consequently, there is a need to educate VA physicians to diagnose the cause of tinnitus and to perform appropriate surgery when indicated. We are unaware of any such effort either under way or forthcoming.

Methods for Evaluating Efficacy of Treatment The patient with tinnitus will always serve as the final arbiter of tinnitus treatment success. There is no consensus, however, regarding outcome methodology for evaluating tinnitus treatment effects.[49,50] Dobie, for example, has suggested the development of a "staging system" to place patients with tinnitus into prognostic categories according to the difficulty in treating them effectively.[51] It is also important to have the clinical capacity to assess accurately the severity of tinnitus for veterans. The "severity" of tinnitus refers to the degree to which tinnitus impacts quality of life. A variety of questionnaires are presently used in the attempt to assess the effects of tinnitus in these different areas,[49] including self-administered questionnaires, for example, the Tinnitus Handicap Questionnaire,[52] the Tinnitus Handicap Inventory,[53] and the Tinnitus Severity Index.[33] There is also the TRT Initial Interview, which is administered verbally by the examiner.[30–32] None of these questionnaires has received universal acceptance. A widely used assessment instrument or "gold standard" that is effective in qualifying and quantifying the aspects of daily living that are affected by tinnitus is clearly needed. Equipped with appropriate information through the use of such a questionnaire, VA clinicians could provide a consistent means of determining the necessity of treatment or tailor treatment to meet veterans' needs. The long-term need is the development of a standardized VA tinnitus assessment instrument.

Evaluation Methods for Disability Determination (Compensation) Like pain, tinnitus is a personal experience that can be indirectly observed only through a patient's behavior and verbal descriptions.[54] No objective test for subjective tinnitus has been discovered in spite of dozens of attempts to do so. Ultimately, the examiner must determine if the patient's report of tinnitus is true "to a reasonable medical certainty" based on the report's plausibility, credibility, and consistency. The best evidence supporting a claim often comes from the results of audiologic testing. Although tests for detecting exaggerated hearing loss are well developed,[55] there is only one known study that has evaluated the differences between individuals with and those without tinnitus.[56] In that study, individuals without tinnitus provided loudness matches at a higher level than actual tinnitus patients, but the reliability of the loudness matches was not significantly different. Thus, there is essentially no evidence from research studies supporting tests to confirm the presence of tinnitus. Testing procedures are generally recommended based on clinical data and experience.[3,57–60]

The findings from our own recent studies (as yet unpublished) suggest that the results from a number of tinnitus psychoacoustic tests should be evaluated in aggregate to optimize the accuracy of determining whether a patient has tinnitus as claimed. These combined psychoacoustic results should then be considered along with other factors that would be relevant in supporting a tinnitus claim. Those factors, summarized by Dobie,[54] include a plausible and consistent history, the credibility of the patient, early documentation, unsolicited complaint, and hearing loss that is not exaggerated.

Research Needs

In the field of tinnitus, as in all medical disciplines, there is a growing awareness of the need for evidence-based treatment methods.[2,50,61] Efforts have increased greatly in the last 25 years to develop effective treatments for tinnitus, but there is little research documenting treatment efficacy.[51,62] An epidemiologic study is greatly needed to define the problem of tinnitus in the veteran population. Basic science studies are also needed to elucidate the neural mechanisms of tinnitus, which currently exist only as theoretic constructs.[63] Ultimately, cures for tinnitus will come about only when there is a clear understanding of the underlying mechanisms.

VA Rehabilitation Research and Development Service Tinnitus has been recognized as a "specific area of interest" by the VA Rehabilitation Research and Development (RR&D) Service. Specifically, the research priorities circular distributed by the RR&D Service states:

> Tinnitus has a high prevalence in the veteran population, but effective treatments have not been developed. Specific topics of emphasis include, but are not limited to, the development and evaluation of the following: (a) Improved instrumentation and techniques for evaluation of patients with tinnitus; (b) Subjective and objective scales of severity and adaptive comparisons to facilitate treatment and rehabilitation; (c) Intervention methodology that may include wearable devices, behavioral modification and medication. (p. 7)

It is thus clear that the RR&D Service has an expressed commitment to funding projects that will result in improvement in clinical care for veterans with tinnitus.

The RR&D Service, in addition to funding individual investigator-initiated research, presently sponsors 12 Centers of Excellence. Each of these RR&D centers focuses on a specific area of rehabilitation for medical problems that are prevalent among veterans. The RR&D NCRAR has been in existence at the PVAMC since 1997. The NCRAR is a multidisciplinary, multisite resource that is dedicated to improving rehabilitative care for veterans with hearing and tinnitus disorders. Development of programs for the remediation of tinnitus in veterans is a continued focus of work at the NCRAR. There is a need, however, for far greater resources to address efficiently the concerns delineated in this chapter.

Factors Associated with Problematic Tinnitus To improve clinical services for tinnitus management, it is important to understand the factors that dictate why so many people with permanent tinnitus seem to be largely unaffected by it, whereas a relatively small percentage require clinical intervention. These factors most likely consist of some complex combination of personality traits, psychological state, and life circumstances of the patient with tinnitus, in addition to the characteristics of the tinnitus sound itself. To evaluate veterans to determine which factors are associated with tinnitus severity, it will be necessary to conduct a large-scale epidemiologic study. Such a study would administer questionnaires that would profile veterans with regard to personality and life-experience factors that could influence the impact of tinnitus on their lives. Additionally, each patient's tinnitus perception should be carefully described and correlated with physical stimuli using sophisticated instrumentation and techniques.

COST IMPLICATIONS TO VA OF ADDING TINNITUS SERVICES

The need to add clinical tinnitus services at VA medical centers raises the inevitable concern about the impact of these services on budgets that are already strained. The implementation of tinnitus services must be prudent and cost-effective. There will be costs associated with providing training to perform these services and to provide the services on a continuing basis. Some of the cost implications can be inferred from the data provided by the VBA regarding compensation benefits. As mentioned above, tinnitus is now the most common new service-connected disability, and tinnitus claims are in an exponential growth stage. Public Law 107-330 (Veterans Benefits Act) mandates a study of the costs of tinnitus compensation and treatment. The costs would obviously be affected by changes in regulations pertaining to tinnitus (eg, compensation allowable for one or both ears) and procedures for tinnitus assessment (eg, level of handicap, subjective scaling).

With regard to professional training, at least one audiologist at each VA medical center should be trained to perform all levels of tinnitus treatment. Basic training can be conducted on-line, and live training should also be available at a more advanced level. Adequate training could probably be accomplished using a week or less of an audiologist's time. The initial training should be supplemented on an ongoing basis, which would also fulfill the need for continuing education credits.

Use of a progressive intervention approach, as described earlier, should result in the most cost-effective method for the DVA to provide tinnitus management. This approach would address different levels of tinnitus severity, and only veterans with the most problematic tinnitus would actually enter clinical treatment on an individualized basis. Through efficient methods of screening, support groups, and group education sessions, the numbers of veterans requiring individualized services would be minimal.

The two clinical trials presently under way through the NCRAR should play an important role in the formation of VA policies affecting implementation of tinnitus services. Both studies are using screening methods to identify veterans with clinically significant tinnitus. These screening methods are being refined and could be useful at all VA medical centers as the "first tier" of progressive intervention. The "second tier" is being addressed by the study that is evaluating the efficacy of both group educational sessions and a support group format. Completion of this study will document the effectiveness of these two forms of intervention that are expected to address the needs of most veterans with problematic tinnitus. Veterans who need individual services would enter the "third tier." This highest level of service is addressed by the second study, which is comparing the relative efficacies of tinnitus masking and TRT. The study was recently concluded, and a brief summary of results is provided below.

CLINICAL TRIAL TO ASSESS EFFICACY OF MASKING VERSUS TRT IN VETERANS

As referred to variously above, a controlled, prospective study was conducted at the PVAMC to evaluate the clinical efficacy of masking and TRT in veterans. The last veteran participant completed treatment in August 2003. Although the results have not been published at the time of this writing, the study is described briefly herein because it represents the type of research evidence that is needed to justify the implementation of clinical services for veterans with severe tinnitus.

After screening more than 800 veterans who called about the study, 124 were enrolled for treatment. Veteran participants were placed into one of the two treatment groups pseudorandomly, that is, the first qualifying veteran was placed randomly, and each successive qualifying veteran was placed alternately into one of the groups. The study audiologist (T. Zaugg) conducted all audiologic and tinnitus evaluations and obtained outcome data. Treatment with TRT was performed by the first author and masking by the second author. Follow-up appointments were scheduled at 3, 6, 12, and 18 months. Self-administered (written) questionnaires included the Tinnitus Severity Index,[33] the Tinnitus Handicap Inventory,[53] and the Tinnitus Handicap Questionnaire.[52] At every visit, subjects completed the written questionnaires and were interviewed by the study audiologist using the TRT Interview Forms.[30–32]

Of the 124 original participants, 111 (53 in masking, 58 in TRT) completed the 18-month treatment protocol. Figure 25-3 shows mean scores from the Tinnitus Severity Index, a 48-point (maximum) index of tinnitus severity.[33] These data are reasonably representative of results obtained across the different outcome instruments: both treatment groups experienced comparable improvement through 6 months of treatment. At the 12- and 18-month visits, however, the TRT group showed significantly greater improvement relative to the masking group.

Figure 25-4 shows mean responses to the question on the TRT Interview, "What percent of your total awake time, over the last month, have you been *aware* of your tinnitus?" These responses were particularly important with respect to the degree that tinnitus habituation was accomplished during treatment, which is the primary goal of TRT. The figure shows that both groups reported that they were aware of their tinnitus, on average, over 70% of their waking hours at the start of treatment. By the end of treatment, the mean response dropped to 32% for the masking group and to 19% for the TRT group. It would thus appear that veterans in both groups experienced significant habituation to their tinnitus, with the TRT subjects showing the greatest effect.

Although this study provides important evidence concerning tinnitus treatment in veterans, the findings cannot be considered definitive. Numerous factors might have contributed to the results, which will be described

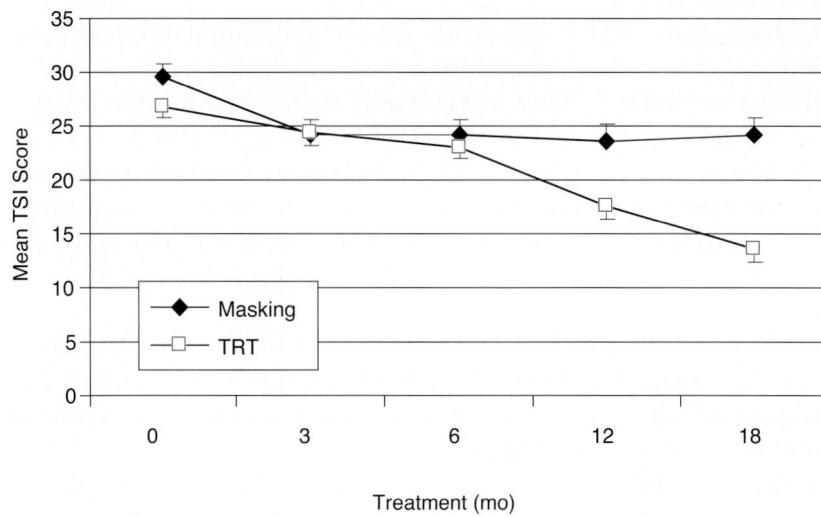

FIGURE 25-3. Mean scores from the Tinnitus Severity Index (TSI) administered at baseline and at follow-up appointments. Means include all completed subjects who provided data at any of the five outcome visits. Error bars represent standard error of the mean. TRT = tinnitus retraining therapy.

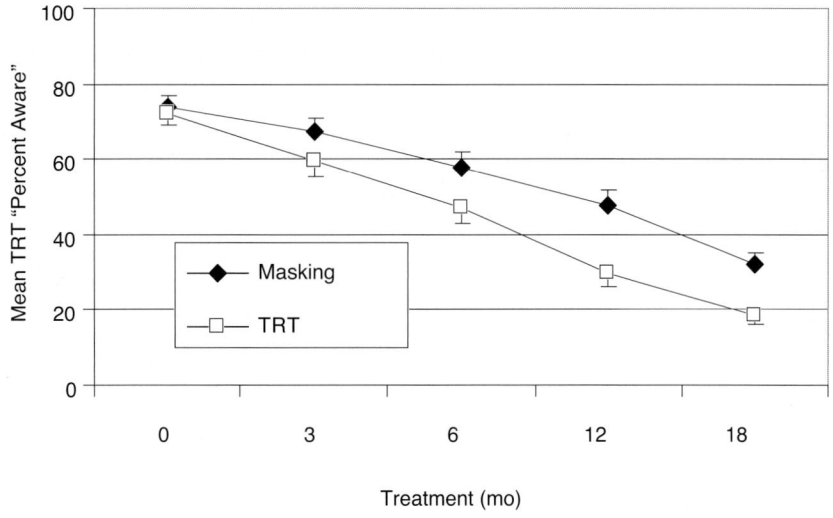

FIGURE 25-4. Mean scores from the Tinnitus Retraining Therapy (TRT) Interview question, "What percent of your total awake time, over the last month, have you been *aware* of your tinnitus?" Means include all completed subjects who answered this question at any of the five outcome visits. Error bars represent standard error of the mean.

in a forthcoming publication. Taken alone, however, these findings are highly encouraging that individualized treatment can be provided effectively to veterans with the most severe tinnitus. The study has been approved for expansion to four VA audiology clinics, which will evaluate the effectiveness of these two methods of treatment under more typical VA clinical conditions.

CONCLUSION

Although many thousands of veterans nationwide suffer from tinnitus, relatively few have access to formalized and effective tinnitus treatment within the VA Healthcare System. It seems clear that the majority of these veterans would experience significant benefit through interaction with clinical professionals who are properly trained in tinnitus management. The challenge is to create a network of such professionals across the VA Healthcare System.

Tinnitus is, of course, a problem that extends beyond the VA Healthcare System. The lives of millions of individuals in the United States are significantly impacted because of intractable tinnitus. Because of our increasingly noisy society, as well as broader segments of the population taking different types and combinations of medications and the increased number of individuals living to advanced ages, the prevalence of tinnitus will increase. As with the VA Healthcare System, adequate and readily accessible treatment for tinnitus is not available in most locations. Some forms of treatment for this condition are promising, and there are clinicians who are qualified and sincere in their efforts to improve the lives of tinnitus sufferers. These clinicians (as well as administrators) are hindered, however, by the absence of outcome data that should be available to make informed judgments regarding treatment efficacy. With a focused and systematic effort to develop a comprehensive tinnitus management program for veterans, such a program could serve as a model for providing tinnitus services beyond the VA Healthcare System.

This chapter outlines the problem of tinnitus for veterans and for the VHA. In the attempt to provide solutions, a number of projects are proposed that, if implemented, could result in VA-wide clinical programs to manage veterans with tinnitus. The objective is to develop cost-effective forms of treatment that will benefit the majority of veteran patients and contain useful methods to screen for patients requiring more extensive treatment. Further efforts are required to disseminate information about tinnitus to veterans and to VA health professionals.

The number of veterans with service-connected tinnitus is high, and these numbers are increasing rapidly. Tinnitus may also be concurrent with or exacerbated by other problems, such as posttraumatic stress disorder, depression, or chronic pain. It is vitally important to provide effective therapeutic services for these veterans and to be able to demonstrate treatment success with valid and reliable measurement tools. If effective tinnitus treatment techniques are available, it is a moral imperative to provide these services to the veterans who are entitled to them.

APPENDIX A

Tinnitus-Impact Screening Questionnaire

1. Do you have tinnitus that is constant? (ie, it's usually or always there, whether you are consciously aware of it or not)
   YES   NO
2. How much has tinnitus annoyed you, on average, over the last month? ("0" would be "not annoying at all"; "10" would be "as annoying as you can imagine")
   0   1   2   3   4   5   6   7   8   9   10
3. How much did tinnitus affect or impact your life, on average, over the last month? ("0" would be "not at all"; "10" would be "as much as you can imagine")
   0   1   2   3   4   5   6   7   8   9   10
4. Does tinnitus affect your sleep?
   Always / Often / Sometimes / Never
5. Does tinnitus affect your concentration?
   Always / Often / Sometimes / Never
6. If your tinnitus is a problem for you, what is the major reason your tinnitus is a problem?

ACKNOWLEDGMENTS

The authors acknowledge helpful contributions from Michael R. Wells, statistician, Data Management and Analysis Service, Veterans Affairs Office of Policy, Planning and Preparedness; Susan Griest, MPH, research investigator, NCRAR; Doug Ohlin, PhD, program manager, Hearing Conservation Program, US Army; and Rachel Wray, director of advocacy and support, American Tinnitus Association. Funding for this work was provided by Veterans Affairs Rehabilitation Research and Development Service (C2300R, C2887R, C2760R, and RCTR 597-0160).

REFERENCES

1. Census 2000 veteran data. Available at: http://www.va.gov/vetdata/Census2000/ (accessed April 15, 2004).
2. Feussner J. Clinical research in the Department of Veterans Affairs: using research to improve patient outcomes. J Invest Med 1998;46:264–7.
3. Vernon JA. Is the claimed tinnitus real and is the claimed cause correct? In: Reich GE, Vernon JA, editors. Proceedings of the Fifth International Tinnitus Seminar 1995. Portland (OR): American Tinnitus Association; 1996. p. 395–6.
4. Schechter MA, Henry JA. Assessment and treatment of tinnitus patients using a "masking approach." J Am Acad Audiol 2002;13:545–58.
5. Henry JA, Fausti SA, Mitchell CR, et al. Computer-automated clinical technique for tinnitus quantification. Am J Audiol 2000;9:36–49.
6. Henry JA, Flick CL, Gilbert AM, et al. Reliability of tinnitus loudness matches under procedural variation. J Am Acad Audiol 1999;10:502–20.
7. Henry JA, Flick CL, Gilbert A, et al. Comparison of manual and computer-automated procedures for tinnitus pitch-matching. J Rehabil Res Dev 2004;41:121–38.
8. Henry JA, Schechter MA, Nagler SM, Fausti SA. Comparison of tinnitus masking and tinnitus retraining therapy. J Am Acad Audiol 2002;13:559–81.
9. Brown SC. Older Americans and tinnitus: a demographic study and chartbook. GRI monograph series A, no. 2. Washington (DC): Gallaudet Research Institute, Gallaudet University; 1990.
10. Hinchcliffe R. Prevalence of the commoner ear, nose and throat conditions in the adult rural population of Great Britain. Br J Prev Soc Med 1961;15:128–40.
11. Leske MC. Prevalence estimates of communicative disorders in the U.S. Language, learning and vestibular disorders. ASHA 1981;23:229–37.
12. Davis AC. Hearing in adults. London: Whurr Publishers, Ltd.; 1995.
13. Office of Population Census and Surveys. General household survey: the prevalence of tinnitus 1981. OPCS Monitor, Reference GHS83/1. London: Office for National Statistics; 1983.
14. Davis A, Refaie AE. Epidemiology of tinnitus. In: Tyler RS, editor. Tinnitus handbook. San Diego (CA): Singular Publishing Group; 2000. p. 1–23.
15. Beck L. Perspective and national office report. Presented at the Annual meeting of the Association of VA Audiologists; Philadelphia, PA; 2002.
16. VetPop2001 adjusted to Census 2000 (Vetpop-2000Adj). Available at: http://www.va.gov/vetdata/Demographics/index.htm (accessed April 15, 2004).
17. Reich GE. The costs of tinnitus. Tinnitus Today 2002;27:18–9.
18. Annual benefits report, fiscal year 2002. Washington (DC): Veterans Benefits Administration, Department of Veterans Affairs; 2003.
19. VBA annual report, 2001. Washington (DC): Veterans Benefits Administration, Department of Veterans Affairs; May 2002.
20. Data report: VA Office of Policy and Planning. Washington (DC): VA Central Office; September 2002.
21. Veterans Benefits Administration. Disability examination worksheet (#1305). Available at: http://vbaw.vba.va.gov/bl/21/rating/Medical/exams/disexm05.htm (accessed April 15, 2004).
22. Dennis K. Development of tinnitus handicap battery. Technical report, HSR&D project 42-054, Health Services Research and Development Midwest Field Program. Washington (DC): Department of Veterans Affairs; 1993.
23. Kirsch CA, Blanchard EB, Parnes SM. Psychological characteristics of individuals high and low in their ability to cope with tinnitus. Psychosom Med 1989;51:209–17.
24. Wilson PH, Henry J, Bowen M, Haralambous G. Tinnitus Reaction Questionnaire: psychometric properties of a measure of distress associated with tinnitus. J Speech Hear Res 1991;34:197–201.
25. Schechter MA, Henry JA, Zaugg T, Fausti SA. Selection of ear level devices for two different methods of tinnitus treatment. In: Patuzzi R, editor. Proceedings of the Seventh International Tinnitus Seminar. Perth: University of Western Australia; 2002. p. 13.
26. Axelsson A, Barrenas M-L. Tinnitus in noise-induced hearing loss. In: Dancer AL, Henderson D, Salvi RJ, Hamnernik RP, editors. Noise-induced hearing loss. St. Louis: Mosby-Year Book, Inc.; 1992. p. 269–76.
27. Penner MJ, Bilger RC. Psychophysical observations and the origin of tinnitus. In: Vernon JA, Møller AR, editors. Mechanisms of tinnitus. Needham Heights (MA): Allyn & Bacon; 1995. p. 219–30.
28. Statement of The Honorable Robert H. Roswell, MD, Under Secretary for Health, Department of Veterans Affairs, before the Committee on Veterans' Affairs, US House of Representatives, on the State of VA Health Care, January 29, 2003. Available at: http://veterans.house.gov/hearings/schedule108/jan03/1-29-03/1-29-03hearing.html (accessed April 15, 2004).

29. Jastreboff PJ, Hazell JWP. Treatment of tinnitus based on a neurophysiological model. In: Vernon JA, editor. Tinnitus treatment and relief. Needham Heights (MA): Allyn & Bacon; 1998. p. 201–17.
30. Henry JA, Jastreboff MM, Jastreboff PJ, et al. Guide to conducting tinnitus retraining therapy (TRT) initial and follow-up interviews. J Rehabil Res Dev 2003; 40:157–78.
31. Henry JA, Jastreboff MM, Jastreboff PJ, et al. TRT Interview Form: an expanded version. In: Patuzzi R, editor. Proceedings of the Seventh International Tinnitus Seminar. Perth: University of Western Australia; 2002. p. 330–9.
32. Jastreboff MM, Jastreboff PJ. Questionnaires for assessment of the patients and their outcomes. In: Hazell J, editor. Proceedings of the Sixth International Tinnitus Seminar. London: The Tinnitus and Hyperacusis Centre; 1999. p. 487–91.
33. Meikle MB, Griest SE, Stewart BJ, Press LS. Measuring the negative impact of tinnitus: a brief severity index. In: Ryan AF, editor. Midwinter Meeting of the Association for Research in Otolaryngology. Des Moines (IA): Association for Research in Otolaryngology; 1995. p. 167.
34. Zaugg T, Schechter MA, Fausti SA, Henry JA. Difficulties caused by patients' misconceptions that hearing problems are due to tinnitus. In: Patuzzi R, editor. Proceedings of the Seventh International Tinnitus Seminar. Perth: University of Western Australia; 2002. p. 226–8.
35. Jastreboff PJ, Jastreboff MM. Tinnitus retraining therapy. Semin Hear 2001;22:51–63.
36. Vernon JAE. Tinnitus treatment and relief. Needham Heights (MA): Allyn & Bacon; 1998.
37. Henry JA, Jastreboff MM, Jastreboff PJ, et al. Assessment of patients for treatment with tinnitus retraining therapy. J Am Acad Audiol 2002;13:523–44.
38. Sweetow RW. Cognitive-behavior modification. In: Tyler RS, editor. Tinnitus handbook. San Diego (CA): Singular Publishing Group; 2000. p. 297–311.
39. Henry JL, Wilson PH. The psychological management of chronic tinnitus. Needham Heights (MA): Allyn & Bacon; 2001.
40. Axelsson A, Sandh A. Tinnitus in noise induced hearing loss. Br J Audiol 1985;19:271–6.
41. Chung DY, Gannon RP, Mason K. Factors affecting the prevalence of tinnitus. Audiology 1984;23:441–52.
42. Meikle MB, Griest SE. Gender-based differences in characteristics of tinnitus. Hear J 1989;42:68–76.
43. Phoon WH, Lee HS, Chia SE. Tinnitus in noise-exposed workers. Occup Med 1993;43:35–8.
44. Ohlin D. Let's hear it for our troops. Saving hearing—and money—in the military. ASHA 1998;40:50–3.
45. Ritter DC, Perkins JL. Noise-induced hearing loss among U.S. Air Force cryptolinguists. Aviat Space Environ Med 2001;72:546–52.
46. Bohnker BK, Page JC, Rovig G, et al. U.S. Navy and Marine Corps Hearing Conservation Program, 1995-1999: mean hearing thresholds for enlisted personnel by gender and age groups. Mil Med 2002;167:132–5.
47. Bohnker BK, Page JC, Rovig G, et al. Navy Hearing Conservation Program: threshold shifts in enlisted personnel, 1995-1999. Mil Med 2002;167:48–52.
48. Perry BP, Gantz BJ. Medical and surgical evaluation and management of tinnitus. In: Tyler RS, editor. Tinnitus handbook. San Diego (CA): Singular Publishing Group; 2000. p. 221–41.
49. Tyler RS. Tinnitus disability and handicap questionnaires. Semin Hear 1993;14:377–83.
50. Meikle MB, Griest SE. Tinnitus severity and disability: prospective efforts to develop a core set of measures. In: Patuzzi R, editor. Proceedings of the Seventh International Tinnitus Seminar. Perth: University of Western Australia; 2002. p. 157–61.
51. Dobie RA. Randomized clinical trials for tinnitus: not the last word? In: Patuzzi R, editor. Proceedings of the Seventh International Tinnitus Seminar. Perth: University of Western Australia; 2002. p. 3–6.
52. Kuk FK, Tyler RS, Russell D, Jordan H. The psychometric properties of a tinnitus handicap questionnaire. Ear Hear 1990;11:434–45.
53. Newman CW, Jacobson GP, Spitzer JB. Development of the Tinnitus Handicap Inventory. Arch Otolaryngol Head Neck Surg 1996;122:143–8.
54. Dobie RA. Medico-legal aspects of tinnitus. In: Patuzzi R, editor. Proceedings of the Seventh International Tinnitus Seminar. Perth: University of Western Australia; 2002. p. 25–8.
55. Martin FN. Pseudohypacusis. In: Katz J, editor. Handbook of clinical audiology. Baltimore: Williams & Wilkins; 1994. p. 553–67.
56. Jacobson GP, Henderson JA. Toward the development of a subjective measure of the presence of tinnitus: preliminary observations [abstract]. In: Popelka GR, editor. Association for Research in Otolaryngology Abstracts. Mt. Royal (NJ): Association for Research in Otolaryngology; 1999. p. 172.

57. Coles RRA. Medicolegal issues. In: Tyler RS, editor. Tinnitus handbook. San Diego (CA): Singular Publishing Group; 2000. p. 399–417.
58. Hinchcliffe R, King PF. Medicolegal aspects of tinnitus. III. Assessment of claimants with tinnitus. J Audiol Med 1992;1:127–47.
59. Meikle M, Walsh ET. Characteristics of tinnitus and related observations in over 1800 tinnitus patients. In: Shulman A, Ballantyne J, editors. Proceedings of the Second International Tinnitus Seminar. Ashford (UK): Invicta Press; 1984. p. 17–21.
60. Tyler RS. Considerations when evaluating a tinnitus patient for compensation. Aust N Z J Audiol 2003;24:85–91.
61. Darby M. Clinical practice guidelines. Boston: Management Decision and Research Center; Washington (DC): VA Health Services Research and Development Service in collaboration with Association for Health Services Research; 1998.
62. Dobie RA. A review of randomized clinical trials in tinnitus. Laryngoscope 1999;109:1202–11.
63. Vernon JA, Møller AR. Mechanisms of tinnitus. Needham Heights (MA): Allyn & Bacon; 1995.

EDITORIAL COMMENTARY

Henry and colleagues provide an entirely new perspective of the societal cost of tinnitus by acquainting us with an annual and growing expenditure of over 285 million dollars for disability compensation for American veterans. Their carefully articulated and logically integrated plan for prevention of tinnitus and improving clinical care of our veterans and, by extension, of all patients with tinnitus deserves careful study and support. These authors advocate a three-tiered, cost-effective management plan of progressive intervention to treat patients. Telephone screening is used as the lowest tier to separate those suffering from tinnitus from those who simply experience tinnitus. Group education and support are the second tier for those who require minimal intervention, and comprehensive individualized management is provided to tinnitus sufferers depending on the severity of the impact of tinnitus on their lives.

James B. Snow Jr

Index

A

Aberrant internal carotid artery, *See* Dehiscent carotid artery
Abbreviated Profile of Hearing Aid Benefit, 310
Acoustic neurinoma, 58
Acoustic neuroma, 58
Acoustic reflex, 223
Acoustic reflex decay, 223
Acoustic tumors, 4
Acetylcholine, 45, 62
Active extinction of conditioned reflex, 301
Activity-dependent plasticity, 193
Acupuncture, 272
Acute tinnitus, 142
Adaptation, 146
Addison's disease and hyperacusis, 12
Adrenergic innervation of the cochlea, 62
Age and tinnitus, 21t, 24–29, 28t, 31–34, 32t, 33t, 35t, 36–38, 37f
Age-related hearing loss, 1
Alexander's law, 211
Alpha-amino-3-hydroxy-5-methyl-4-isoxazole propionic acid, 193
Alpha1-selective adrenoreceptor blocking agents, 108
Alprazolam, 269, 273, 275
Alternate binaural loudness balance, 222
Alternating current, 327
American Speech-Language-Hearing Association, 342
American Tinnitus Association, 286
Aminoglycoside antibiotics, 144

Amino-oxyacetic acid, 273
Amitriptyline, 274
Amygdala, 162–167
    basolateral nucleus of, 166, 167
    lateral nucleus of, 164, 165, 167
    medial nucleus of, 165
Anemia, 257
Angiography, 213, 216, 216f, 217f, 257f
Angiotensin-converting enzyme inhibitors, 108
Animal models of tinnitus, 80–95, 271
    Bauer procedure. *See* Bauer animal model of tinnitus
    Guitton procedure. *See* Guitton animal model of tinnitus
    Heffner procedure. *See* Heffner animal model of tinnitus
    Jastreboff procedure. *See* Jastreboff animal model of tinnitus
    Moody procedure. *See* Moody animal model of tinnitus
Annual income and tinnitus, 25t, 28t, 29–31, 32t
Annoyance
    caused by tinnitus, 4, 321
Anodal stimulation, 327
Anxiety, 278–285
Anxiety Sensitivity Index, 281, 282
Anterior auditory field, 147, 148, 150, 167, 175–179, 177–179f
Anterior olfactory region, 162
Antiarrhythmics, 273
Anticonvulsants, 273
Antidepressants, 274

Anxiety disorder, 5
Anxiety sensitivity, 281
Aortic stenosis, 257
Arousal, 164, 165
Arrhythmias, 207
Arteriosclerosis, 1
Arteriovenous malformation, 216, 216f, 257
Arthritis, 1
A scale, 2
Ascending pharyngeal artery, 216
Attention, 164, 321
Attention control, 280, 317, 318
Audimax Theraband, 327
Audiologic assessment, 212, 213
Audiologist, 220
Auditory association cortices, 164
Auditory brainstem response, 9, 213, 256
    stacked, 256
Auditory cortex, 151
Auditory deafferentation, 256, 259, 260, 260f, 261f
Auditory nerve disorders, 58
Auscultation, 210, 257
Autoimmune inner ear disease, 56
Automatic gain control, 97, 303
Autonomic nervous system, 8, 96–105, 165, 300
    sympathetic part of the, 96, 98, 103, 301
Axis I disorders, 283
Axis II disorders, 283

B
Baclofen, 274
Bandstop noise, 145, 146
Basal ganglia, 163
Basilar membrane, 59, 60
Bauer animal model of tinnitus, 86–89, 87f, 88f, 94
Bayesian probability theory, 11
Beaver Dam, Wisconsin Hearing Loss Study, 20
Beck Anxiety Inventory, 281–283
Beck Depression Inventory, 244, 278–280, 283
Behavioral psychotherapy, 282

Behavioral therapy, 273, 317, 318
Bell's palsy and hyperacusis, 12
Benzimidazole inhibitors of gastric acid secretion, 108
Benzodiazepine, 273, 274
    withdrawal from and hyperacusis, 12
Betahistine, 274
Bilateral contralateral routing of signal, 303, 306
Bing tuning fork test, 209
Biofeedback therapy, 272, 278, 280, 281
Blinding, 267
Blood-labyrinth barrier, 55
Body mass index and tinnitus, 29t, 30
British Tinnitus Association, 81, 281
Brodmann's areas 21 and 41, 168
Bruxism, 109
Bupropion, 285, 288
Burst firing of auditory neurons, 150, 157, 172, 173, 175, 182–185, 190

C
Calcitonin gene-related peptide, 62
Calcium, 147
Calcium homeostasis, 58
Calcium response element binding protein, 47
Carbamazepine, 273
Carboplatin, 144
Carotid artery aneurysm, 257
Carotid artery stenosis, 257f
Caroverine, 274
Cartwheel cells of the dorsal cochlear nucleus, 119, 128, 157
Categorization of patients with tinnitus, 297–299, 298t
Cathodal stimulation, 327
Cerebellar vestibular tests, 211
Cerebellum, 102
Cerebral cortex, 163, 164
Cerebrospinal fluid hypertension and hyperacusis, 12
C fibers of the cochlea, 63

C-fos, 148, 149, 167
Characteristic frequency, 145–148, 151, 173, 173f, 174f, 176, 177–184f
Children and tinnitus, 37, 38
Chloroquine, 144
Cholinergic system, 195
Chronic tinnitus, 1, 142–144
   definition of, 17
Ciba Foundation, 222
Cingulate gyrus, 162, 163
Cinnarizine, 274
Cisplatin, 57, 144, 155
Classical auditory pathway See Lemniscal auditory pathway
Clinical Interview Schedule, 279, 283
Clinically significant tinnitus, 98
Clonus of the tensor tympani muscle, 57
Cochlear amplification, 60, 62, 63, 73
Cochlear blood flow, 63
Cochlear implants, 272, 327
Cochlear motor theory of tinnitus, 60
Cochlear nucleus, 118, 119, 125, 157
Code for silence, 329
Cogan's syndrome, 56
Cognitive restructuring, 280, 317
Cognitive therapy, 251, 273, 281, 315, 317
Combination instrument, 311, 312, 342
Common spinal tract of the facial, glossopharyngeal and vagus nerves, 118f, 119, 119f
Computed tomography, 213, 214f, 217f, 255
Computer-automated tinnitus assessment, 222
Concentration, 4, 6, 165
Conditioned reflex, 98–100, 103, 301
   extinction of, 101, 103–105
Conditioned stimulus, 81, 165, 167
Conditioned suppression, 81
Conductive hearing loss, 1, 2, 57
Confidence interval, 269, 271
Connexin 26, 44
Connexin 31, 44

Contralateral routing of signal, 303, 306, 312
Control group, 268
Corticosteroid treatment, 56
Cost-effectiveness, 251, 252
Cost-utility analysis, 252
Costen's syndrome, 116
Counseling, 315
   in tinnitus retraining therapy, 299–301
Counterdemand instruction, 279–281
Cranial nerve testing, 207–209
Craniomandibular disorder, 57, 116
Cronbach's alpha, 239
Crown Crisp Experimental Inventory, 278, 279
Cyclandelate, 274

D

Deafferentation, auditory, See Auditory deafferentation
Decreased sound tolerance, 8–12, 60
   prevalence of, 10, 11
   triggering factors, 11
Definition of tinnitus, 1
Dehiscent carotid artery, 215, 215f, 257
Dehiscent jugular bulb, 215, 215f
Department of Veteran Affairs, 337
Depression, 4, 5, 165, 278–280
Depressive disorder, 6
Description of tinnitus, 3
Developmental plasticity, 191
Diabetes, 207
Diagnostic and Statistical Manual of Mental Disorders, Third Edition-Revised, 283
Diazepam, 273
Diencephalon, 163
Diplacusis, 224
Direct current, 327
Directive counseling, 316
Discomalleolar ligament, 57
Discordant dysfunction theory of tinnitus, 96, 97
Disco tinnitus, 101

Disequilibrium, 207
Disinhibition, 120
Dizziness Handicap Inventory, 244
Dopamine B-hydroxylase, 196
Dopaminergic system, 195, 196
Dorsal cochlear nucleus, 114, 119–123, 132f, 149–158, 152f, 154–156f, 167, 171, 172
Dorsal column of the spinal cord, 125
Double blind, 267, 268
Double-dissociation principle, 165, 166
Doxepin, 286
Drinking alcohol and tinnitus, 24, 29t, 30, 207
Dynamic balance principle, 102, 103

E

Ear diseases and tinnitus, 55, 56t
Edge effect theory of tinnitus, 53, 61, 146
Educational level and tinnitus, 25t, 28t, 29–31, 32t
Effect size, 321, 321t
Egyptian papyri, 326
Electrical stimulation, 272
Electrical suppression, 331–333
Electroacoustic cochlear implant, 329
Electromagnetic therapy, 272
Electromyography, 213, 272
Electronystagmography, 212
Electrophonic activation, 328
Embolization, arterial, 216
Emotion, 4, 6, 162–169
Endocochlear potential, 56, 59, 60
Endolymphatic hydrops, 55
Endolymphatic potential, 55
Endoscopy of the middle ear, 215f
Endoscopic surgery of the posterior cranial fossa, 218f
Entorhinal area, 162, 164
Eperisone, 274
Epidemiology
    definition of, 16
Epithalamus, 163

Ethacrynic acid, 57, 144
Eustachian tube occlusion, 57
Ewald's second law, 211
Excitotoxicity of neurons, 157
Existential therapy, 318
External auditory canal occlusion, 57
Extralemniscal auditory pathway, 125, 164
Extroversion, 279
Eysneck Personality Questionnaire, 278, 279

F

False-negative error, 267
False-positive error, 267
Faradization, 327
Fasciculus cuneatus, 119, 120
Fear conditioning, 165–167
Fear learning, 165
Feasibility of a tinnitus questionnaire, 240
Fibromuscular dysplasia, 257
Final common path of tinnitus, 52, 53, 57, 58
Flunarizine, 270, 274
Fluoxetine, 274, 285, 288
Free-floating anxiety, 279
Freezing, 165
Frenzel lenses, 211, 212
Furosemide, 57, 144
Fusiform cells of the dorsal cochlear nucleus, 157

G

Gallaudet Hearing Scale, 27
Galvanization, 327
Gamma-aminobutyric acid, 45, 46, 62, 193
Gamma knife radiation therapy, 256
Gaze-evoked tinnitus, 259, 262, 262f
General health and tinnitus, 25t, 27, 30, 32t, 33t, 35t
General Health Questionnaire, 278, 282
Gentamicin, 144
Ginkgo biloba, 85, 270, 274

Glomus jugulare tumor, 216, 217f, 257, 258f
Glomus tympanicum tumor, 216, 216f, 217f
Glutamate, 45, 46, 157, 193
Glutamate decarboxylase, 47
Glutamate-induced excitotoxicity, 61
Glycine, 46, 48
Golgi tendon organs, 113, 114, 119, 123
Grading of tinnitus, 19
Granular layer of the dorsal cochlear nucleus, 122, 136
Granule cells of the dorsal cochlear nucleus, 119, 121f
Granule layer of the ventral cochlear nucleus, 126
Guitton animal model of tinnitus, 91, 94
Gustation, 165

H

Habituation, 104, 105, 301, 302
Hamilton Rating Scale for Anxiety, 281–283
Hamilton Rating Scale for Depression, 279, 283, 288
Head injury and hyperacusis, 12,
Head injury and tinnitus, 19, 19t, 22, 22t, 33t, 35t, 207
Head shake vestibular test, 209t, 211, 212
Head thrust vestibular test, 209t, 211
Hearing aids, 6, 251, 272, 310–312, 342
Hearing difficulty, 4, 6
Hearing Handicap Inventory for Adults, 244
Hearing Handicap Inventory for the Elderly, 244
Hearing impairment and tinnitus, 25t, 26f, 27, 28t, 30, 32t, 33t, 34, 35t, 37f
Hearing loss
    age-related. *See* Age-related hearing loss
    conductive. *See* Conductive hearing loss
    noise-induce. *See* Noise-induced hearing loss
    rapidly progressing. *See* Rapidly progressing hearing loss
    sensorineural. *See* Sensorineural hearing loss
    sudden. *See* Sudden hearing loss
Hearing protection devices, 2

Heffner animal model of tinnitus, 89–91, 89f, 90f, 94, 152
Hennebert's sign, 212
Heritability of tinnitus, 34
High rate pulse trains, 329
Hippocampus, 162–164, 166
    perirhinal area of, 164
H,K-adenosine triphosphatase, 44
Homeostasis, 165
House-Brackmann scale, 207
Hughson-Westlake ascending-descending audiometric test technique, 225
Humanistic therapy, 318
Hyperactivity of auditory neurons, 149–158, 152f, 154–156f
Hyperacusis, 8–13, 9f, 223, 230, 299
    definition of, 8
    prevalence of, 11
Hyperdynamic states, 257
Hypertension and tinnitus, 1, 38, 207
Hyperventilation-induced nystagmus test, 209t, 212
Hypnosis, 272
Hypothalamus, 163, 167
Hysteria, 278

I

Impact of tinnitus, 4
Imagery training, 280, 317
Imipramine, 286, 287
Immitance, 223
Immune-mediated inner ear disease, 56
Incidence of tinnitus, 20
    definition of, 20
Inferior colliculus, 114, 122, 125, 128, 147, 149–151
    central nucleus of, 122, 128, 135f, 149, 171
    external nucleus of, 128, 171
    pericentral nucleus of, 149
Inclusion criteria, 269
Information about hearing and tinnitus, 318

Injury-induced plasticity, 194
Inner hair cells, 58, 59, 61, 155
Innervation of hair cells, 58
Insula, 163
Interspike interval, 173–175, 173–175f, 177–179f
Intracellular potential of hair cells, 55
Introversion, 279
Isk potassium channel, 44

J

Jastreboff animal model of tinnitus, 81–85, 82–86f, 94
Joint Commission on the Accreditation of Healthcare Organizations, 250

K

Kainate, 45, 157
Kca potassium channel, 46
K-Cl cotransporter, Kcc4, 44
KCNQ1, 44
KCNQ4 potassium channel, 44
Kindling, 299
Kv1.1 potassium channel, 46
Kv3.1 potassium channel, 46–48
Kv4.2 potassium channel, 46

L

Lamotrigine, 274
Laser therapy, 272
Lateral olivocochlear bundle, 58, 61
Lateral inhibition, 146, 192, 329
Lateral parabranchial nucleus, 167
Lateralization of tympanic membrane graft, 57
Learning, 165
Learning-induced plasticity, 193, 194
Lemniscal auditory pathway, 164, 171
Lidocaine, 115, 147, 151, 190, 270, 273
Limbic system, 8, 96, 98–105, 162–169, 300

Lipoid proteinosis, 166
Localization of tinnitus, 53, 54f
Locus ceruleus, 167, 195
Longitudinal Study of Aging Danish Twins, 34
Loudness discomfort level, 9, 10, 10t, 223, 230
Loudness tolerance, 230
Lyme disease and hyperacusis, 12

M

Magnetic resonance imaging, 213, 214f, 216, 255, 256
    functional magnetic resonance imaging, 190
    gadolinium enhanced, 213, 214f, 255, 256, 256f, 258f
Magnetic therapy, 272
Magnetoencephalography, 151, 190
Magnocellular layer of the ventral cochlear nucleus, 126
Major depressive disorder, 282
Mammillary bodies, 163
Mann-Whitney test, 274
Marginal cell region of the ventral cochlear nucleus, 126
Maskability, 222, 223
Maskers, 272
Masking devices, 3, 6, 271
Masking, 3, 221, 222, 310, 311, 315, 350–352
Massage therapy, 272
Matching
    loudness or intensity, 3, 222–228
    pitch or frequency, 3, 222–228
Medial geniculate body, 125, 167, 172
Medial olivocochlear bundle, 58, 60–62, 76
Median nerve stimulation, 109–111, 125
Medullary somatosensory nuclei, 118f, 119, 120
Melatonin, 269, 270, 274
Memory, 163–165, 167
Meniere's disease, 3, 43, 55, 205, 213, 250, 340
Meniere's syndrome, 55
Metropolitan statistical area and tinnitus, 27
Mexiletine, 115

Mianserin, 288
Microvascular compression syndrome, 218f
Military service and tinnitus, 22t, 30, 31, 32t, 205, 337
Minimum masking levels, 223, 228, 229
Minnesota Multiphasic Personality Inventory, 278
Misophonia, 9–13, 9f, 99, 100, 103, 105, 299
Misoprostol, 274
Mitral regurgitation, 257
Mnemonic processes, 163, 166
Modified Somatic Perception Questionnaire, 244
Molecular layer of the dorsal cochlear nucleus, 122
Moody animal model of tinnitus, 91–94, 92f
Multidimensional Pain Inventory, 288
Multiple sclerosis, 58
Multivariate analyses of tinnitus prevalence, 31–34, 32t, 33t
Muscarinic acetylcholine, 45
Muscle spindles, 113, 114, 119, 123
Muscrimol, 171

N
Na,K-adenosine triphosphatase, 43
Na-K-Cl cotransporter, 44
Nasopharyngoscopy, 210
National Academy of Sciences, 222, 338
National Center for Health Statistics, 16
National Health and Nutrition Examination Survey, 18
National Health Examination Survey, 18
National Health Interview Survey, 16
National Institute on Deafness and Other Communication Disorders, 17
National Institute of Mental Health Diagnostic Interview Schedule, 282
National Institutes of Health, 17
Natural history of tinnitus, 1, 5, 267
Negative affect, 321
Neocortex, 163
Neonatal hearing screening, 73
Nucleus basalis, 195

Neurologic model of somatic tinnitus, 117–120
Neuromodulatory systems, 195
   cholinergic. See Cholinergic system
   dopaminergic. See Dopaminergic system
   noradrenergic. See Noradrenergic system
   serotonin. See Serotonin system
Neurophysiological model of tinnitus, 96–105, 295, 310
Neurotic conversion, 278
Neuroticism, 279
Neutral demand instruction, 281
Nicotinamide, 274
Nicotinic acetylcholine, 45, 62
N-methyl-D-aspartate, 45, 46, 193, 195
N-methyl-D-aspartate antagonist, 166, 167
Noise exposure and tinnitus, 19, 19t, 23t, 24, 30, 33t, 34, 35t, 142, 143, 148–150, 152–156f, 157, 172, 180–186, 180–184f, 205, 206, 337
Noradrenaline, 62
Noradrenergic system, 195, 196
Nord Trøndelag Hearing Loss Study, 17, 18, 21t, 22, 22t, 24, 27, 28t, 29–31, 34, 35t, 36–38, 37f
Nord Trøndelag Health Survey, 17
Nortriptyline, 250, 274, 275, 287, 288
Nurturing patient expectations, 314
Nystagmus, 211, 212

O
Objective tinnitus, 1, 2, 70, 255, 255t
Obsessionality, 279
Occupation and tinnitus, 28t, 30,
Octopus cells of the posteroventral cochlear nucleus, 148
Odds ratio
   calculation of, 27
   history and use of, 18
   of having tinnitus, 2, 2f, 28t, 32t, 33t, 35t
Olfaction, 162, 165
Olfactory bulb, 162
Open earmold, 311
Open trial, 270, 271

Oral contraception and tinnitus, 38
Orbitofrontal cortex, 163
Organ of Corti-specific proteins, 46
Oscillopsia, 212
Ossicular disarticulation, 57
Osteitis deformans, 57
Otic tinnitus, 120, 121
Otitis media, 57
Otoacoustic emissions, 69–76, 230, 231
    distortion-product otoacoustic emissions, 69, 71f, 73–75, 74f, 223, 231, 300
    evoked otoacoustic emissions, 69, 73
    spontaneous otoacoustic emissions, 62, 63, 69–73, 76
    transient evoked otoacoustic emissions, 69, 71f, 73, 75f, 76
Otoanchorin, 46
Otosclerosis, 2, 57
Ototoxic agents, 206
Ototoxic drugs and tinnitus, 57
Ototoxicity monitoring, 73
Outcome measure, 271
Outcome variable, 268
Outer hair cell-based cochlear amplifier, 60
Outer hair cells, 58–61, 69, 155, 157, 300
Oxford-Family Planning Association contraceptive study, 38

P

Paget's disease, 57
Palatal myoclonus, 210, 258
Paleomammal, 163
Paraganlioma, 210
Paranoia, 278
Paroxetine, 274
Passive avoidance procedure, 86
Passive extinction of conditioned reflex, 104, 301
Patulous eustachian tube, 210
Pearson product-moment correlation, 239
Periaqueductal gray area, 167
Perilymph fistula and tinnitus, 212
Perilymphatic fistula and hyperacusis, 12
Periodicity, 145
Permanent tinnitus, 6
Persistent stapedial artery, 257
Phantom auditory perception, 96, 300
Phenelzine, 285, 286
Phonophobia, 8, 9
Pink noise, 148
Pitch
    low-pitched versus high-pitched tinnitus, 53, 53f
Placebo
    active, 268
    inert, 268
Placebo controlled, 267, 268
Plasticity, 189–197
    activity-dependent. *See* Activity-dependent plasticity
    developmental. *See* Developmental plasticity
    learning-induced. *See* Learning-induced plasticity
    injury-induced. *See* Injury-induced plasticity
Pneumatic otoscopy, 212, 216
Poisson process, 329
Portland Veterans Affairs Medical Center, 337
Positron emission tomography, 168, 190, 255, 258, 259f, 261f
Power analysis, 269, 270, 271
Prefrontal cortex, 164
Preproenkephalin, 45
Presbycusis, 2
Prestin, 45, 60
Prevalence of tinnitus, 20–30, 21t, 22t, 25t, 26f, definition of, 20
Primary auditory cortex, 147, 148, 150, 164, 167, 171, 173, 175–179, 173–184f
Problems
    caused by tinnitus, 4
Prognostic factors, 6, 267, 270
Prognostic staging system, 271
Progressive intervention model, 344
Proreptile, 163

Pseudohypacusis, 73
Psychasthenia, 279
Psychoacoustic characterization of tinnitus, 98
Psychological treatments, 314–322
Psychoneuroticism, 279
Psychotherapy, 273
Pterygoid muscles, 123
    medial, 110
Pulsatile tinnitus, 58, 205, 213, 213t, 214–216f, 216, 218, 255t, 257, 257f, 258
Pyramidal cells of the dorsal cochlear nucleus, 119
Pyramidal system, 163

Q

Quality of tinnitus, 3
Quality-adjusted life-years, 252
Questionnaire, 243, 244
    feasibility of. *See* Feasibility of a tinnitus questionnaire
    reliability of. *See* Reliability of a tinnitus questionnaire
    validity of. *See* Validity of a tinnitus questionnaire
Questionnaires, 237–252
    Subjective Tinnitus Severity Scale, 242t, 243
    Tinnitus Cognitions Questionnaire, 242t, 247
    Tinnitus Coping Style Questionnaire, 242t, 247, 248
    Tinnitus Handicap Inventory, 242t, 244, 310, 348, 350
    Tinnitus Handicap Questionnaire, 242t, 244, 245, 288, 289, 348, 350
    Tinnitus Handicap/Support Scale, 242t, 246, 247
    Tinnitus Problems Questionnaire, 241, 242
    Tinnitus Questionnaire, 242t, 243, 244, 282
    Tinnitus Reaction Questionnaire, 242t, 246, 280, 281
    Tinnitus Severity Index, 348, 350
    Tinnitus Severity Scale, 242t, 246, 247, 281, 288
Quetelet's ponderal index, 30
Quinine, 58, 85, 172, 175–179, 176–179f, 184–186

R

Race/ethnicity and tinnitus, 22t, 25t, 28t, 29
Radiation, 207
Raphe nuclei, 195
Randomized clinical trial, 6, 266
Rapidly progressing hearing loss, 55, 56
Reaction to tinnitus, 4
Reclassification of tinnitus signal, 104, 105
Recruitment, 9, 11, 222, 224
Reduction of tinnitus-related neuronal activity, 104, 105
Region of the United States and tinnitus, 30, 31
Regression to the mean, 5
Relaxation training, 273, 279, 318
Reliability of a tinnitus questionnaire, 239
Reorganization as a part of plasticity, 151, 190, 263
Residual inhibition, 3, 222, 223, 229, 311
Reticular formation, 125, 128
Rheumatoid arthritis, 56
Rhinencephalon, 162, 163
Right hemisphere association cortex, 190
Rinne tuning fork test, 209, 209t, 210, 210f
Risk factors of tinnitus, 19, 19f, 20
    definite risk factors, 19, 19t
    familial risk factors, 34–36
    genetic risk factors, 34–36
    possible risk factors 19, 19t
    shared environmental risk factors, 34–36

S

Salicylate, 59, 60, 82–85, 83–85f, 87, 91, 142, 146–148, 147f, 150, 151, 172–179, 173f, 175f, 177–179f, 184–186
Sample size, 269
Schizophrenia, 278
Schwabach tuning fork test, 209

Secondary auditory cortex, 147, 148, 150, 172, 175–179, 177–179f
Selective serotonin reuptake inhibitors, 274
    bupropion. See Buprpion
    fluoxetine. See Fluoxetine
    paroxetine. See Paroxetine
    sertraline. See Sertraline
    trazodone. See Trazodone
    venlafaxine. See Venlafaxine
Self-Help for Hard of Hearing People, 342
Self image, 318
Sensation of tinnitus, 1, 4, 6
Sensorineural hearing loss, 1, 2
Septal nuclei, 163
Serotonin, 48
Serotonin system, 195
Sertraline, 285, 289
Service-connected disability, 337
Severity of tinnitus, 6
Sex and tinnitus, 24–27, 31–34
Side effects, 268
Single photon emission computed tomography, 255
Site-of-lesion testing, 73
Sleep, 4, 6, 97, 165, 319
Sleep disturbance, 321
Smoking cigarettes and tinnitus, 24, 29t, 30, 33t, 34, 35t
Somatic anxiety, 279
Somatic modulation of tinnitus, 109, 110, 117–120, 123
Somatic tinnitus 114, 117–120, 122, 123, 125
Somatic tinnitus syndrome, 114–116, 120, 123
Somatosensory modulation, 328
Somatosensory system, 125, 126f, 164, 165
Somatosound, 1, 2, 3, 105
Sound conditioning unit, 342
Sound localization, 119, 120
Sound therapy, 302, 303, 315, 315t
Spontaneous and gaze-evoked nystagmus test, 209t, 211
Spontaneous exacerbation of tinnitus, 5
Spontaneous remission of tinnitus, 6
Spontaneous rate of auditory neuron activity, 59, 146–158, 152f, 154–156f, 172, 173, 174f, 175, 176f, 178–183f, 190, 329
    decreased spontaneous rate theory of tinnitus, 59
    increased spontaneous rate theory of tinnitus, 59
Stapedectomy and hyperacusis, 12
Stapedial muscle spasm, 210
Startle, 165
State anxiety, 281
State Trait Anxiety Inventory, 278, 281
Statistical power, 269
Statistical significance, 270
Stereotactic radiation, 216
Sternocleidomastoid muscle, 109, 110, 114–116, 123
Stratification, 6, 270
Streptomycin, 144
Stria vascularis and tinnitus, 55
Structured Clinical Interview for Diagnosis, 283
Student's t-test, 274
Subaudible tinnitus, 2
Subjective tinnitus, 1, 70, 255
Substance P, 63, 127
Sudden hearing loss, 55, 56
Suffering from tinnitus, 1, 4, 6
Suicide, 5, 165, 284, 297
Superior canal dehiscence, 212, 213
Superior olivary complex, 118, 125, 128
Suppression of tinnitus, 229
Suppression ratio, 81
Symptom Checklist-90 Revised, 278, 282
Synaptic efficacy, 193
Synchrony of auditory neuron activity, 59, 146, 150, 172, 174, 175, 185–187, 190
Systemic lupus erythematosis, 56

T

Thalamocortical dysrhythmia, 190

Thalamus, 164, 171
   anterior part of, 163
   dorsal medial part of, 163
Tectorins, 46
Telephone screening, 344
Temporal lobe, 163
Temporary threshold shift, 61
Temporary tinnitus, 1, 2, 61
Temporomandibular joint disorder or syndrome, 57, 116, 117, 207
Temporomandibular therapy, 272
Tensor tympani muscle spasm, 210
Theory of tinnitus
   cochlear motor. *See* Cochlear motor theory of tinnitus
   discordant dysfunction. *See* Discordant dysfunction theory of tinnitus
   edge effect. *See* Edge effect theory of tinnitus
   spontaneous rate. *See* Spontaneous rate of auditory nerve fibers, decreased spontaneous rate theory of tinnitus increased spontaneous rate theory of tinnitus
   type I and II afferent auditory neuron imbalance. *See* Type I and II afferent auditory neuron imbalance theory of tinnitus
Thyrotoxicosis, 257
Tinnitus
   acute. *See* Acute tinnitus
   chronic tinnitus. *See* Chronic tinnitus
   clinically significant. *See* Clinically significant tinnitus
   disco. *See* Disco tinnitus
   objective. *See* Objective tinnitus
   otic. *See* Otic tinnitus
   permanent. *See* Permanent tinnitus
   pulsatile. *See* Pulsatile tinnitus
   somatic. *See* Somatic tinnitus
   subaudible. *See* Subaudible tinnitus
   subjective. *See* Subjective tinnitus
   temporary. *See* Temporary tinnitus
   transient. *See* Transient tinnitus
Tinnitus instrument, 311
Tinnitus Patient Survey of the American Tinnitus Association, 286
Tinnitus-related neuronal activity, 96
Tinnitus retraining therapy, 13, 105, 228, 251, 295–308, 298t, 302f, 304f, 350–352
   for hyperacusis and misophonia, 13, 297, 298t, 299, 303–305, 304f
Tobramycin, 144
Tocainide, 270, 273
Tonotopic map, 145, 151
Toynbee tube, 210
Trait anxiety, 281
Transient receptor potential superfamily of genes, 44
Transient receptor potential vanniloid type 1 channels, 63
Transient tinnitus, 101
Trapezoid body, 118
Trazodone, 285, 288
Treatment effect size, 271
Tricyclic antidepressants, 274, 285
   amitriptyline. *See* Amitriptyline
   doxepin. *See* Doxepin
   imipramine. *See* Imipramine
   nortriptyline. *See* Nortriptyline
   protriptyline. *See* Protriptyline
   trimipramine. *See* Trimipramine
Trigeminal ganglion, 125, 129, 129f, 130–133f, 137f
   mandibular division of, 125–127
   ophthalmic division of, 125–127
Trigeminal innervation of the cochlea, 63
Trigeminal nuclei, 125, 134f, 135f
Trimipramine, 269, 274, 287
Tuning fork tests, 209, 209t, 210, 210f
   Bing. *See* Bing tuning fork test
   Rinne. *See* Rinne tuning fork test
   Schwabach. *See* Schwabach tuning fork test
   Weber. *See* Weber tuning fork test
Tympanic membrane perforation, 57
Type I afferent auditory neurons, 58–63
Type I or II afferent auditory neuron imbalance theory of tinnitus, 59

Type II afferent auditory neurons, 58, 59, 136, 157
2-deoxyglucose, 148, 149, 167

U

Ultrasound therapy, 272
Unconditioned stimulus, 81, 165, 167
Understanding speech, 4, 5
United Kingdom National Study of Hearing, 20
Urbach-Wiethe disease, *See* Lipoid proteinosis
US Bureau of the Census, 17, 27
US Occupational Safety and Health Administration, 2

V

Validity of a tinnitus questionnaire, 239
    content 239
    criterion-related, 239
    construct, 239
    responsiveness, 239, 240
Valsalva's maneuver-induced nystagmus test, 209t, 212
Varicose veins, 1
Vascular compression of the cochleovestibular nerve, 216, 218, 218f
Vascular lesions, 3
Vascular loops in the internal auditory canal, 58
Vegetarians, 275
Venlafaxine, 285, 288
Ventral cochlear nucleus, 126, 129–131, 129–134f, 137f, 148
    anteroventral cochlear nucleus, 148
    posteroventral cochlear nucleus, 148
Ventral tegmental area, 195
Vernon and Meikle standard procedures, 224–227
Vertigo, 207
Vestibular evoked myogenic potentials, 213
Vestibular schwannoma, 58, 256, 256f
Vestibular tests, 209t, 210–212
    cerebellar. *See* Cerebellar vestibular tests
    head shake. *See* Head shake vestibular test
    head thrust. *See* Head thrust vestibular test
    hyperventilation-induced. *See* Hyperventilation-induced nystagmus test
    spontaneous and gaze-evoked. *See* Spontaneous and gaze-evoked nystagmus test
    Valsalva's maneuver-induced. *See* Valsalva's maneuver-induced nystagmus test
    vibration-induced. *See* Vibration-induced nystagmus test
Vestibulo-ocular reflex, 211
Veterans Affairs Healthcare System, 337
Veterans Benefits Administration, 337
Veterans Benefits Administration Veterans Service Center, 341
Veterans Health Administration, 337
Veterans Affairs National Center for Rehabilitative Auditory Research, 338, 349
Veterans Affairs Puget Sound Health Care System, 338
Veterans Affairs Rehabilitative Research and Development Service, 349
Veterans service organization, 347
Vibration-induced nystagmus test, 209t, 212
Videonystagmography, 212
Vision, 165
Volta, 326

W

Washout, 266
Weber tuning fork test, 209, 209t, 210, 210f
Whiplash injury, 116
Williams syndrome and hyperacusis, 12
Winding up, 299
World Health Organization model for describing consequences of health conditions, 237, 238t

Z

Zinc, 274, 275
Zwicker tone, 144, 192